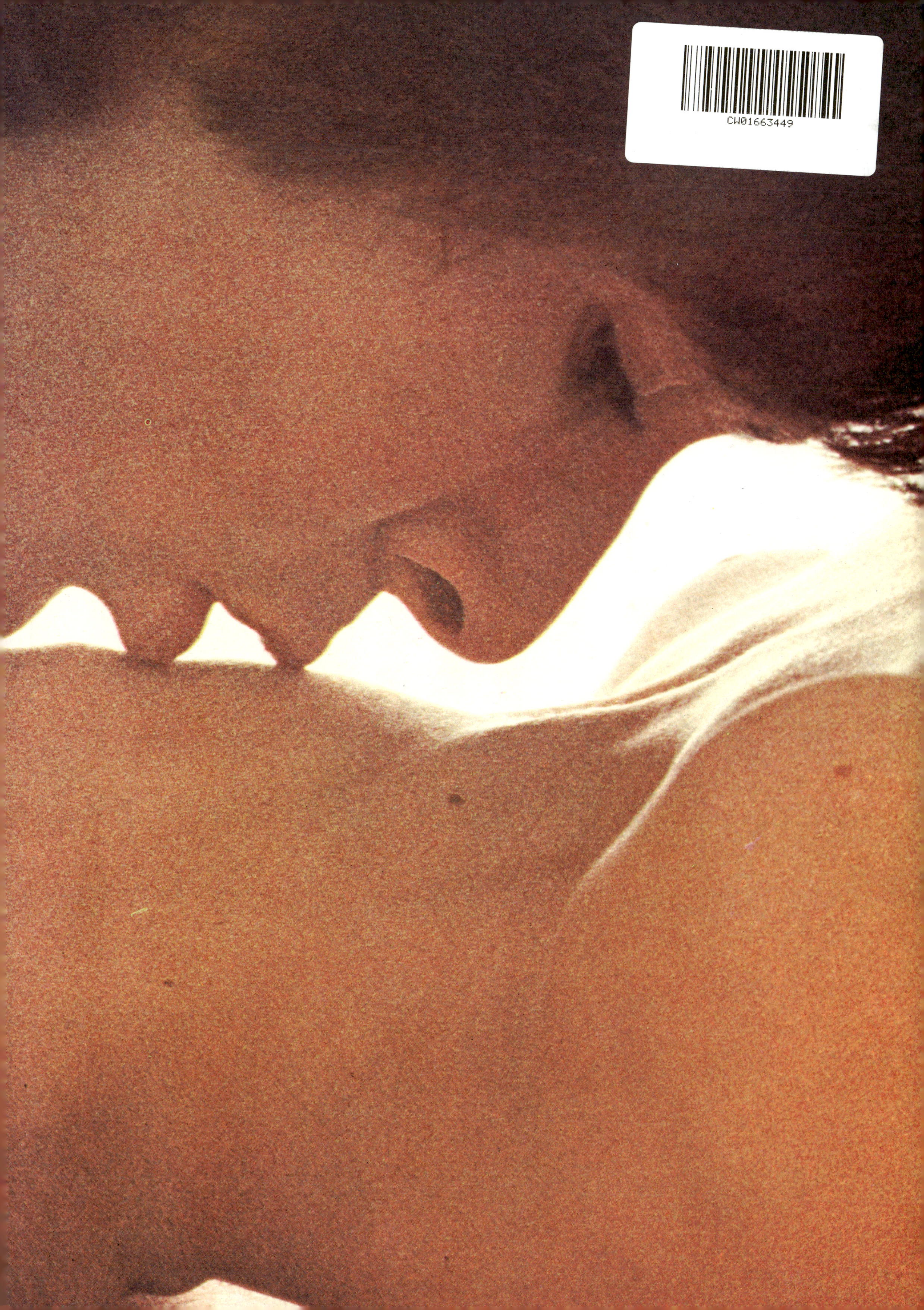

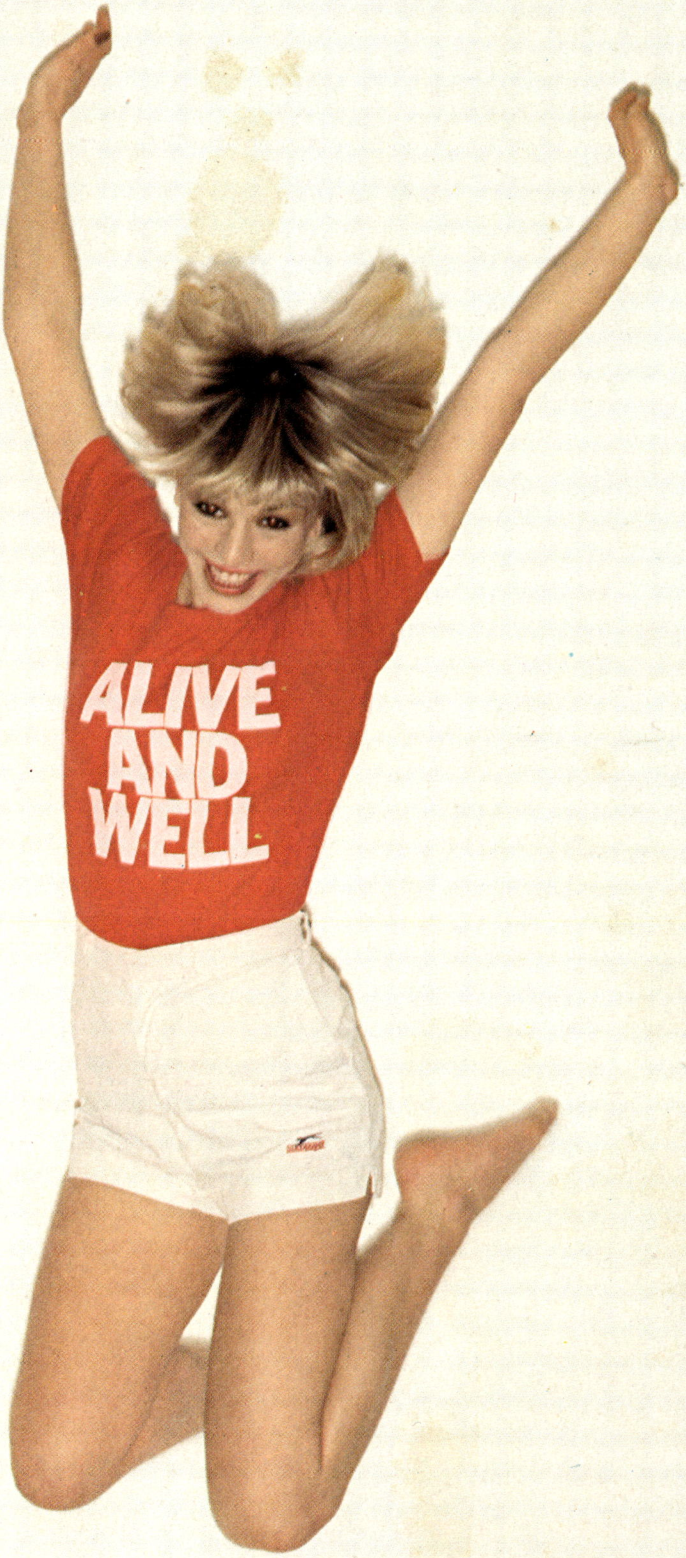
ALIVE
AND
WELL

ALIVE

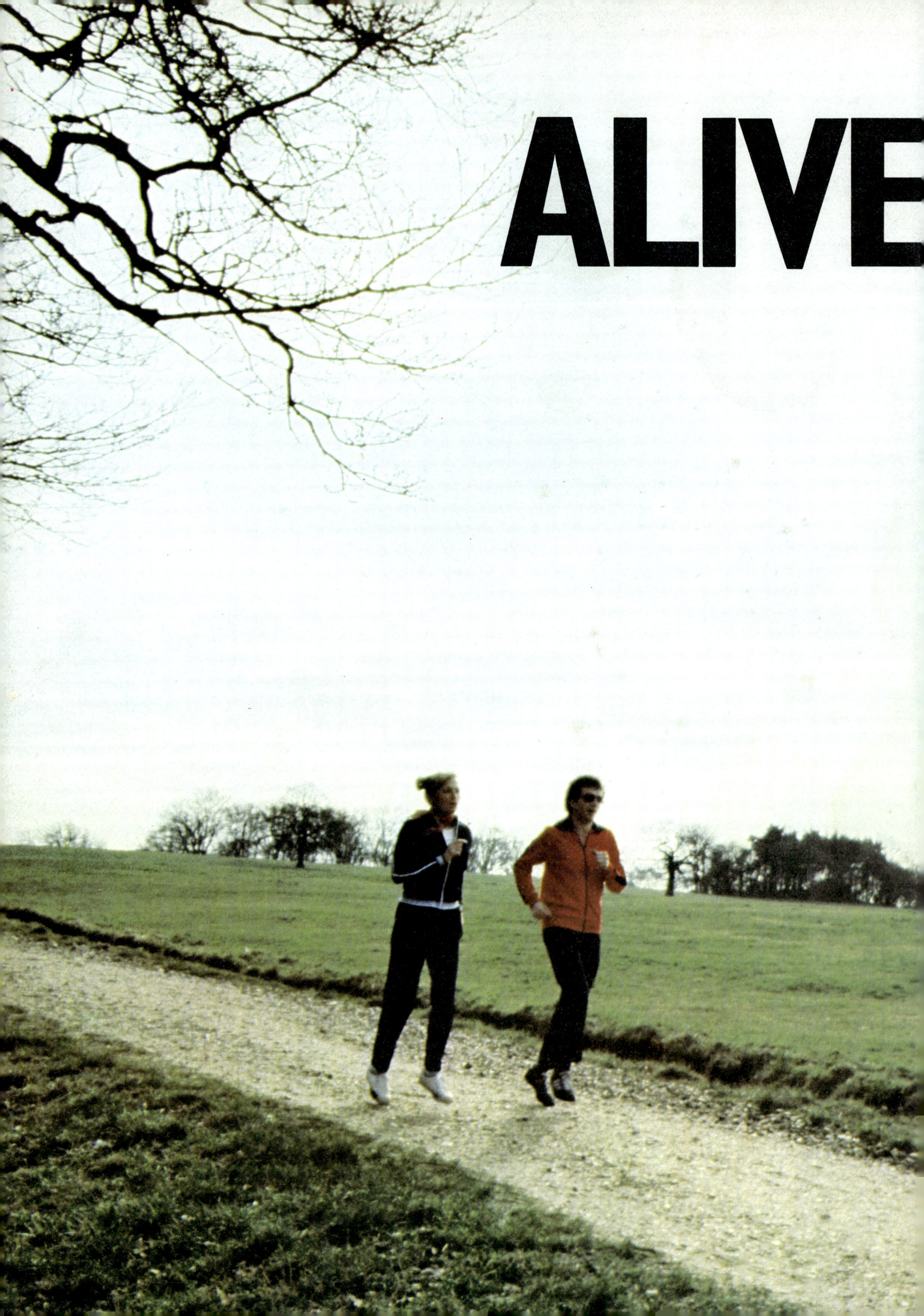

AND WELL

A New Approach to Healthy Living

Consultant Editor
Alan Kingdon MBBS MRCS LRCP

Foreword by Jackie Stewart

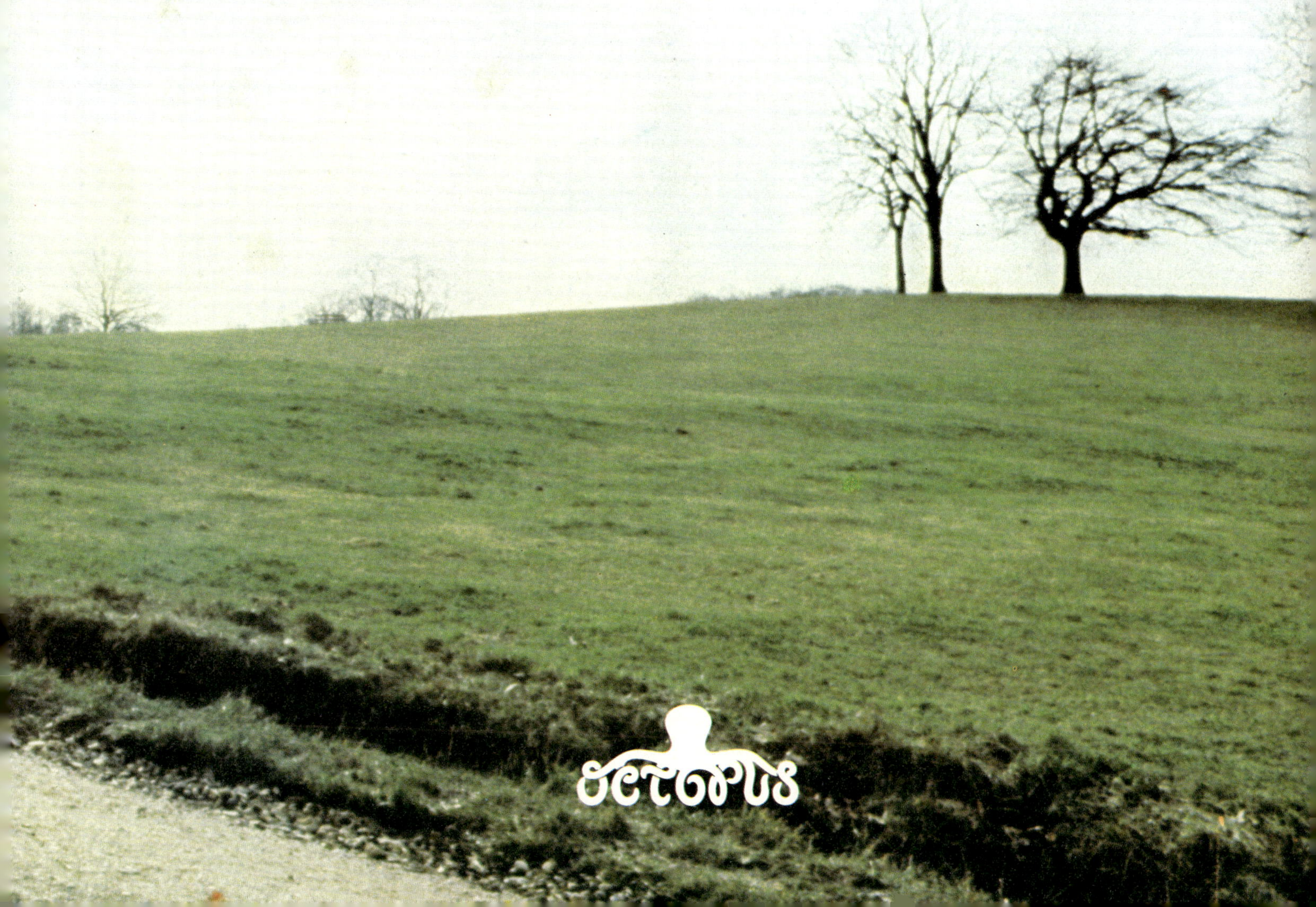

Contents

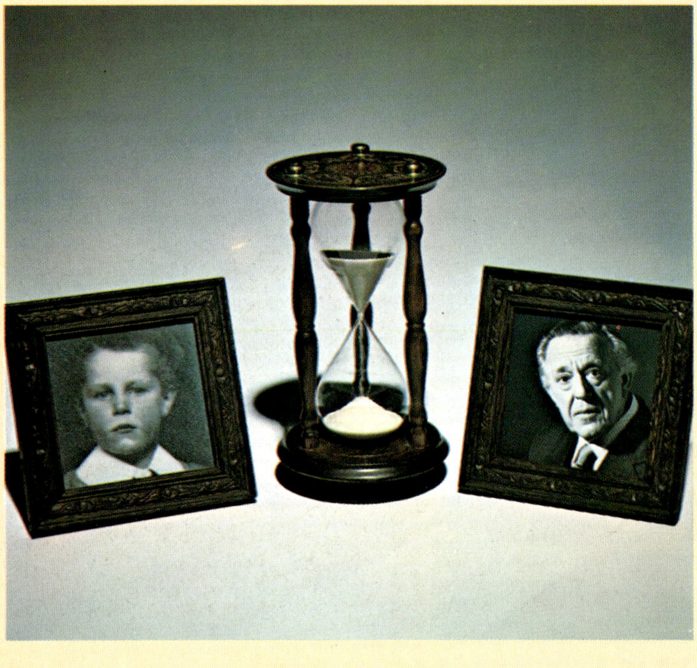

First published 1978 by Octopus Books Limited
59 Grosvenor Street, London W1

ISBN 07064 0913 2

Printed in Italy by New Interlitho SpA

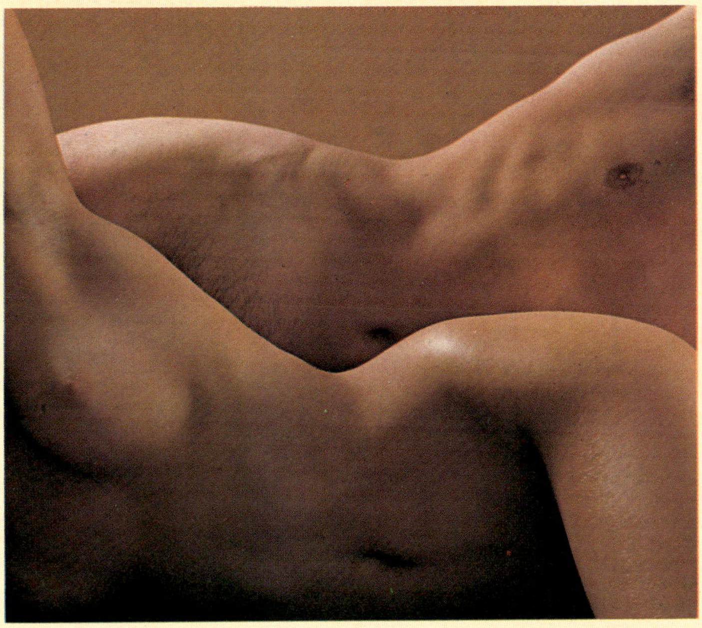

Understanding Your Body 22

Your Working Surface 48

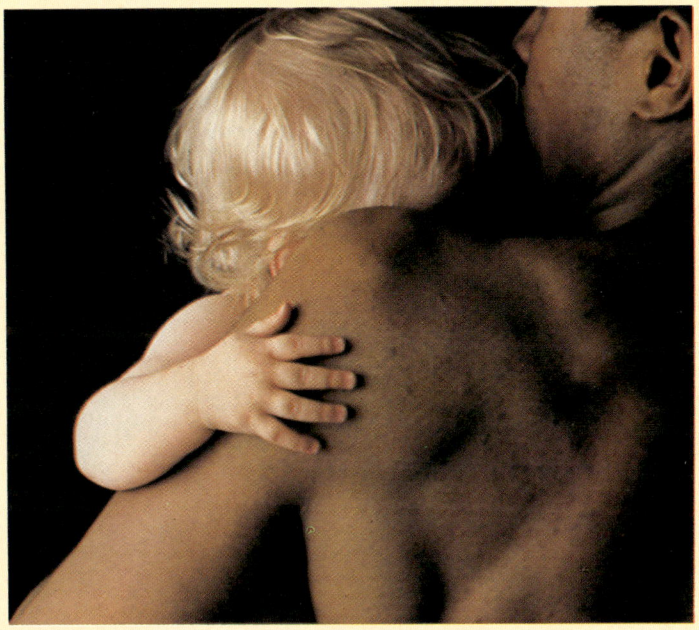

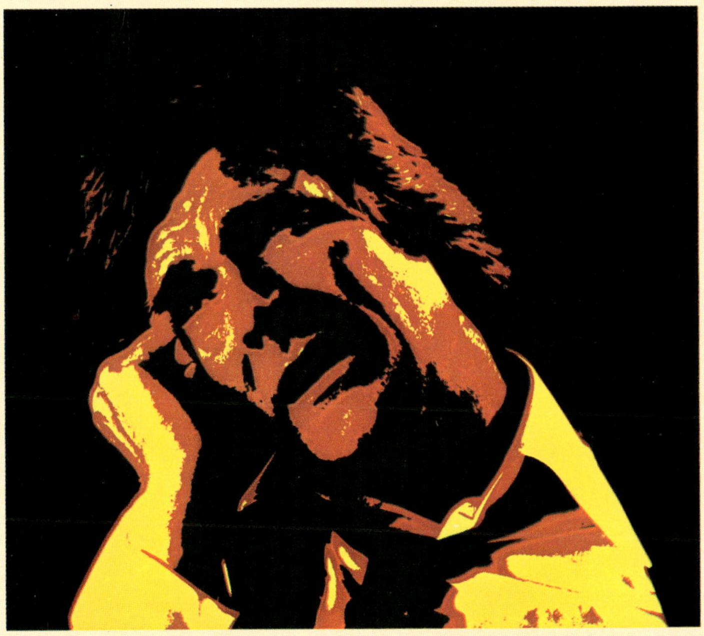

Stress Today 66

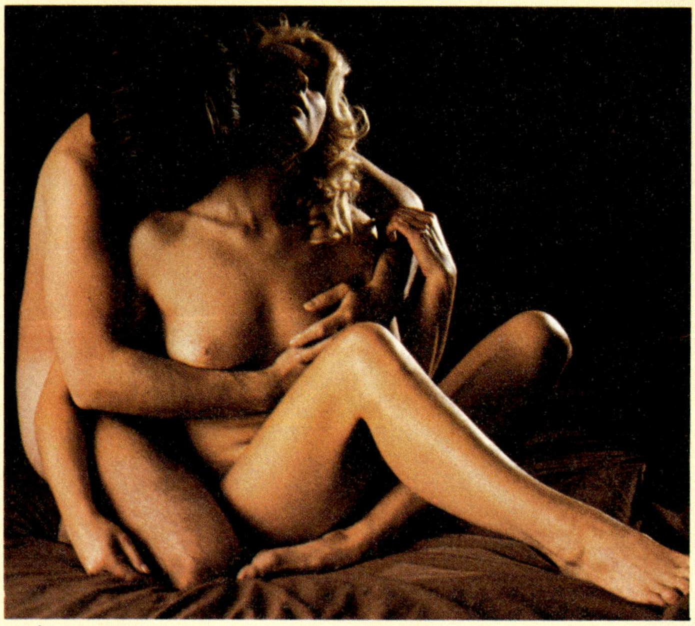

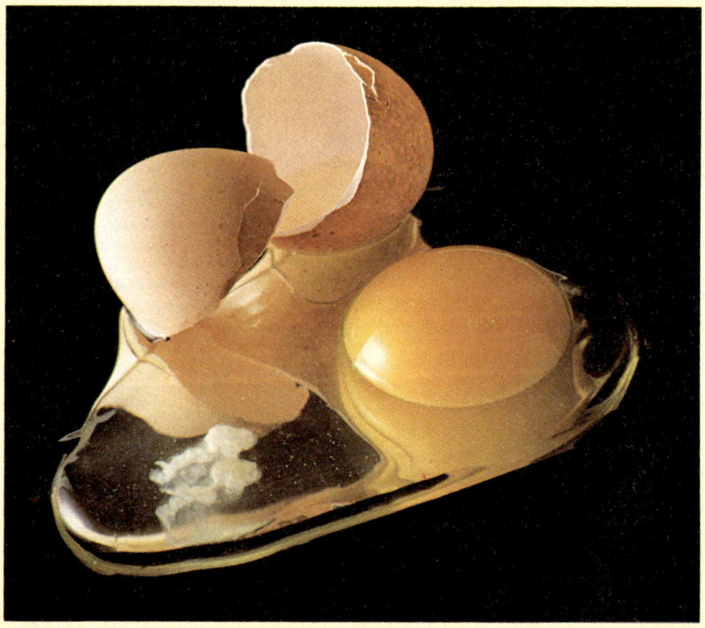

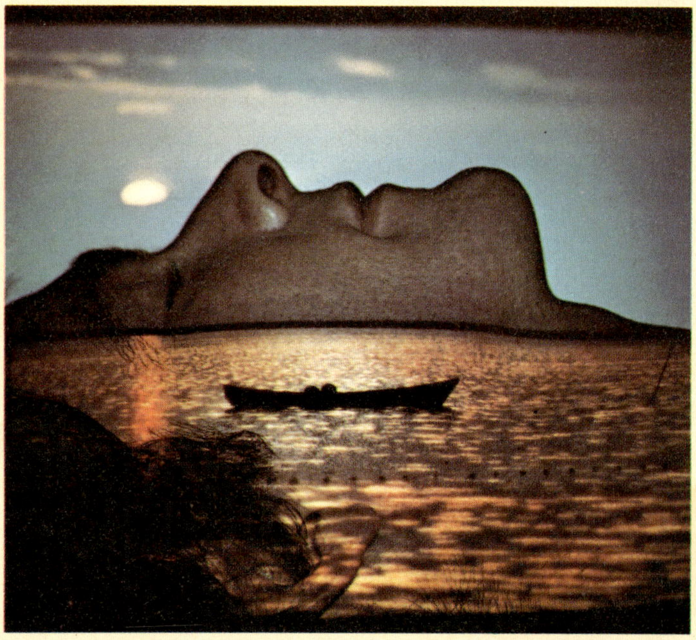

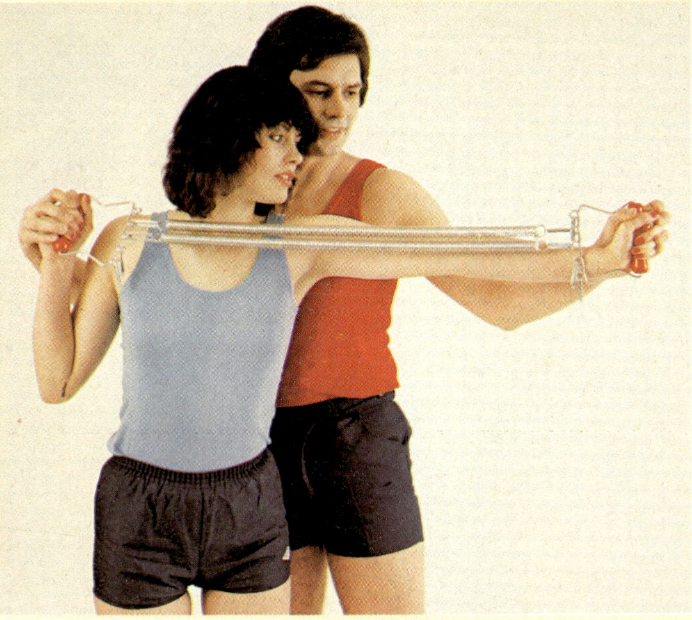

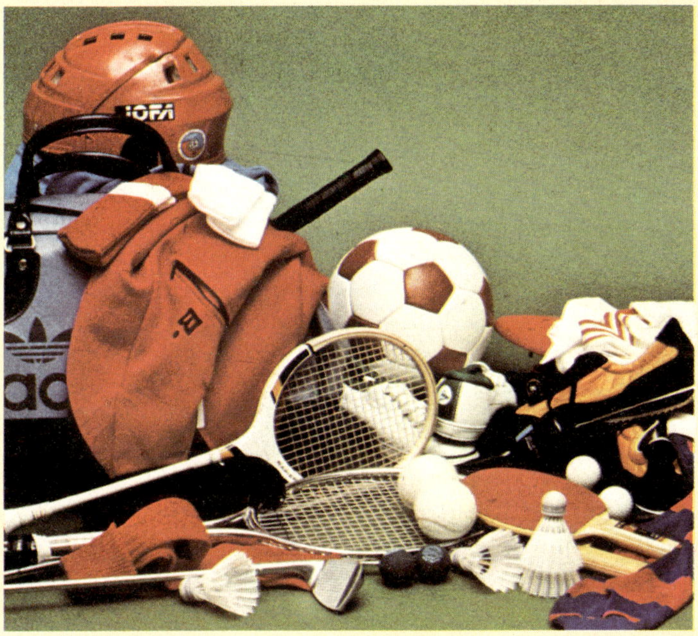

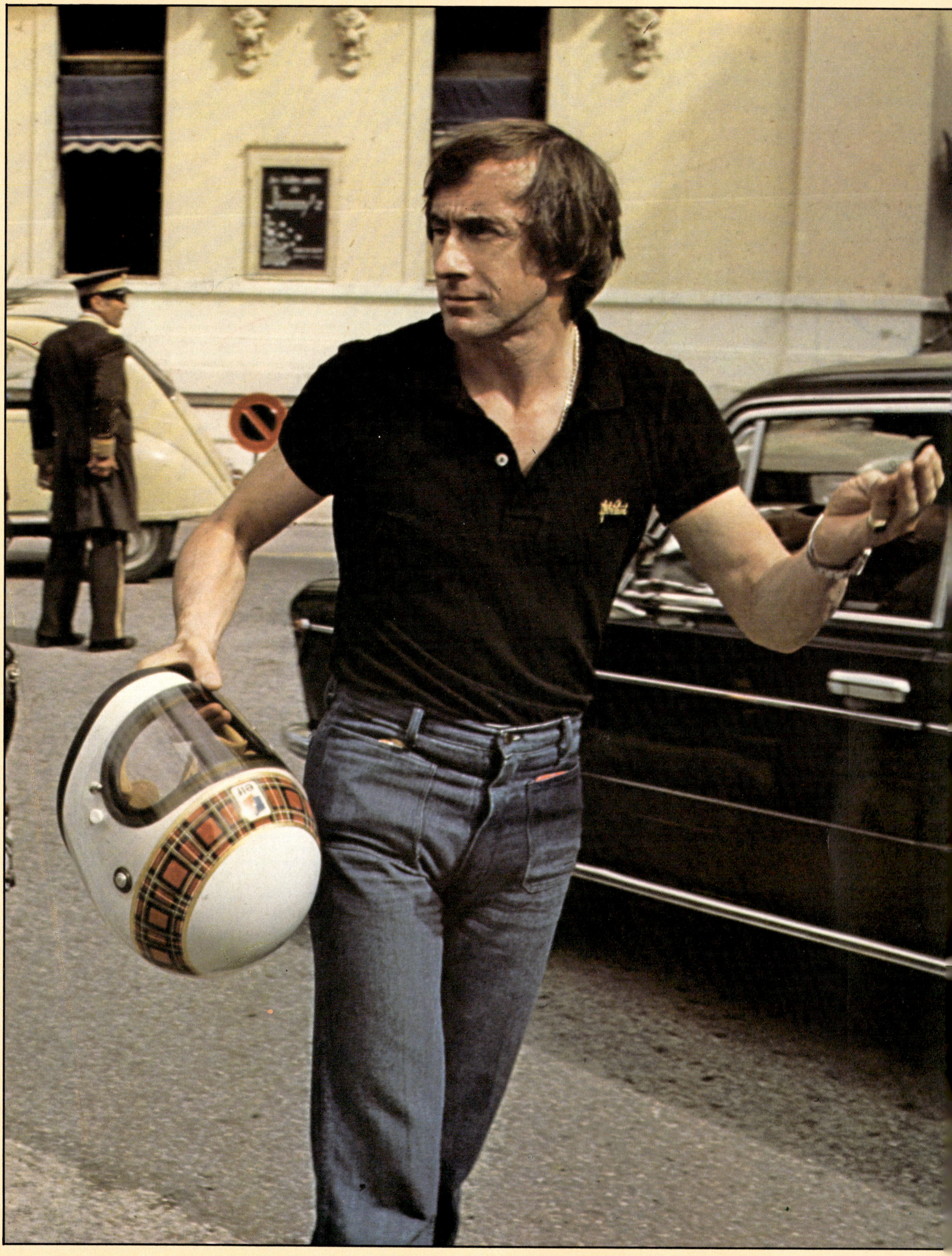

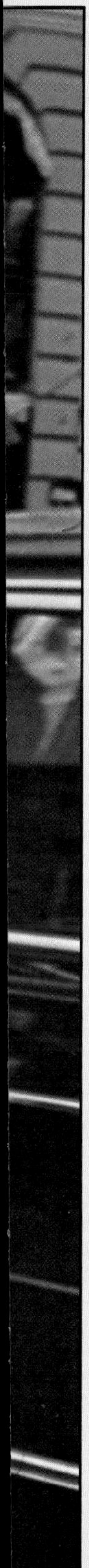

Foreword

As with many people I have always endeavoured to live my life to the full. And, perhaps to some extent I have been fortunate enough to do so. I have been lucky to enjoy some success and hence the opportunity to see many aspects of life often denied to others. One of the deepest impressions made on me is how important it is, for success, to keep physically fit, eat sensibly, understand your own limitations, and know how to relax. Whether driving a formula one car or relaxing with my family it has all been made easier by keeping fit. Concentration, stamina, strength, all greatly help increase one's efficiency and can often reduce the severe demands made on us during our lives. It can, of course, also give you that extra edge.

Nearly all sports are useful in keeping fit and certainly play an important role in relaxation and leisure.

I have always felt that physical fitness means mental fitness, and from my own experience I know that I am certainly more able to make quick positive decisions when in physically good shape.

On the odd occasion when I have allowed my body to gain unnecessary weight, I have certainly found life sluggish and I become easily bored. Agility of mind seems to be parallel with agility of body. And certainly when I have needed reserves of strength both mentally and physically, it has been to my distinct advantage to be in good condition.

This is certainly true in times of accident or illness where the recuperation powers are necessary. I have many friends in varied lives who share my views. Some of them are not directly concerned with sports – I can think immediately of the astronauts, many of whom I have had the good fortune to become friends with, and while there sometimes is no great physical exertion required their mental conditioning prior to their journeys into space has been very closely linked to their physical training programme.

I am impressed that the authors of this book feel it necessary to include references to every aspect of life. Mixing health and beauty with exercise, sex and stress. I am especially pleased to see a comprehensive section on food and nutrition which reinforces my own feelings on the importance of a good balanced diet. Diet plays a vital part in everyone's life and so often seems to be unnecessarily abused in today's world.

This book really does cover all the most important parts of our lives and I am sure it will help many readers to improve the quality of their lives.

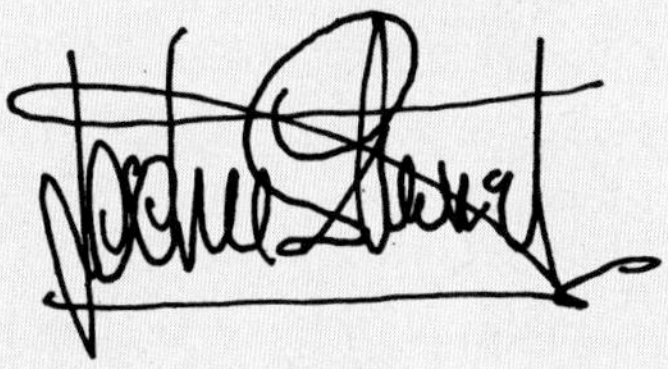

Jackie Stewart

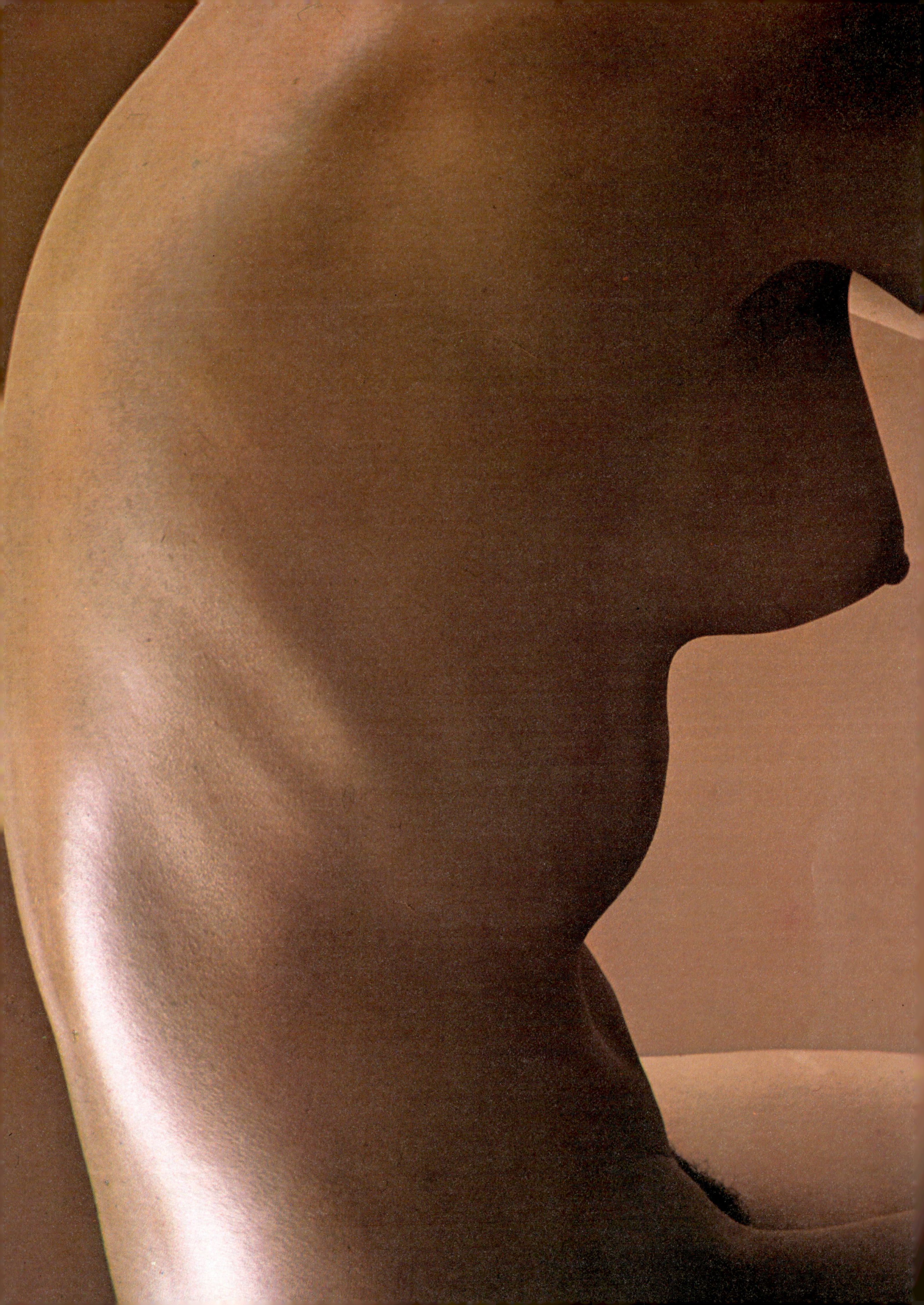

Contributors and Consultants

Alan Kingdon MBBS MRCS LRCP
Lionel Bender BSc
Philip Cauthery MB ChB DPH
John Davies MBBS MRCS LRCP DPhysMed
Elizabeth Fenwick PhD
John Goodbody BA
Christopher Knight BChD LDS
Christine Pickard MB ChB FRSM
Geoff Tansey BSc
John White MD FRCP

North American Consultant
Elliott M. Goldwag PhD
Executive Director of the
Renaissance Revitalization Center, Nassau
and a founder of the Holistic Health Association

Australian Consultants
John Watson MBBS D (obst) RCOG
Fellow of the Royal Australian
College of General Practitioners

Anthony Millar OBE MBBS FRACP
Director of Research,
Institute of Sports Medicine, Sydney

WHAT KIND OF LIFE DO YOU LEAD?

Modern living tends to be unhealthy because it provokes mental stress, the tendency to eat too much over-refined food and to take far too little exercise. Life may be more pleasurable than ever before, but it does not automatically lead to longevity. Our bodies seem to rapidly deteriorate due to the benefits they receive. Careful examination of our life styles is imperative.

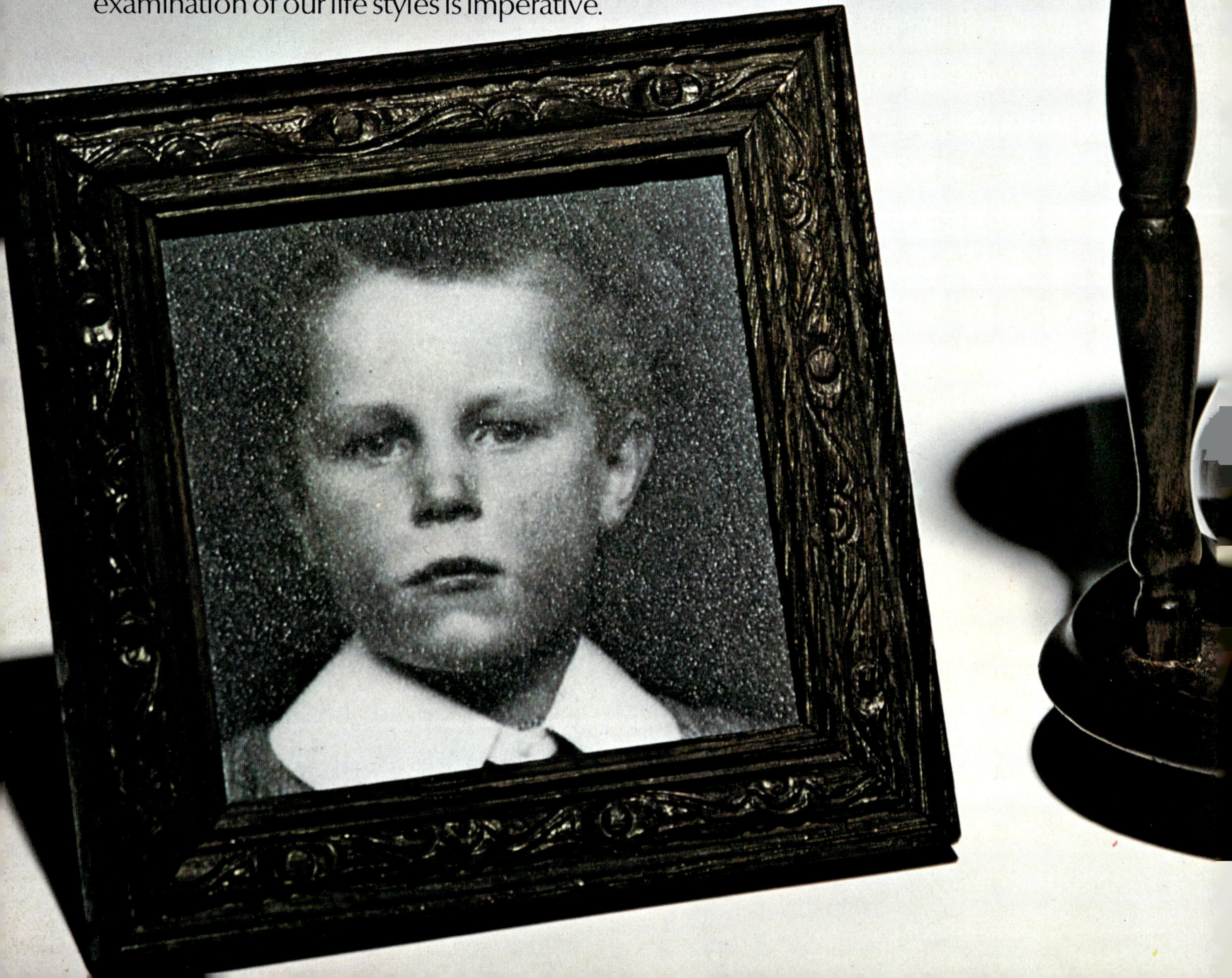

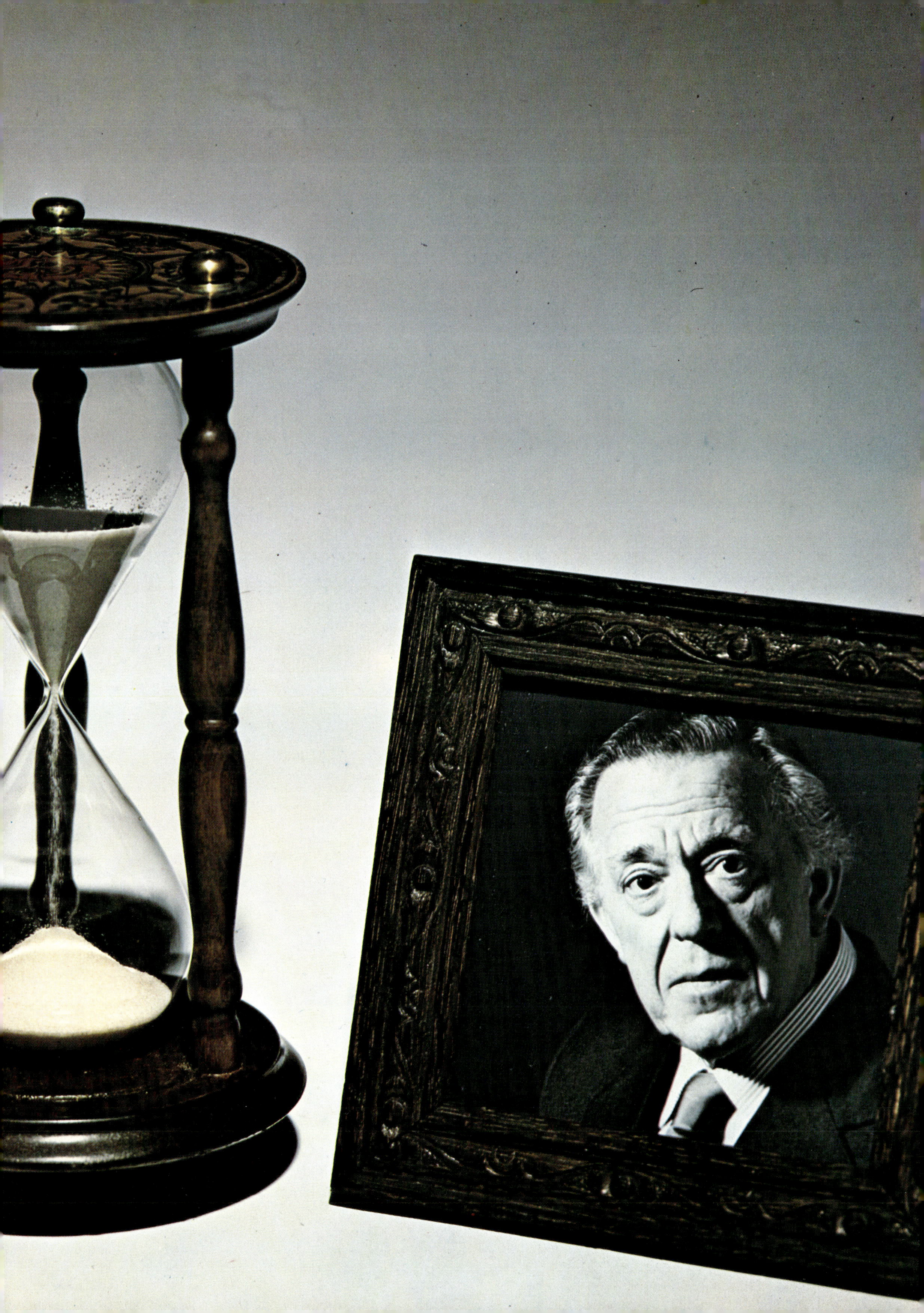

Designs for Living

This book is designed to help you to improve the quality of your life, to help you to look and feel good. It is aimed at everyone including the chronically sick, the average person, the super-fit athlete and the elderly. This is not a diet book or a fitness manual, there are already plenty of those around. Most of them are inadequate and many of them inaccurate. All of them, I think, are rather boring. This book is different. It is going to look at living *in toto*: examine the harmful aspects to see if we can eliminate them, look at what we are stuck with and what, realistically, we have to accept. We will also look at the things we are not doing, but ought to be doing. The dos will put more excitement into your life, the don'ts will take away the lethargy.

You may ask why bother, though I feel that if you are reading this book you already have your own answers. However, it is interesting to speculate on our motives. I think that the sexual motive is important. It may even be the only motive. Consider the clothes we wear and how they are advertized and marketed. It is all about making ourselves attractive to the opposite sex, or for some people to the same sex. The cars we drive are extensions of our aggression and sexuality and are sometimes unfortunately substitutes for these qualities. Sex is beautiful: not only does it motivate, it's fun, it's good exercise and it's relaxing, but of course to get the very best out of it, you need a healthy body and an alert mind. And if that isn't a reason to bother, what is?

The Dangers of Modern Living

Modern living tends to be unhealthy because it provokes mental stress, the tendency to overeat over-refined foods and to take too little physical exercise. Largely because of these three simple factors *one third* of deaths in the USA are from coronary thrombosis and the rest of the world is fast catching up. This book is more concerned with quality of life than longevity, but the latter nearly always follows as a consequence of the former.

However, life expectancy is increasing statistically, and this makes people ask whether the so-called diseases of civilization are really just a myth. The answer, unfortunately, is no. Life expectancy might have increased more, but for rubbish foods and highly sedentary occupations with no physical outlet. Modern technology has conferred enormous benefits but refined processed food is not one of them. We have eliminated many diseases that were fatal 20 years ago. Modern surgical techniques, antibiotics and other modern drugs have equipped us doctors to deal effectively with almost all known illness. So remarkable has been the progress in medicine and surgery that life expectancy has increased in spite of our unhealthy habits.

But we are concerned with the quality of life, and the fact is that civilization is here to stay. Guided missiles, polaris submarines, fast-breeder reactors, Concorde, Watergate, inflation, unemployment, noise, pollution, traffic jams, mugging, high rise flats, terrorism .... this is our heritage. We are stuck with what we have got, but do we need any more benefits of civilization? Perhaps we should listen to the conservationists. In the future the side-effects of progress could outweigh its advantages. Politicians become progressively more pragmatic and are usually concerned with the very short term. Individuals should therefore pay very careful consideration to any potentially harmful innovation, and object according to their conscience.

On the other hand we do not want to stagnate just because we already have women's lib., holidays in the sun, central heating, blue movies, Jimmy

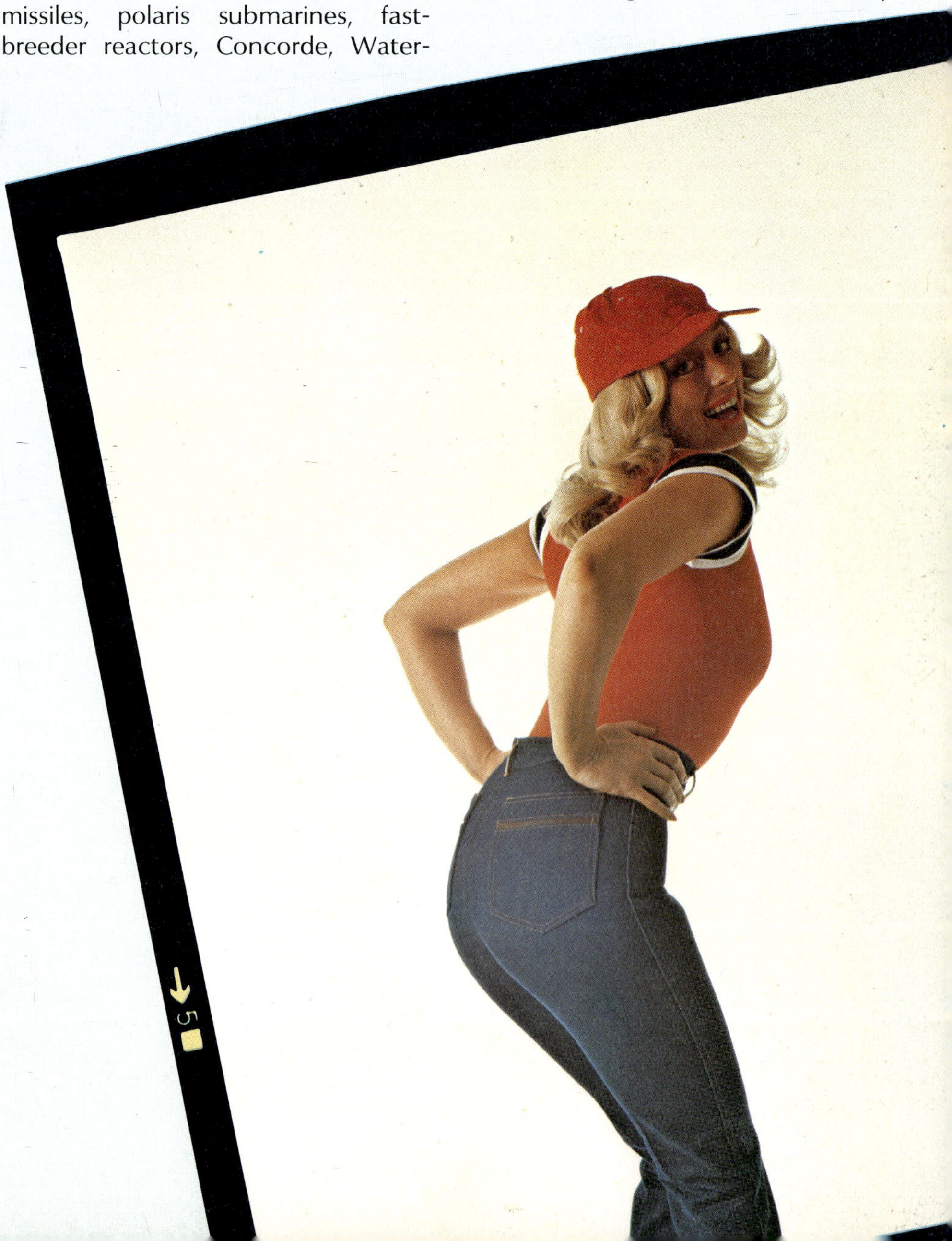

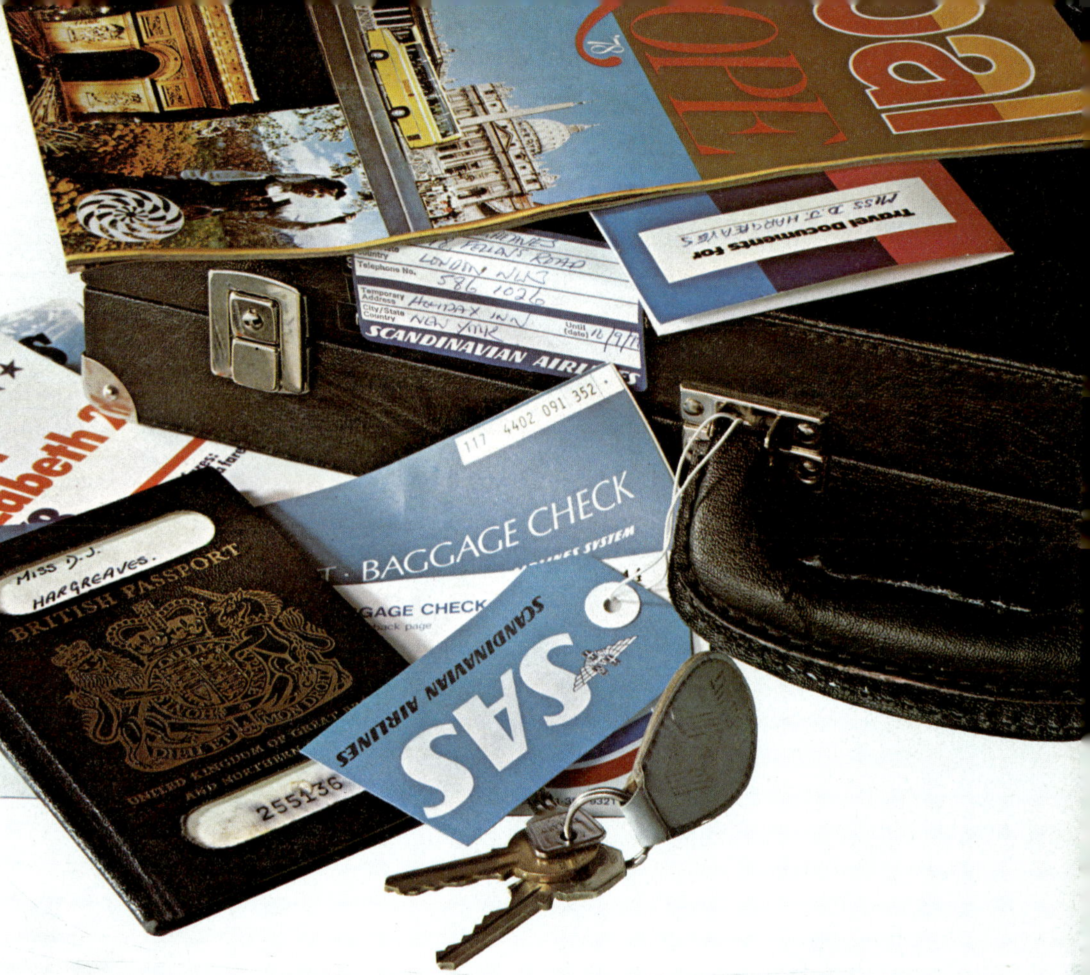

Practically no part of the globe is inaccessible these days. We can experience tropical nights, palm-fringed beaches, exotic cities. Seeing other ways of life is stimulating as well as entertaining

Carter, valium and vibrators. There is nothing wrong with the good life. Use technology where it can help you to make the most of yourself. Hair transplantation did a lot for Frank Sinatra; if it would help you, go to a reputable clinic. Modern dentistry alone can transform your appearance, but remember that carious teeth are again a reflection of poor diet. Let the dentist repair the damage, but save on your future payments by eliminating sugar. Plastic surgery can get rid of your bat ears, improve your bust, or give you a face lift.

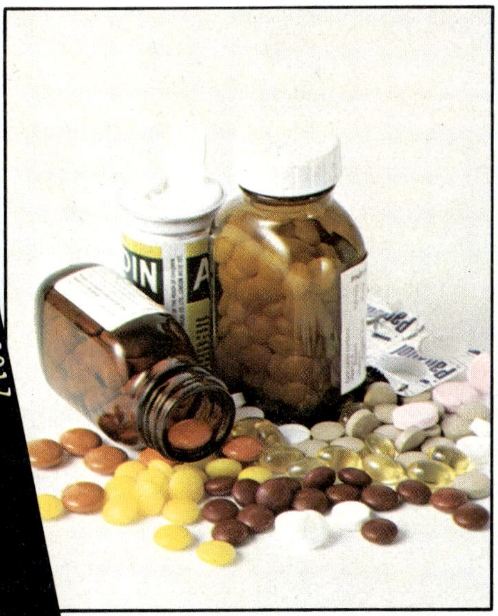

Tight jeans and T-shirts outline the body, (left) emphasizing those parts currently considered sexually attractive. Pills may cure life's minor ills, but will not give you a body bursting with health

These are valuable techniques for people with real problems, but they are never the complete answer. They can solve a specific deformity, but overall fitness reflects in the face and physical carriage and this is more important. Modern transportation means that we can have fresh fruit and vegetables from anywhere in the world and these things are good for us and well worth having. There is nothing wrong with home comforts and gadgets that take away some of the tedium from life. It is interesting to be able to travel and live for a short time amongst other cultures; it broadens one's intellectual horizons and increases understanding.

The acquisition of modern home comforts and freedom to see the world implies material success. How much do you need? There is a tendency these days for younger people in careers to consider the quality of the whole of their lives, turn their backs on ambition to some extent and settle for a middle level of responsibility. They feel, rightly, that there is more to life than work. However, there is a natural instinct to try to succeed for its own sake, and relating ambition to fulfilment must be a personal decision depending on many factors. But, no matter how devoted you are to reaching the top of your chosen career *you must find time for some form of exercise, eat the right diet and find some time for relaxation.* Otherwise, however hard you work and however clever you are, you will not fulfill your potential.

Of course it must be remembered that we are all genetically different and have different potentials. Some of us look like Robert Redford or Sophia Loren, and seem fit and successful without apparent effort. Most of us are not so lucky, but we all of us have some features of physique or personality which we can exploit, and some defects which we can eliminate. The most important message of this book is *Realize Your Potential.*

Your Physical Fitness

In the first section of this book Lionel Bender and Dr Elizabeth Fenwick will give you an awareness of your physical potential, and you will see that you can be super-fit ... if you want to be. The advice given is based on widely accepted scientific fact, although of course there are still big gaps in man's knowledge. The medical profession has a comprehensive knowledge of pathology; the understanding of illness which might be affecting 5 per cent of

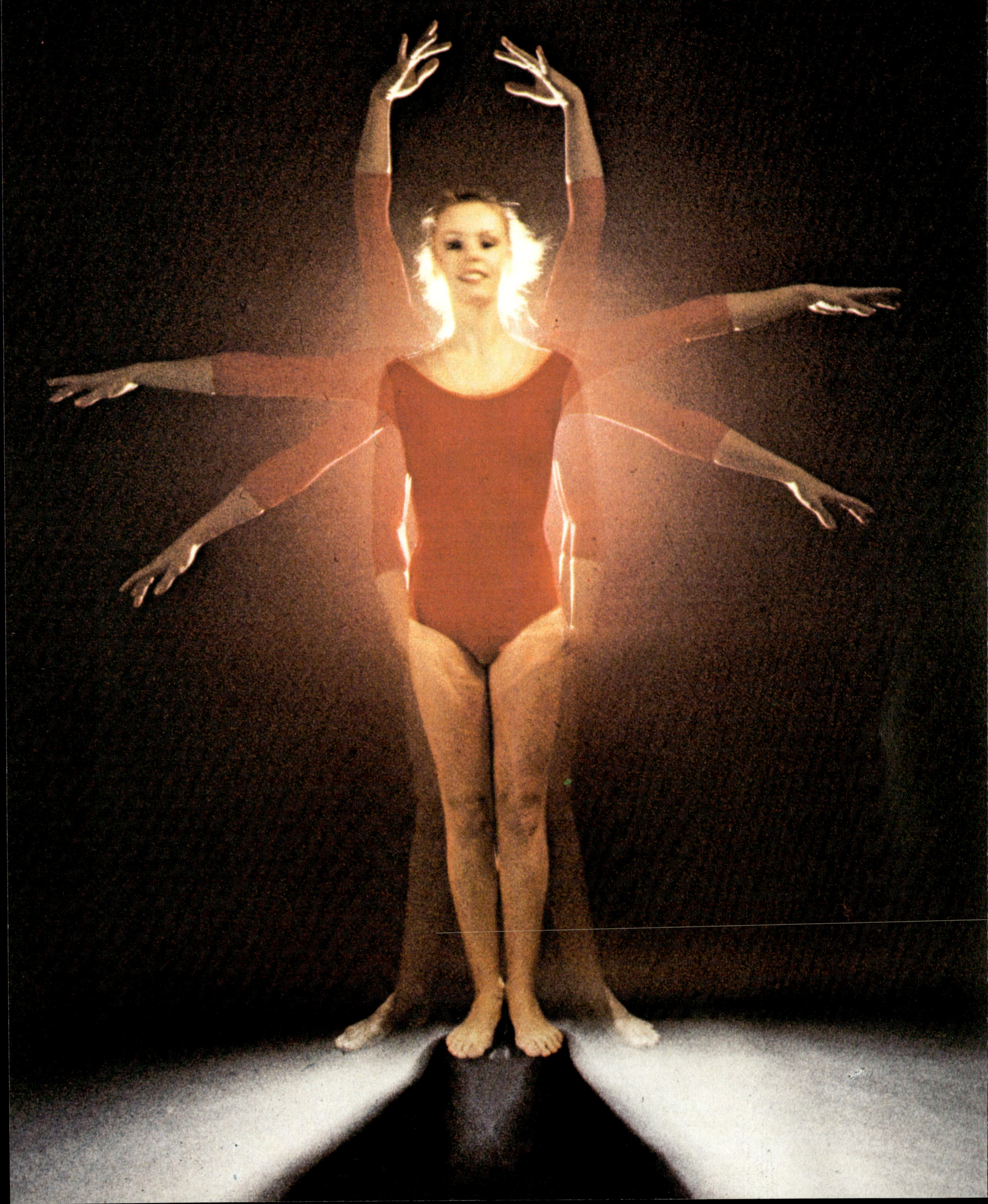

us at any one time. Similarly, there is a wealth of knowledge now concerning the fitness and training of the super-athlete, perhaps the 5 per cent at the other end of the spectrum. We are concerned primarily with the middle 90 per cent. Preventive medicine is now becoming a trendy phrase and rightly so. We want to eliminate as much illness as possible before it happens and leave the average man and the average woman in the middle of the spectrum free to move into the super-fit bracket if they feel so inclined.

Such is the variety of sporting events available to most people today that in my view everyone can excel at something. It is largely a question of motivation and the will to win. Few of us have the competitive instinct of the top-class athlete, or the inclination to spend several hours a day in training. We may prefer to spend these hours indulging in some of the other pleasures that life has to offer . . . and why not? However, it is nice to feel we could do it if we really wanted to.

Your Appearance

Looking good is feeling good is looking good. We therefore include an account of the skin, how to look after it and what can go wrong with it. This is written by a dermatologist, Dr John White, and aptly reminds us that the skin is our shop window and merits looking after. Expensive skin preparations are not necessarily the best, and he rightly emphasizes fundamental skin procedures which are basic and easy to follow for everyone.

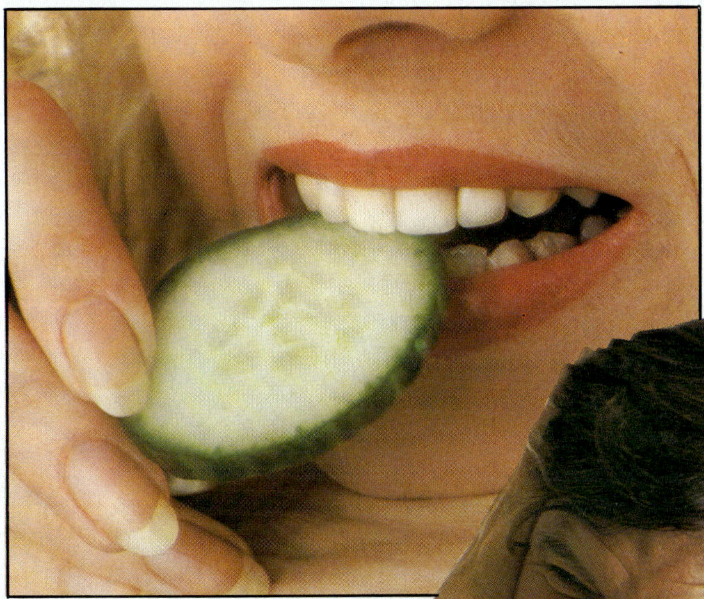

Beautiful skin, hair, teeth and eyes are the rewards of a correct diet, with lots of fresh fruit and vegetables, as well as exercise

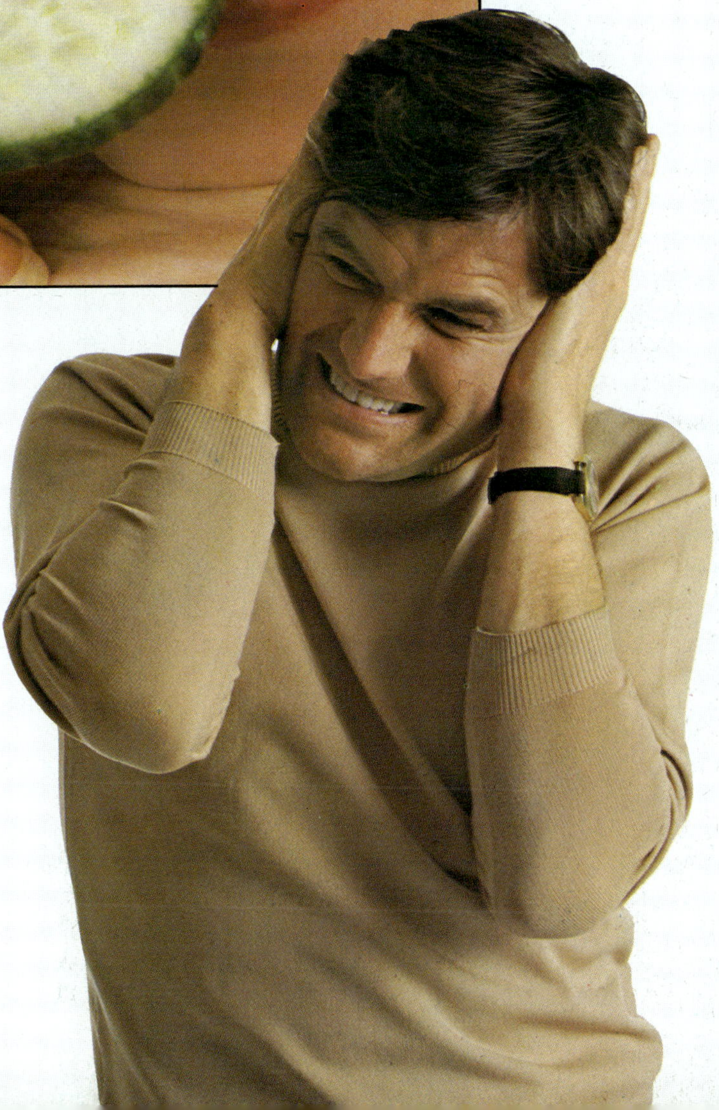

A healthy body, not too fat or too thin, with supple muscles contributes to an attractive appearance. Mind and body interact very closely. Improving one improves the other. Stressful problems can affect our health, so it is essential to think of the body as a whole

Remember that the skin tends to reflect the overall state of health, physical and mental, so pay attention to the basic principles of body care and the skin will tend to take care of itself. Healthy attractive teeth are tremendously important, more so in my view than the cut of a suit or the label on a dress. As with the skin the help of the dentist is sometimes useful for dealing with the problems that can still occur in spite of a healthy vigorous life. Therefore we also include a section concerned with dental care and an account of what modern dentistry can perform to overcome even the most disfiguring of problems.

Your Mental Fitness

In another section on mental pressure, Dr Christine Pickard discusses the all-too common complaint: stress – what causes it and what alleviates it.

Stress can be defined briefly as the psychological effects of the pace of life which in turn affect our physical well-being. This will be discussed more fully later. Stress has always been a part of man's life though today it takes different forms – noise and financial worry rather than defence from other animals. However, the physiological effect is the same. Lipids or fats are mobilized from the body's stores and released into the bloodstream in order to provide a source of energy for the muscles and heart. This is sometimes referred to as the 'fight or flight mechanism'. It is well illustrated by looking at the serum of a racing driver after a race when it appears turbid and milky, while under normal circumstances it is a clear straw coloured fluid. If these fats are not used by the body's muscles they get laid down in the arteries in the form of atheroma. This impairs the arteries' ability to carry oxygen-loaded red corpuscles. It most often involves the coronary arteries and can precipitate a coronary thrombosis. In this frequently fatal condition a part of the heart muscle dies because of lack of oxygen due to inadequate blood supply.

This is where *exercise*, the modern equivalent of fight or flight, is so important. The fats in the bloodstream are used to provide energy, preventing the build-up of atheroma.

Your Sex Life

Perhaps the best, and to my mind the most relaxing, form of exercise is sex. 'After-glow' is a beautiful phrase and describes the feeling perfectly. It is the ultimate relaxation. Many people complain of feeling irritable after long periods of abstinence. They deserve to be fulfilled and for both sexes it should be a mutual pleasure, not a duty. Physical and emotional wellbeing will always enhance the act of love.

For many sex is a delicate subject. Whatever your feelings Dr Philip Cauthery's dissertation should prove illuminating. The best advice is not to let sex worry you and not to get caught up in a performance phobia. Some people's needs are smaller than others. If you are one of those people, that is no problem; you do not have to exceed the natural average. Relax and do it when you want to and how you want to. One of my gynaecology teachers remarked to me years ago that nothing two people in love do can ever be regarded as perverted. In our progressive times the two could be three or more. You have the full range of sexual expression at your disposal, make the most of it and do not let indifferent health and vigour interfere with your capacity to enjoy it.

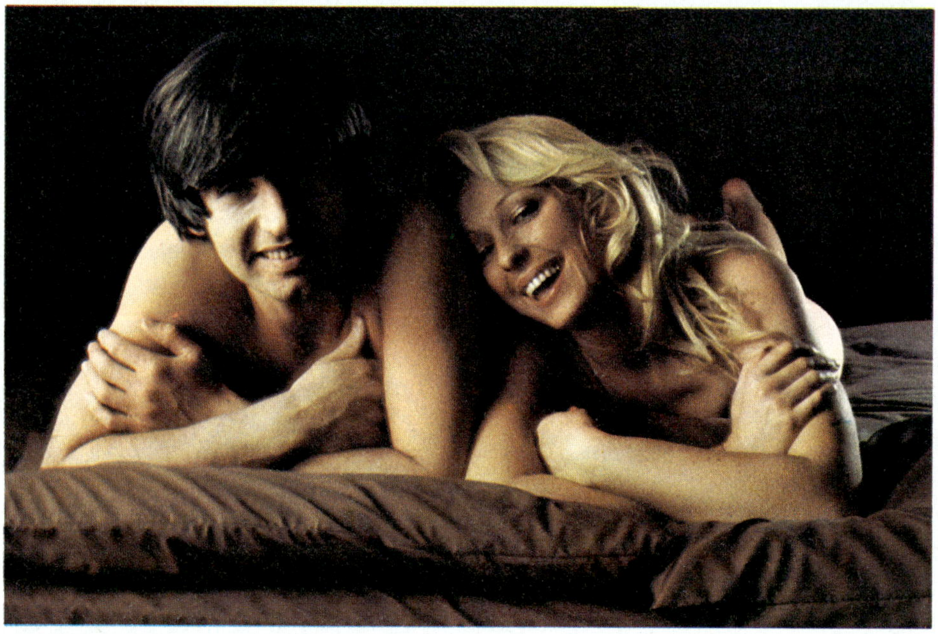

Sex is good for you, and a healthy body increases the capacity to enjoy and perform, as well as attract.

What you should eat

The expression: you are what you eat overstates the case a little. But there is no denying that a healthy diet is the cornerstone of a healthy and fulfilled existence. In a later section Geoff Tansey will explain the biochemistry of nutrition and discuss diets.

Your main objective should be to avoid over-refined food. The evidence of an over-refined diet as a contributory factor to heart disease is largely drawn from studies of other cultures. Our knowledge in this field is due to the enormously important work of Dennis Burkitt and Surgeon Captain Cleave RN. Both men noticed that the diseases of civilization did not occur in many parts of primitive Africa. There were no varicose veins or haemorrhoids. There was no diverticulitis, appendicitis, bowel cancer or peptic ulcer. No coronary heart disease and yet immigrant Africans to America and Europe began to develop these conditions.

Clearly diet is largely responsible, because in Africa the diet is mainly one of wholemeal – that is unrefined – cereals. This observation has been confirmed on the whole by many scientific studies and has completely changed our approach to the treatment of diverticular disease. It would seem that a refined diet slows the transit time of food from mouth to anus to as much as 80 hours, while for the indigenous African it is less than 30 hours. With the more rapid transit time there is less absorption, hence less of a tendency to obesity. Some of the end-products of the process of digestion would appear to be carcinogenic so that the less time they are in contact with the lining of the bowel the less chance there is of bowel cancer. Slow transit times are associated with increased pressures within the bowel impeding circulation within the veins and thereby encouraging varicose veins and haemorrhoids. Refined carbohydrates, which are largely sugar and white flour, are easily absorbed and often consumed in excess of energy requirement. They are therefore stored in the body in the form of *fat*. Unrefined carbohydrate in the form of fibre is less easily absorbed and passes through the bowel.

Some other dietary factors are also important. Our closest evolutionary relatives tend to be vegetarians and there is considerable evidence that ascorbic acid (Vitamin C), large amounts of which are contained in fresh fruit and vegetables, confers some protection against colds and influenza. Remember that such illnesses might have been fatal for man in his wild state, interfering with his ability to hunt and defend himself. I do not wish to suggest that we should become vegetarians but that we should eat more fresh fruits, salads and vegetables, and that if we have to cook vegetables, they should be cooked lightly. They taste better that way anyway.

There is also evidence that there is less tendency to obesity when small meals are eaten often. The common habit of one large meal a day is not the healthiest approach and the large meal is even more damaging if it is eaten late in the evening. A walk after a meal, an instinct for some, is definitely a good thing. Where food is taken infrequently it becomes necessary to store it for energy, and food or energy can only be stored in the form of fat. In the case of infrequent eaters metabolic processes are set up to achieve this, resulting in an increased tendency to fat.

I doubt if many under fives will be reading this book, but if you are a parent remember your children's future physique and be aware of another important factor. *Fat children tend to become fat adults.* Fat children who become fatter before the age of five increase their number of fat cells, the total number of body fat cells remaining fixed thereafter. Although it is subsequently possible to reduce the amount of fat in each cell, the number of cells cannot be reduced and this makes losing weight more difficult.

Here is some basic dietary advice. We have already said that natural is best, and this is the important guideline. Health foods are gradually becoming more popular and this is particularly true in the USA. This is a healthy trend, though some health foods are rather faddish. A healthy diet should include wholewheat, cereals, pastries and breads, fresh fruit and vegetables and should exclude white refined flour and sugar products.

In order to produce one teaspoon of sugar it is necessary to process two pounds of sugar beet. Sugar beet itself would be a highly nutritious food giving the bowel the volume that it is designed to handle. The dietician Yudkin's phrase describing sugar is very apt: pure, white and deadly. Cut out sugar completely if you can; if you can't cut down and dilute its effect by adding wholewheat cereals to your diet. I regard sugar almost as addictive. It is generally used as a form of bribery for children, thereby laying down a lifelong habit that is difficult to give up, but it can be done. Many people use sugar substitutes which I would not encourage. The use of some substitutes is banned in the USA because of a risk of bladder cancer, but more important than that the sweetening effect panders to the sweet tooth, and as long as you have a sweet tooth you will find it difficult to resist sweets and cakes. You should try to re-educate your palate, learn to appreciate the healthier foods and in a surprisingly short time you will come to prefer them.

Many people instinctively feel that they should have at least one hot meal a day. This is quite unnecessary. In general raw vegetables are preferable. In addition to the quality of diet those with weight problems will be concerned with quantity. In most cases eliminating sugar is sufficient, but if it is not then eliminate the foods with high calorie values such as potatoes.

Remember that if you are overweight dieting for a few weeks is not enough, you have to make a permanent modification to your dietary habit. The type of diet I am suggesting is not dull or anti-social, quite the reverse, it is varied and interesting. Fresh fruit and cereals or yoghourt make a delicious breakfast. I recommend salad at lunch with wholemeal bread, which can also be used at teatime in the form of sandwiches. I make no apology for our quaint, rather

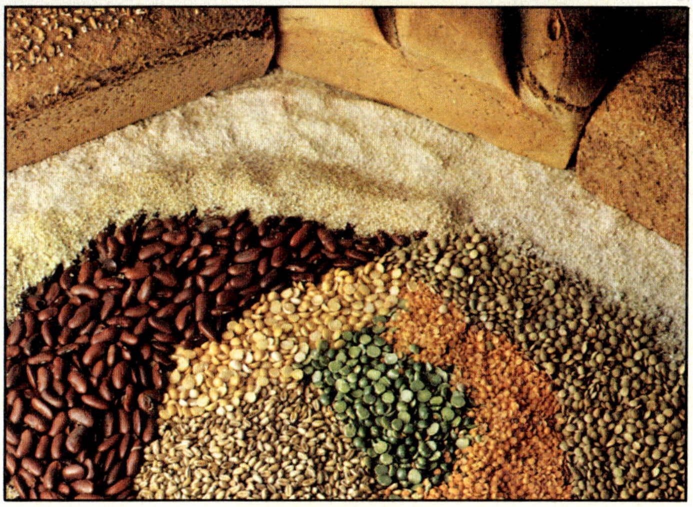

Refining flour removes the wheatgerm and fibre. Wholemeal bread, peas, beans and lentils all provide essential fibre for good digestion and protein to build a beautiful body

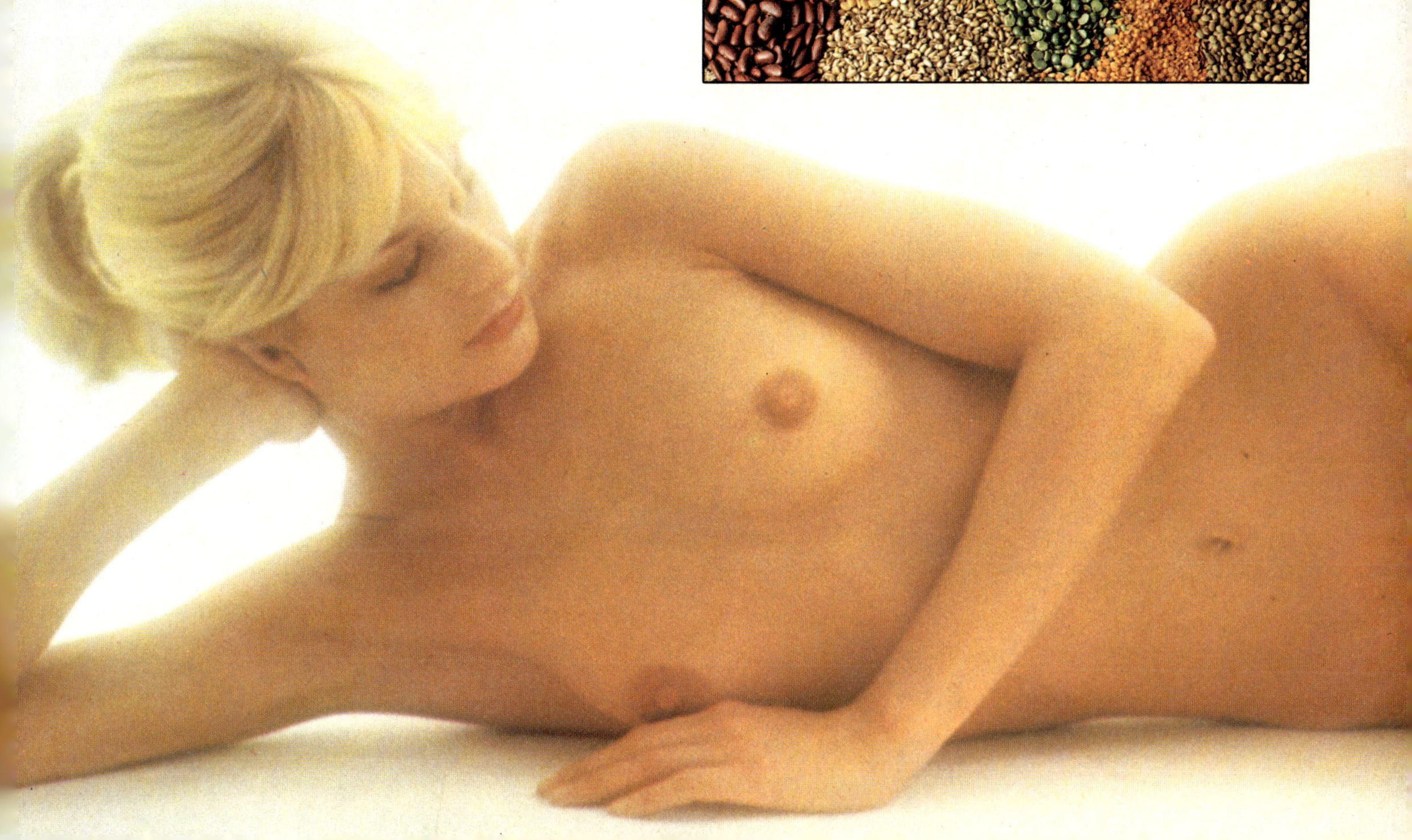

charming British habit of tea because it is so important to eat a little often. Dinner can be any combination of meat and vegetables again with salad if possible. These basic meals can be varied enormously. The reader can of course design his own diet based on this simple advice with the help of a calorie chart if necessary.

Now to lay a few dietary ghosts. First of all garlic is actually good for you. It seems to reduce blood pressure so if you suffer with hypertension forget your breath and enjoy Mediterranean food. People with good taste enjoy it and do not object to the smell anyway. Perhaps that is not always true, but 'What the hell!' Onions confer a similar beneficial effect, but rather less so. The Mediterranean peoples enjoy their food so much more than other countries and have a lesser incidence of civilization diseases, so a healthy diet does not have to be dull.

Secondly, additives and preservatives are not killers. They are numerous in so many of our packaged foods, and a certain amount of controversy surrounds all of them. The evidence is not terribly convincing but a degree of suspicion rightly exists. Remember the irrefutable generalization that natural is best but don't worry: monosodium glutamate will not kill you or make you impotent.

Thirdly, alcohol, in moderation of course, is not harmful and may even be good for you. I enjoy a drink, perhaps because I was once a medical student, or maybe because I am inadequate in some way. In excess of course alcohol is disastrous, both socially and physically, but moderate drinkers live longer than teetotallers. They do! It always seems to help at parties anyway despite Shakespeare's words in *Macbeth*.

Fourthly, many of us like coffee after a meal, but some people say it causes coronary heart disease. The evidence is unconvincing, so don't worry about it.

Lastly, cholesterol is a highly controversial topic in medical circles, but at the present time there is no convincing evidence indicating cholesterol in the aetiology of coronary heart disease. This will be more fully discussed in later chapters on nutrition.

How to Relax

Although relaxation follows naturally from strenuous exercise and from sex, it is also important in itself. It is an important attitude to acquire. It will not always be appropriate to go for a run or play a game when the pressure of work or difficult personal relationships bear down. Some people are 'laid back' and have no need of gimmicks. For others yoga, various forms of meditation, psychoanalysis, and so on, are important triggers in aiding relaxation. A sauna has the same effect; some people ascribe more to it, but its only real benefit is that it is relaxing. Remember that, used in the wrong way, saunas can be dangerous. They sometimes cause dehydration and even death for people taking large doses of diuretics.

The ability to relax is important in so far as it implies negative stress but unlike exercise it does not have a positive effect. As with other important topics the various forms of relaxation merit a separate section in the book. Transcendental meditation, yoga and so on have become fashionable for various reasons, partly perhaps because of the influence of the Beatles. Other less dramatic, more mundane, things such as religion, a family meal, a drink with friends, music or the cinema are perhaps more worthwhile for the less trendy majority. By mentioning religion in this group I do not imply any disrespect for sincere beliefs, but from a strictly medical scientific viewpoint, faith and its associated ceremonies and music have the same relaxing effect as some of the baser pleasures I have mentioned. Whatever you believe in or makes you feel good, relaxed and happy works in this respect.

Though modern society produces the stress it provides many of the

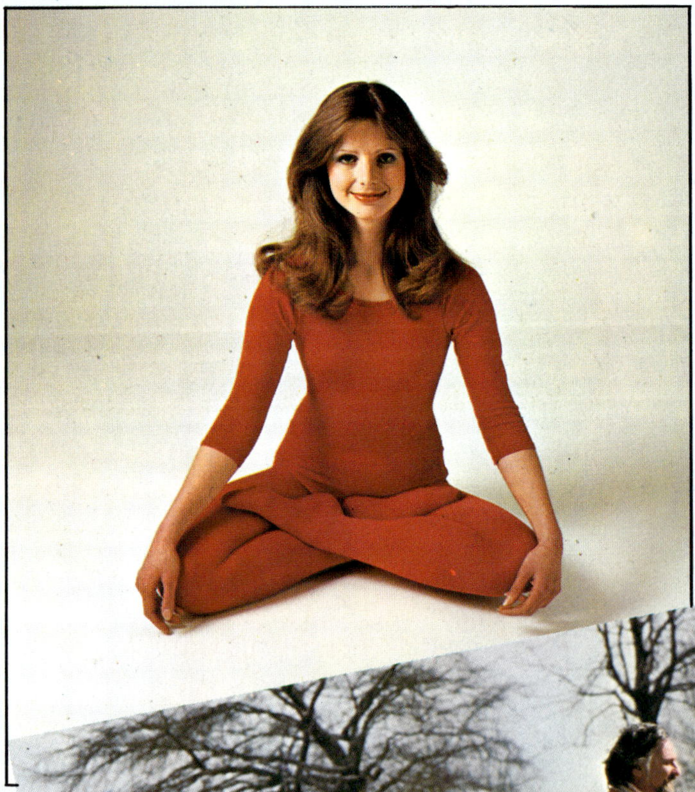

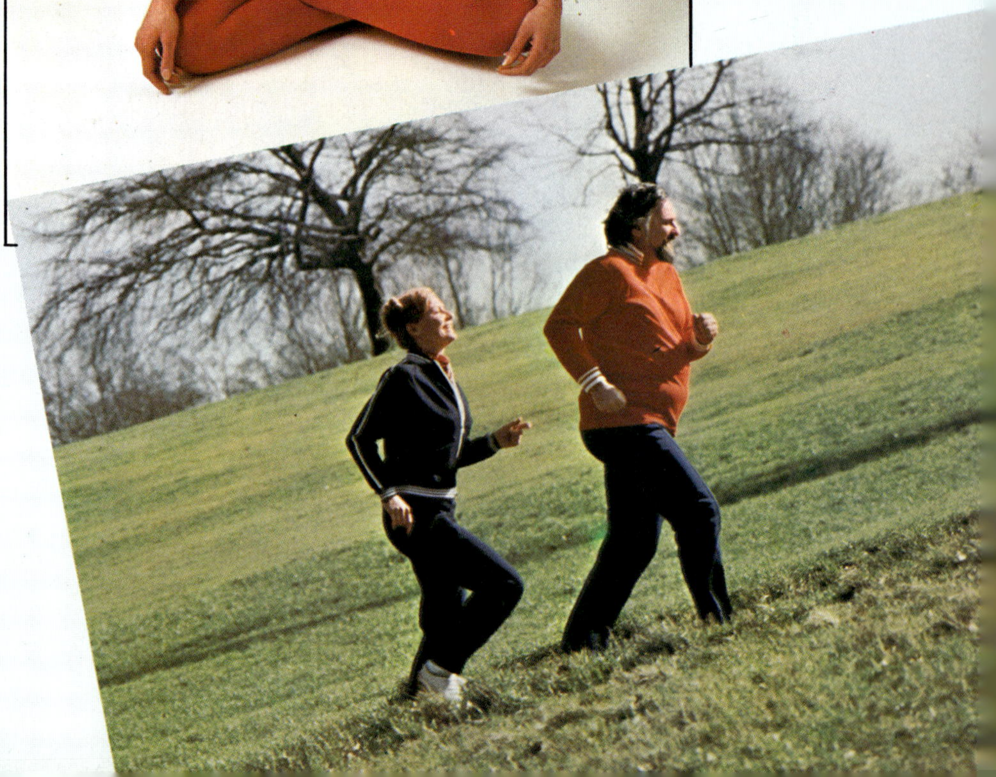

Jogging (below) and workouts in the gym (right) both provide good balanced exercise. The heart and lungs are made to work and so strengthened, and the muscles developed. Exercise brings healthy physical tiredness, but learning to relax properly is also important. Yoga (left) is one of many ways we can relax, and it also keeps the body supple

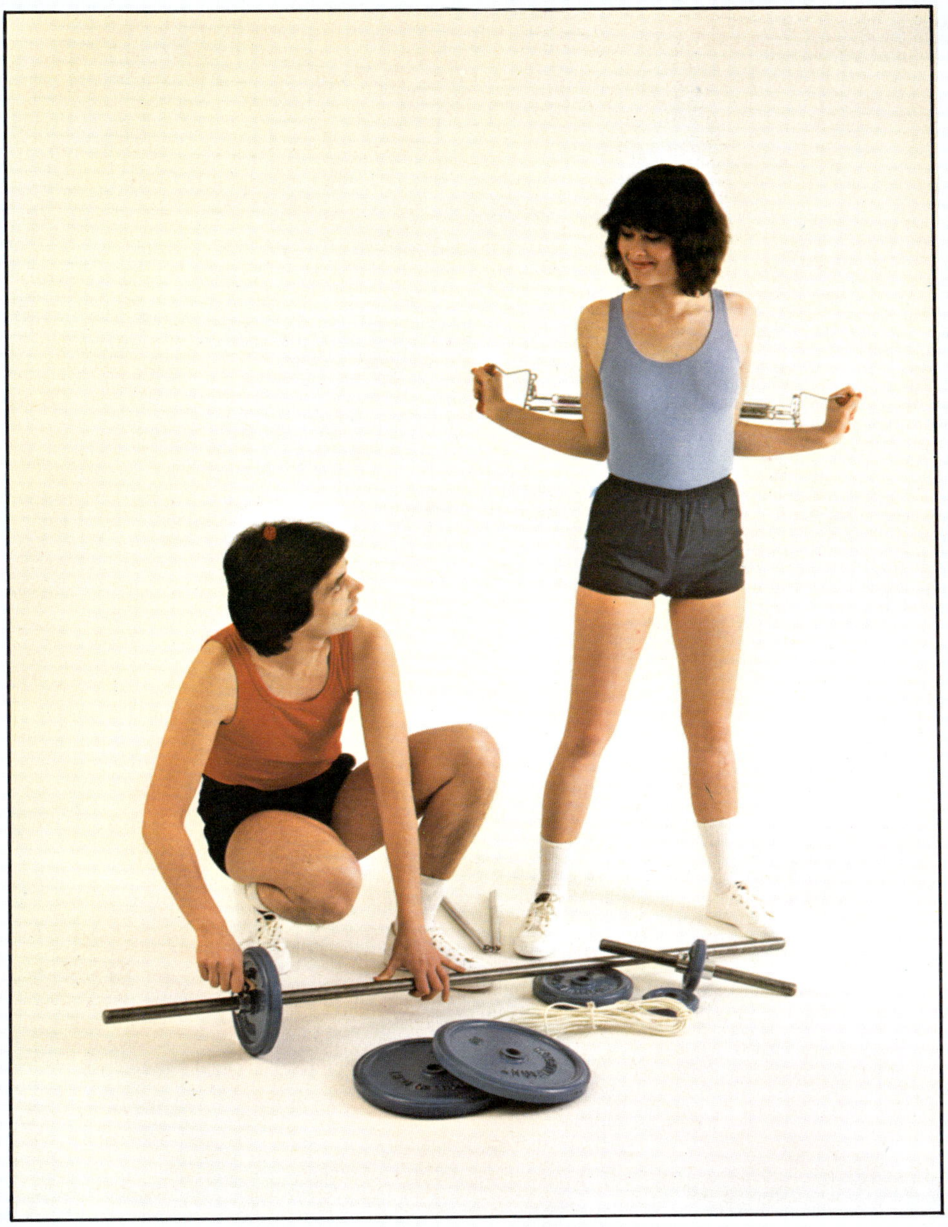

antidotes including the much maligned television. Do not let the part of your life which should provide the relaxation produce more stress, and avoid the temptation to get into the rat-race of social climbing. Be yourself and do the things you enjoy, not the things you think others might expect you to do. In this way you will attract friends you will genuinely like and who like you and friendship of this sort is one of the most valuable aids to relaxation.

Exercise and Sports

Having established a healthy diet and discovered the value of relaxation we must also exercise. Though we use energy (calories) in exercise it is difficult to lose a significant amount of weight by exercise alone. However, a good programme of exercise will certainly help to redistribute that weight and make you look and feel better. This important topic also merits two separate sections in our book where we discuss exercise and specific forms of sport. We will also be explaining the sort of injuries you might sustain in the pursuit of these activities.

Complicated repetitive exercise programmes, although beneficial, are boring. If you find them boring then there is a good chance that you will default so pick a game or sport that will interest you and involve you socially. Taking exercise should be fun and such is the enormous range of sports and sports facilities open to us now that it would be easy to make it so.

As John Goodbody will point out, it may be preferable for you to supplement your chosen sport with some other form of training, such as running or jogging. Having established the habit of a regular run it becomes enjoyable particularly if you get out of town in good weather. This does require some self-discipline particularly after a tiring day at work, but the time when it is most difficult is when it is most beneficial.

Remember my earlier remarks about exercise offsetting the potentially harmful effects of stress. The feeling of relaxation in the bath after a run is magic, the cares of the day are washed away. It is almost like the feeling after sex . . . not quite so good, after all sex is good exercise too. It has been observed that a common habit, particularly amongst American males, is the late night visit to the fridge. Missing out on the midnight snack and making love instead could save him more than 300 calories as well as being enjoyable.

A word of warning: if you are starting a fitness programme from scratch, take care. Do not overdo it. Start slowly and build up gradually. Squash is very much a growth sport in the UK, well established in Australia and starting to gain popularity in the USA. It is an ideal sport in many ways, exciting and easy to learn, enjoyable no matter what the level of skill, very physically demanding which of course makes it highly beneficial. However, squash carries a high mortality rate because of the explosive type of physical exercise it entails. In people over 30 not accustomed to physical exercise it could precipitate a coronary thrombosis. At this age if you are thinking of taking up squash or starting any other form of rigorous training see your doctor for a thorough physical check-up, which should include an ECG. This warning of course applies particularly to those suffering from a chronic medical condition such as angina or high blood pressure.

This warning must not discourage you from taking exercise if you do come into this category, for it is particularly important for patients with a heart condition to get fit, but strict medical supervision is essential in these cases. Routine care for patients who have had a coronary thrombosis generally includes advice regarding diet (losing weight is generally appropriate), and should always include advice about exercise. After a period of complete rest you can start walking short distances, building up to longer distances, then jogging, and away you go.

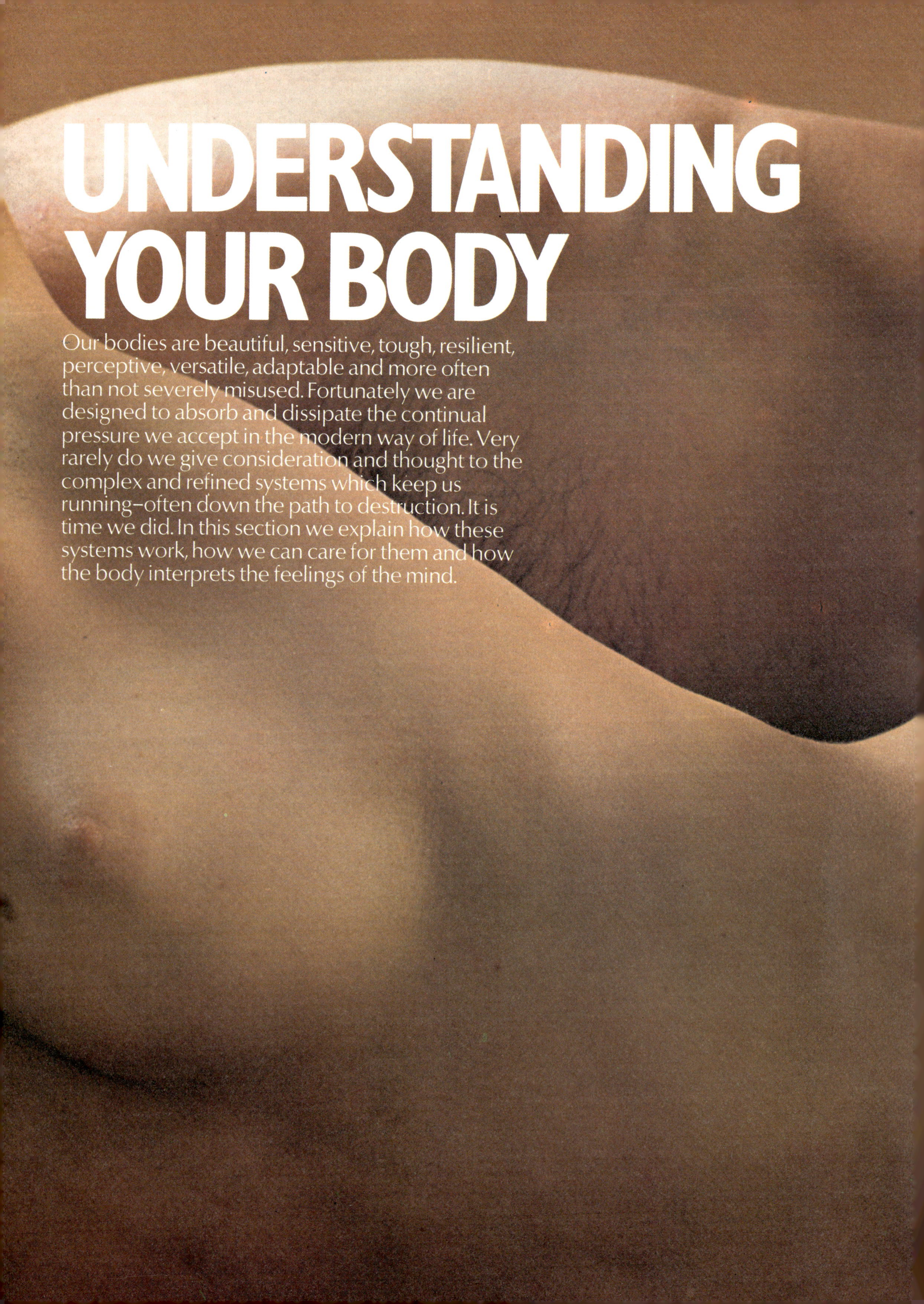

UNDERSTANDING YOUR BODY

Our bodies are beautiful, sensitive, tough, resilient, perceptive, versatile, adaptable and more often than not severely misused. Fortunately we are designed to absorb and dissipate the continual pressure we accept in the modern way of life. Very rarely do we give consideration and thought to the complex and refined systems which keep us running–often down the path to destruction. It is time we did. In this section we explain how these systems work, how we can care for them and how the body interprets the feelings of the mind.

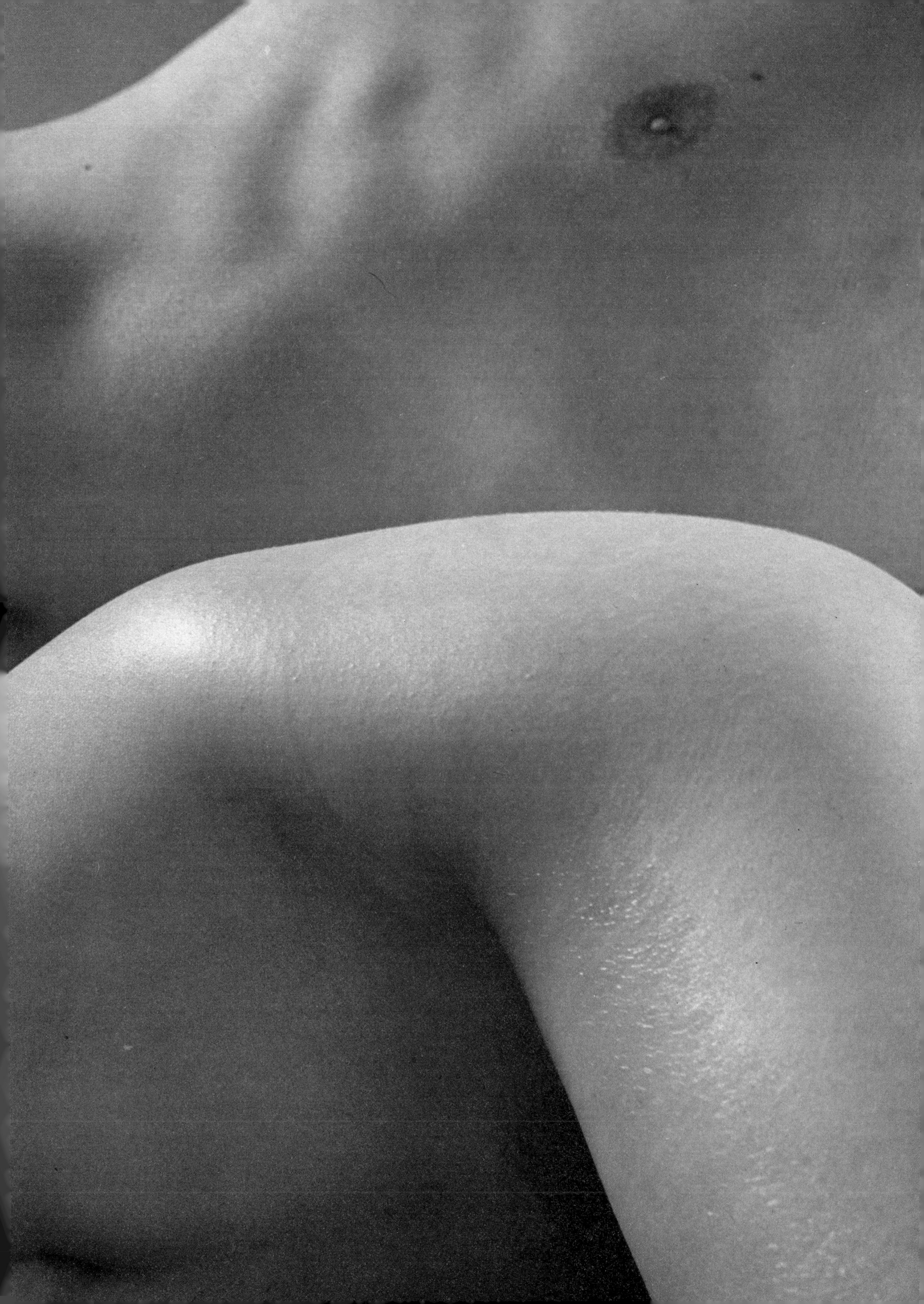

The Body Beautiful

The nineteenth-century English satirist, Samuel Butler, once described the human body as 'a pair of pincers set over a bellows and a stewpan and the whole fixed upon stilts'.

Medical science has since progressed considerably. With X-ray and ultrasonic machines, and with brain scanners, one can now photograph the body as if it were transparent. With fibre optic techniques one can film inside the body, within such organs as the heart, lungs and womb. Radioactive tracers injected into a gland can be used to determine the fate of the hormones it secretes into the bloodstream. With electron microscopes even the mysteries of the cell – the basic unit of all living creatures – have, to a large extent, been solved. Equipped with this knowledge, a present-day counterpart would undoubtedly regard Butler's description as too simple and too crude, preferring rather to compare the human body to a complex machine than to an assembly of limbs and guts.

In attempts to explain how the organs of the body function, doctors (and medical textbooks alike), often make comparisons with mechanical objects; 'the brain', for example, 'acts like a computer'; 'the heart functions as a pump'; 'the eye works like a camera'; and even 'the lungs act like bellows'. Such analogies are quite valid, but they are also potentially dangerous for they influence your attitude toward your own body. Most of us do, indeed, treat our bodies as machines; we use (and abuse) them, assuming that, given a regular and adequate supply of food, kept warm (but not too hot), and allowed several hours rest each day, they will give us about seventy years of trouble-free service.

Happily, the majority of us will reach the mythical 'three score years and ten' without serious upset, for the human body has an amazing capacity for coping and adjusting to the ups and downs of everyday life and for self-repair should minor faults develop. Nevertheless, when serious illness or injury does occur, our bodies never miss the opportunity to point out the error of our ways; unlike a car, for example, repair, replacement of spare parts or a major overhaul of the body is rarely possible, let alone successful.

Whether by God's design or as the product of millions of years of evolution, the human body is built and functions on a level far more sophisticated, more intricate, and often more efficient (and more mysterious) than any many-made machine. Yet, the comprehension and acceptance of such a fact has only recently been adopted by doctors let alone by popular body books and health guides.

In schools, libraries and bookshops one can still find 'workshop manuals of the human body' in which the traditional western view of man as a machine, and as a living creature composed of two units – 'mind' and 'body' – is perpetuated. Such books describe the activities of organs or body systems in terms of 'structure and function'. The 'body' – the blood and guts of man – is viewed as that part concerned with the maintenance of life, with growth and with reproduction. With reference to the 'mind' – the source of all mental functions – doubt as to its nature is invariably expressed; the link between the structure of the brain's grey-matter and its functions is still a little unclear. 'Fault-finding and treatment sections' within these books probably recommend cures of a mechanical nature (surgery) for problems of the 'body'.

A comparable eastern 'body manual' or a folklore family health guide, would undoubtedly express a more metaphysical view. Free from the logical, scientific approach of western medicine and its formal methods of teaching and practice, such books would describe the body as a single entity (and with little or no reference to machines). The 'problem pages' here would recommend such treatments as herbal cures, hypnotism, group therapy and faith healing (rather than surgery), most of these methods exploiting and emphasizing the close interaction between 'body' and 'mind'.

Whereas, in the past, stories of people who would stick knives through their skins without drawing blood; who would attain health and cure from illness through meditation; or even of people who 'worried themselves sick' or 'died of a broken heart', were ignored or rejected by the medical world, present theories of how the body works are continually being revised and adapted to include explanations of such phenomena.

With the birth of the sciences of biochemistry, genetics, physiology, histology and pharmacology, many of the secrets of life and of the human body have been revealed. It is now known, for example, that the endocrine system – the collection of glands in the body which secrete hormones – is involved in many 'mind' over 'body' situations. (Emotion, such as fear, affects the body's physical state as a result of the action of the hormone adrenaline). Furthermore, many cases of asthma, ulcers and heart disease are almost certainly brought on by emotional stress or strain; remove the emotional or social pressures or reduce the pace of life and the symptoms are suppressed or even disappear completely.

The achievement of peak fitness and health therefore requires an awareness of the complexity and essentially non-mechanistic nature of the human body and an appreciation of the strong interaction between 'body' and 'mind'.

By treating one's body with the corresponding respect, one should indeed attain a long and healthy life.

Although the physical appearance of the sexes is so different and yet so attractive, the physiological make up of both male and female is virtually identical. Except for the sex organs, all other components are found within each framework

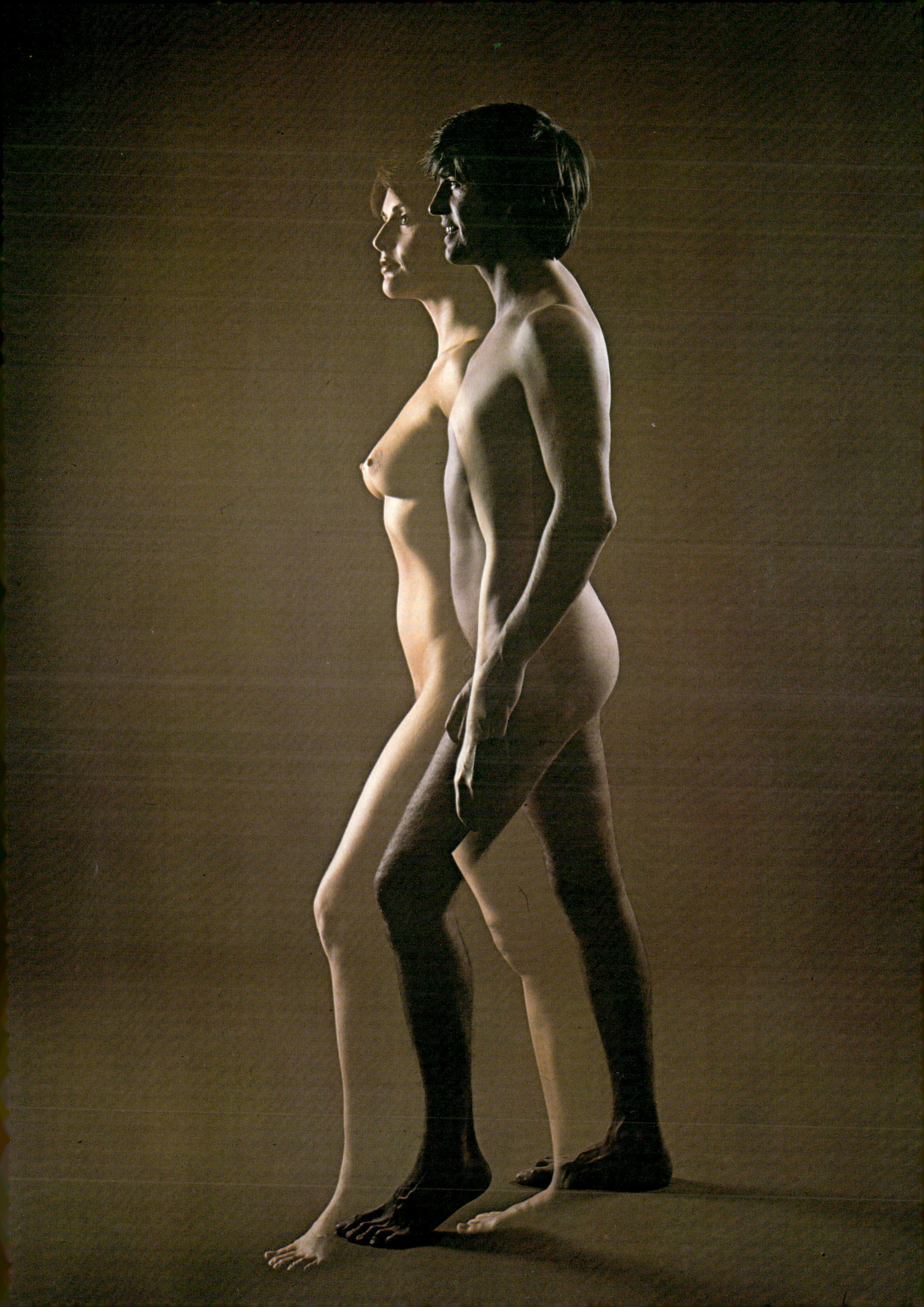

Control Systems

The human body is a highly complex and intricate assembly of cells, tissues and organs. Simply for convenience, however, we can consider the body to be made up of a number of different systems (or functional units) each responsible for a specific range of activities. To introduce these systems, let us take an imaginary journey through the body discussing each in turn as we encounter it. Let us follow, first of all, the path of food, starting from the moment it enters the mouth.

The *digestive system* is concerned with the breakdown of complex food materials into simple chemicals that can be readily absorbed into the body. In the *mouth,* food is subjected to both chemical and mechanical attack. Saliva, from the *salivary glands,* starts the chemical breakdown of sugars, while the *teeth* cut, tear and grind up large pieces of food. With the chewing movements of the *cheeks, tongue* and lower *jaw,* food is rolled into a small ball. In swallowing, this ball is forced into the *oesophagus,* the first section of the 30-foot-long muscular tube, popularly referred to as our guts, extending from the mouth to the rectum. Waves of contraction passing along the length of the tube – an action stimulated by that part of the nervous system beyond our conscious control – churn the food up and push it through the *stomach* and *intestines*. Digestive juices released from the stomach walls, from the *pancreas* and from the walls of the *small intestine,* bring about an almost complete breakdown of fats, carbohydrates and proteins. All that remains is a semi-solid mass of undigested food (combined with unwanted chemicals released by the *gall bladder,* and with millions upon millions of bacteria – offspring of the normal bacterial inhabitants of the intestines). These waste materials are subsequently eliminated by the body; the whole process of digestion from intake of food to defaecation ideally takes twenty-four hours but is usually far longer.

Digested food materials are absorbed into the body's two major transport systems. Fat soluble substances pass into the *lymphatic system* – a network of vessels draining fluid from tissue spaces and later returning it to the bloodstream. Water soluble substances – mainly vitamins, simple sugars and digested protein material – are absorbed directly into the *blood circulatory system*. They are carried in the first place to the liver.

Although regarded as an accessory to the digestive system, *the liver* is, nevertheless, essential to the processing of food in the body. It deals with such activities as the interconversion and storage of proteins, fats and carbohydrates; with the conversion of toxic materials into harmless ones; with the production of bile salts, essential for the digestion and absorption of fats; and with storage of some vitamins. (It is also responsible for the destruction of worn out blood cells and with the manufacture of blood clotting materials). The liver is a chemical factory.

From the liver, food materials are distributed to each and every cell by the *blood circulatory system* – the body's plumbing system. (If joined end to end the pipes – arteries, veins and capillaries – would stretch almost 60,000 miles.) At its centre, and acting as the driving force of the system, is the *heart*. This is a muscular bag, no bigger than our fists and weighing less than a pound. The heart functions as a double pump. The right hand pump receives blood from the general body circulation and pushes it through the lungs and on to the left hand pump. From the latter, blood is pushed around the body returning to the right hand side of the heart once more. Beating about 70 times a minute and ejecting about a cupful of blood with each beat, the heart pumps the nine pints of blood in the system around the complete circuit approximately once every minute. It does so incessantly (and automatically) throughout our lives.

What do cells do with their supply of food materials? Some – the proteins and fats in particular – are used as structural components to build, maintain and repair tissues; cells such as those of the skin, blood and intestinal wall are continually dying off or are lost and must be replaced. Most products of digestion are used to provide energy; this is the most important use of carbohydrates. Cells burn up complex materials in the presence of oxygen to produce chemical energy with the formation of carbon dioxide and water as waste products (a process similar to the combustion of petrol and air in a car engine to produce mechanical energy with carbon monoxide and oxides of nitrogen as wastes!).

But what is the source of this oxygen? Here the *respiratory system* comes into play. Oxygen is transported from the *lungs* – the respiratory organs – to tissues by red blood cells. As blood flows through the lungs, gaseous exchange occurs. As we breathe in – brought about by the simultaneous contraction of the *diaphragm* and muscles of the *rib-cage* – fresh, oxygen-rich air is drawn into our lungs. Circulating blood in the lung walls gives up unwanted carbon dioxide (plus a little water) and in exchange, picks up the oxygen. A relaxation of the diaphragm and rib-cage muscles allows the elastic walls of the lungs to force out the carbon dioxide-laden air.

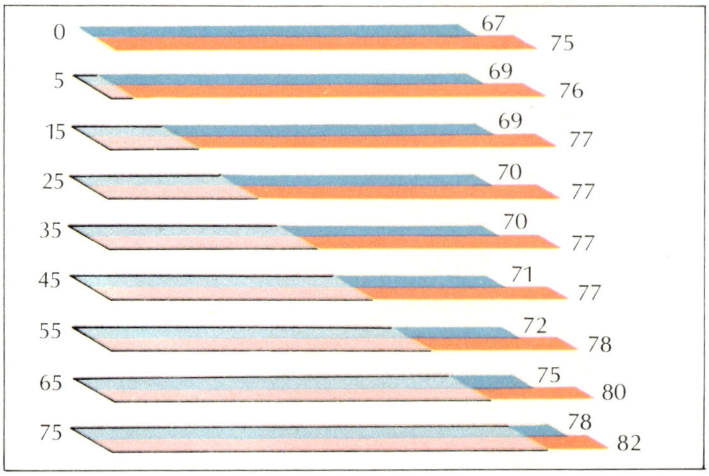

The chart (left) shows how life expectancy increases with age, and that women generally live longer than men. At birth men can expect to live to 67, women to 75, however by 55 the life span has increased to 72 and 78 respectively

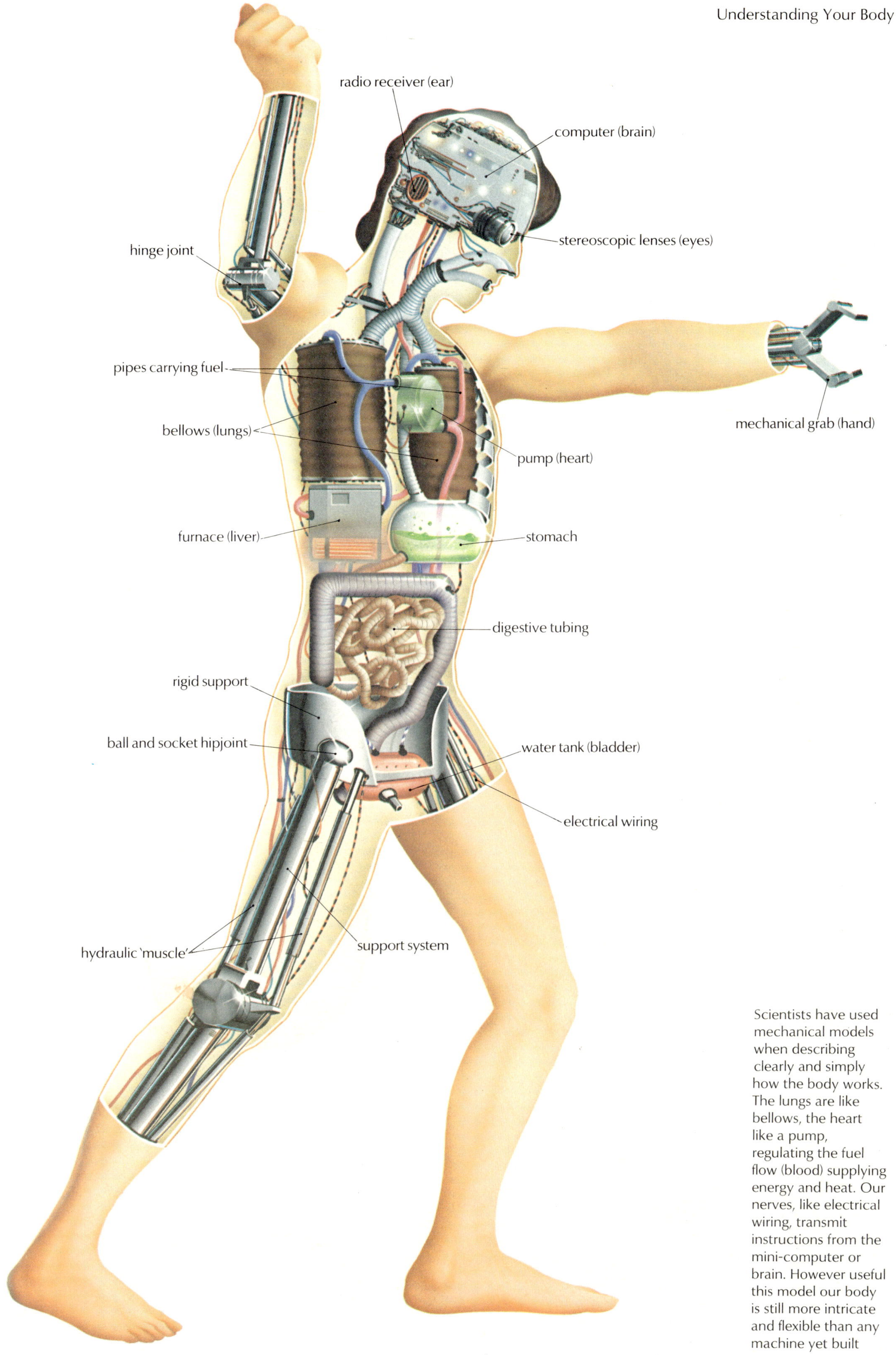

Scientists have used mechanical models when describing clearly and simply how the body works. The lungs are like bellows, the heart like a pump, regulating the fuel flow (blood) supplying energy and heat. Our nerves, like electrical wiring, transmit instructions from the mini-computer or brain. However useful this model our body is still more intricate and flexible than any machine yet built

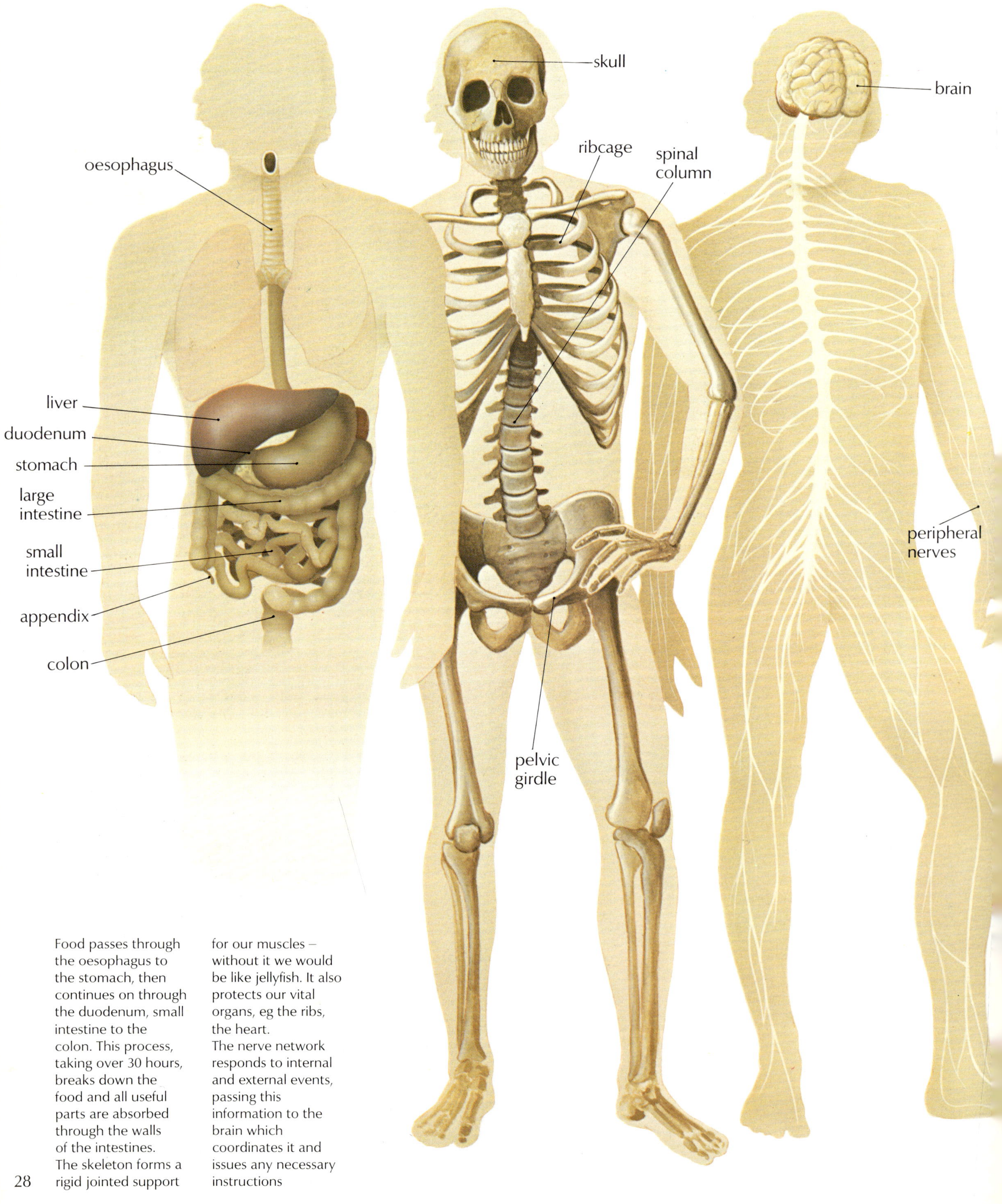

Food passes through the oesophagus to the stomach, then continues on through the duodenum, small intestine to the colon. This process, taking over 30 hours, breaks down the food and all useful parts are absorbed through the walls of the intestines.
The skeleton forms a rigid jointed support for our muscles – without it we would be like jellyfish. It also protects our vital organs, eg the ribs, the heart.
The nerve network responds to internal and external events, passing this information to the brain which coordinates it and issues any necessary instructions

Cells use up their energy reserves in a variety of ways; just to maintain life; to carry out their specific roles – muscle cells to contract and nerve cells to transmit impulses, for example; and for growth, repair and reproduction.

The body system consuming most energy is almost certainly the *locomotor system;* it is concerned with movement. The *skeletal system,* in addition to providing support, giving shape to the body (together with the *skin*), and protecting such organs as the lungs, heart and brain, provides a series of levers. Pairs of *muscles* attached to bones function in an antagonistic manner – one contracts as the other relaxes – operating these levers to produce movement of limbs and changes in posture. Muscles act by converting chemical energy into mechanical energy, but the system is only 25 per cent efficient; much of the energy is lost as heat (a situation again comparable to a car engine). With over 600 skeletal muscles in the body, a considerable amount of food material must therefore be consumed to perform any actions; should one's work involve prolonged physical activity one may need to eat twice as much as a sedentary worker to maintain one's stamina and strength.

Of all the constituents of our diet, carbohydrates are the most important source of energy. Whenever the body burns up protein for energy, waste materials containing nitrogen are produced. These are toxic to cells and furthermore, cannot be excreted as a gas like carbon dioxide. Removal of such substances is the function of the *excretory system;* this incorporates the kidneys, the ureters and the bladder.

Each of our kidneys contain more than a million tiny filter units which remove almost all the non-cellular material from the blood as it circulates through them. Together the kidneys sieve some 50 gallons of fluid from the bloodstream each day. More than 99 per cent is returned, being essential to the body to maintain a constant level of salts and liquid. The remaining 1 per cent – two or three pints perhaps – is excreted as urine, a fluid which consists mostly of water, toxic wastes and unwanted salts.

Although the body lacks true *systems* for growth and repair – these are conducted on a cellular level – it does possess a *reproductive system.* A man's testes continually produce sperm – several million each day. A woman's ovaries produce a single egg at approximately monthly intervals. Following coitus from the fusion of sperm and egg, one cell – the fertilized egg – grows into a multi-million cell new individual.

The role of coordinator of the body's actions, whether digestion, excretion, respiration or reproduction is shared by the *endocrine system* and the *nervous system.* The former consists of a number of glands which secrete hormones, or chemical messengers, into the bloodstream. Hormones stimulate or inhibit the action of specific target organs. Under the influence of the master endocrine gland – the pituitary – the adrenals, pancreas, thyroid, parathyroids, thymus and testes or ovaries, secrete their respective hormones which control such slow, long-term processes as growth, reproduction and the maintenance of stability of the body's internal environment. They may also be responsible for establishing circadian rhythms – the body's inherent biological clocks – which influence our physiology and mental and physical abilities on a daily (or even a weekly or monthly) basis.

The nervous system is concerned both with the coordination of actions and with the reception and response to messages from the environment. The eyes, ears, nose and tongue, and touch, temperature and pressure receptors in the skin, transmit information to the brain relating to your surroundings. Conditions within the body – blood pressure, oxygen and carbon dioxide levels in the blood, and body temperature for example – are similarly monitored by internal receptor cells. Information received from all these sensory organs or cells is processed and interpreted by the brain which reacts by relaying messages to effector organs such as muscles or endocrine glands. These, by virtue of their actions, together minimize the effects of environmental changes to maintain stability both internally and between the body and its surroundings.

In addition to its life supporting role, the brain – the control centre of the nervous system – is concerned with the functions and abilities of memory, judgement, imagination, creative and conscious thought. Quite which part of the brain deals with each of these faculties is still uncertain; the mysteries and complexities of the mind are proving somewhat more difficult to solve than those of the body.

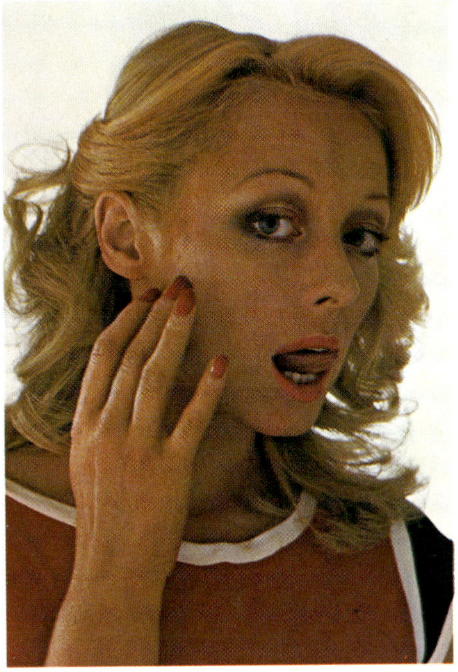

Sight, smell, touch, hearing and taste are the five senses with which we recognize the world around us and which help us distinguish between pleasure and pain

A description of the human body such as this must inevitably make many simplifications. Here the body has been viewed as a collection of systems. But no biological unit – cell, tissue, organ or even animal as a whole – operates in isolation. Each interacts, interrelates (and often communicates) with all the others; some are almost totally dependent on others. The digestive system, for example, functions only with the aid of the nervous system, the muscular system, and such organs as the liver and pancreas. The respiratory and blood circulatory systems work in harmony with each other to provide cells with a continuous supply of fuel and oxygen and to remove many of their wastes. Movement is a product of the combined action of the skeletal and muscular systems; these, in turn, are operated and controlled by the nervous system. The list of computations is endless. In truth, the human body is so complex, intricate and sophisticated in makeup and in mode of operation, as to almost defy any attempt at description.

Heart and Lungs

Arteriosclerosis and coronary artery disease are now the major killer diseases of the western world and much can be done by the individual to avoid factors which contribute to the disease. Age and sex are contributory factors and women seem more protected than men in their pre-menopausal years. Obesity, high cholesterol intake in susceptible individuals and smoking, add up in the stakes against the individual. A low-carbohydrate, low-cholesterol diet lessens the risk of obesity and in the laying down of artheromatous plaques in arteries. Exercise combined with care over diet, can help maintain an individual at the optimum weight for his height and age, and graded exercise will improve the stroke volume and thus the cardiac and pulmonary efficiency.

The heart is a hollow muscular organ about the size of a clenched fist and its function is to maintain a constant circulation of blood throughout the body by regular rhythmic contractions. It consists of four chambers, the two small chambers called atria, and two larger chambers called ventricles. Blood which is returned to the heart from the lungs having been oxygenated is received into the left atrium, then passes into the left ventricle where it is pumped into the aorta and then through the arterial network to all tissues of the body. Now deoxygenated the blood returns to the right atrium of

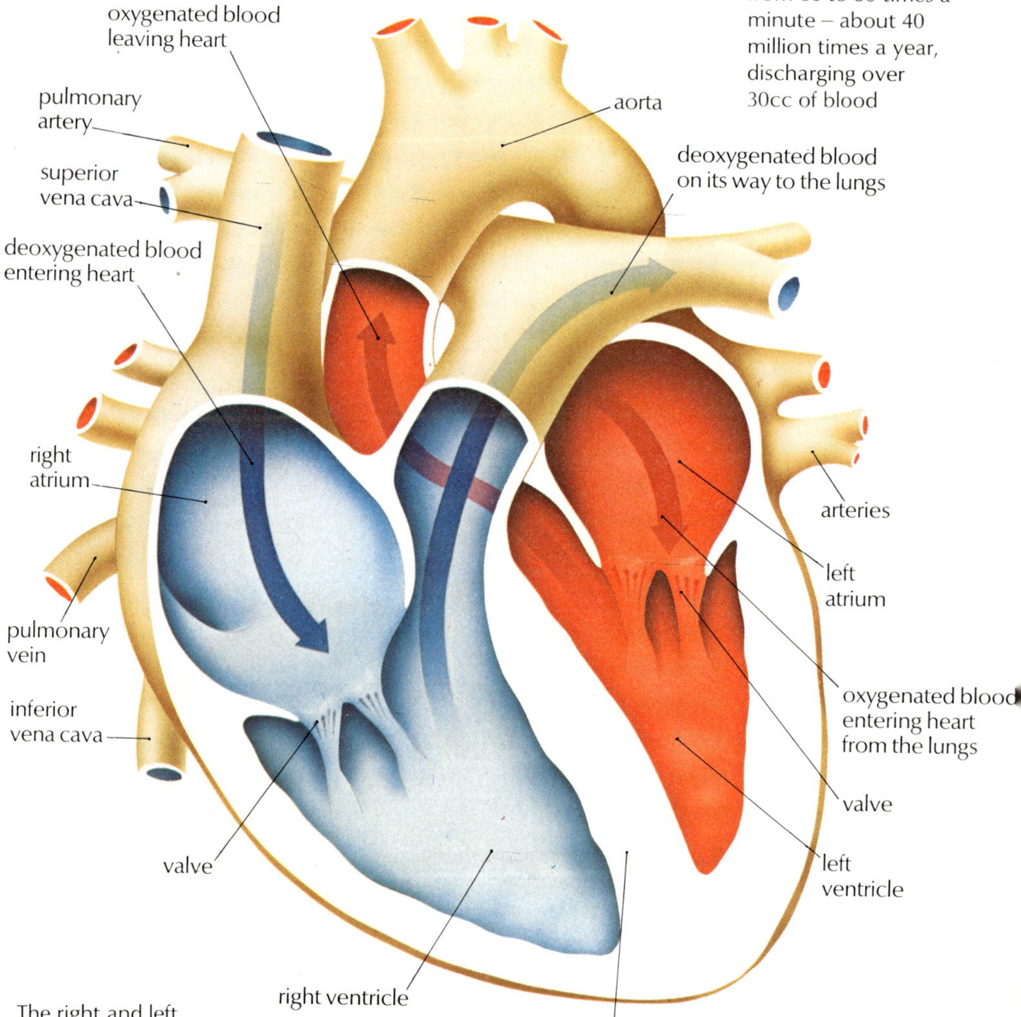

The adult heart beats from 60 to 80 times a minute – about 40 million times a year, discharging over 30cc of blood

The right and left atria, below, fill with blood simultaneously and pump it on to the respective ventricles where it is pumped to lungs and the rest of the body, a process involving ·3 second work, ·5 second rest

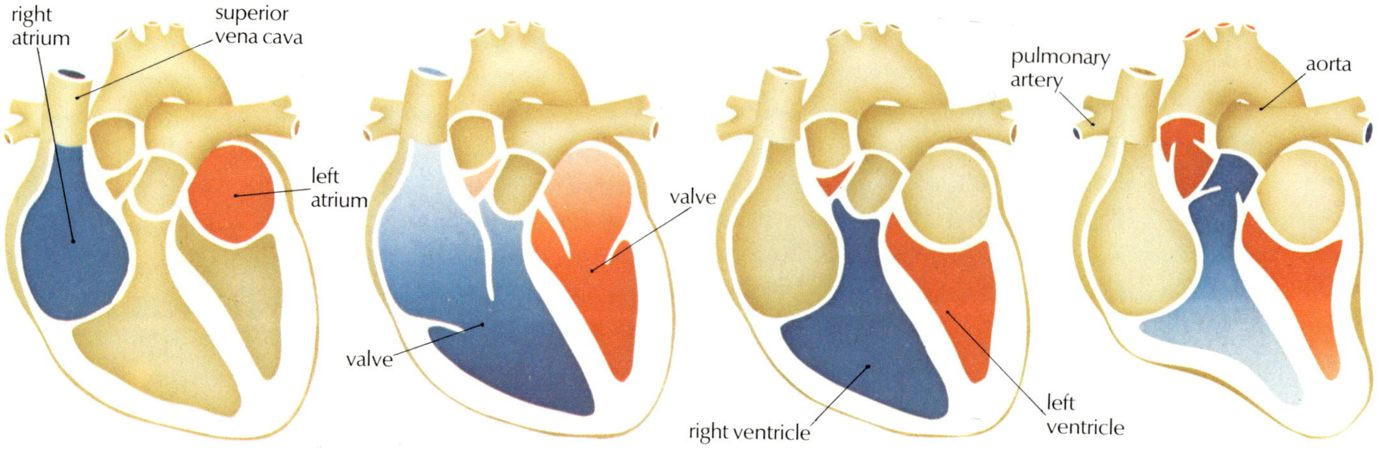

the heart then passes into the right ventricle where it is pumped to the lungs via the pulmonary artery.

The heart consists of three layers. The myocardium is the middle layer consisting of special cardiac muscle. There is a smooth inner layer of endothelium called the endocardium; and an outer inelastic layer called the pericardium which prevents over-distention of the heart. Non-return valves separate the atria from the ventricles and in turn the ventricles from the pulmonary artery and the aorta. These valves allow blood to flow in one direction only, thus ensuring that the heart is an effective pump.

The cardiac muscle has a special property in that it is able to contract spontaneously and rhythmically without nervous stimulation. The heart's pacemaker is called the sino-atrial node. It is situated in the right atrium and beats at about 70-80 beats per minute. The ventricles have a natural rate of 20-40 beats per minute. As the sino-atrial node naturally beats faster then other heart muscle fibres and therefore forces the other part of the heart to follow its rhythm under normal circumstances, it is called the pacemaker. Each contraction starts at the pacemaker and spreads along a special bundle of conduction fibres known as the bundle of His. Although the heart has the power to beat rhythmically without nervous stimulation, the autonomic nervous system regulates rate of beating and the force of contraction.

The heart beat is the contraction of the ventricles and the rate is the number of heart beats per minute. This varies from individual to individual, but is about 70-80 beats per minute in an adult at rest. The rate is raised in exercise when the heart has to pump more blood to active muscles, and also in emotional states, fevers and in some diseases. A slow rate is found in trained athletes, in the elderly and again in some diseases. In stress and anxiety, the adrenal gland releases the hormone adrenaline which also causes the heart rate to rise.

Like other muscle tissue, the cardiac muscle needs an oxygenated blood

The lungs, below, are made up of hollow, sponge-like organs, the alveoli, which air enters through the alveolar ducts

Oxygen in the air passes through the moist wall of the alveolus into the deoxygenated blood in the capillaries

Excess carbon dioxide passes from the deoxygenated blood through the alveolar wall into the lungs and then out

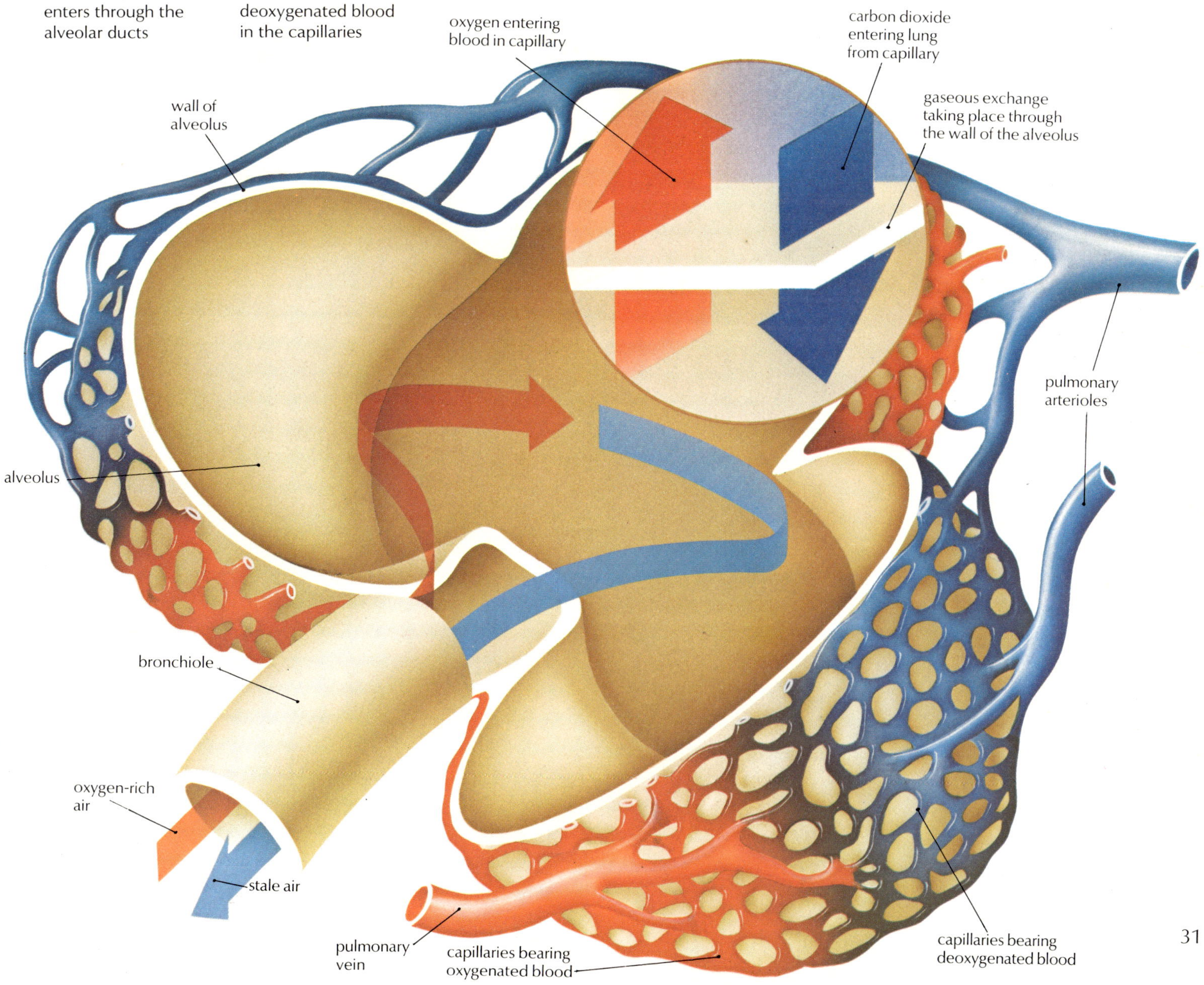

supply and this is supplied by the right and left coronary arteries; these are the first arteries branching off from the aorta. It is these arteries which, if narrowed or blocked by the disease process arteriosclerosis or hardening of the arteries, cause angina or a coronary thrombosis or heart attack.

Blood pressure is the systemic arterial blood pressure, that is, the pressure exerted on the walls of the arteries by the blood ejected from the left ventricle. The blood pressure varies according to the needs of the body; it falls with rest and rises with activity. Exercise, excitement, anxiety, fear all cause the blood pressure to rise. An adequate blood pressure is needed to ensure the flow of blood to the tissues and it depends on several factors. It depends on the cardiac output, that is, the volume of blood ejected by each ventricle in a minute, the elasticity of the arteries and the total amount of circulating blood. If there is blood loss, then the blood pressure falls and the subject may go into a state of shock or collapse. Now, the blood pressure is controlled at various centres. It is under the control of the central nervous system and at sensitive receptor sites which automatically, on sensing a raised blood pressure, slows the heart rate until the blood pressure falls. Chemicals such as metabolites, hormones and adrenaline, influence the blood pressure and it is also affected, like the heart rate, by emotion, anxiety and fear.

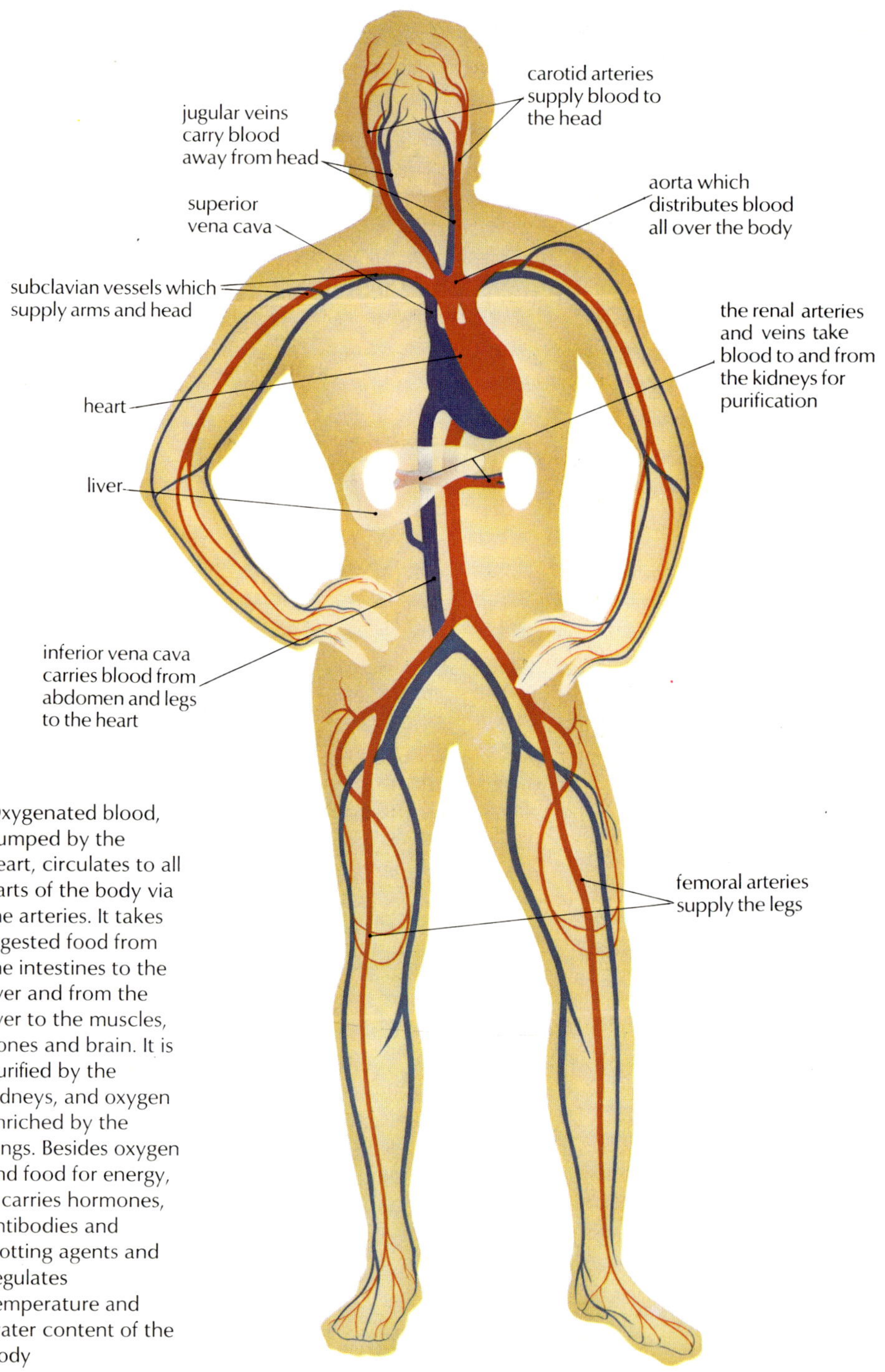

Oxygenated blood, pumped by the heart, circulates to all parts of the body via the arteries. It takes digested food from the intestines to the liver and from the liver to the muscles, bones and brain. It is purified by the kidneys, and oxygen enriched by the lungs. Besides oxygen and food for energy, it carries hormones, antibodies and clotting agents and regulates temperature and water content of the body

Circulatory system

The aorta arises from the left ventricle of the heart and it in turn branches into arteries, dividing into arterioles and finally capillaries. The interchange of oxygen, nourishment and waste products takes place by osmosis through capillary walls. The capillaries in turn lead into venules which become veins and these return the carbon dioxide loaded blood to the right side of the heart and then to the lungs where the carbon dioxide is expelled. Arteries are structured like the heart, in that they have three coats. An outer fibrous coat to give strength and protection to the vessel, a middle coat of plain muscle fibres with some elastic fibres which are circular and therefore contract and relax altering the calibre of the vessel. The inner layer has again some elastic fibres supporting the lining cells from the middle muscular layer. Smaller arteries and arterioles are more muscular than elastic; therefore the blood supply to an organ or tissue is mainly controlled by the variation in calibre of smaller arteries or arterioles. The veins have correspondingly three coats but are much thinner. Many veins have valves to assist the venous return to the heart and prevent a back flow. Any disfunction of these valves gives rise to back flow of returning blood causing varicose veins in the lower limbs. Moderate to mild varicose viens are easily dealt with by a course of injections.

Cardiovascular fitness

The degree of cardiac activity is expressed by the cardiac output which is the volume of blood pumped by each ventricle per minute. Stroke volume is the volume of blood ejected from each ventricle in one beat and therefore one can see that cardiac output equals heart rate times stroke volume. Athletes increase their stroke volume and the more highly trained the individual, the greater is the contribution of an increased stroke volume to the elevated cardiac output of exercise which reduces the heart rate, thus making a more efficient pump.

Muscles and Action

In man, muscle performs the function of converting chemical energy into mechanical energy. This in turn serves many useful functions and because our muscles are often underused in today's society they may give us discomfort too.

Posture and balance

The posture of the body depends on the tone of its muscles. In standing upright, the head must be carefully balanced on the trunk, the trunk on the legs and the legs on the feet. This is at first far from easy, and it takes an infant many months to learn to stand unsupported. The force of gravity tends constantly to cause the body to fall forwards and muscles which act against gravity in this way are called anti-gravity or postural muscles.

The tone in the different groups of muscles which control balance varies according to the needs of the moment. The tone is regulated reflexively by impulses coming from stretch receptors in the muscles themselves, from the eyes, from the balance mechanism in the inner ear and from pressure receptors in the skin, especially the skin of the soles of the feet.

In health all muscles, even when at rest, are in a continuous state of slight contraction, i.e. muscle tone. If any part of the nerve supplying the muscle is severed, or part of the spinal cord to which the nerve is connected, tone is lost and the muscle becomes flaccid. Muscle tone is lessened during sleep.

Muscular pain and stiffness

Untrained people, during and following strenuous muscular exercise, may experience pain and stiffness. The pain usually occurs during exercise, whereas stiffness appears a few hours later.

It is thought that the pain of strenuous exercise is the result of an accumulation of lactic acid which is a product of muscle metabolism. This initiates the pain receptors localized in the muscle and the pain disappears on ceasing exercise, as the lactic acid diffuses from the muscles to the bloodstream.

During exercise, fluid accumulates in muscles and a number of hours may be required for its reabsorption into the bloodstream. This gives rise to a sensation of stiffness when the muscle is stretched.

Heat production

The chemical reactions which occur in the muscle cells during contraction result in the production of heat. This is one of the important ways in which heat is produced to keep the body warm. Indeed, if the body cools down, the involuntary contractions we call shivering start to produce more heat.

During exercise, more heat is produced than the body needs and sweating is one method of readjustment that takes place to increase heat loss.

Smooth muscle

This kind of muscle is designed for comparatively slow contraction over relatively long periods of time, with little expenditure of energy, so that it does not tire easily. Its action is not under voluntary control, hence it is also known as *involuntary muscle*.

In the smooth muscle system of the intestine, the circular and longitudinal muscle fibres act in a co-ordinated manner to produce the action known as *peristalsis*. By means of these rhythmic contractions, the contents of the intestine are mixed with digestive juices and slowly move down the alimentary canal.

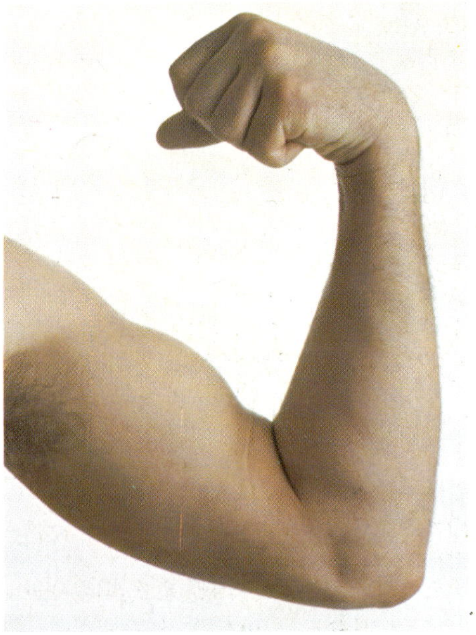

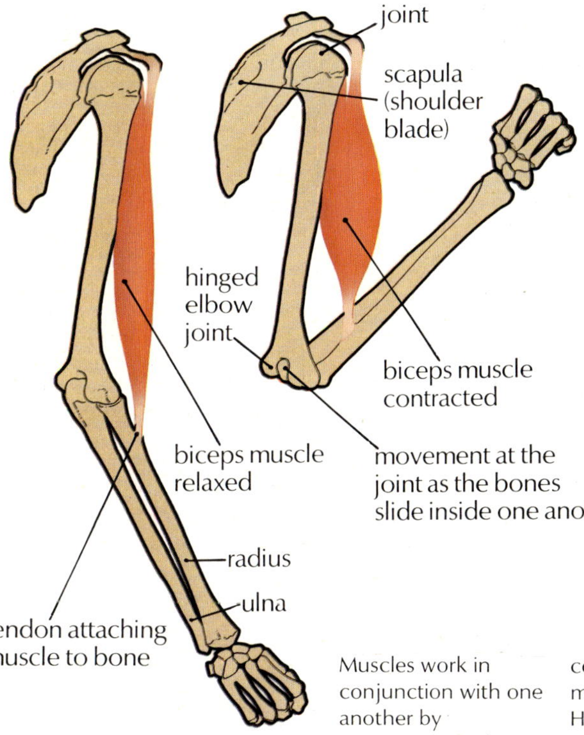

Muscles work in conjunction with one another by contraction and relaxation, and the more a muscle contracts, the more movement there is. Here a command from the brain causes the biceps to contract, lifting the forearm

Cardiac muscle

The heart starts beating three or four weeks after conception and goes on beating until death. Thus it can never 'rest' and in addition, it must be able to conduct impulses in such a way that the various parts of the heart contract in the correct sequence to produce an ordered and effective heart beat. There are special conducting muscle fibres called Purkinje fibres which carry out this particular work.

Skeletal muscle

Striped or skeletal muscle is designed for strong contraction over relatively short periods of time and its contractions involve a considerable expenditure of energy. It needs, therefore, a rich blood supply to bring food materials and oxygen to it and to dissipate the heat generated as well as to dispose of waste products, i.e. metabolites. Skeletal muscle tires very quickly and contraction of this type of muscle is under voluntary control, hence it is called *voluntary muscle*.

The skeletal muscle system in man is elaborately organized. The performance of a simple movement such as the raising of the arm, requires elaborate control, regulation and participation of many muscles, nerves and sense organs.

Each individual muscle in the system is usually described as having an *origin* and an *insertion*. Upon contraction, it exerts a force tending to draw origin and insertion close together.

The shortening of a muscle against a load or resistance, results in the performance of work, while the development of tension without shortening, serves to prevent movement as in the maintenance of posture.

The contraction of a muscle involves three distinct but interrelated events which are: stimulation of the muscle by impulses from the central nervous system; chemical changes in the muscle that furnish the energy for contraction; and rearrangement of some of the structural elements of the muscle fibres into a shorter form.

The system of skeletal muscles

Skeletal muscle fibres are connected together to form muscles by what is known as connective tissue. Each fibre is surrounded by a delicate sheath, the *endomysium;* the fibres are bound into bundles by the *perimysium* and the bundles form the muscle itself which is surrounded by the *endomysium*.

A muscle is sometimes attached directly to bone but very often it is attached by means of a thick bundle of strong white shiny collagen fibres called a

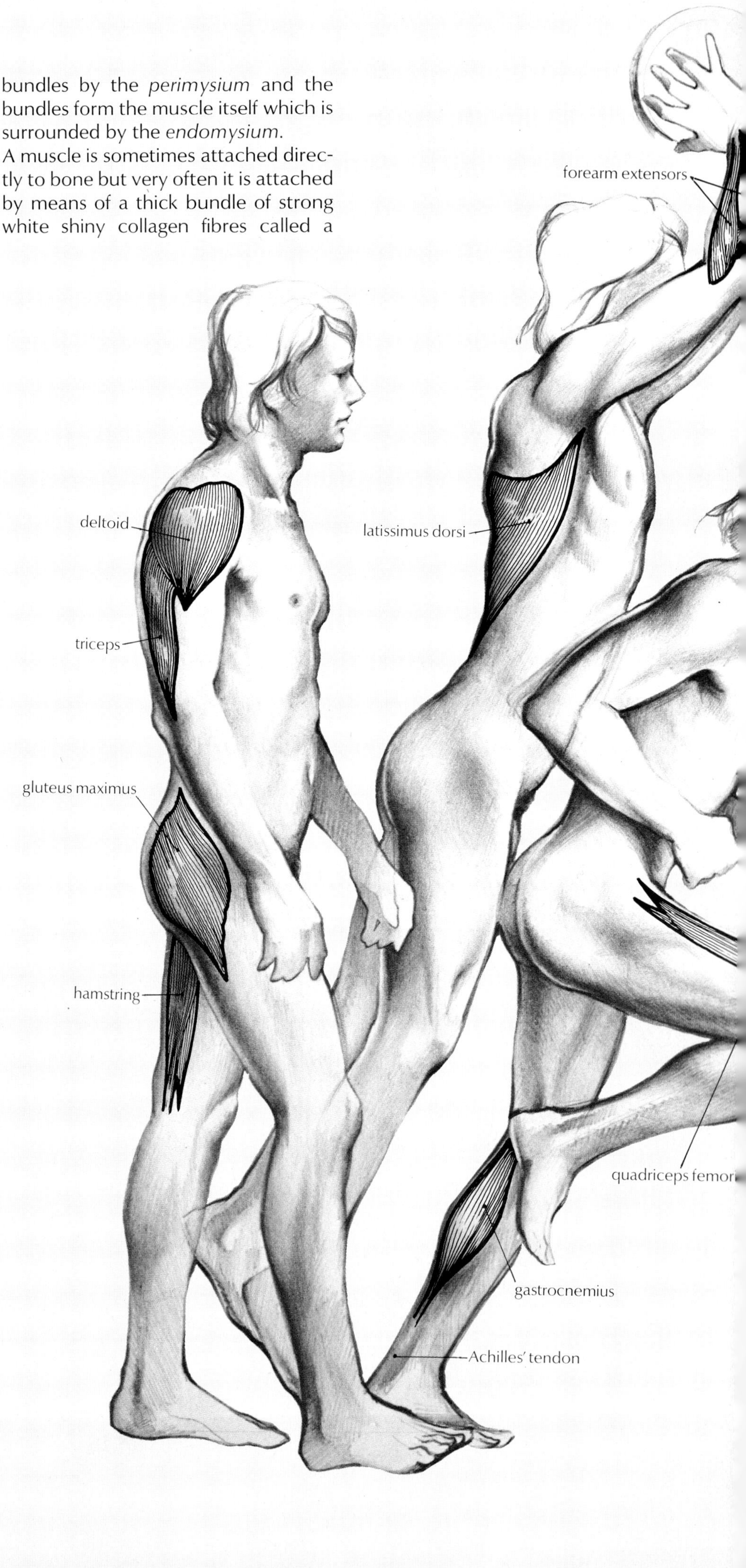

tendon. Muscles may have tendons of origin and tendons of insertion.

Different kinds of muscles

Skeletal muscle fibres range in length from 1mm to 30cms. They are arranged in a number of different ways to form six different kinds of muscle. The structure of a muscle reflects its function, because when a muscle fibre contracts, it shortens to approximately half of its relaxed length. The longer the muscle fibres, the greater the range of movement the muscle produces; the parallel and fusiform types are most effective in this respect. The greater the number of muscle fibres in a muscle, the more power it can exert. The multipennate type is specialized in this direction. Also some muscle groups, such as the hamstrings, or the back of the thigh, act over two joints, the hip and knee joints.

Muscle strength

Strength may be defined as the ability to exert tension against resistance, and this depends essentially on the power of contraction of muscular tissue.

The state of training plays a very important role in the power of contraction of muscular tissue. In a muscle weakened by lack of exercise or disuse, for example bed rest, gains in strength due to a tailored exercise regime commonly exceed 50 per cent during the first two weeks.

When a muscle is repeatedly contracted under overload conditions several times weekly, as in weight-training, it responds by undergoing hypertrophy, i.e. increase in muscle bulk. It is possible to increase the power of muscles three times or more without increasing the volume and this is accomplished by training with near maximal loads and using few repetitions. Hypertrophy without an accompanying significant gain in strength, results from training with moderate loads and using many repetitions.

Strength is related to age and sex. Strength scores of males increase rapidly from 12-19 years of age and at a rate proportional to weight increases.

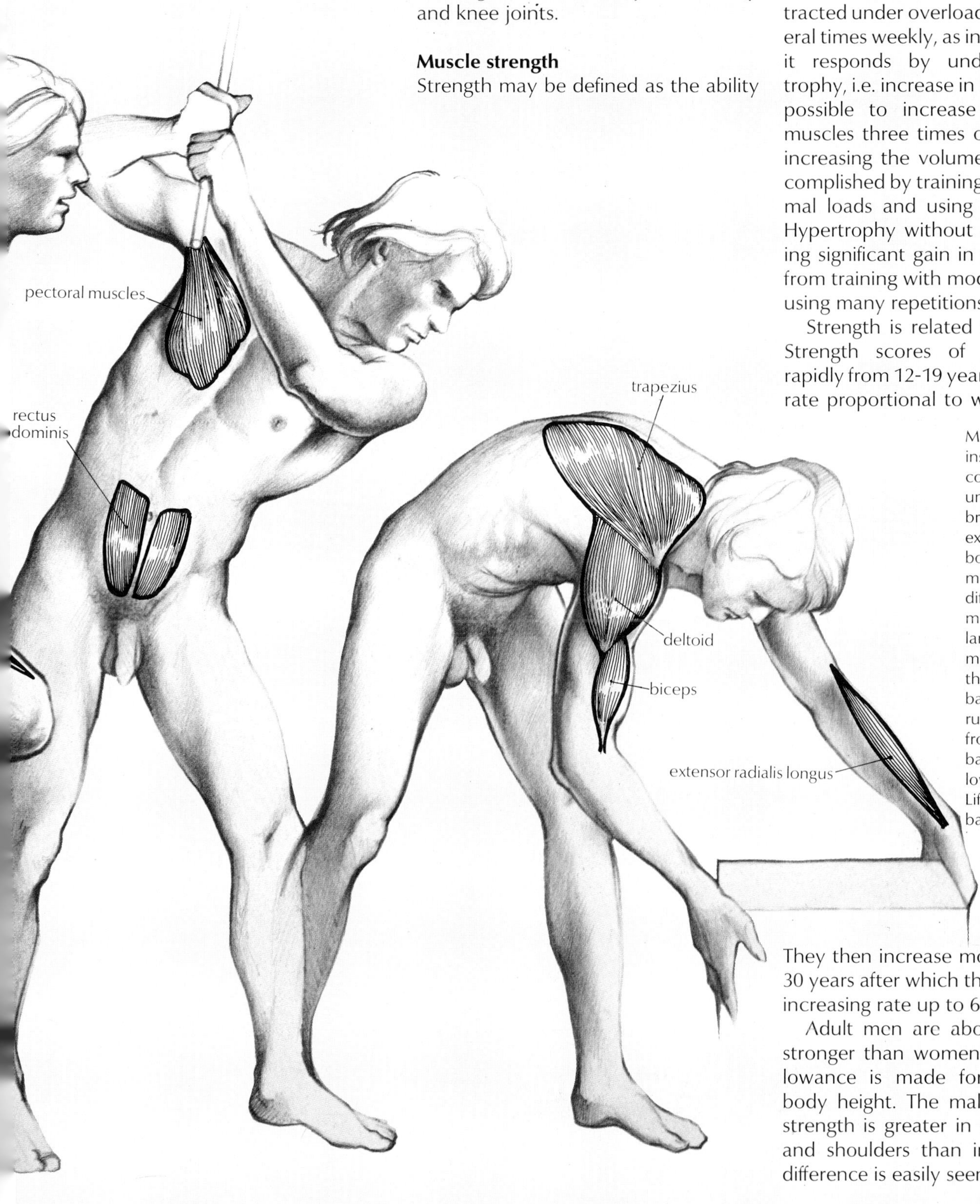

Muscles when instructed consciously or unconsciously by the brain contract or expand, making our body move. Each movement involves a different group of muscles – walking largely uses the thigh muscles, catching those of the side, back and forearms, running those of calf, front thigh, and batting, chest and lower abdomen. Lifting involves the back and upper arm

They then increase more slowly up to 30 years after which they decline at an increasing rate up to 60 years of age.

Adult men are about 45 per cent stronger than women even when allowance is made for differences in body height. The male superiority in strength is greater in the trunk, arms and shoulders than in the legs. The difference is easily seen in physique.

The Back

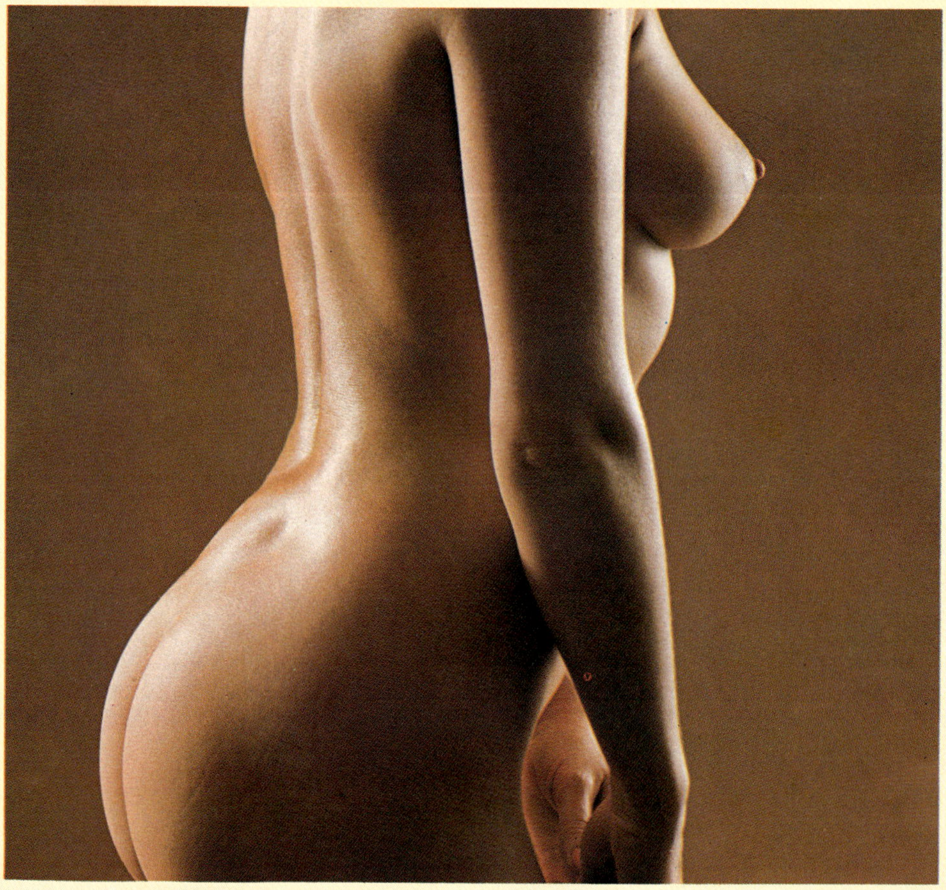

The spine is not naturally a straight line, but curves in an 'S' shape from neck to bottom

The bad back is almost a music-hall joke, so common that most of us will suffer from it at some time in our lives. In Britain a million and a half people go to their doctors each year with back pain, and 13 million working days are lost because of it. And yet it is largely our own fault. The 24 separate vertebrae, held together by ligaments to form the flexible S-shaped spinal column, are probably the most misused bones in our bodies.

Back pain is not usually serious – nobody ever died of backache – but it has a disproportionate effect on the sufferer. The days you wake up with a bad back you feel irritable, incapable and about ten years older than you actually are. Although a 'slipped disc' is the most widely quoted source of back pain, it is by no means the most common one. If your back aches, the chances are that it is due simply to muscle strain, brought about because you habitually put the muscles of your back in unnatural positions, or subject them to the effects of cumulative stress. Although it is flexible, your spine can be, and often is, thrown out of shape by bad posture, or strained from carrying heavy weights awkwardly. The man who habitually suffers from a bad back on Monday mornings has probably spent too much of the weekend carrying his children around: his wife probably has one the whole week through as well. Whatever it is you are lifting, aim to keep your back as straight as possible – bend your knees, not your spine.

But it is not only weight-lifters who tend to get back trouble. Most chairs and car seats are badly designed, giving no support to the lower back, so you may suffer backache even if your job involves sitting behind a desk for most of the day, or driving long distances. Keep a cushion handy to tuck behind the base of your spine and give it the extra support your seat may not provide.

Even a simple activity like washing up in a sink which is too low may cause

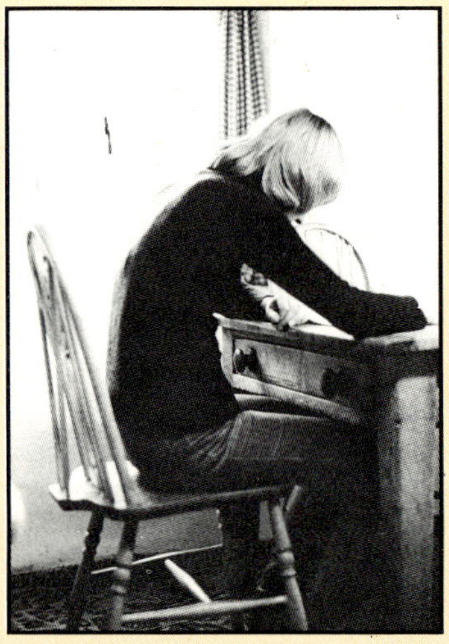

Sitting badly can cause back strain

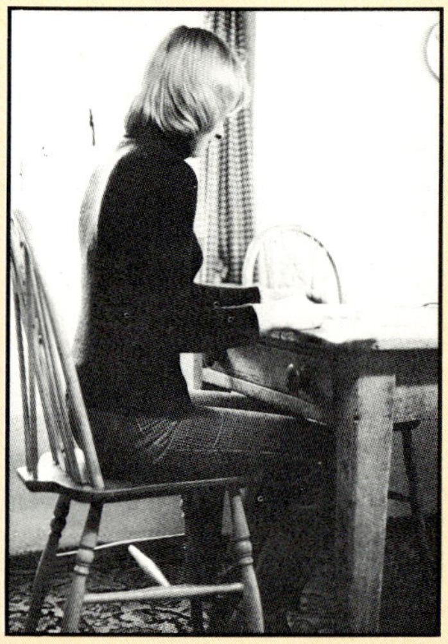

Correct posture: back and legs supported

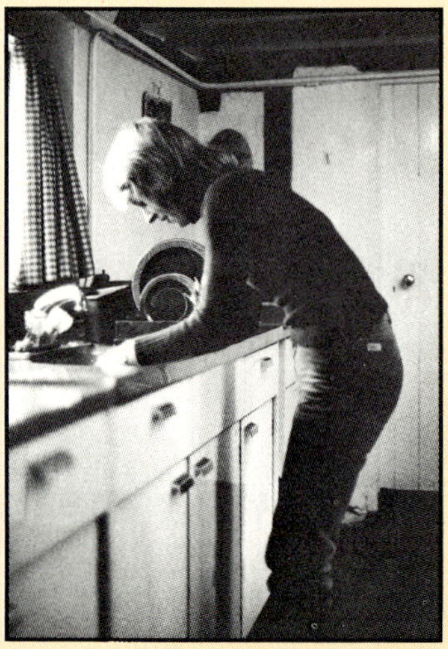

Sinks at wrong height cause stooping

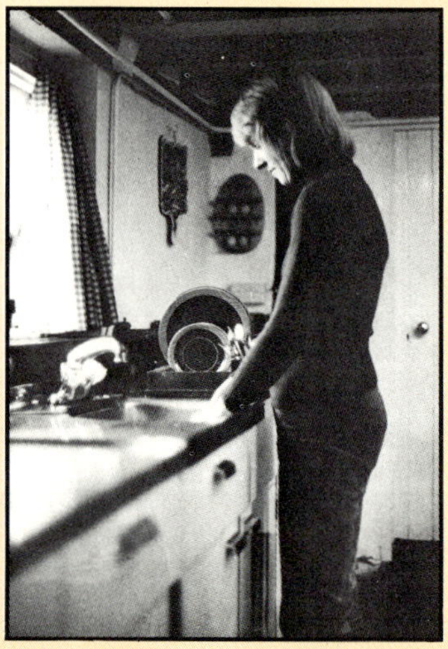

Vary your height or that of the bowl

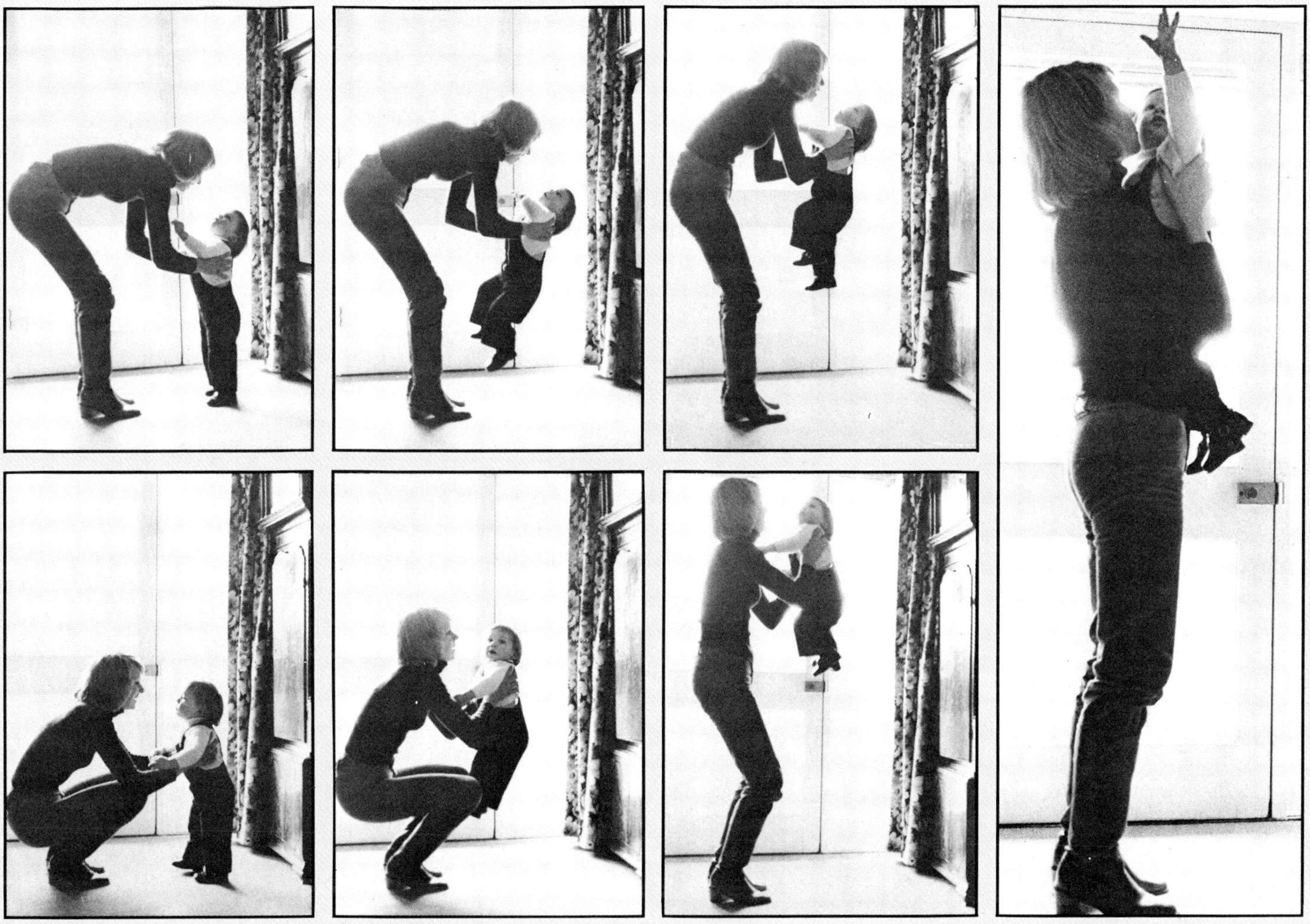

Lifting an object, a baby, suitcase, typewriter and so on can strain back muscles or cause a 'slipped disc'. Always crouch, never bend from the waist, when lifting. *Far right:* correct standing posture

incapacitating backache because it involves prolonged stooping. Most kitchens are designed for people of average height. If you are tall it is worth putting a couple of bricks under a washing-up bowl in the sink, in order to raise it a few inches.

The heavier you are, the more prone to back problems you are likely to be. If you are carrying a couple of extra stone around, it is your back muscles that will take the strain. If you are particularly worried or upset about something you may find that this leads to back trouble too, because the emotional strain you are under can cause muscle tension.

A goose-feather bed may have been romantic, but disastrous for the spine. If your mattress is too soft it means you will be spending all night with an unnaturally curved back. If you are planning to buy a new mattress anyway, you may like to try a specially designed orthopaedic one. A cheaper solution that works very well is simply to use an ordinary, firm mattress, with a sheet of board underneath it.

Pregnant women are particularly liable to back troubles, because the shift in their centre of gravity causes them to lean slightly backwards, putting extra strain on their muscles.

A true 'slipped disc' occurs when one of the cartilaginous discs which lie between one vertebra and the next and which act as the shock absorbers of the backbone, gets pushed slightly out of place so that it causes pain by pressing on adjacent nerves. Usually this results from some sudden, awkward movement, and typically it happens when the vertebrae of the spine are misaligned and heavily loaded at the same time – stooping down and forwards to lift a suitcase out of a car boot, for example, or to push up a heavy window. But it may be caused by some movement so apparently harmless that it is not even noticed at the time. Unlike muscle strain, coughing, sneezing or straining worsens the pain from a slipped disc, and in severe cases it may spread down one or both legs.

There is no specific treatment for a slipped disc, and no sure-fire cure. Most doctors will advise you to rest, and they may give you drugs to relax the back muscles which go into spasm after the injury and prevent the disc slipping back. Sometimes a doctor will recommend you to wear a rigid supportive strait-jacket. Your doctor will probably not recommend an osteopath, but a great many people go to them all the same and claim that their results are at least as good as any conventional treatment. If you do go to an osteopath, don't leave it too late. Manipulating a disc back into place is easier if it is done two or three days after the injury. Most methods work in time – because most discs slip back eventually of their own accord. But a disc which has slipped once is always more likely to slip again, so once you have suffered one, regard your back as especially vulnerable and take extra care especially when lifting. The only sensible advise for guarding against back pain is to ensure that back muscles are regularly exercised.

Posture and Balance

Few of us can walk across Niagara on a tightrope, but we are all very successful at maintaining our balance in less demanding circumstances. We can right ourselves if we trip or if somebody jolts us off balance, we can walk along the corridor of a moving train; we know, even in the most disastrous circumstances, which way up we ought to be and manage, on the whole, to stay that way. Most of us can master even more complex feats of balance and coordination – ice skating, mountaineering, skateboarding or surfing. Even the most poorly coordinated can learn to ride a bicycle.

We do not normally have to think about staying upright. Our brains are 'programmed' to keep our bodies in balance. Watch a child learning to walk though, and you will see that he is still laying down these basic programmes and building up the reflexes. He walks with his legs wide apart to give him an extra-secure base, and a trip that an adult would recover from immediately will send him flat on his face. But once the basic movement patterns and reflexes have been laid down we don't have to think consciously about posture until we are learning some new activity which needs new postural skills.

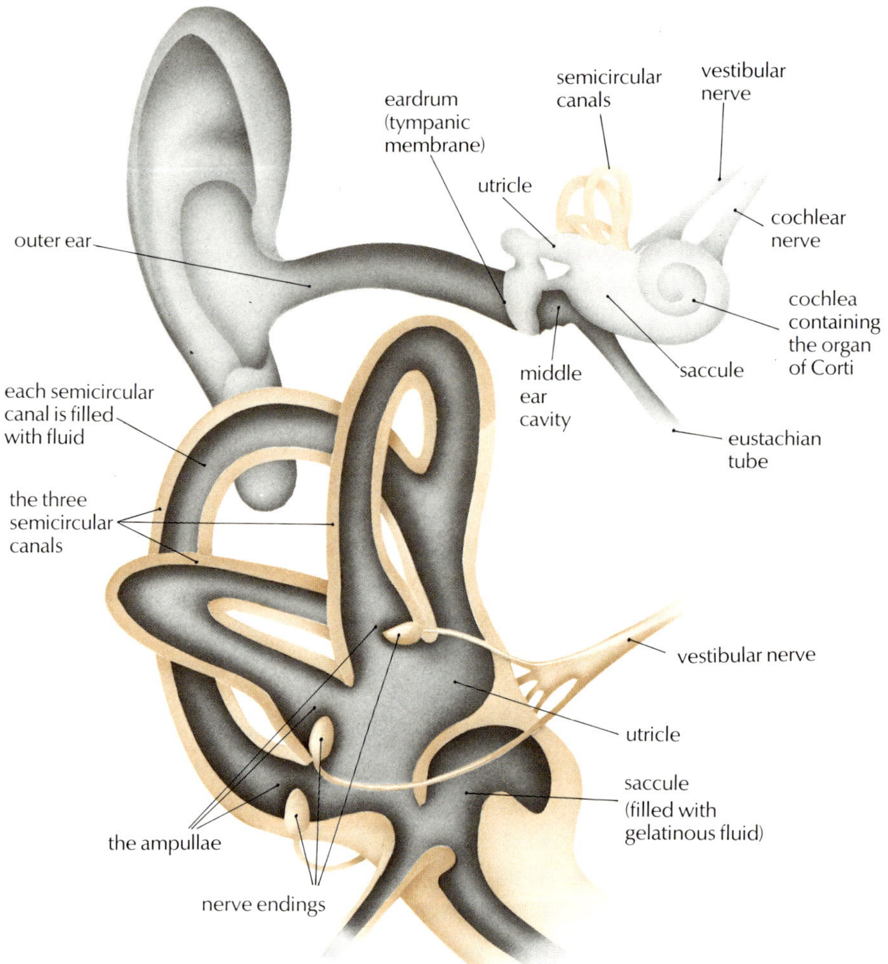

The ampullae contain fine hairs which are attached to nerve endings. When the head moves, the fluid in the canals moves the hairs, and this information is carried to the brain, where it is interpreted, telling us if we are moving. A similar arrangement in the utricle and saccule responds to gravity, telling us which way up we are

Our main organs of balance are in the middle ear. They are sensitive to any movements or changes in the position of the head and send the information they receive to the hind part of the brain which deals with posture and movement. During the first two years of a child's life, when he is learning the basic patterns of movement, this part of the brain grows so rapidly that by the time he is two it has almost reached adult size. The brain receives messages about changes in position not only from the organs of balance but from the muscles themselves, together with visual signals from the eyes. It can occasionally misinterpret these signals. For some time after we have come off a merry-go-round, for example, the organs of balance in the ear are still affected, and override the messages from our eyes and muscles which tell us we are on *terra firma* once more, so we feel dizzy. The ghost train whose track runs through a turning cylinder gives us such strong visual cues that we are tilting sideways that we lean the other way, making totally unnecessary adjustments to a purely illusionary change in position. And the visual cues our brains receive when we watch a moving train pass our own stationary one convince us that we ourselves are moving.

But usually the system works well and the brain continually monitors our movements, making small but constant adjustments to our posture by damping down some groups of muscles so that others can act more strongly until the correct movement or position is achieved.

A great deal of muscular activity is involved even when we are only standing still. The muscles are continually under tension and are having to adjust to maintain balance. So standing upright all day, even though we are apparently 'doing' nothing, can still be tiring.

The 'best' posture, whatever we are doing, is the one which puts least strain on muscles and backbone. For most of us, our natural posture is disastrous – we slump and stoop, over our desks, our books, the washing-up, the typewriter. Test your posture by standing with your back against a wall, your weight resting evenly on your feet. Your shoulder blades and buttocks should touch the wall. If only your shoulders touch, you are round-shouldered; if only the middle of your back touches, your spine is curved too much and your posture is bad.

If you sit for any length of time, make sure your chair does not make an awkward posture (and its consequent back problems) inevitable. Choose a chair which will support the base of your spine – if necessary use a cushion. The seat should slope slightly backwards and be deep enough to support your thighs. It should adjust for height so that your knees are not bent to an angle of more than 90°. Anyone who spends much of the day copytyping should try to change the work from one side to another, to avoid continual twisting of the spine, or better still, clip the copy directly in front of them.

If you are driving a car, the same rules apply – keep your back upright and supported, with a cushion if necessary. Ideally you should be able to rest your head against the seat-back. In practise, this means a head-support, which should be high enough for your head to rest comfortably against.

Never bend from the waist – remember if you are lifting anything that your leg muscles are much stronger than your back muscles, so use them. Keep your spine as straight as possible, and the load as near your body as possible.

Body Language

The subtle language of the body, conveyed by posture and position of head, legs and arms, adds to our verbal messages. Subconsciously we recognize the confidence radiated by upright posture, hands behind head, chin up. Hands on hips, legs spread wide, head jutting forward denotes aggressive confidence, while crossed legs and the head touched or supported shows thoughtfulness. When depressed we enfold our body with our arms and cover our faces. A row brings invasion of territory as the man grabs the woman's clothes. Initial sexual encounters entail little eye or body contact. A dominant man makes the woman look down, while the flirting couple show similar body posture, expression

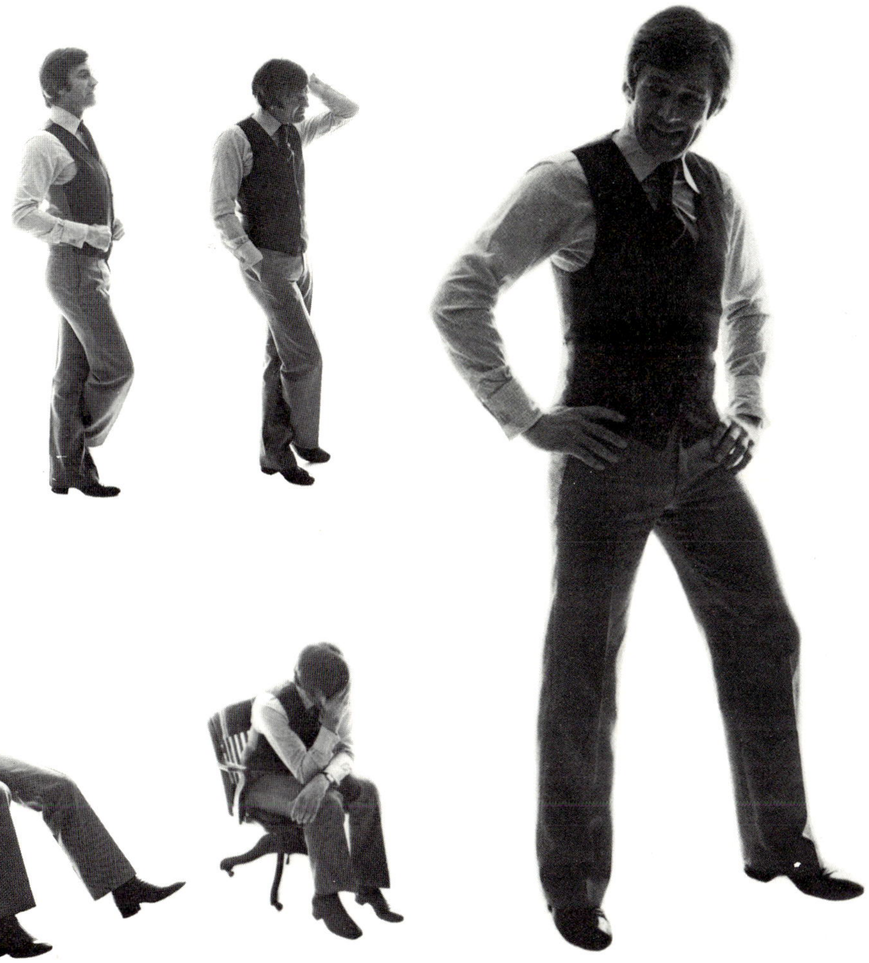

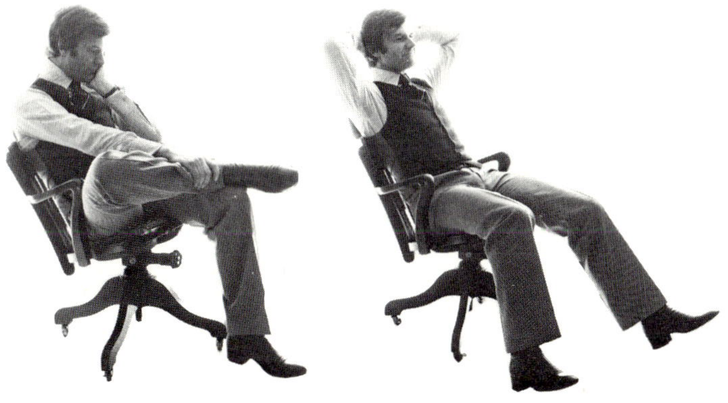

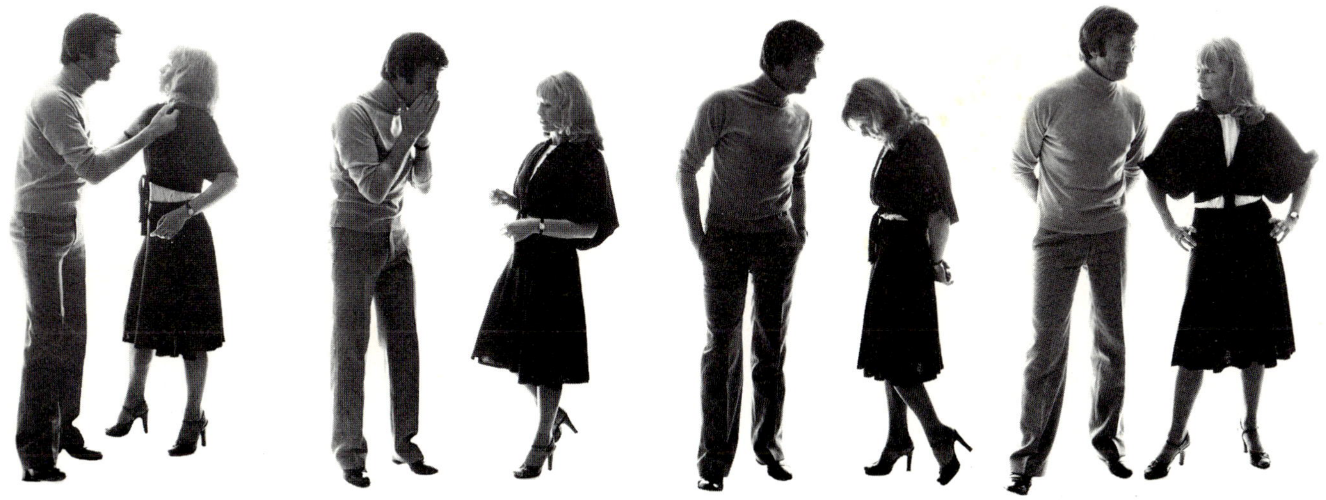

Sex Roles

No drive towards a unisex world can eradicate the differences between men and women, however it may try to minimize or ignore them. They are inevitable, based as they are on nature's expectation that women will bear and rear children, and that men will support and protect the family while it is still dependant. But what is being rapidly eroded is the long-held assumption that such differences inevitably operate to the advantage of the male, that to say a woman is 'different' is an admission not simply of difference, but of inferiority. The more women take part in the traditional preserves of a man's world the more it becomes apparent how much the sexual differences have been overlaid by social influences, how many of what we have always thought to be physical limitations are really cultural ones. Once the expectations and aspirations of women started to rise, so did the number of achievements.

Our gender is determined by the two sex chromosomes which each body cell contains. The normal male has an X and a Y chromosome in every cell, the normal female has two X chromosomes. It is our particular chromosome combination – XX or XY – which is responsible for the most obvious sexual differences, our sex glands and organs; the ovaries, womb and vagina of the female, the testes, sperm ducts and penis of the male.

Our chromosomal gender is usually, but not always matched by what is called our 'core gender', which is what we actually *feel* ourselves to be. This feeling of maleness or femaleness develops around the age of three to four and may be influenced by what is called our 'gender of assignment', which is what our parents lead us to believe we are. Again, we may not be assigned the 'right' sex – there are plenty of cases of parents desperate for a son and who have brought their daughter up as if she were a boy, and vice versa. Another possible cause is due to bad learning enforced upon the child and this is one of the most pertinent theories put forward to explain bisexuality. It can indeed lead to great mental confusion during later life, often manifesting itself at an unconscious level causing erratic and inappropriate behaviour.

Other sexual differences are apparent even from birth. Boys tend to be slightly heavier at birth and remain larger throughout childhood. But girls learn to talk earlier and start to mature sooner, both physically and emotionally. As a result of their earlier growth spurt at puberty, girls from about twelve to fifteen are, for the first and last time, both bigger and stronger than boys of the same age. At puberty the secondary sexual characteristics appear in both sexes; breast development and the onset of menstruation in girls, rapid growth and deepening of the voice in boys, while in both sexes characteristic patterns of body or facial hair develop and the genitals enlarge.

As adults, women are lighter and usually have less muscle but more fat than men. They tend to be weaker than men, but to have more stamina, perhaps because child care in the early years is a day and night affair. Their bones are lighter and smaller, their pelvis wider and shallower for easier childbearing. Their legs are shorter, their shoulders narrower and they have a lower centre of gravity. They burn up energy more slowly than men and their heart, lungs and brain are all smaller in proportion to their body size. Women have a smaller number of touch-sensitive nerve-endings too, which gives rise to the belief that they can bear pain better than men.

If you are a man, your larger brain capacity does not necessarily mean that you are more intelligent. No significant differences have been found between male and female IQs, but what does seem to be true is that men and women excel in different mental fields and approach problems in different ways. Women on the whole tend to do better in the spheres of language, logic and memory, while men, contrary to popular opinion, are more intuitive, more likely to be good at music and painting and are visio-spatially oriented to the world around them. The man is more likely to recognize a face, the woman to remember the name that goes with it. A woman will tend to settle an argument with words, a man with action. Women tend to be more cautious, to think ahead, as befits their prime role in caring for the young; men are the risktakers, the adventurers.

But a woman need not be limited, even physically, by the mere fact of her sex, nearly as much as was once thought. The difference in male and female records in track athletics, for example, has been declining steadily ever since women started to take part in these events. The performance of female athletes is improving faster than that of men even in the long distance events which they were always thought to be incapable of running without distress. The current unofficial women's marathon record, for example, would have won the gold medal in all the Olympic games up to and including 1924 and would have won the bronze medal at the 1948 Olympics.

In swimming, women's records are catching up with men's even more quickly than they are in athletics, in fact women already hold the speed record for swimming the English Channel in both directions. Perhaps in long distance events particularly, superior female stamina may make up for superior male muscular power. If women's future achievements follow the same trend, their best performances could equal the best men's within the next three or four decades.

Unisex may be the trend of the moment, but the differences between men and women cannot be removed or disguised. Even the jeans 'uniform' cannot hide the swell of female hips, the crotch gap, while the man's more angular shape shows little difference between waist and hips

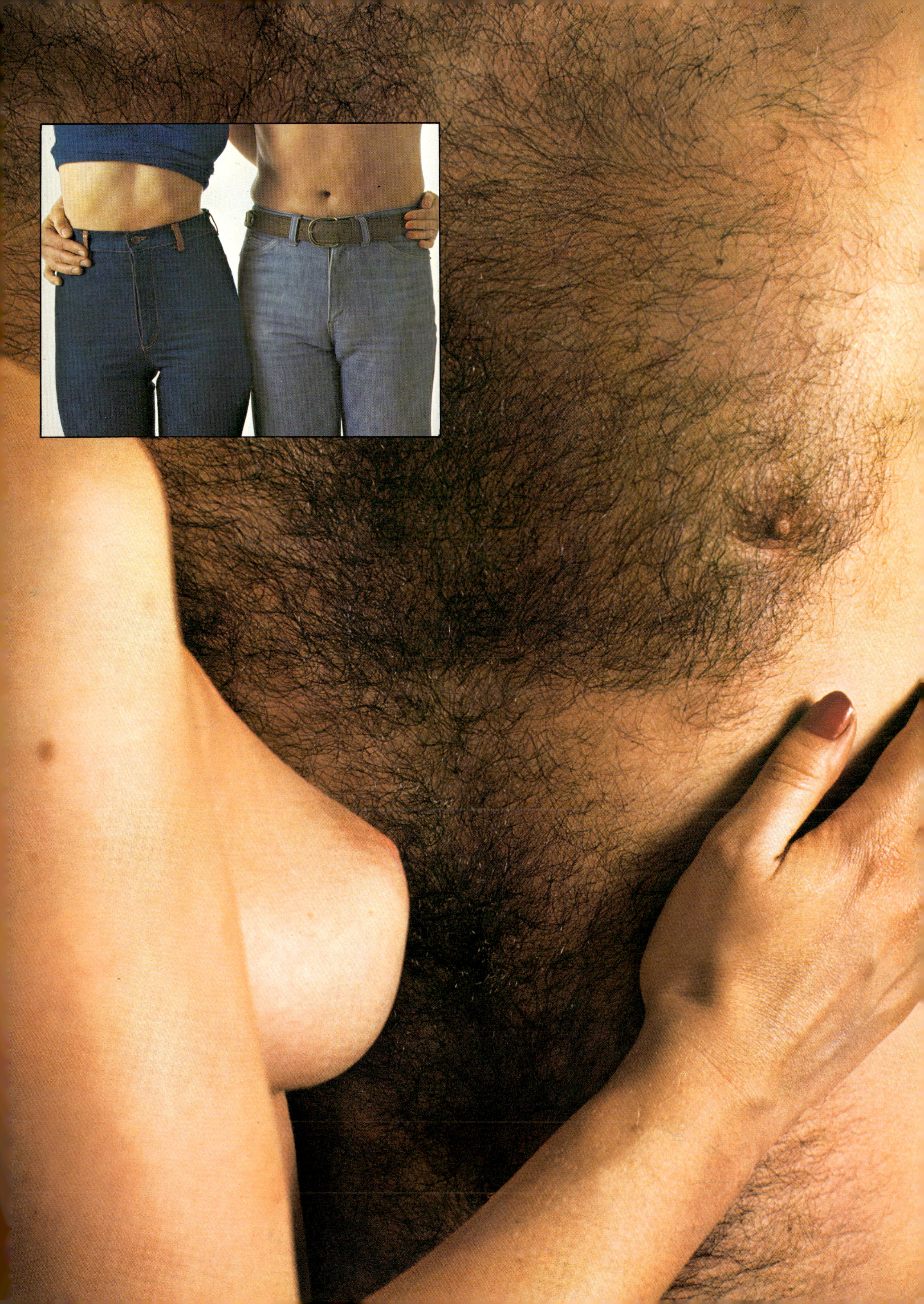

Body Types

Not all women, however hard they try, will end up with a body like Brigitte Bardot's. And the seven-stone weakling is very unlikely indeed to become Charles Atlas, no matter how many hours a day he spends building up his body. We can all improve our shapes, reduce (or increase) our weights to some extent, trimming bits off here and there, improving our health and fitness, but by and large we are limited by our own body type.

We all vary greatly in build – within the 'normal' range of men and women, not taking account of excessive thinness or obesity, there can be variations of 30 per cent in height and 60 per cent in weight. But three basic constitutional types are recognized: endomorph, mesomorph and ectomorph. Most of us are a mixture of them all, but with one predominating. Our body type seems to influence our behaviour, too – we come to expect certain personality traits in people of a certain physical type, and very often we are right.

The typical endomorph is smooth-skinned, rounded, heavily built, even tubby. He has a long body, small hands and feet. He is likely to have fine hair and go prematurely bald. He is a friendly fellow, popular, outgoing and relaxed – the 'pure' endomorph may be rather too relaxed, to the point of virtual inertia. His body movements are slow and deliberate, his breathing and heart-beat slow, full and regular. He is not impulsive, tends to deliberate and works things out before he acts. He is tolerant and easy going – the sort to make the best of things as they are, rather than move heaven and earth to change them. He may be self-indulgent and have a tendency to depression. He may suffer from gall-bladder trouble, over-eating and drinking, possibly even alcoholism or addiction to hard drugs.

The mesomorph is a more rugged fellow, strong, large-boned and athletic, the classic Olympic champion, needing lots of exercise. He has springy hair but he too may go bald, though usually receding from the front, while the endomorph starts thinning at the crown. He is aggressive and driving, liking to wield power, to dominate. His ambition, drive and aggression are likely to carry him to the top – the stress diseases are the ones he is most likely to suffer from.

The ectomorph is slight and thin – little muscle and less fat. He looks fragile but in spite of his lack of physical strength may be surprisingly tough, in fact his health is the best of the three and he is likely to live the longest. He is sensitive, maybe over-sensitive, tend-

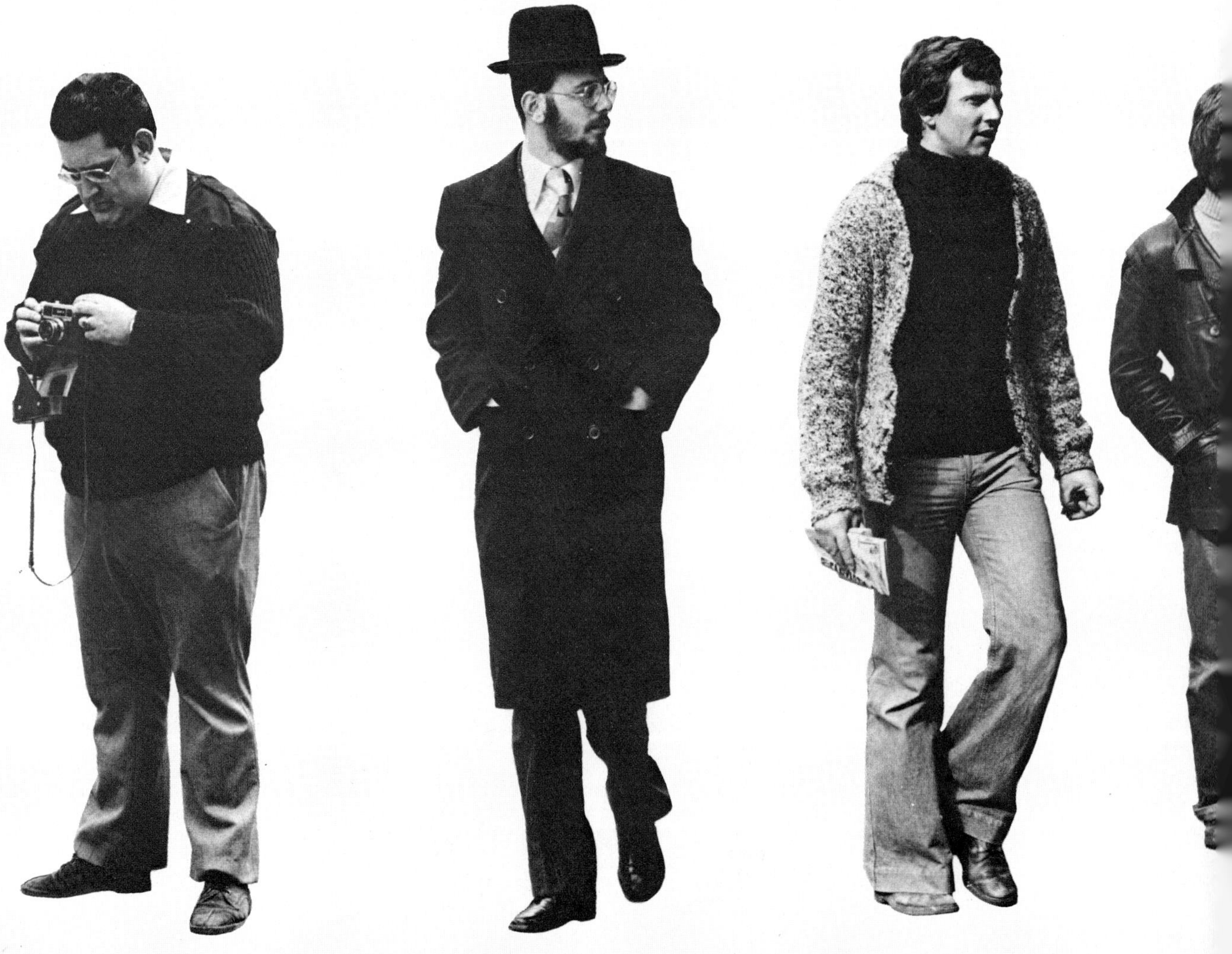

ing to be fussy about his food. He likes a high-protein diet but otherwise has a smallish appetite. In spite of his innate good health he can be something of a hypochondriac, may suffer from constipation and have a low pain threshold. He is very aware of what is going on around him, intelligent, thoughtful, something of an intellectual, but because he is not as outgoing as the classic endo-and meso-types he may not be able to put himself across as well, or sway others to his point of view. He is likely to be a loner, an orderly person who likes a fairly rigid routine in his life.

Obviously few of us conform absolutely to any of these basic stereotypes. But anyone's physique can be classified fairly accurately by using a seven-point scale for all three shapes and describing them in terms of their score on the scales. Thus a high mesomorph might be 1-7-1, with only traces of endo and ecto characteristics. The person equally balanced between the three types would be described as 4-4-4 – average for endomorphy, mesomorphy and ectomorphy. If we know our basic constitution we know at least what it is reasonable for us to aim at; if you are a plump endomorph you may never be as slim as you would like, but you can at least comfort yourself that nature intends you to be that way. It is the fat ectomorph who really needs to go on a diet.

But within the limits which nature has imposed we manage to alter and adapt ourselves amazingly well. The small waists of the Victorian ladies, their be-whiskered men, the bosomy Edwardians, the flat-chested flappers of the twenties and their boyish, centre-parted, smooth-faced escorts all demonstrate how subtly we superimpose a culturally acceptable structure on nature's basic framework.

We use make-up and clothes both to project a desired image of ourselves and also to conform to other people's expectations of us – your doctor, for example, will wear a white coat rather than blue denims to give you confidence by reinforcing your idea of him as a conventional and (by implication) reliable member of a dependable profession. The modifications we made ourselves can influence the final image we present to the world far more than the imperfections we were born with.

How do we see ourselves? We tend to measure ourselves against an 'ideal' shape which may bear very little resemblance to the real thing. Extremely fat and extremely thin people, asked to estimate their size, may do so with surprising inaccuracy. The very overweight tend to underestimate their girth while anorexics (sufferers from a disease in which the victim is convinced he is overweight and diets often to starvation level) see themselves as very much fatter, and less attractive than they really are.

From left to right: A typical endomorph, ectomorph and mesomorph. Most people are combinations of body types – like the ecto-mesomorph and two meso-endomorphs below. Women are usually more ectomorphic than men of similar age

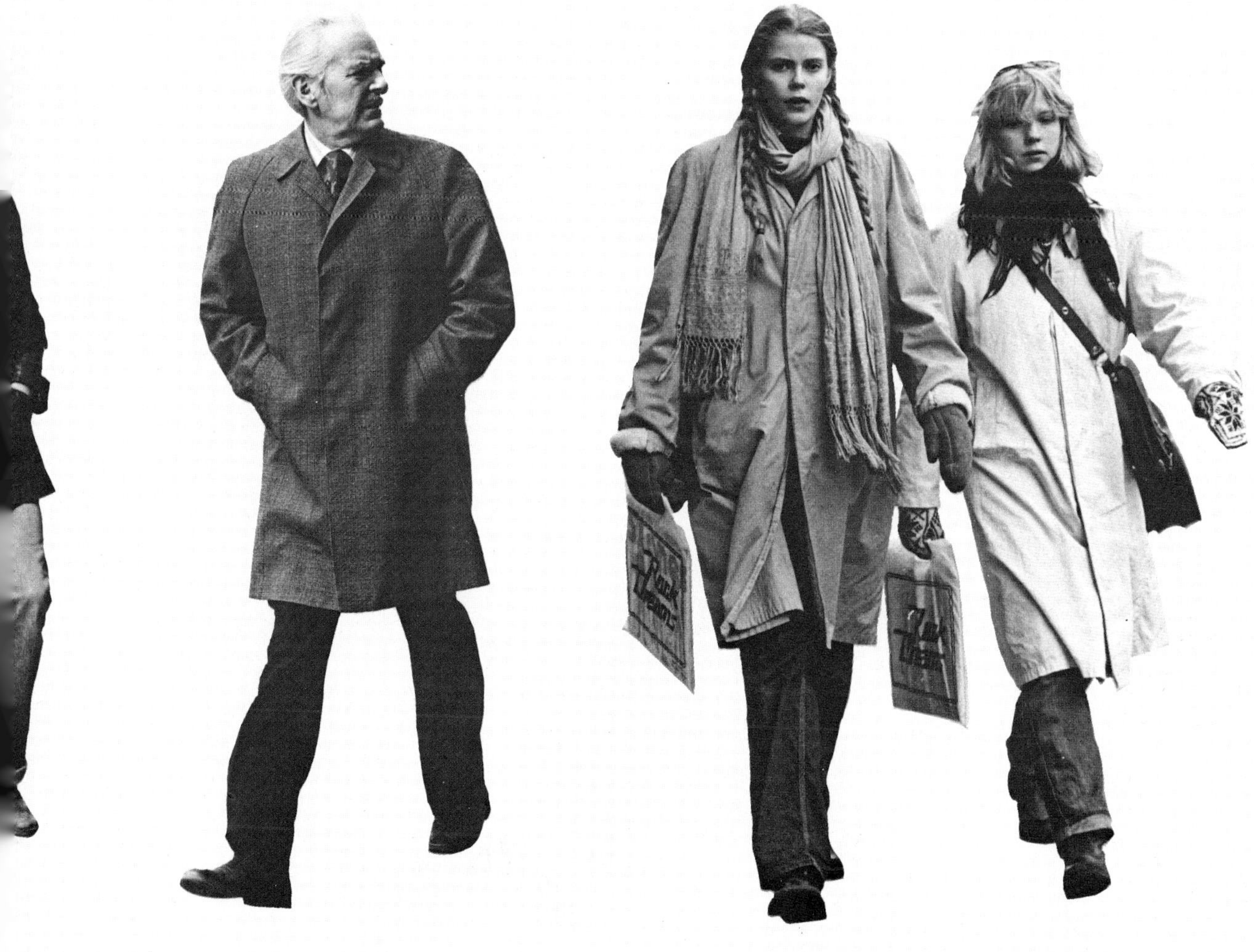

Use and Abuse

Although the average person's lifespan has lengthened dramatically (39 years in the early nineteenth century, 71 now), too many of us still die sooner than we need and virtually everyone is less healthy than they should be. Things are worse if you are a man – a woman usually has at least another six years of life ahead of her when her partner dies. For a reasonable life-span and a healthy old age you need to care for your body as you do for your car – rather better in fact, as there is very little second-hand value in a worn out body and no chance of a replacement.

The safest way to a ripe old age is to eat little, drink less, smoke not at all and stray from one's own hearth-side only for periods of unstressful work and regular exercise. An unappealing regime which, while it might keep our bodies young and beautiful, would make us mentally middle-aged before our time. The natural order of decay produces a middle-aged outlook in most of us by our mid-twenties, that is to say we become stable, settled, resistant to change, predictable, cautious about new ideas. To keep mentally young we need new interests, new challenges, a few risks, a little fun. It is sensible to treat your body with respect, but to be over-cautious or obsessional can be self-defeating. It may pay to live a little dangerously.

If you want to be over-cautious about anything, choose smoking, the most widely practised and dangerous form of bodily abuse. Men are heavier smokers than women – 19 per cent of men but only 5 per cent of women smoke more than 20 a day. Lung cancer, bronchitis, coronary disease, emphysema, peptic ulcer and stroke are all associated with heavy smoking. There is only one encouraging thing to say to smokers – some of the damage can be undone if you give it up. Now.

For every 10 per cent over the ideal weight for your age, sex and height your life expectancy decreases by 13 per cent. The fatter you are, the harder your heart has to work to pump blood around your body and the higher will be your blood pressure. Fat deposits which narrow your arteries make the heart work even harder and raised blood pressure puts the kidneys at risk too. The list of diseases and conditions which seem to be exacerbated by fatness if not caused by it, is legion – chest infections for example, diabetes, gallstones, even cirrhosis of the liver. But fat people are much less likely to commit suicide. Maybe they are happier, or more placid, or perhaps they just can't summon up the energy.

If you need to slim, don't skip meals – food speeds up the body's metabolism and increases the rate at which it burns up food or fat, so eating little and often is better than one enormous binge. Exercise after a meal increases the burn-up rate too – the old nanny-based advice to rest after a meal is absolutely wrong. Worst of all is a large meal late at night; your body will convert it into fat, not energy or warmth which are unneeded in bed.

Alcohol, in small doses, is the ideal social lubricant, a wonder-drug which makes us smarter, wittier, friendlier and less inhibited than we would be without it. Remember that alcohol is actually a brain depressant, though we all regard it as a relaxant – it makes you feel better, but you probably won't be

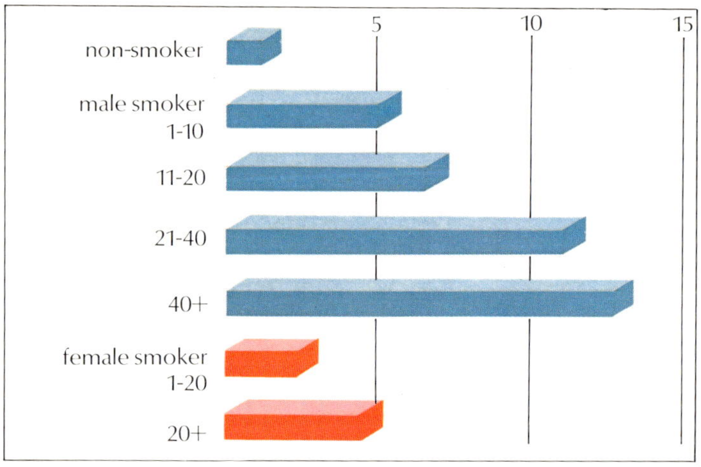

Cigarette smokers are twice as likely to die of a heart attack than non-smokers. Nicotine stimulates the release of cholesterol into the blood, clogging the arteries. If you smoke more than 40 a day, your life may be reduced by 12 years, and even as few as 10 a day can curtail life by as much as 5 or 6 years

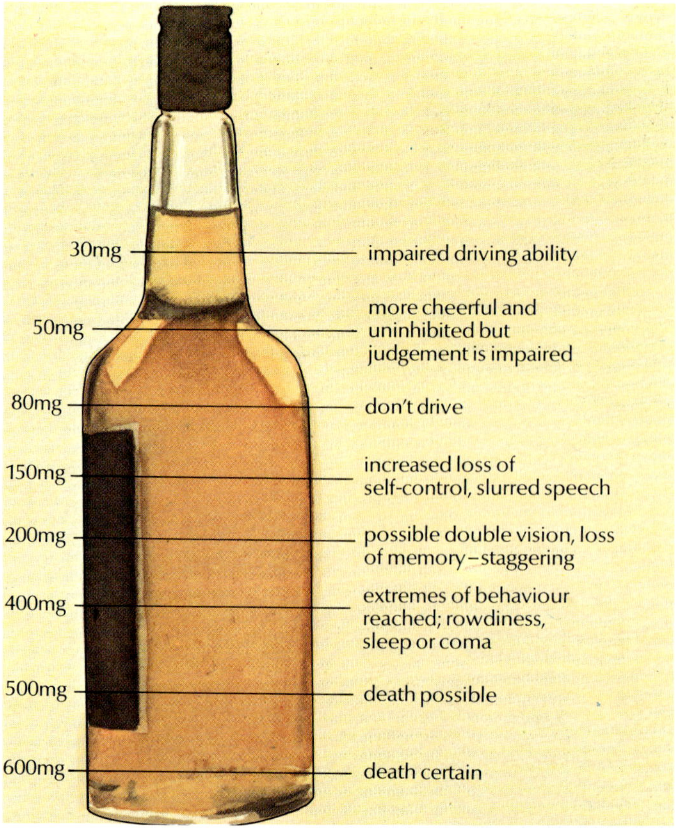

Drinking may lubricate the wheels of social pleasure, but taken in excess it is very dangerous. As the amount of alcohol consumed leads to a greater concentration in the blood, so disastrous changes occur. Only 30 mg can increase the possibility of an accident, and 50 mg impairs judgment, removes inhibitions. 150-200 mg brings slurring of speech, forgetfulness and sometimes rowdiness. 400 mg in the blood usually brings sleep or a coma. At 600 death is certain

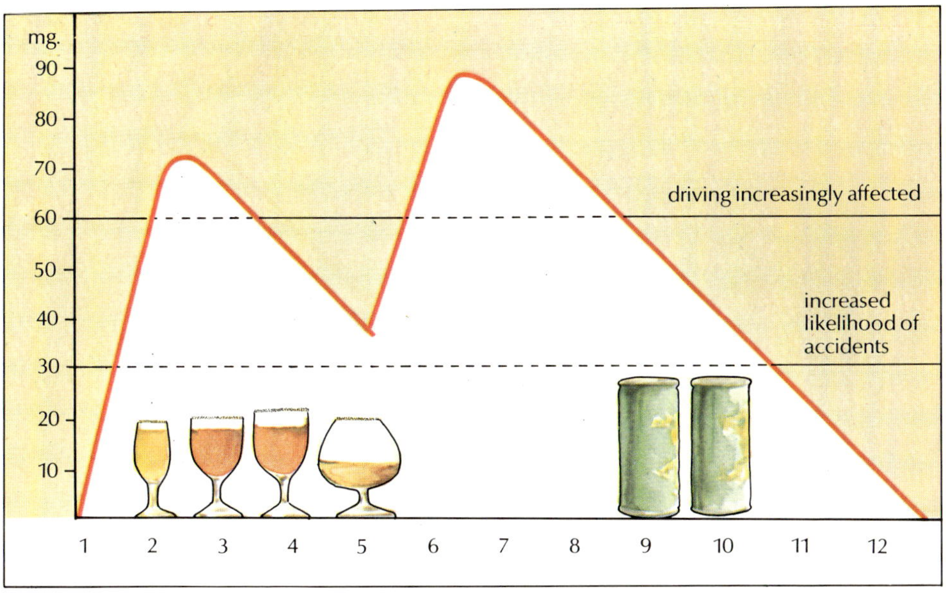

Even though a glass of sherry, two of wine and one of brandy with a meal at lunchtime may not raise the alcohol content of the blood over the legal limit, driving is still much impaired. Alcohol has a cumulative effect many people are not aware of. If you follow these drinks with just 2 pints of beer several hours later after work, the alcohol content of your blood will exceed the legal limit for dangerous driving

functioning quite as well. Moderate drinking won't harm you – your body can take an occasional hang-over – chronic over-drinking will, leading to chronic gastritis, mental deterioration, cirrhosis of the liver. If you are overweight, make allowance for the high calorie value of alcohol; a whisky rates the same as a poached egg, a glass of champagne has as many calories as a piece of bread and butter. It's up to you which you'd rather have.

While we take too little exercise, most of us aim for too much sleep, and underestimate the amount we actually do sleep. Seven hours sleep is plenty and many of us could manage on less. Most of us don't really know whether we have slept or not. Studies which have recorded the electrical brain waves of people throughout the night have found that most of the people who claimed the following morning not to have slept a wink had been indisputably asleep most of the night. Not sleeping won't hurt you. Worrying about not sleeping will.

Travel can be a strain or a relaxant, depending how you take it. If you are a competitive driver, fuming in traffic jams, setting yourself impossible arrival dead lines, you will be doing your heart and blood pressure no good at all. Jet travel has problems of its own. Jet-lag is a real condition, something to make allowances for if you have to travel, particularly if you have important business to do. It takes time for your bodyclocks to adapt to a new timezone. Try to travel by day, go to bed as soon as you arrive, no matter what the local time is. Don't overeat or overdrink on the way and wait 24 hours before making any decisions or taking any actions that really matter.

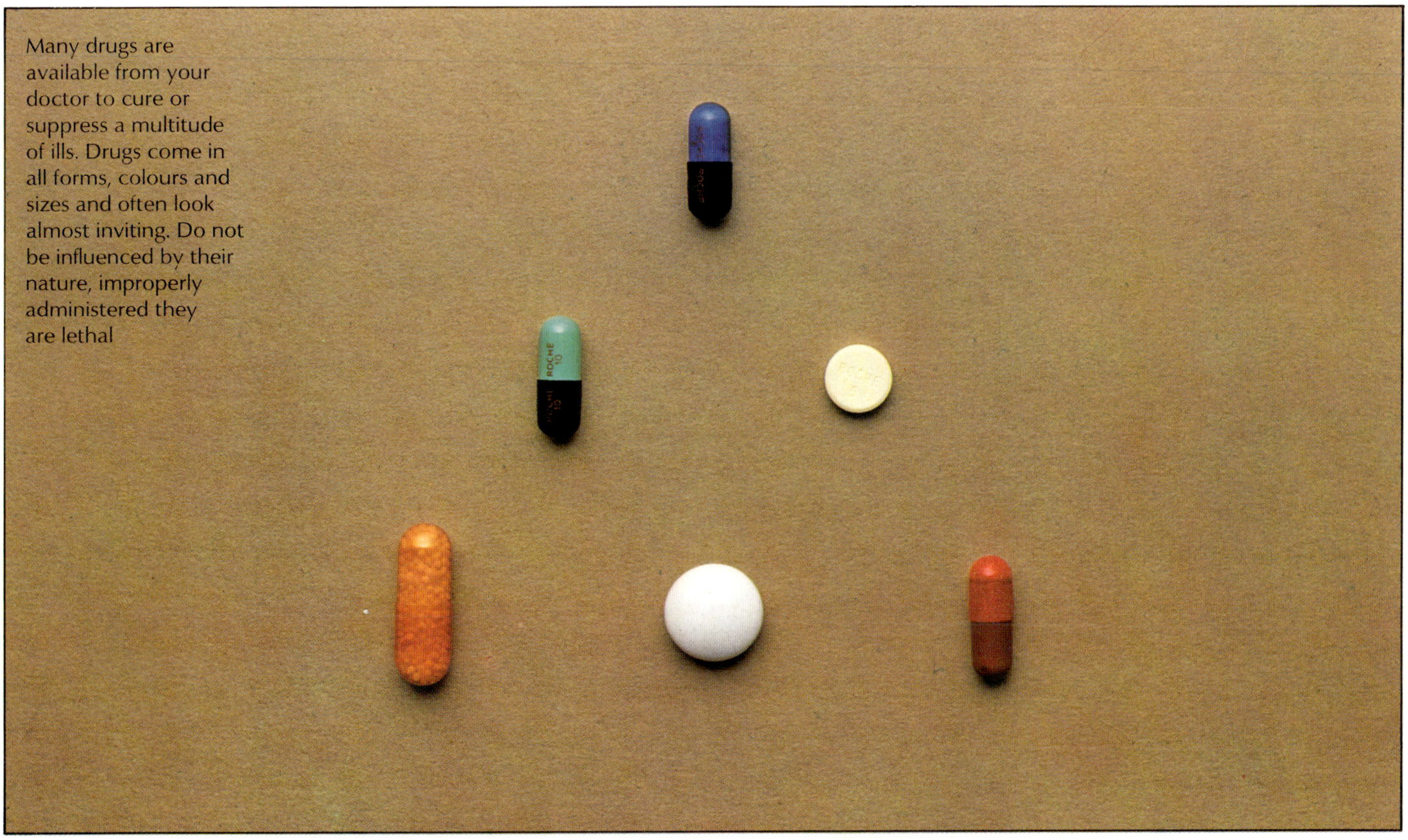

Many drugs are available from your doctor to cure or suppress a multitude of ills. Drugs come in all forms, colours and sizes and often look almost inviting. Do not be influenced by their nature, improperly administered they are lethal

Drugs

TYPE OF DRUG	USED FOR	POSSIBLE SIDE-EFFECTS	COMMENTS
1. Anti-infective agents			
Antibiotics (Penicillin, ampicillin tetracycline)	Bacterial infection of all body systems, e.g. pneumonia, middle ear infections, gut infections, skin eruptions	Risk of allergy to penicillin, producing skin rashes, fever, mouth sores at first dose, more severe reactions with subsequent doses	Tetracycline should not be used in pregnancy or on children up to 12 – it discolours developing teeth
Other anti-bacterial agents eg sulphonamides (Septrin)		Skin eruptions, damage to kidneys and urinary tract, blood disorders	Less potent than antibiotics may be combined with them in cases of drug resistant organisms
2. Drugs acting on brain and nervous system			
a) Tranquillizers			
Major (Largactil)	Serious psychiatric disturbances requiring sedation	Lack of muscular co-ordination, slowed reflexes, mental sluggishness. Drowsiness, blurred vision, slurred speech	Risk of dependance of addiction. Effects of tranquillizers may be increased if they are taken with alcohol or other drugs
Minor (Valium, Librium)	Anxiety, tension		
b) Anti-depressants Monoamine oxidase inhibitors (Nardil)	Depression and anxiety states	Constipation, skin rashes, sweating, headaches, dizziness, palpitations	Less frequently used because of adverse effects when used with other drugs, alcohol and some foods, such as cheese, marmite
Tricyclics (Imprimine, Triptizol)	Depression	Headaches, palpitations, blurred vision, sweating	Takes effect therapeutically after 2-3 weeks
c) Sedatives and Hypnotics Barbiturates (Seconal, sodium amytal)	Used in small doses for anxiety states in larger doses for insomnia	Drowsiness, vertigo, mental confusion, slurred speech	Barbiturates can be lethal if taken with alcohol, and are now prescribed with caution because of the dangers of addiction
Non-barbiturates (Mogadon, Mandrax)	Used in small doses for anxiety states in larger doses for insomnia	Hangover symptoms, drowsiness, mental confusion	Brain functioning does not return to normal for a considerable time (up to 3 months) after taking sleeping pills
d) Analgesics and anti-pyretics			
Aspirin	Fever reduction, headache, toothache, menstrual pain, rheumatic disorders	Bleeding from stomach wall. Occasional allergic reactions	Should never be used by sufferers from stomach or duodenal ulcers, or asthma.
Codeine	Headache etc.	Constipation	Addictive in large quantities
Paracetamol	As for aspirin	Anaemia and liver damage	
Phenacetin	As for aspirin	Anaemia, kidney damage	
Opium derivatives (morphine, heroin)	Relieving severe pain	Anaemia, kidney damage	Addictive
e) Anti-emetics (Dramamine, Avomine)	Motion sickness, vertigo, nausea and vomiting	Drowsiness	Sedative effect increased by alcohol. Do not drive or perform any task needing alertness after taking them
f) Anti-convulsants (Phenobartitone)	Epilepsy	Drowsiness, unsteadiness	
3. Drugs acting on digestive system			
a) Antacids	Heartburn, indigestion, flatulence	None	Antacids containing bismuth can cause bismuth poisoning in a few people who take it for a long time
b) Laxatives and purgatives (liquid paraffin, senna preparations, cascara)	Constipation	Over-purgation can lead to loss of salts from body	Do not take in cases of severe abdominal pain. Roughage added to diet is a better solution for constipation – all laxative drugs taken regularly can rob the gut muscle of its ability to contract
c) Anti-diarrhoeals Kaolin preparations	Non-infective diarrhoea	None	See anti-infective agents
Antibiotics (Neomycin)	Bacterial infections of the gut	Vitamin deficiencies	See anti-infective agents
Sulphonamides		Skin rashes	

TYPE OF DRUG	USED FOR	POSSIBLE SIDE-EFFECTS	COMMENTS
4. Drugs acting on Cardiovascular system			
a) Heart regulators (Digitalis preparations, procaine)	Heart failure and arrhythmias	Vomiting, blurred vision	Must be taken in correct dosage to avoid side-effects
b) Coronary vasodilators (Glyceryl trinitrite)	Angina	Can produce a drop of blood pressure in too high dosage	Must be taken in correct dosage to avoid side-effects
c) Hypotensive drugs	High blood pressure	Fainting attacks on standing	Must be taken in correct dosage to avoid side-effects
5. Hormone preparations			
a) Oral Contraceptives (Anovlar, Conovid)	Preventing pregnancy, regulating menstrual cycle	Nausea, weight gain, headaches	The main risk, of thrombosis, not yet fully assessed, but seems to be highest in women over 35 years who have been on the pill more than 5 years
b) Corticosteroids	Rheumatic conditions, asthma allergic skin conditions	Taken in high doses 'Moon' face marks, (striae) on skin, weakening of bones	Should be taken only in low dosage for short periods of time
6. Drugs acting on genito-urinary system			
Diuretics (induce urination)	Heart failure, high blood pressure, pre-menstrual tension	Salt depletion	Because they rid the body of water, diuretic drugs produce a dramatic weight loss and are sometimes taken as a 'short cut' by slimmers. But they are ineffective as the weight is quickly regained
7. Anti-allergic drugs			
Antihistamines	Skin rashes, hay fever, conjunctivitis, travel sickness	Drowsiness, loss of appetite, dry mouth dizziness, blurred vision	Alcohol can make the sedative effect more pronouced. Phenergan is sometimes used as a mild sedative for children
8. Drugs affecting appetite			
a) Appetite stimulants	Anorexia (loss of appetite)		Central nervous system stimulants e.g. amphetamine are now no longer prescribed as appetite suppressants because of the danger of addiction
Tonics (caffeine, vitamin preparations, irons, strychnine)	Mild debility, convalescence, loss of appetite	Iron preparation may cause constipation	Should be taken only for a short time
b) Appetite suppressants Bulking agents (methyl cellulose preparations)	Obesity	a) Some danger of intestinal obstruction if bulking agents are used in high doses	
Anonectic drugs (Ponderax)		b) Depression, vomitting, diarrhoea, skin rashes	
9. Drugs affecting respiratory system			
a) Bronchial relaxants	Asthma, bronchitis, emphysema	Dry mouth, palpitations	a) Some bronchial relaxants contain adrenaline and tolerance to these may develop after repeated use
b) Expectorants	Chest congestion	May cause drowsiness	
c) Cough suppressants	Severe or unproductive cough	Some contain codeine, may cause drowsiness, constipation	c) Should only be used for a 'dry' cough, where no fluid is being brought up from chest
d) Nasal drops or sprays	Nasal congestion or inflammation; hay fever		d) Only occasional use recommended – not more than about five times daily
e) Cold cures			e) Cold cures are usually a mixture of drugs designed to relieve the symptoms of, but not to cure, the common cold

YOUR WORKING SURFACE

Imagine a material that is waterproof, like tarpaulin, yet can let out water and oil, that can protect, like a suit of armour, and yet is infinitely sensitive to touch, that remains firm yet is more flexible than rubber. It is also a beautiful material – whether pink and white, suntanned, brown, black or yellow. That substance is your skin. Because it protects us, can transmit pleasure and can look very beautiful we should give it the very best of care and maintenance we can. Diet, exercise and relaxation all contribute to a healthy, glowing skin but correct cleansing and grooming are essential as well.

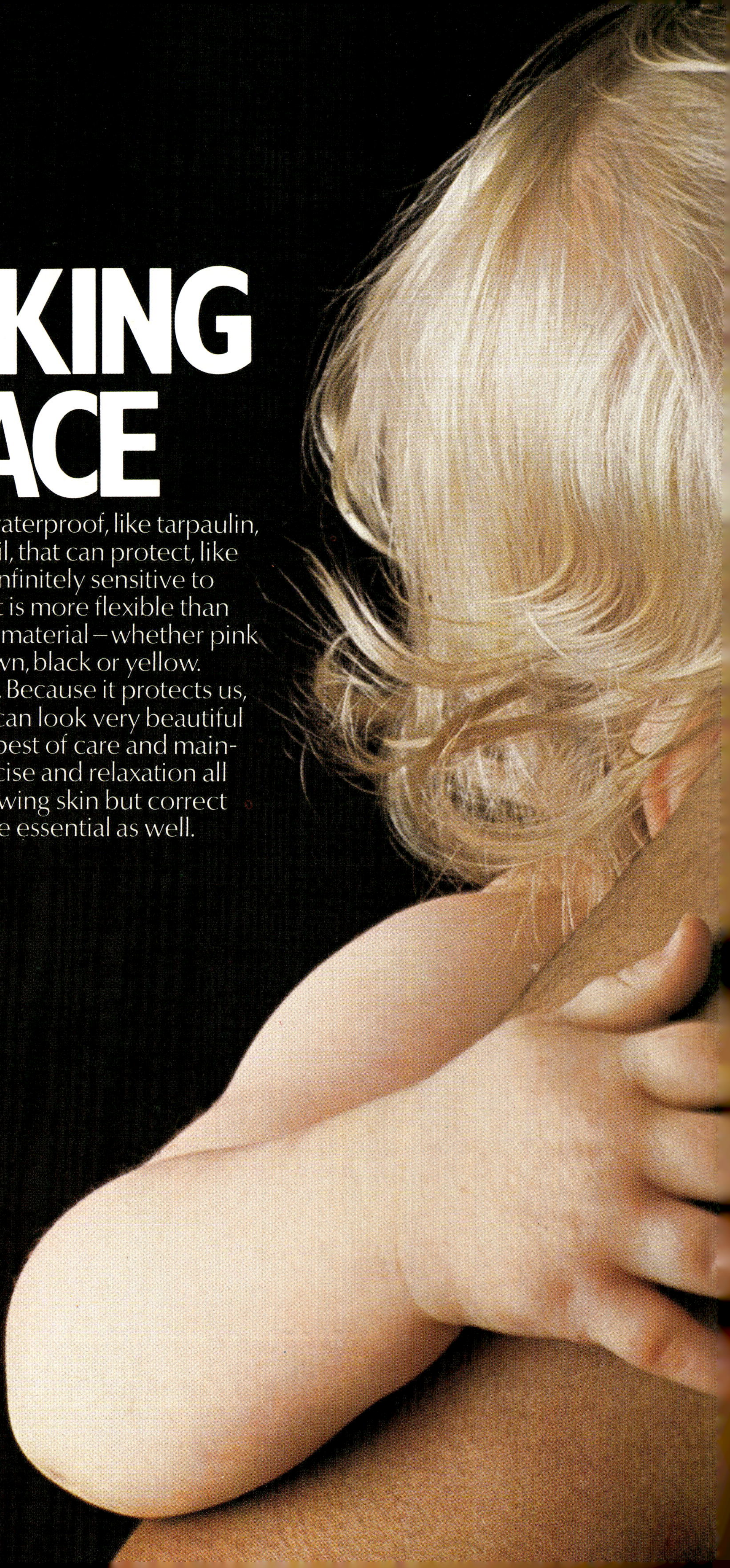

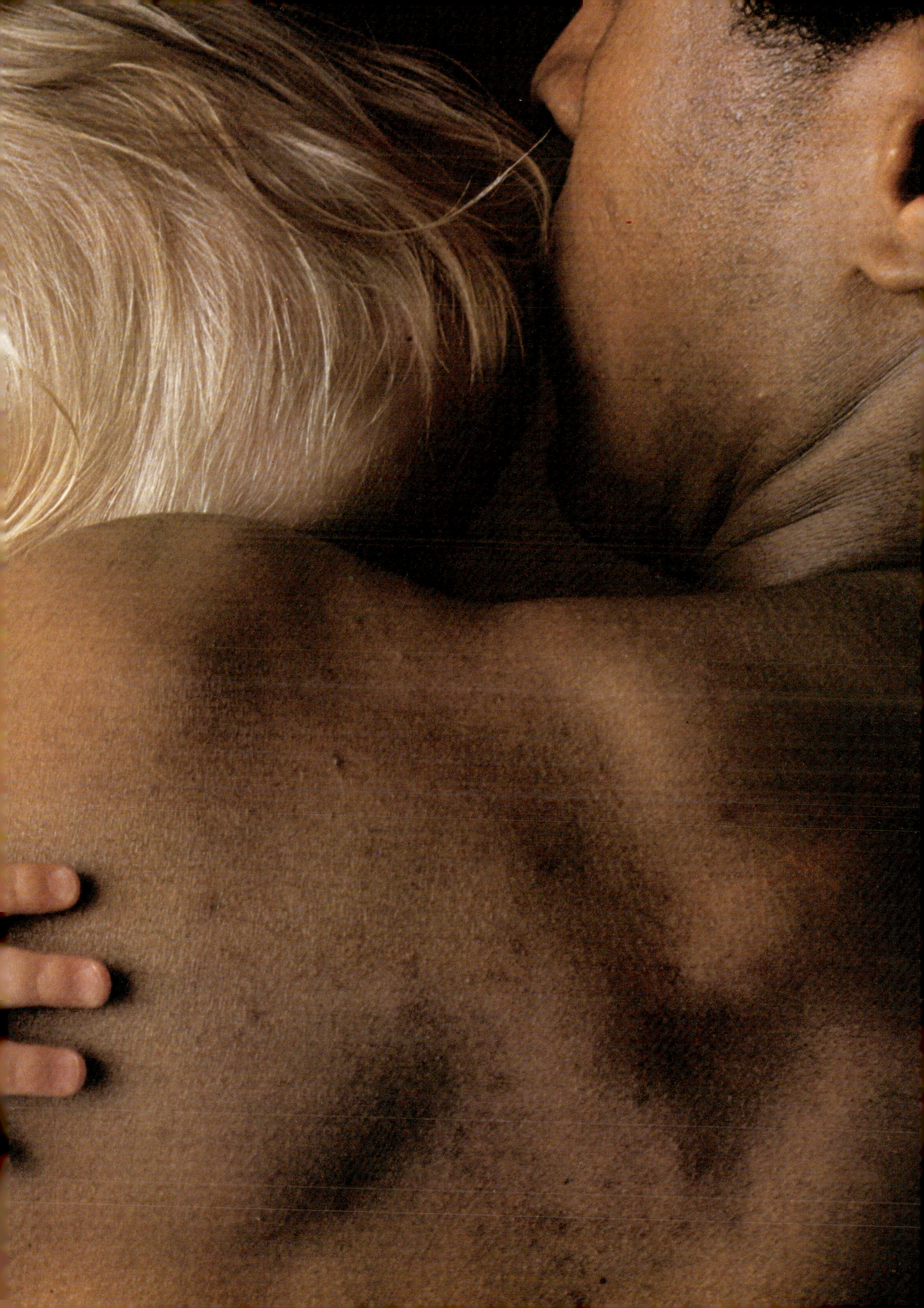

The Outer Covering

Skin covers the entire outer surface of your body and forms a protective coat that is nearly 19 square feet in area. It is a remarkable material, protecting us as it does from wind and rain, keeping out bacteria, sustaining injuries, helping to regulate body temperature and giving us information about our environment. It also prevents us from losing the water that makes up about 70 per cent of our bodies. The skin is a strong, leathery covering which withstands stresses and strains that would tear many other materials. In areas that are particularly subjected to friction it is especially hard and thick – compare your palm to your face, for example and feel the different textures. And then compare your palms to the soles of your feet, particularly the heels.

Skin is basically made of two layers, an outer layer known as the epidermis and the inner layer or dermis. The epidermis has an outer membrane made of protein called keratin, which provides the skin's basic protective barrier. Keratin also forms our hair and nails. The surface of the epidermis is made up of dead cells which are constantly being worn away and replaced by cells from the deeper layers. The 'wearing away' is very evident on the scalp when you have dandruff.

The colour of skin is determined by the amount of melanin it contains. Melanin is a pigment found in the deepest layer of the epidermis, which functions to absorb and protect us from ultraviolet light. A negro skin contains much more melanin than a white skin. If a white skin is subject to strong sunlight, as in suntanning, the epidermis responds by producing more melanin. Tanning is the skin's method of protecting itself. An excess of ultraviolet light can easily cause sunburn and what is not always realized is that long standing exposure to ultraviolet light in poorly pigmented skin may cause skin cancer. Ultraviolet light damages the molecules of deoxyribonucleic acid (DNA) which carry the genetic code of the cell. Negro skin is unaffected by ultraviolet light because of the amount of protective melanin that is present which absorbs this light. Unfortunately, however, albino negros do occur in Africa and because they have no protective melanin they tend to develop skin cancers.

It is important that the epidermis contains a certain amount of water which is held in by an outer layer of grease or fat called sebum, produced by sebaceous glands in the skin's dermal layer. It is easy to wash away this outer layer of sebum by constantly subjecting the skin to too much soap, strong detergent, or to dry atmospheres and wind. If this happens the skin dries out, cracks and fissures appear as in 'chapped hands'. A moisturizing cream helps to replace lost water and also contains a lipid (or fat) to keep the water in the keratin. The skin's inner layer, or dermis, contains an inelastic protein called collagen. This substance is extremely strong and

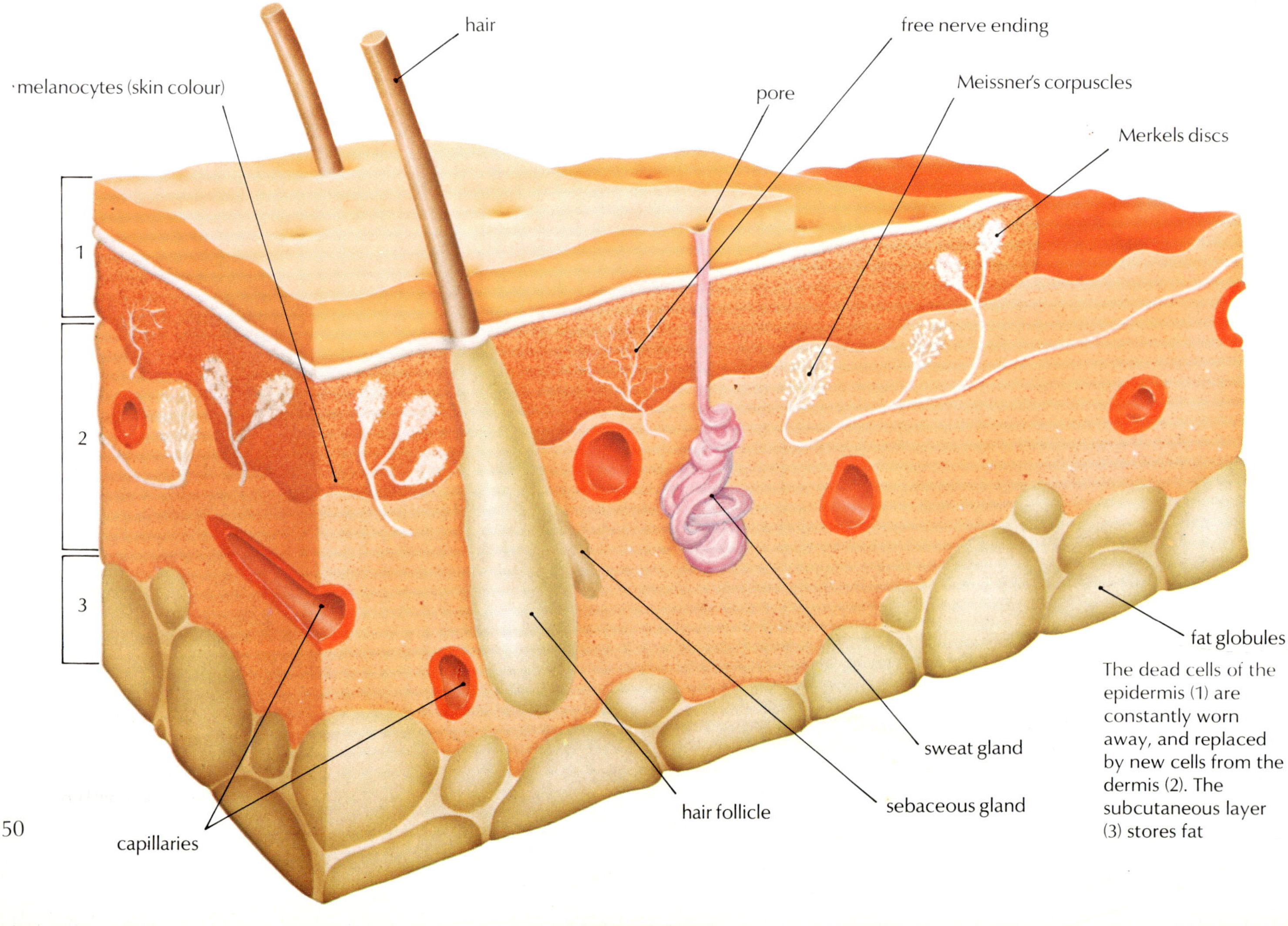

The dead cells of the epidermis (1) are constantly worn away, and replaced by new cells from the dermis (2). The subcutaneous layer (3) stores fat

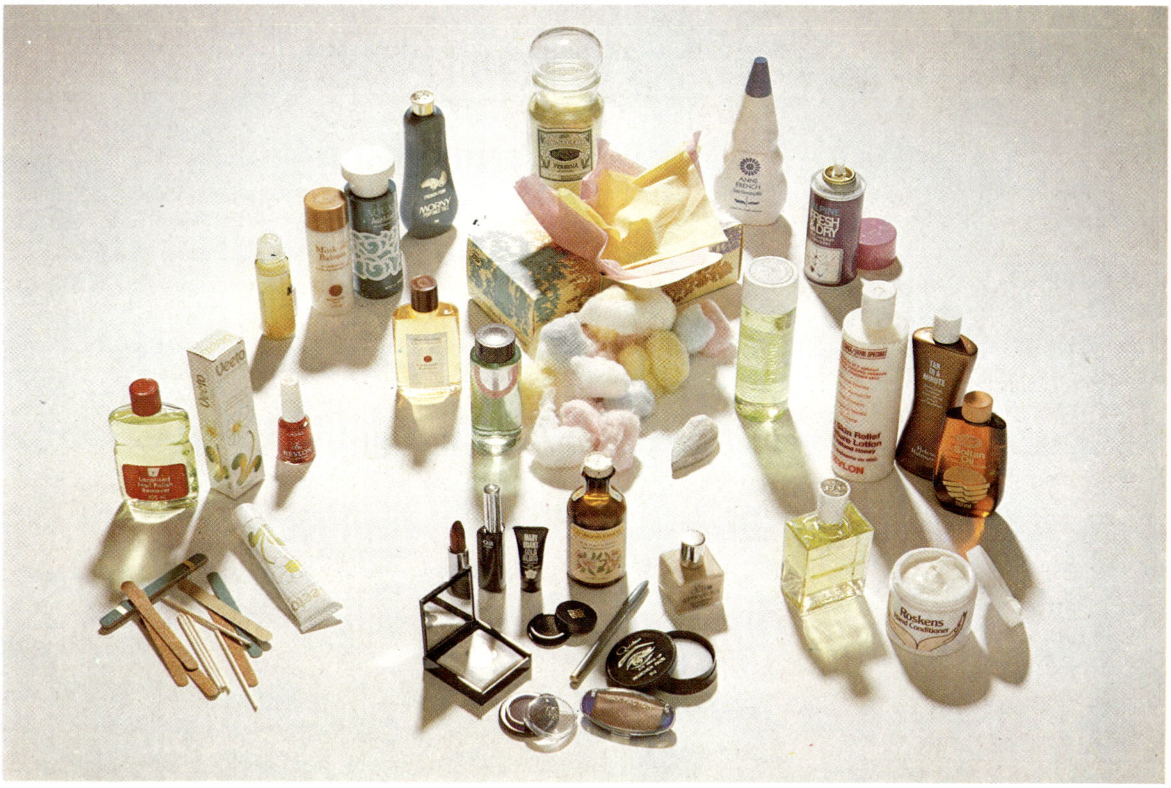

We apply a wide range of cosmetic products to our skin and hair; cleansing creams, make-up, moisturizers, talcum soap, shampoo etc. We hope to compensate for the dryness of central heating and pollution in the air. These products are very useful, but serve to camouflage basic deficiencies caused by an unhealthy life-style. They cannot cure them

because of this the dermis from animal skin is dried to make leather. Another protein called elastin makes the dermis elastic and resilient. As the skin ages it loses its elasticity and becomes wrinkled. Over-exposure to ultraviolet light from the sun can also cause the skin to lose its elasticity. The face develops 'crow's feet' and the back of the neck becomes cobblestoned in appearance – sometimes known as 'farmer's neck'.

Beneath the collagen and elastin is a layer made principally of fat cells. This subcutaneous layer insulates us against the cold and cushions us. Women have more subcutaneous fat than men and therefore have a more curvaceous body compared with the more angular outline of the male.

The living cells of the dermis must be supplied with oxygenated blood, which is carried from the heart by arteries which break down into tiny capillaries in the dermal layer. Through the permeable walls of the capillaries, fluid is released into that surrounding the skin cells. Waste products pass back by the same process and are carried away by the capillaries to the veins. If an artery supplying the skin is blocked then that part of the skin will die and an ulcer will develop. If veins fail to carry the blood away, as in varicose veins, then stagnation, and ultimately ulceration, may also occur. A second system of tubes – the lymph vessels – also drain away waste products from the skin. If these are obstructed for any reason the skin around them swells from an excess of fluid. An excess of sunlight can cause capillaries to break – hence the broken veins in the cheeks of older people.

Nerve endings in the skin enable us to sense pressure, temperature and pain. Pain acts as a protector, warning us of impending danger. Loss or damage to the nerves of the skin makes it anoetic and liable to excessive damage and sometimes can even cause ulceration.

The nerves in the dermis also control the skin glands, which open into the epidermis but are sited in the dermis. They are the hair follicles, the sebaceous or oil glands and the sweat glands which help keep the skin cool.

The sebaceous glands not only oil the surface of the skin but also coat the dead hair produced by the hair tubes or follicles. It has never been known for sebum to be totally absent but sebaceous activity is much reduced in eczema and this contributes to the dry, scaly skin seen in this skin problem.

Man, relative to other mammals, is hairless. The hairs on his body are erected by muscles at their base when it is cold producing 'goose pimples', but are ineffective in insulating the body. The hair on the scalp is, however, a very good sunscreen. Loss of hair or baldness is cosmetically troublesome but more importantly it can allow chronic solar damage.

The sweat glands, under the control of nerves, regulate body temperature. When we are too hot we produce a watery secretion which draws heat from the body as it evaporates from the surface of the skin. Some parts of the body such as the armpits and the genital areas contain special sweat glands, called apocrine glands, which produce a milky fluid associated with arousal and sexual attraction.

Care must be taken to keep these areas clean as here bacteria can breed on stale sweat and produce an offensive odour. Deodorants contain an antibiotic which kills the odour-producing bacteria, and antiperspirants are even more effective because they contain substances which block sweat ducts and slow down the rate at which bacteria multiply. Blocking the sweat ducts is quite harmless as thousands of other ducts at other sites help keep the balance. In rare conditions bacteria can be absent and in hot climates the inability to sweat means that the person must take a dip in cold water in order to cool down.

Care of your skin depends on keeping it free from dead skin cells, dirt and grease. Perhaps even more important, it depends on eating a varied balanced diet, because the skin is fed from within not from without.

Scalp and Hair

A good head of hair is not only a sign of good health, it is a tremendous boost to the morale. Small wonder that we spend so much of our time, money and effort on keeping it in good condition.

We have between 100,000 and 200,000 hairs on our heads. Each is produced by a division of cells at the base of a tiny sheath called a hair follicle. The cells become filled with keratin, the nitrogenous compound that also forms the outer layer of skin. The hair that we see is simply dead protein which is oiled by sebaceous glands connected to the hair follicle. The hair follicle goes through a definite growth cycle each follicle's cycle being quite independent of the next. Growing at the rate of about 0.35mm a day, the growth phase lasts for about three years. After a transitional phase of three weeks during which the hair becomes loose there is a resting phase of three months when the old hair falls out. The hair follicle then begins to produce another hair. Each of us probably loses about 300 hairs a day. Contrary to popular belief cutting or shaving does not make hair grow any faster but if the hair is in a resting phase, then plucking stimulates the follicle and it will move into a growing phase.

The colour of the hair is determined by pigment granules injected into each hair cell. The shade depends on the amount of the brown-black pigment, melamin and the yellow-red pigment phaemelanin there is present. When production of these pigments dwindles and air bubbles form in the hair shaft, the hair goes grey or white. The hair can be dyed with a rinse, which coats the outside of the hair, or by a semi-permanent dye which will survive about six shampoos. Neither of these dyes penetrate the keratin and combine with the hair. Permanent dyes do, however, combine with the keratin and may cause skin allergies.

It is therefore important to carry out skin tests each time you use this type of dye. Care must also be taken with removal of these dyes or with frequent bleaching with hydrogen peroxide. Both of these may make the hair very brittle so that it breaks off a short distance from the scalp. As the living roots are not damaged the hair will regrow but of course this takes time. Regular use of hair conditioners which coat the hair with a layer of wax and discriminating use of bleaches will help avoid excessive hair damage and loss. All in all, the less chemical treatment your hair receives the less damage it will sustain and the stronger it will be.

Whether your hair is straight or curly depends on the arrangement of chemical bonds between sulphur atoms in the hair. By using certain chemicals to break these bonds so that they reform in a different pattern, straight hair can be 'permanently waved'. The 'permanent waves', however, grow out as the hair grows. Again, some people are sensitive to the chemicals used in perms, and dyed or bleached hair may be too brittle to withstand the further chemical onslaught. Always remember how long each hair takes to grow.

Just as straight hair can be permed so very curly hair can be straightened. Negroes have solved the problem of straightening their hair by using a hot steel comb and vaseline. The hot vaseline is combed through the hair, and the heat makes the hair straighten. The disadvantage is that the vaseline runs down the hairs and damages the upper part of the hair follicle.

Men and women alike can style or colour their hair in any way they choose but there is little that men can do about losing their hair. Baldness occurs as a matter of course due to the amount of the male hormone androgen released into the bloodstream. Less androgen – less hair. The hair first recedes from the crown and temples and this gradually extends until the top of the head is bald. The age at which men start to bald is genetically determined and it is quite normal for hair to start receding during adolescence. The only cure for baldness is castration before puberty. Castration after puberty will not 'bring back' any lost hair but the baldness will not 'get worse'. There are several other causes of baldness in both sexes which may be due to general health, or to local diseases of the scalp. In these cases medical advice is needed. One interesting cause of hair loss which may occur after severe illness or after pregnancy is a partial synchronization of the hair follicle growth phase. This means that a lot of hair comes out at the same time, but there is no cause for concern as the hair will regrow together. Rolling hairs tightly onto rollers can cause baldness

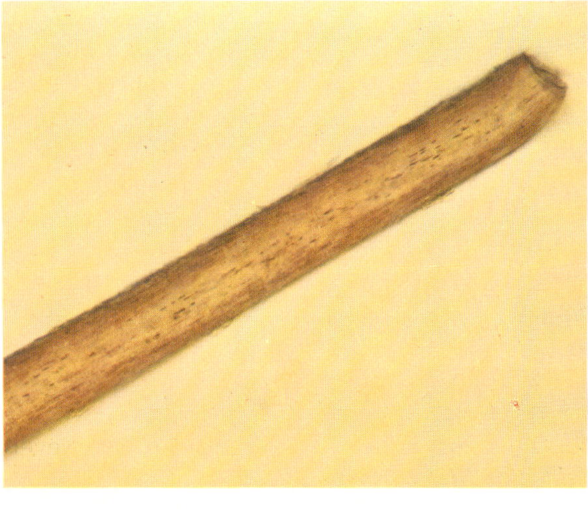

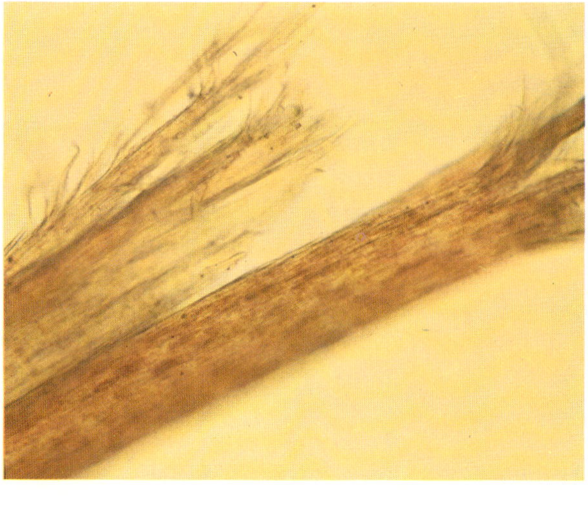

Keeping your hair in good condition is vital to your appearance. The hair (far left) shows the ideal situation; strong, straight, firm and healthy. The hairs (left) show exactly the reverse; bad condition and damaged ends

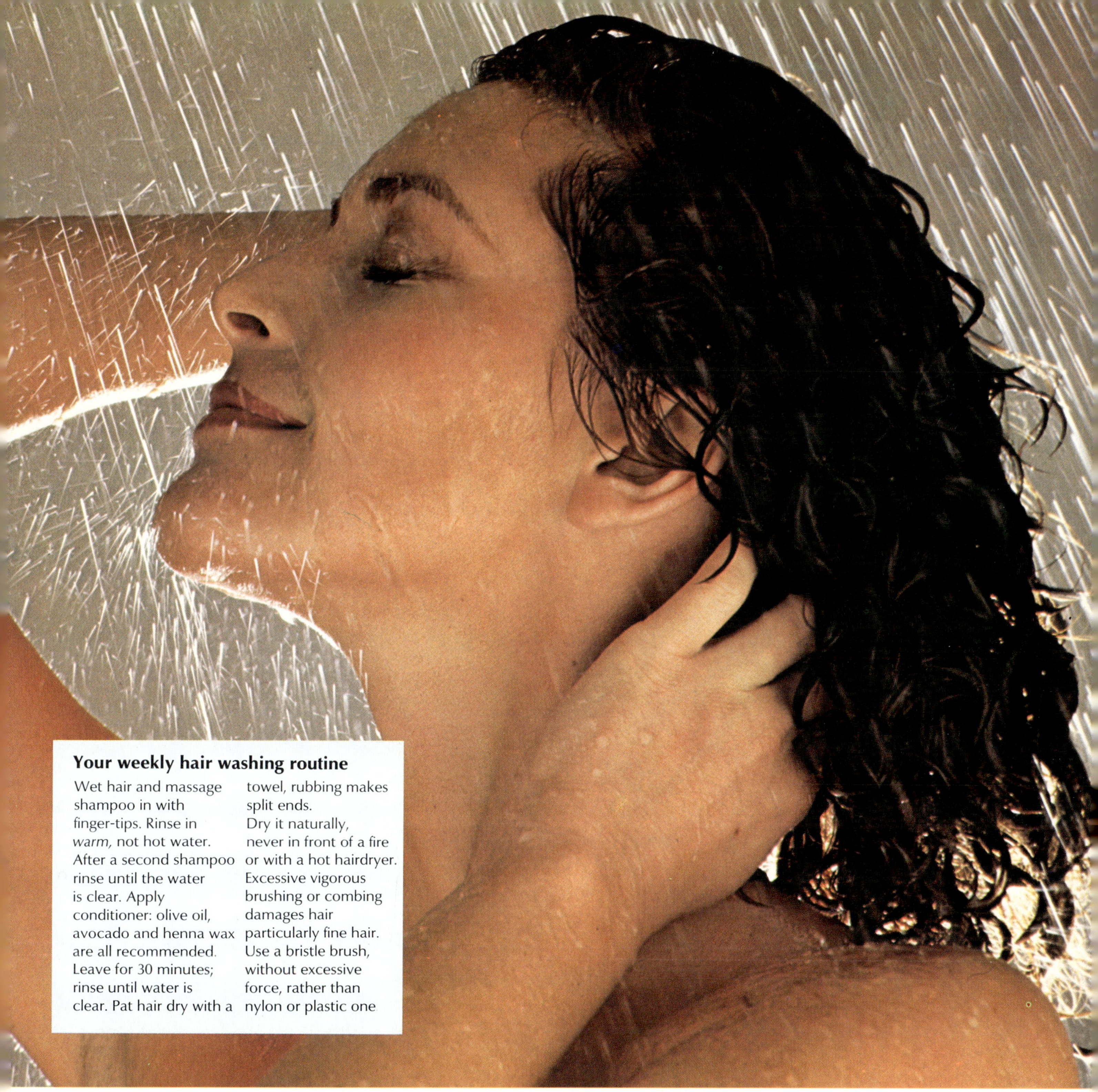

Your weekly hair washing routine

Wet hair and massage shampoo in with finger-tips. Rinse in *warm,* not hot water. After a second shampoo rinse until the water is clear. Apply conditioner: olive oil, avocado and henna wax are all recommended. Leave for 30 minutes; rinse until water is clear. Pat hair dry with a towel, rubbing makes split ends. Dry it naturally, never in front of a fire or with a hot hairdryer. Excessive vigorous brushing or combing damages hair particularly fine hair. Use a bristle brush, without excessive force, rather than nylon or plastic one

by constant traction and damage of the hair follicle, similarly over-vigorous back-combing and tightly pulling the hair into a pony-tail are to be avoided. Many people vigorously massage the scalp or rub-in hair tonics when they think that they are 'going thin'. The scalp is well supplied with blood vessels which 'feed' the hair follicles but massaging the scalp will not increase the blood supply but will probably break off the hairs and do more harm than good.

Another popular misconception is that dandruff heralds baldness. This is quite untrue. The surface of the scalp loses small pieces of epithelium every day just as the rest of the skin does. Usually these are microscopic and quite unnoticed. In dandruff however they appear much larger and cause a fine shower of scales on the shoulders. Dandruff can be caused by both over-activity and under-activity of the oil-secreting sebaceous glands and in both cases the best treatment is the use of a medicated shampoo. Brilliantines and hair creams can clog the hair follicles and encourage dandruff, as can hair lacquers which should be used sparingly and not too close to the hair.

The secret of maintaining a good head of hair is to eat a balanced diet to give correct nourishment to the living cells producing the hair, and to keep the hair clean. It should be shampooed about twice a week, certainly no more, because each time you wash your hair you remove its natural oil. Excessive shampooing can also damage the surface of the hairs which then become prone to tangling and matting. The shampoo you use depends on the greasiness of your scalp. If very greasy a strong shampoo is needed and frequent washing is necessary. Avoid cheap shampoos as they contain a mild alkali that may irritate the scalp.

You should either dry your hair naturally or gently with a towel. Never use a hot hair drier or direct heat.

The Face

Your face is your shop window so look after it. With a little extra care and attention, most make-up can be made redundant so that if the natural look is 'in fashion' you will have no need to worry about your skin's condition.

The skin of your face is similar to the skin elsewhere on your body but it is adapted so that it can convey expression. There are numerous sets of muscles in the deeper part of the skin, or dermis, which can be moved voluntarily. Non-verbal communication is extremely important. It is also exciting when used, for example, to signal 'come hither' looks between people attracted to each other.

Another form of facial expression is blushing. The blood vessels of the face are quite responsive to various emotions. As the outer epidermis of facial skin is extremely thin it is hard to hide the embarrassment or excitement that has caused the blood vessels to dilate and the person to blush. Of course we may also blush because we are hot. In extreme heat we sweat profusely on the face because the skin here contains many sweat glands. These may also respond when we eat spicy food.

There are also a large number of glands in the skin of the face producing the grease called sebum. These supply enough grease to keep the skin of the face as well as that of the hands in good condition. It is a surprising fact that we readily convey grease to our hands by constantly touching our faces.

Over-production of sebum, or grease, from the sebaceous glands can bring about two unpleasant and very widespread facial problems, blackheads and acne. Blackheads are formed when a pore becomes blocked by dirt or dust or excessive oil. If the pore is open to the air, the surface oxidises and turns black (if it is closed it becomes a whitehead). If the affected pore is not cleaned the sebum, unable to come out through its normal exit, ruptures and the surrounding demis becomes inflamed and infected. If touched at this stage, the trouble will spread. Blackheads affect the face, neck and shoulders. A diet of fresh fruit and vegetables, and little greasy food, the use of antiseptic soap and avoidance of greasy cosmetics along with sunlight and fresh air can all help keep black-heads at bay and produce a glowing healthy skin.

A recent survey in southern England revealed that about 80 per cent of teenagers were troubled by acne. This may not be very reassuring to teenagers, who are very often self-conscious and can be depresssed by this problem on top of all the others they may be experiencing. Acne nearly always disappears when puberty and growth are completed, though. Acne in adolescents is usually produced by the hormonal unbalance of puberty, and does not usually respond to washing and changes of diet, although cutting down on sugar intake can sometimes help. Acne is an infection of the hair follicle and sebaceous gland and consists of inflamed boils which produce pus and scar when they heal. It is confined to the face, neck, chest and back. There are some medicated lotions containing mild irritants which produce peeling and so unblock the pores. Sunlight has the same effect, and a suntan helps conceal the scars. If the condition is very bad a low dose, long term antibiotic which can be obtained from your doctor can bring a dramatic improvement.

The face is capable of conveying many expressions from glee to gloom. It is also often the first indicator of good or bad health

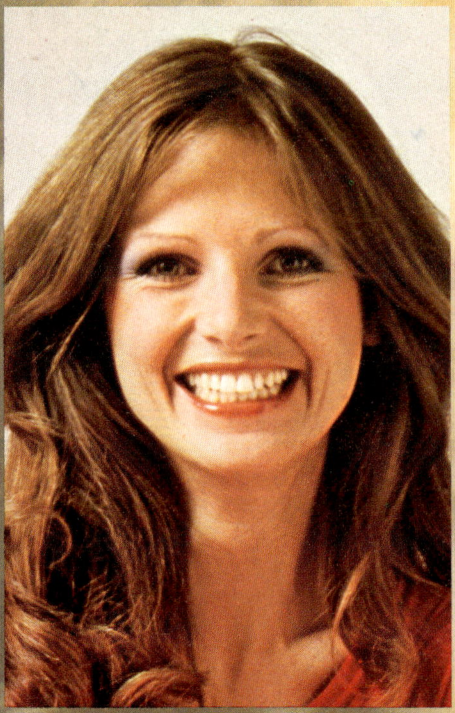

If you have greasy facial skin it will need frequent and thorough washing with soap and water. It is also a good idea to use a strong astringent, for this causes the skin to contract and the pores to close after washing your face. If you have dry skin then cleansing with an aqueous cream, which is available from the chemist without prescription, is excellent. Apply it with a damp flannel, and then wipe it off. The cream can also be used for removing make-up. Dry facial skin will also benefit from the use of moisturizers, which form a waterproof barrier to prevent the skin losing too much moisture.

Dry skin, like greasy skin, can benefit from moderate amounts of sunlight, but whatever your skin type and especially if you lack much pigment in the skin always remember to protect your face against excessive amounts of sun. This produces sunburn in the short term and in the long term the normal workings of the epidermis can be upset so that it does not produce a smooth, outer surface but a red, scaly area. If these areas are left long enough they can develop into skin cancers. Another important change occurs in the dermis which will give rise to more of the skin creases or 'crow's feet' of old age.

If you keep your face clean and eat a healthy balanced diet then probably your best make-up is none apart from a sunprotective cream against harmful ultraviolet rays. However, fashion often demands a brightly coloured face and the cosmetic chemists provide the material with which the fashion editors fill their magazines. Most cosmetics are relatively harmless and extensive testing ensures that most problems are elminated before the products are marketed. Rashes said to be caused by cosmetics are usually found to be coincidental and not due to the cosmetic. If you do use make-up, however, always remember to remove it carefully and thoroughly each night.

The only other problem likely to be

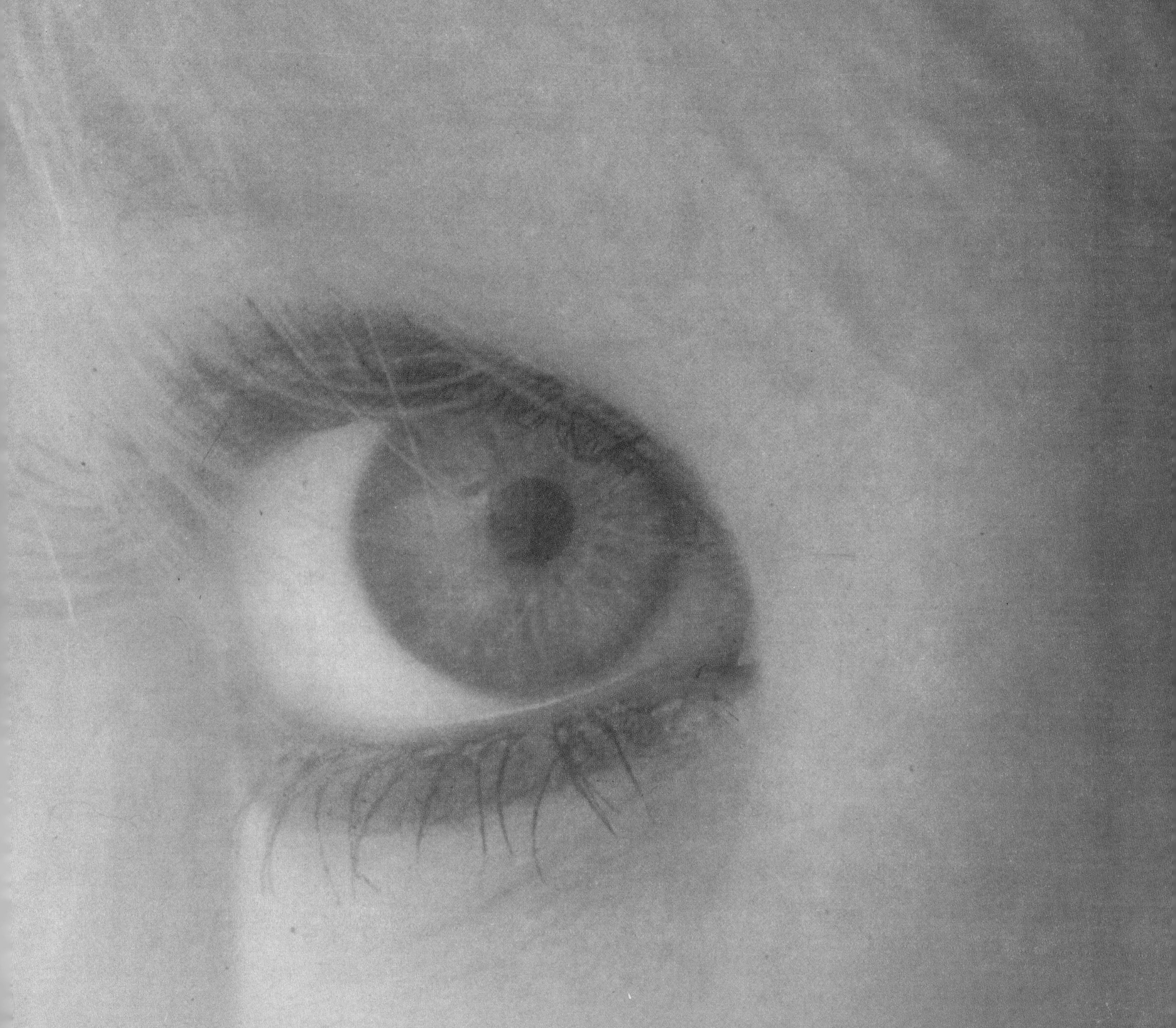

encountered by women is that of facial hair. Men produce a beard from puberty onwards, which can be light or heavy, and can choose whether or not they shave it off. Women sometimes have a mild growth of facial hair. They sometimes resort to plucking it, which only causes further growth of the hair and may cause infection. If the hair is thin it is better to cut it with scissors and if it is dark it can be bleached. A permanent removal of hair is often required, however, if growth is heavier, and the usual method is by electrolysis. It is essential that you receive treatment from properly trained operators otherwise scarring can result. It is therefore advisable to consult a practitioner who is a member of one of the recognised societies of electrolysis.

Care of your eyes

Vibrant, sparkling eyes are essential if your face is to look healthy. The most important way to ensure this is to get plenty of sleep. But avoid eye fatigue caused by inadequate lighting and work in daylight whenever you can. If your eyes feel tired you can refresh them by splashing them with cold water, or by bathing them with diluted salt water or a medicated eye-bath. After washing your face always pat your eyes dry and never rub them. This will not only irritate them but will damage the delicate skin around the eyes and may encourage wrinkles. Remove your eye make-up very gently with oily cotton-wool pads and even though it is difficult try to remove all the makeup.

Always remove particles of dust or grit from your eye with great care as you can easily damage the cornea. If constant blinking fails to move the particle then gently lift your upper eyelid outwards and downwards over the lower one and move your eye under the closed lid. If the particle fails to come away easily then you must see a doctor. A stye is simply inflammation around an eyelash caused by an infection of the hair's oil gland. Constant bathing with hot water should clear it up but antibiotics prescribed by your doctor may be necessary.

The Hands

Human hands are remarkably specialized pieces of machinery, purpose built not only for tough manual jobs, but also for delicate precision work. As they are one of the most crucial parts of the body and often the most harshly treated it is especially important to give them good care and attention.

Their adaptability and functional success is in part due to the adaptations that have occurred in the skin. The skin on the palms is much harder and more than twice as thick as it is on other parts of the body. The epidermis has an extra layer and is considerably thicker, especially in manual workers. Its outer surface is subtly ridged in more or less parallel curves to make it non-slip. The fascinating things about these line patterns or 'finger-prints' is that everyone has a different one. There are no hairs and no sebaceous glands on the palms. The grease that is needed to keep them pliable comes however, from the face for one is frequently subconsciously touching one's face and transferring facial grease to the hands.

The deeper layer of skin, the dermis, is also thickened for use in hard work. It contains increased amounts of elastic tissue integrated with the fatty and fibrous tissue so that the pad of fat returns to its normal size and shape after it has been compressed.

The nails protect the ends of the fingers from a large amount of trauma. Like hair they originate from the skin and are made of hard keratin. They rest on a nail-bed or 'quick' formed from the epidermis and which looks pink because of the underlying blood vessels. The white half-moon at the base of the nail is where the nail is actively growing and appears white because it is only loosely attached to the tissue beneath it. Some people enjoy eating their nails. The bitten nails are traumatized but although they are small they will grow faster than the other nails. It is probably the sheer stress on the nail plate which stimulates the increased growth of the nail. Simple trauma induced by manual work may well stimulate the growth of nails. Nails, if lost, will be replaced if the growing root is not damaged. Nails can give clues to one's general health. Healthy nails are pink and firm yet flexible. Spoon-shaped nails which will hold a drop of water denote anaemia. Nails that are bent right over or clubbed are associated with chest diseases. And if the nails are very distorted this can be due to a fungal infection or a skin disease of the epidermis called psoriasis. White spots on the nails are as yet thought to be unrelated to any disease and, therefore, quite harmless.

The colour of one's hands depends on a variation in the amount of blood flowing through the superficial blood vessels. Intense heat for example, will cause the vessels to expand, blood flow to increase, and the hands to turn red. A sudden noise can cause the flow to fall. Sometimes people are abnormally sensitive to the cold, as seen in 'milkmaids' white hands which may first go blue or red then back to white. Excess yellow pigment may be the result of a jaundice known as carotenaemia which is confined to the palms and which is associated with eating lots of carrots! A problem sometimes found with vegetarian diets.

Considering the extremes of environment to which the hands are exposed, both in industry and at home, it is remarkable how well they survive. The most common abuse to which we subject them is washing-up. Detergents, and especially 'biological' washing powders, by their very nature are extremely good at washing out fat and grease. It is only logical that they will do the same to unprotected hands. The skin becomes scaly and cracked and eventually typically red and inflamed in the condition known as 'housewife dermatitis'. Detergents also make the nails brittle. The best protection is to wear gloves for washing-up, and to make use of mops for floor cleaning and tongs for lifting out wet

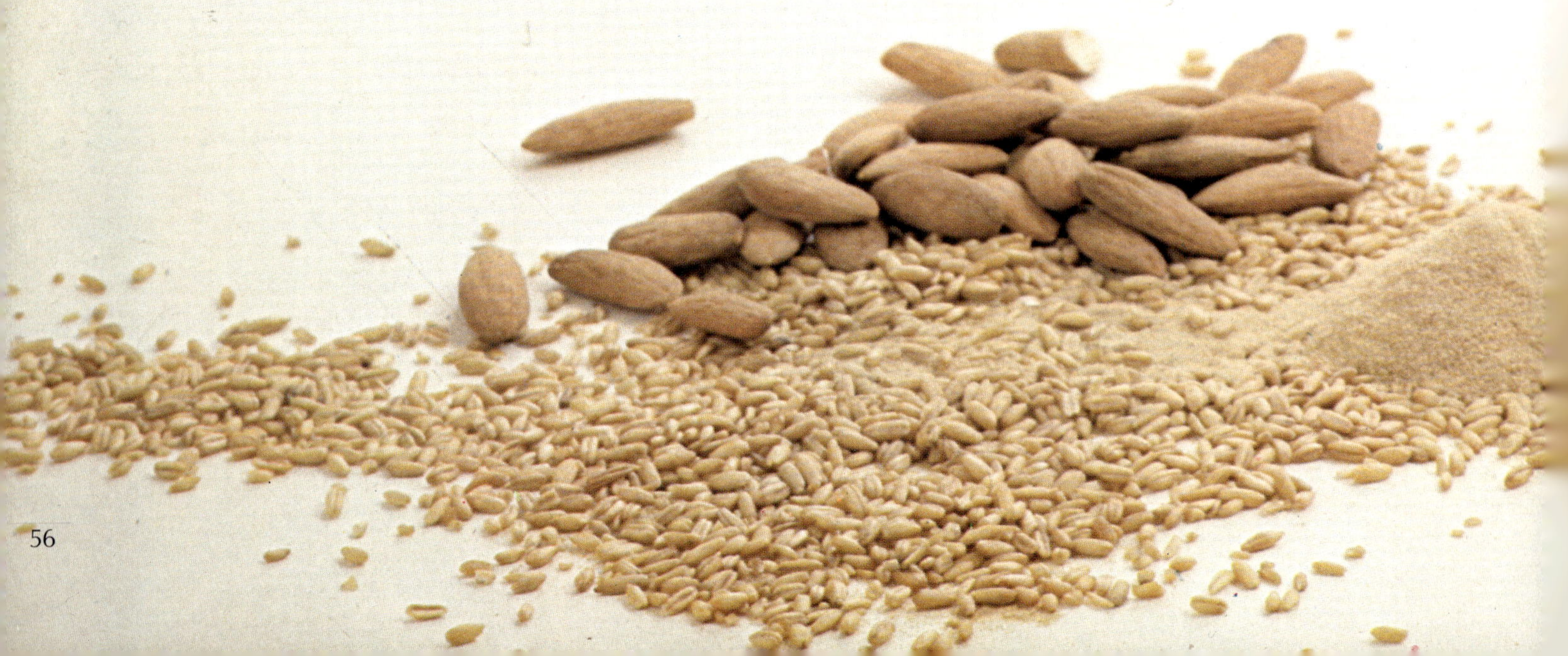

washing. On occasions when you do not use gloves make sure that you rinse your hands with clean water and dry them carefully before you go outside. As soon as you detect any dryness or chapping liberally apply handcream.

Modern detergents are also used extensively in industry in order to mix oil and water to make cooling fluids. When dealing with these it is essential to use gloves, or at second best barrier creams which help to provide a wall against these corrosive substances.

Soaps not only clean the hands but also wash out natural oils. White soft paraffin and vaseline are both excellent and cheap ways of replacing the lost grease. Emulsifying ointment which is easily obtained from your chemist is especially useful for dry skin for it combines a cleansing agent with a grease and will keep the hands both soft and dry. However careful you are to keep your hands clean and well looked after, it is possible to pick up infections. Warts, for example, are a virus infection which can be spread by human contact. The wart virus causes

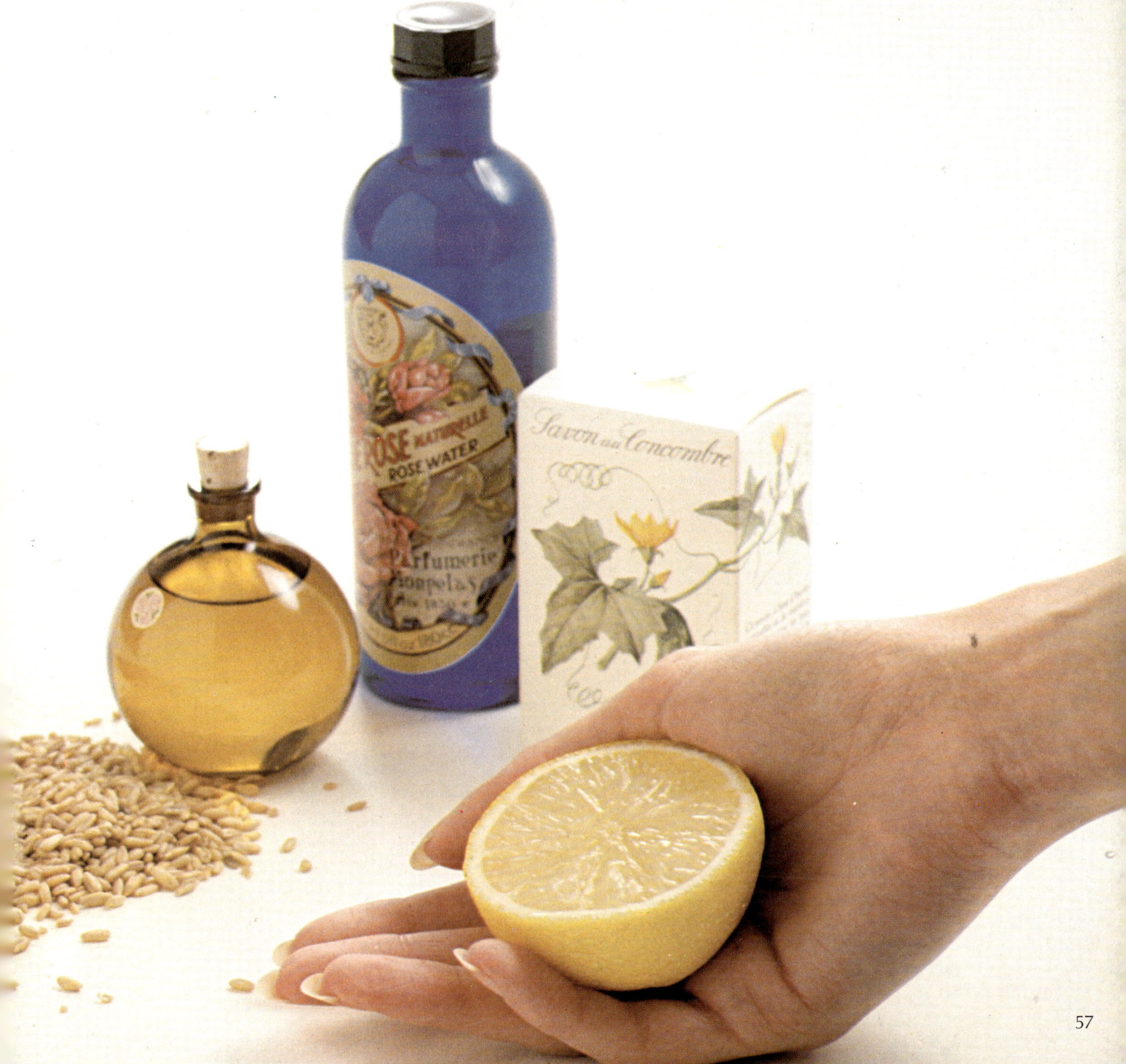

Our hands are exposed to heat, cold, dryness, detergents and at the same time we expect them to be beautiful. Nature provides perfect natural elements to compensate for the way we abuse our hands. Almond essence, grain and wheatgerm blended form a moisturizer, lemon soothes red and rough 'washday' hands. There are numerous soaps available today manufactured from herbs and vegetable extracts. Rosewater is a gentle perfume for the wrists, and can be a non-abrasive face wash

an outgrowth; or tumour, of the epidermis which can become unsightly and more important, painful. Sometimes the blood vessels supplying the wart cells become obstructed, or thrombose, and appear as black dots. This is an excellent sign for it usually means that the wart will disappear. In fact 80 per cent of warts go within three months but if they persist the best treatment is a daily application of a mixture of salicylic acid, lactic acid and colloidon, obtainable from the chemist. Never try to remove them yourself by cutting them out as this may cause the virus to spread, bringing new warts and adding to the discomfort and unattractiveness.

Manicure

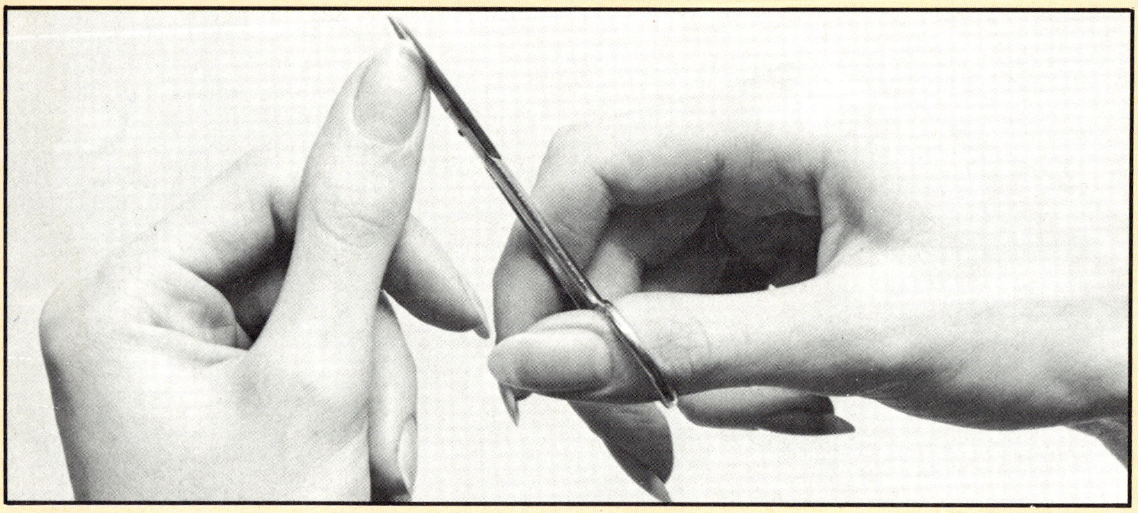

Correct cutting of finger-nails not only makes them more attractive, but strengthens them and reduces chipping. They should be cut straight and square with nail scissors only, and the rough edges then filed with the light side of an emery board. To remove dead skin at the base of the nail, push cuticles back

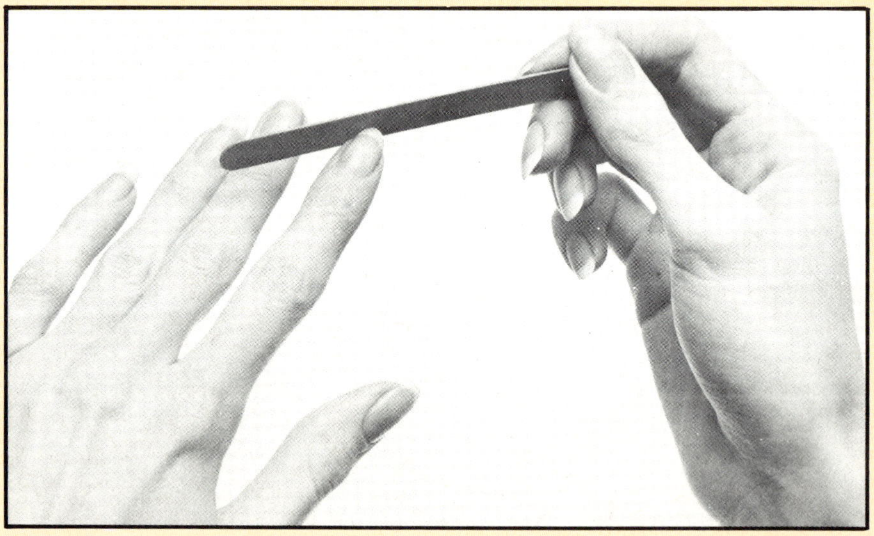

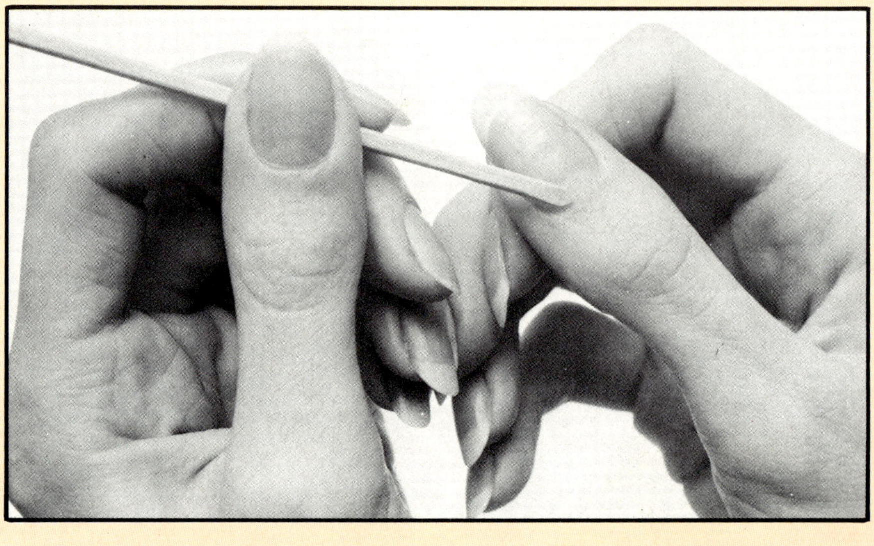

Your general state of health is often clearly seen in the condition of your finger-nails. If you are 'run down' and eat a poorly balanced diet your nails can be brittle and ugly. Careless filing will split your nails and so too will constant exposure to detergents and the over-use of nail polish. Nail hardeners only 'pickle' the nails. The only way to keep them strong and healthy is to eat sensible nutritious food and give them constant attention.

On average finger-nails grow about half a millimetre a week and quicker in summer than winter. They grow about four times faster than your toe-nails and growth is most rapid in the middle finger nail and slowest in that of the little finger.

If you are prone to biting your nails try coating them with white iodine which is available from chemists. This makes the nails so hard that it becomes unrewarding to bite them. As a nail care routine first cut your nails with a pair of sharp scissors. Then file them carefully with an emery board, in one direction only to avoid them splitting. If your cuticles have grown over the white half-moon at the base of the nail soften them with a cuticle cream before immersing them in warm water and then gently push them back with a blunt-ended wooden stick.

Legs and Feet

On average we walk about 75,000 miles during our lifetime. Most of us, however, spare a little time for the care of our feet. Not only do we neglect them but we force them into ill-fitting shoes because these are 'in fashion' and then wonder why we suffer from painful corns, bunions and ingrowing toe-nails. It is essential that foot care begins in childhood when the foot bones are growing and that the feet are always given as much attention as the rest of the body.

The skin on the soles of the feet is like that on the palms of the hands, highly specialized. The outer layer is harder and thicker and lacks hairs and oil glands. It has a print pattern on its surface similar to that on the hand. Often a footprint is taken on newborn babies for identification. The inner layer, or dermis, is well supplied with cushioning fat and elastic tissue to resist compression. The toe-nails grow extremely slowly – about four times slower than finger-nails – and take about a year to be totally replaced.

Take care of them by cutting them short and straight across and by removing any dirt lodged under the nails.

Skin and nails and sometimes the legs and body suffer from the effects of badly fitting shoes. Fashion determines curious shoe shapes which can compress and distort the feet and bring unnecessary pressure and friction on the skin. The skin responds by thickening especially in the epidermis and the result is the well-known corn. If you develop corns try to alleviate the pressure with sensible padding and then go to a chiropodist to have them removed. Corns can also develop as a result of flat feet, the sole of the foot rests on the ground, instead of being arched, so that abnormal pressure is put on the balls of the feet. Appropriate padding or specially constructed shoes will reduce the pressure and help to alleviate the trouble. Shoes that are too small or that are the wrong shape for your feet can also cause bunions. The big toe is forced to bend inward towards the others and the toe-nail is pushed sideways. The joint between the 'bent' big toe and the rest of the foot often becomes painfully inflamed and if this is not relieved by more comfortable shoes you should consult a chiropodist or your doctor.

Uncomfortable shoes can also squeeze the sides of toes against the edges of the nails so that the nails 'ingrow' and become swollen and painful. Avoid this problem by wearing roomy shoes and by cutting your toenails short and straight across. Rounding them off at the sides encourages them to ingrow.

The wrong height of heel for your particular kind of foot and arch can bring great discomfort. Too low a heel may strain the calf muscles; carried to its extreme the calf can overdevelop and become unsightly. If the heels of your shoes are too high your posture may be affected, producing back-ache or even a tilted pelvis. Varicose veins and swollen ankles may result from the constant wearing of stiletto heels, as these have such a small area in touch with the ground that the ankle and leg overwork to keep the body stable.

Verrucae, or plantar warts, are the equivalent of warts on the hands. They are caused by an infective virus which

Pedicure

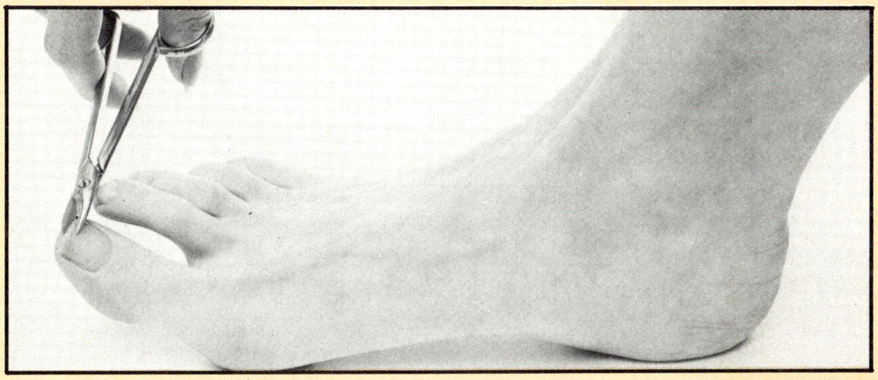

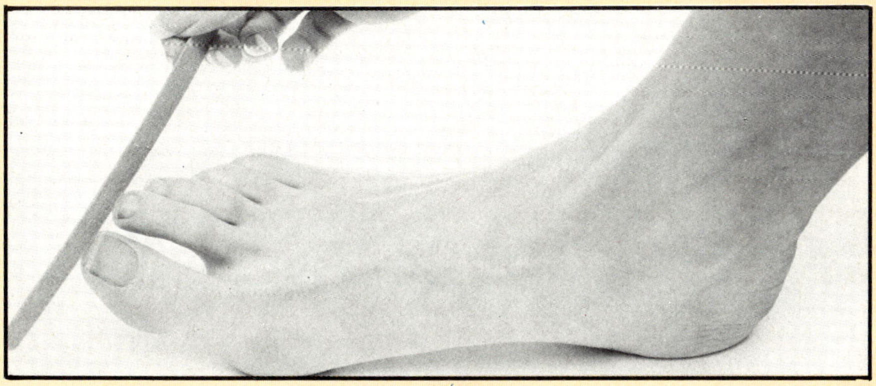

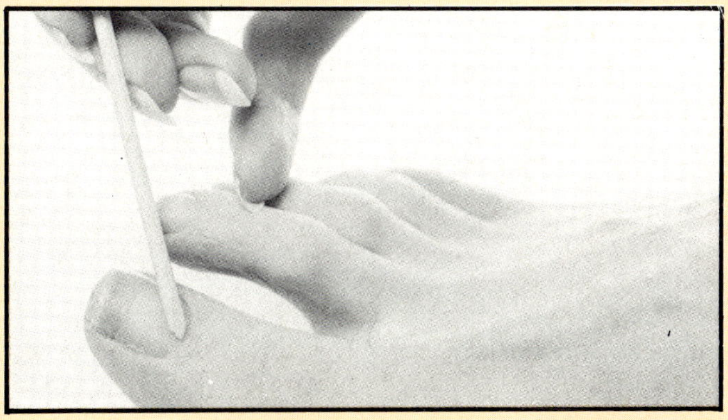

Feet can be as beautiful as hands, if you follow the same simple steps of cutting, filing and cuticle care. It is important to cut toenails straight across as cutting into the corners encourages ingrowing toe-nails

grows on the epidermis and produces a rough swelling. At sites of pressure such as the sole they are pressed into the foot and become very painful. If you discover that you have a verruca, seek advice immediately because they are much easier to treat early in their development. A chiropodist can relieve the pain by paring down a verruca but never try to do this yourself. It is best to avoid catching them in the first place. This can be done by protecting your feet in places such as swimming pools and showers which are likely places to pick up the infection. Here, rough floor surfaces have spicules of silica which dislodge skin bearing the verruca virus and in turn inject it into the foot of another person. Six weeks later this person will have a verruca. It is possible to obtain a plastic covered sock which, as well as protecting your feet from infection, also prevents an infected foot from spreading the virus. Sports halls are also places where verrucae are spread. Splinters carrying the virus can penetrate the skin of bare feet and the infection will be spread. Therefore, if the activity permits, it is sensible to wear gym shoes.

Another foot infection to beware of catching in a communal shower room is athlete's foot. It is caused by a fungus that is especially adapted to living on the human skin. Athlete's foot starts as a scaling between the toes but it may spread to the sole of the foot, or to the groin or, in fact, to anywhere on the body. As the fungus likes moisture it is most important to dry your feet well after showering, especially between the toes, and to use a fungicide powder if you are using communal showers.

It is important to wash your feet at least once a day. Dirty, sweaty feet provide a fertile environment for infections as well as producing an unpleasant odour. The odour is produced by harmless bacteria which live on the oil in the normally odourless sweat. Although foot deodorants may 'cover up' unpleasant foot odour, cleanliness is the only really effective measure. Socks too should be changed regularly for the same reasons.

As well as looking after your feet by keeping them dry and clean and by wearing comfortable roomy shoes, it is important to look after your legs especially if your job requires many long hours of standing.

Blood reaches the legs easily enough through the arteries but it has an uphill struggle to return via the veins to the heart. In healthy legs the uphill struggle is aided by one-way valves at intervals along the veins which prevent backflow of blood. The squeezing action of the calf muscles and the pumping of nearby arteries, together called the venous pump, further helps to push the blood towards the heart. Sometimes this efficient pump breaks down or the valves fail, the veins become swollen, the blood stagnates, the legs ache and the ankles swell. The swollen veins in this condition, called 'varicose veins', are easily seen as they are near the surface of the skin. If there is bad stagnation of blood the leg can become ulcerated. It is therefore very important to seek advice about varicose veins when you first suspect that you have them. If the treatment of leg ulcers is necessary, it involves treating the malfunctioning veins. Veins may be removed or injected with a clotting solution so that blood is redirected to healthy veins, and some compressed with the familiar elastic stockings.

Clothing your feet

To avoid problems with your feet always wear shoes that give you adequate support under your instep and heel and which allow you to spread your toes freely.

It is children's feet that are most easily damaged by ill-fitting shoes. Soft growing bones need plenty of room in which to lengthen and change shape. Children's feet should, therefore, be measured for width and length about every two months and their shoes should have a growing pace of about $\frac{3}{4}$in. Shoes take on the shape of your foot as you wear them so that one

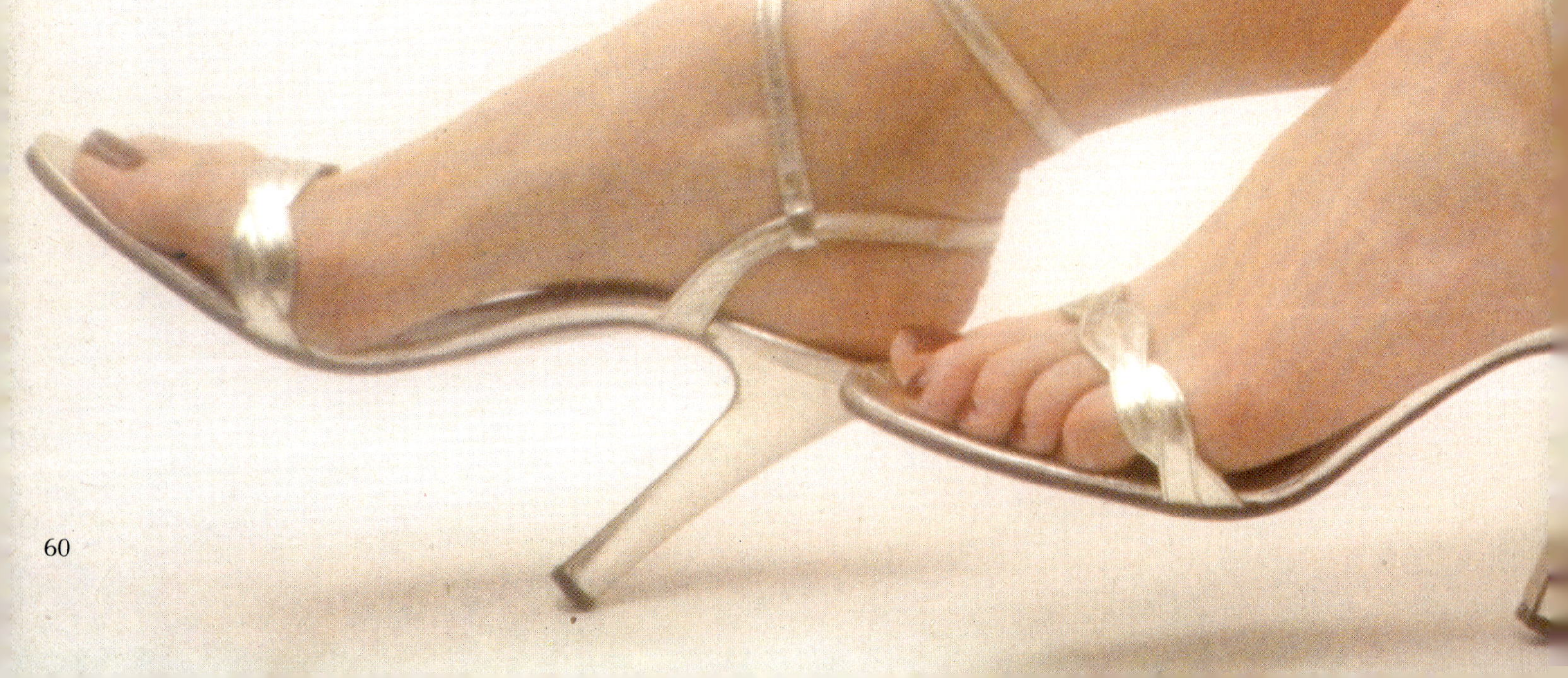

persons shoes should never be worn by another. This is especially important in the case of children.

Although it is now difficult to do, try to find a shoeshop in which your feet are measured and in which you can seek sound advice. Remember that suede or leather shoes will 'give' as they are worn in, but plastic shoes will not. Although suede or leather shoes are more expensive they are preferable to plastic ones. They are warmer, they allow your feet to 'breathe' and unlike plastic shoes they absorb sweat. Finally try to avoid shoes with extremely high heels and those with 'platform' soles.

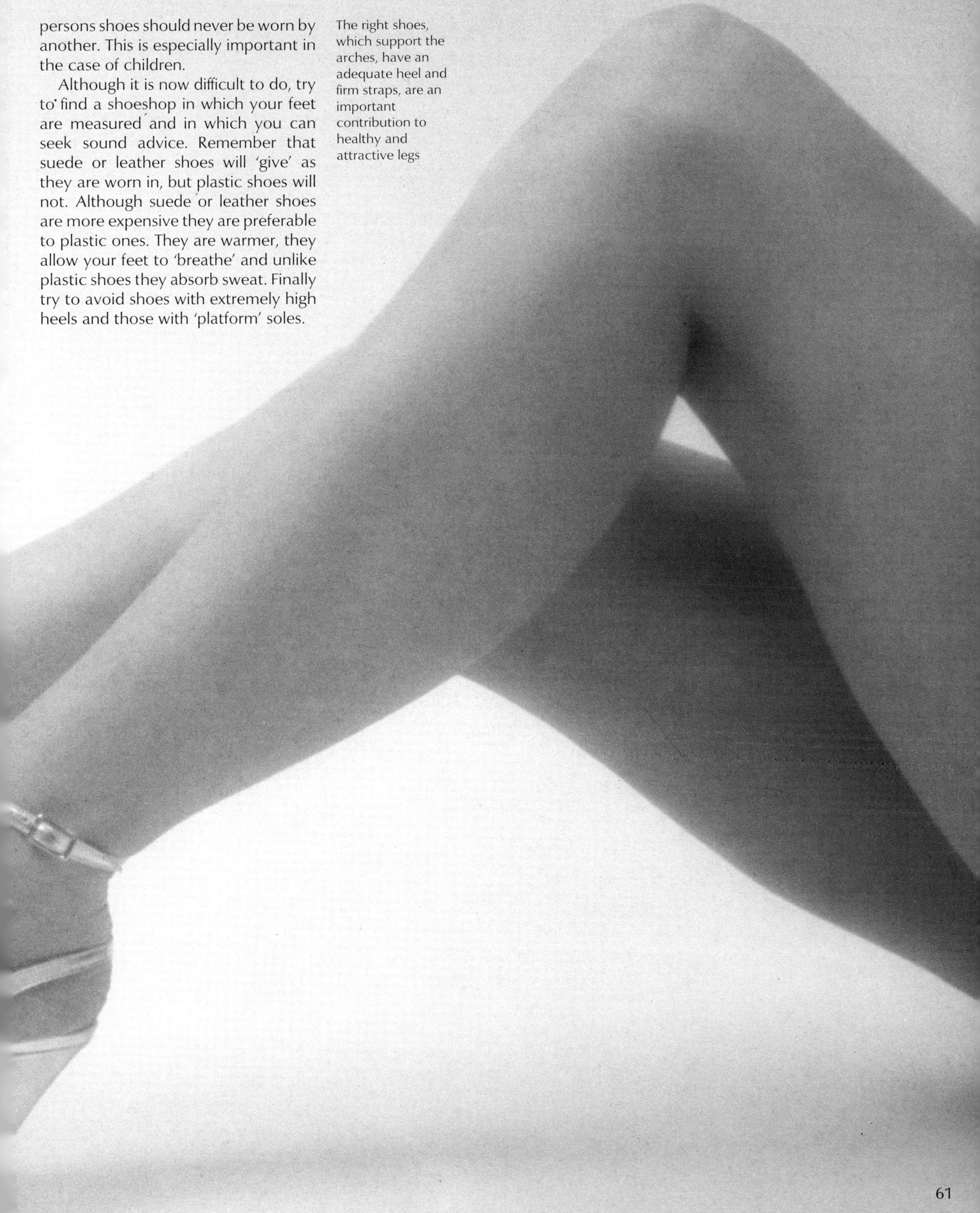

The right shoes, which support the arches, have an adequate heel and firm straps, are an important contribution to healthy and attractive legs

Modern Dentistry

Our teeth are important for various reasons. They enable us to chew our food, they aid pronunciation and form an important part of our appearance. Modern dentistry is constantly improving so that people have a greater understanding of what is happening in their mouths, and these days a far stronger emphasis is being laid on prevention of dental decay, as well as new ways of making a trip to the dentist less frightening.

The teeth are present deep inside the developing jaws within a few weeks of the foetus being formed and from that time they continue to grow and develop until they erupt into the mouth. The first teeth to arrive, the baby teeth or deciduous teeth, begin to erupt six months after birth and after two years there should be a full set of 20 baby teeth. These last until the age of six and at that stage the permanent teeth begin to erupt and to take the place of the deciduous teeth, which of course loosen and are shed. This process of gradual replacement of the primary or deciduous teeth by the permanent teeth takes some seven years in all and is known as the period of mixed dentition.

It is important to realize that although the deciduous teeth are not to last for many years it is not good if they are lost too early, due to decay for example. First, because a child cannot eat successfully without all or at least most of his teeth and secondly because the deciduous teeth actually guide the permanent teeth into their proper position. The deciduous teeth perform this function right up to the age of 12 or 13. Early loss of the deciduous teeth – for example at the age of six or seven, very often leads to a mouth with crossed or crooked teeth in later life. It is for this reason that your dentist will pay great attention to filling and preserving the baby teeth even though they are soon to be lost.

Modern dentistry is responsible for the supervision of the jaws and teeth and is concerned that all goes according to plan. Various disorders can affect the teeth during life – disorders of the development of the jaws and teeth arising out of complications during teething or structural defects, either of the enamel layer, or of the body of the tooth itself, which is called dentin. The jaws and teeth can be affected as well by disease in other parts of the body. In our affluent society the dentist is concerned with fighting two principal diseases which seem to advance and destroy our teeth in a quite horrifying way. These are dental decay, or caries, and periodontal disease, which attacks the gums.

Out of the total adult population of the UK, more than 30 per cent have lost *all* of their permanent teeth; up to the age of 35 the teeth are ravaged by dental decay (caries). After the age of 35 periodontal or gum disease is the major cause of tooth loss. In one study 99 per cent of secondary school children were found to have some degree of periodontal disease, by 17 years 36 per cent were seriously affected, by 35–39 years of age 46 per cent of adults in the UK were about to lose their teeth

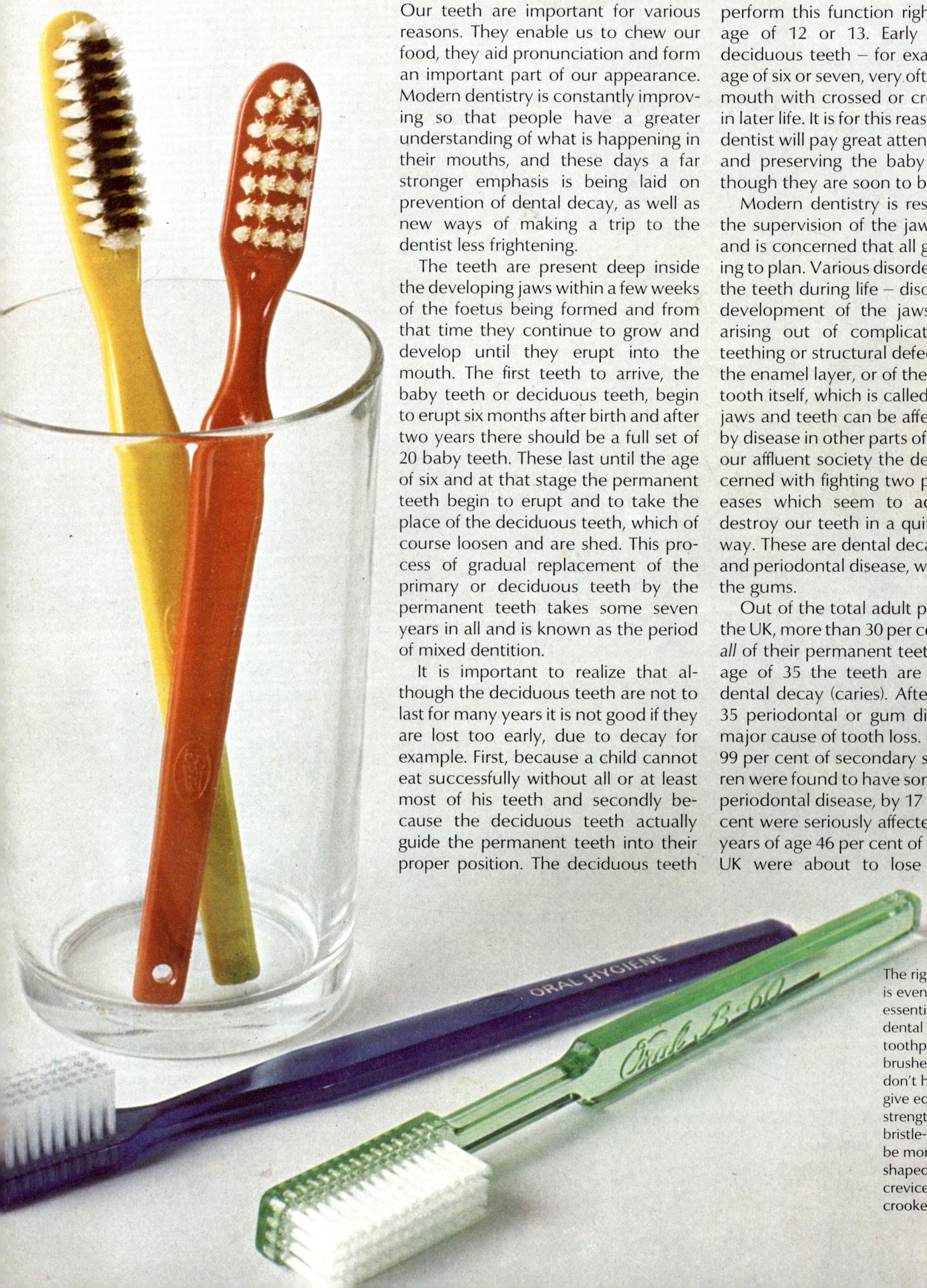

The right toothbrush is even more essential to good dental hygiene than toothpaste. Nylon brushes are firmer, don't harbour germs, give equal bristle strength and, unlike bristle-brushes can be more easily shaped for the crevices between crooked teeth

because of periodontal disease and between 55–59 years of age the percentage had risen to 95. (Shieham 1969 and Shieham 1971).

The major factor in these two main dental diseases is plaque. Plaque is a thin film which coats the surface of the teeth and contains a multitude of bacteria. Carbohydrates and sugars are somehow absorbed into this microscopically thin layer and form the ideal environment for the bacteria. This combination is then perfect for the onset of dental decay in the body of the tooth. At the neck of the tooth the plaque develops further and eventually forms a hard scale which is called calculus or tartar. The supporting structures are attacked by the bacteria which live in the plaque and scale and this begins periodontal disease.

The more advanced society becomes, for example in the United States of America and in Western Europe, the greater the amount of dental decay. This has for a long time been attributed to the fact that the more civilized we become then the more over-refined becomes our diet; we are eating a diet rich in sugars and with an excessively purified carbohydrate element. Modern research tends to suggest that unknown protective factors have been removed from the diet by over-refining and this over-refining of the present day diet produces an environment round the tooth overwhelming in its power to cause decay.

The Eskimos' natural diet is virtually carbohydrate and sugar free, consisting almost exclusively of animal and fish protein and fat. Surveys show that on this diet fewer than 1 per cent of the teeth of these people are decayed. In other primitive communities such as the Bantu the diet consists mainly of

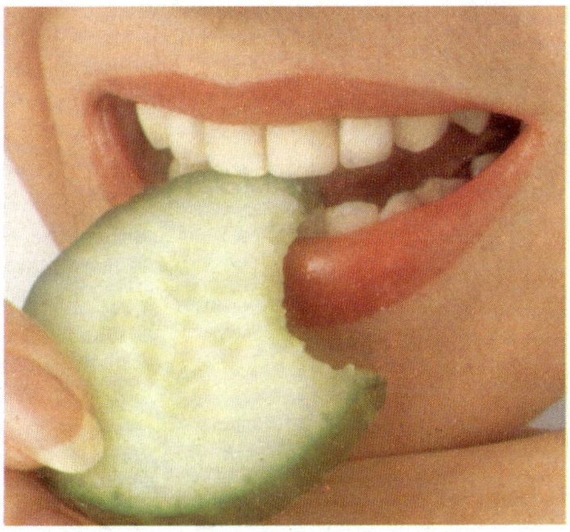

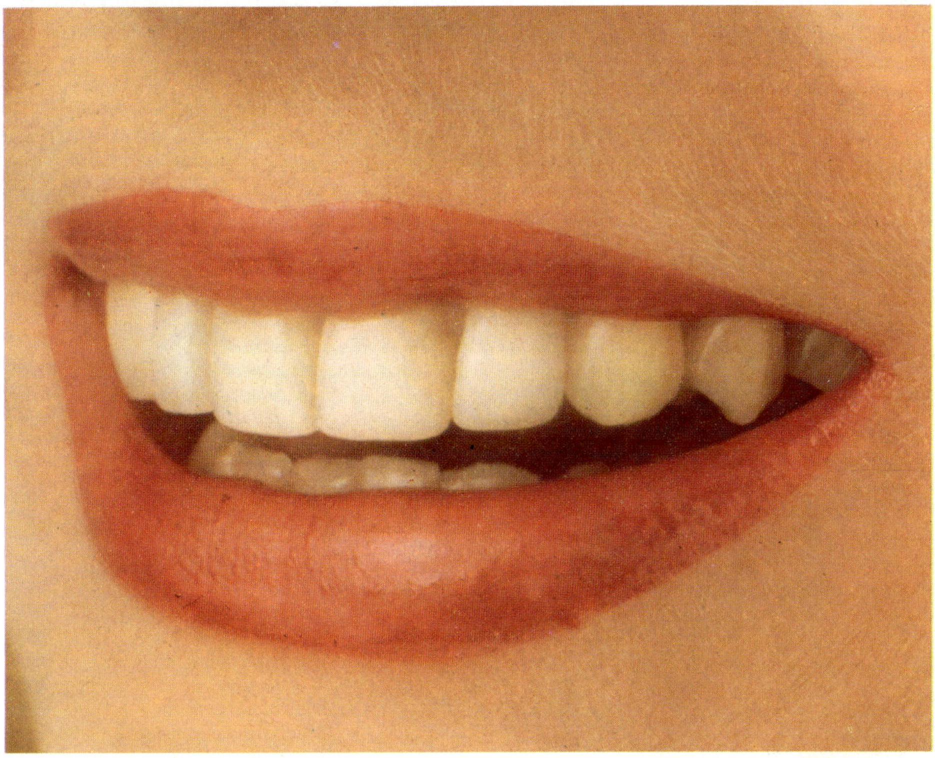

Correct brushing of teeth – up and down – for at least five minutes each day helps remove the built-up plaque which causes tooth decay and forms the ideal environment for gum disorders

coarsely ground cereals. Again the individual decay is very low. Conversely, in the more civilized societies it is clear that the baby teeth are decayed soon after eruption and the disease spreads rapidly and widely.

For many years the dentist's answer to these problems has been to repair the ravages of decay by the traditional methods of cleaning out the decayed parts of the tooth and placing fillings. Using various materials and various different techniques the tooth can be built up and fully restored to its original shape and once more brought into function. Any teeth which are considered to be so decayed that they are beyond repair would be extracted; and the spaces so created eventually filled by artificial means, such as dentures. However, modern medicine and modern dentistry are both increasingly concerned not only with the repair of damaged organs but with prevention. The modern dentist thus emphasizes more and more preventive dentistry.

One factor which is proven to cause a dramatic reduction in decay is the presence of fluoride in the diet. The normal and natural way in which fluoride is ingested is via the water supply and a succession of detailed studies has shown that the incidence of dental caries is reduced in areas where fluoride levels are at least at a level of one part per million. Protection of the enamel layer is conferred by fluoridated water only if there is continuous exposure during the development of the teeth. Where there has been fluoride added to the water supply to a level of about one part per million the reduction in the number of teeth affected by decay was more than 50 per cent. (Backer Dirks 1974). Artificial fluoridation has produced no detected ill effects on the general health of the community in towns where the water has been treated with fluoride.

For those persons who do not consume fluoridated drinking water during the period of tooth development, fluoride can be provided as a supplement in various ways. Fluoride tablets can be taken during the period of development of the teeth, or topical fluoride applications at regular intervals, e.g. twice yearly. These fluoride preparations are applied by the dentist to the surface of the tooth. Also significant reduction in decay has been observed using fluoride-containing toothpaste in conjunction with topical applications of fluoride.

In the USA preventive dentistry is practiced to the extent that special sessions are held with the patient

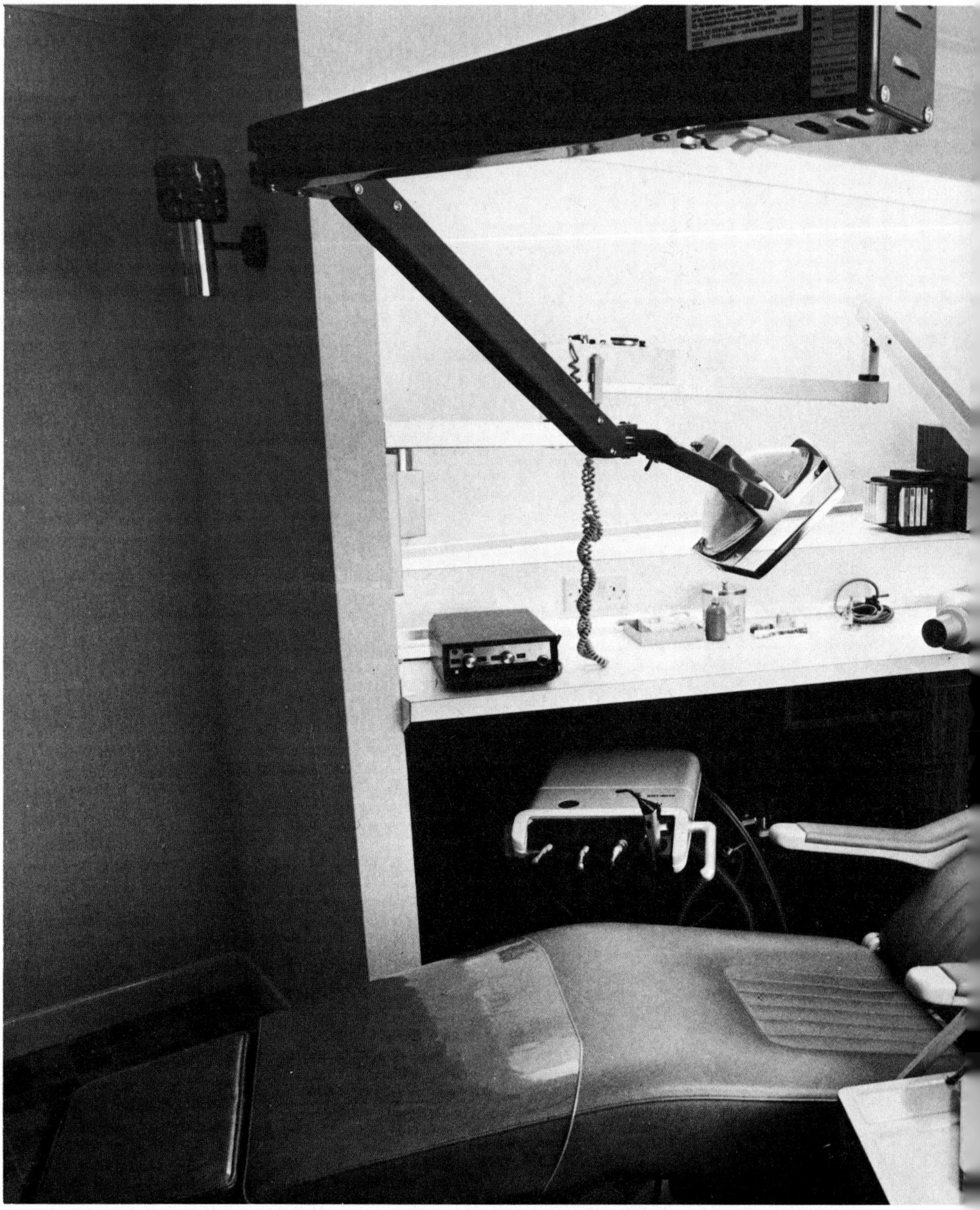

The modern dental surgery aims to remove the dread and fear most people feel when going to the dentist. Reception rooms are bright and cheerful. In the surgery itself, the 'chair' is reclining, rather like a couch, with comfortable arm and head rests. Music from a stereo or radio is soothing and contributes to a more relaxed atmosphere. Attractive decor and indoor plants are further elements that nowadays help to alleviate apprehension

devoted to dietary counselling. This takes place in a patient education room equipped with audio-visual aids etc. The patient is equipped with a diet sheet aimed at providing a proper balanced diet and restricting the intake of refined carbohydrates. Finally, preventive dentistry is aimed at educating the patient to improve personal oral hygiene by more effective toothbrushing. It is better to clean the teeth thoroughly and effectively once a day rather than quickly and superficially three or four times a day.

Half a century ago most people would not think of going to the dentist unless they had a serious problem, such as dental pain or a broken tooth, an abscess or, in the case of the wealthy, for the provision of artificial teeth. Today people are more and more interested in the preventive aspect of medicine and dentistry. Just as jogging is becoming popular, and people are becoming concerned about their weight and their diet, people now hope and expect to maintain full health and of course full dental health for the whole of their lives. In the UK and the United States people keep a regular check on their teeth and gums by visiting their dentist much in the same way as one would provide one's car with a 5,000 mile service.

Because of modern design techniques, the dentist can now present an

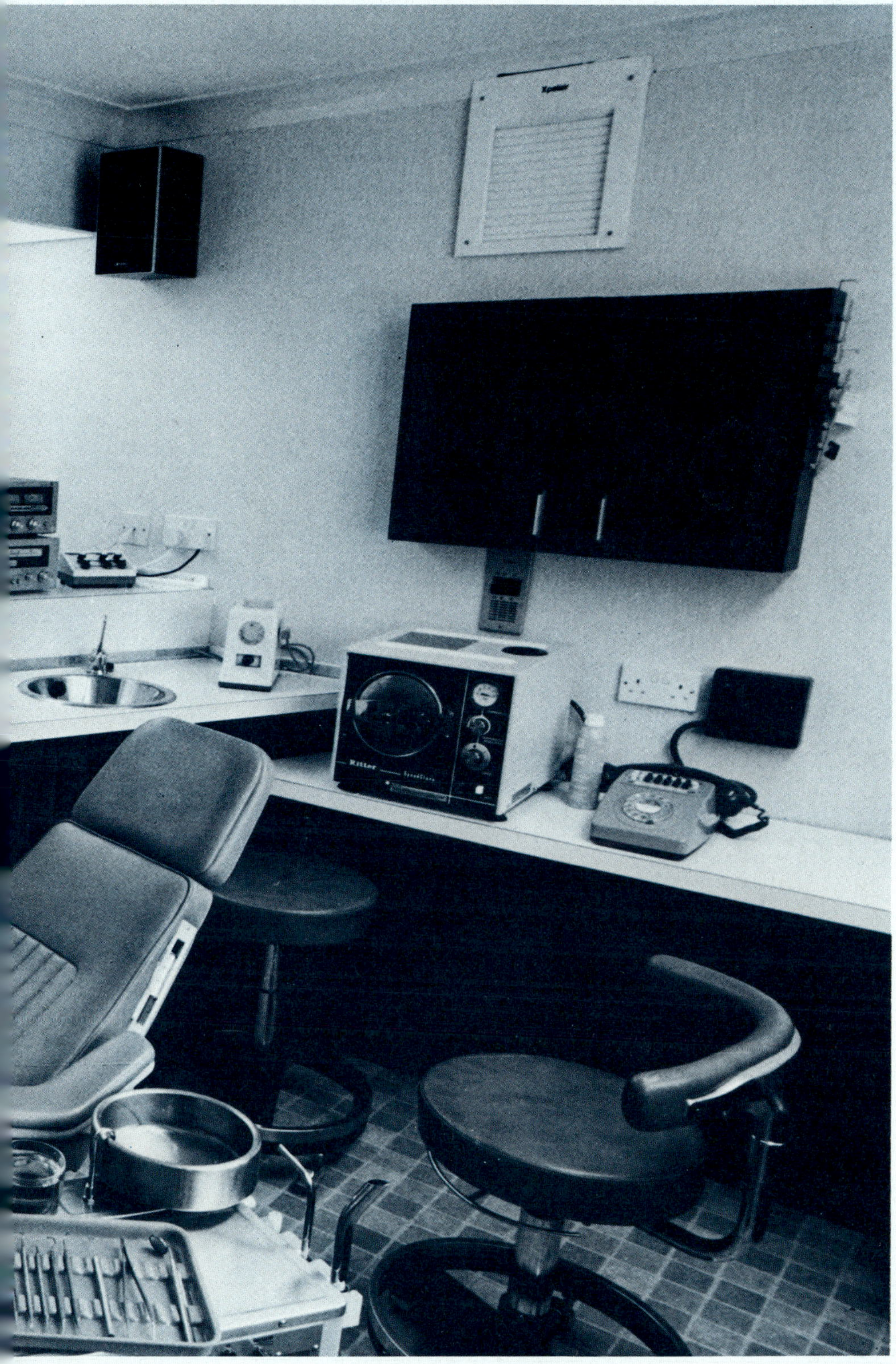

image which provides an outward aura of calm and confidence. Thus a cheerfully designed reception and waiting area, cheerful staff and perhaps piped music all help to alleviate the dread which traditionally has always accompanied us on our trip to have our teeth checked. Surgery areas are now often carefully designed to achieve this effect too. Because of today's technology the design of the present day dental surgery helps the dentist to be able to perform work of the highest technical standard and at the same time to promote the comfort and reduce the apprehension of the patient.

For many years the anxious patient has been in the forefront of the dentist's consideration and one of the biggest advances made in treating patients has been towards reducing apprehension. In many surgeries a technique called Relative Analgesia is used. The patient is relaxed, seated in the dental chair, which takes the patient to a supine position and is then asked to breathe a mixture of oxygen and gradually the patient becomes a little drowsy, perfectly relaxed and happy and quite cooperative and any feeling of pain which may have been there is greatly reduced. This of course is a great help to the dental team and it becomes possible to perform work and produce results which otherwise might not have been possible.

Some dentists use a drug which is called diazepam (valium). This drug is slowly injected into a vein in the patient's arm, and within a very short time, i.e. 15 minutes, the most nervous patient becomes relaxed and cooperative. I have seen patients so tense and so full of dread that they could hardly speak – and indeed had to be helped into the surgery. Such patients have been treated with diazepam and the results have been quite dramatic. Within a short time the patient tends to become relaxed, a little drowsy and quite happy and cooperative. These patients can then be provided with whatever treatment they need and indeed most of them are fully prepared to come back and undergo a further course of treatment.

So modern dentistry is increasingly concerned with prevention; patients are helped with all the advantages of fluoride, and sound advice with respect to their dietary habits; and we are all (as patients) encouraged to have regular dental check-ups so that any problems can be sorted out, the earlier the better. The dentist himself, equipped with modern techniques, machinery and materials, can provide the solution to so many problems, both functional and aesthetic. Indeed with the development of modern porcelains discoloured, broken or badly decayed teeth can all be made to look attractive, healthy and brand new again.

We can see that prevention is better than cure. In fact the same healthy diet that protects your heart protects your teeth. Other more specific preventive measures include fluoride and good dental hygiene; regular brushing of teeth after meals, the use of toothpicks or water picks, dental floss and sugarless chewing gum. Where prevention has not been effective modern dental techniques can reconstruct teeth that are excellent in appearance.

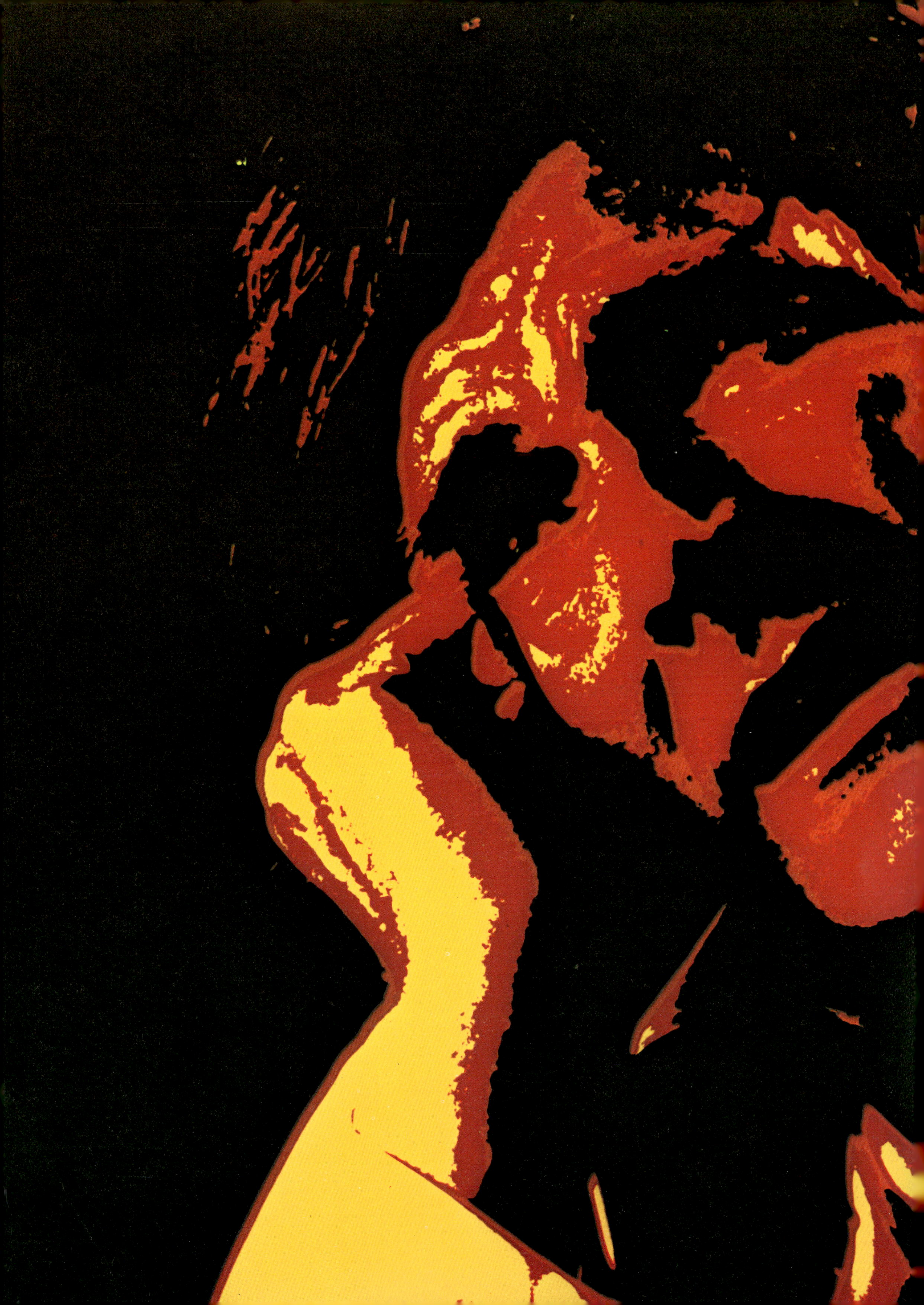

STRESS TODAY

We live in a highly organized society. Survival is no longer a physical response to danger of fight or flight. The problems that confront us have to be dealt with in other, more socially acceptable ways. Our bodies begin to conflict with our minds. Once the problems begin to build up, the stress on our body can actually cause illness. How do we recognize this pattern, and how can we break out of it? This section pinpoints the areas of stress in our lives and helps us break the spiral.

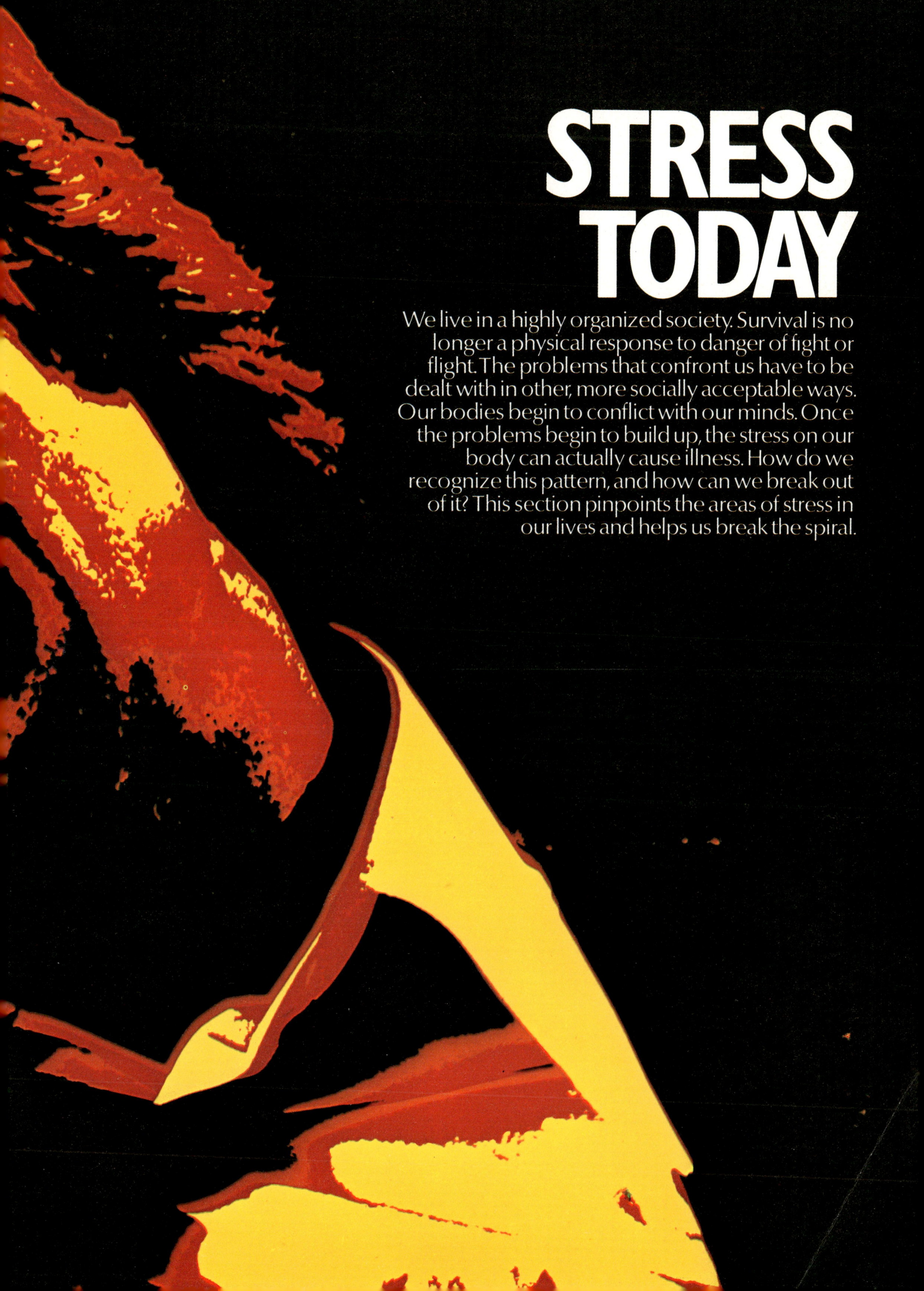

What is Stress?

Stress is a word with which we are all very familiar. We have all heard experts talking about the 'stresses of modern life', and we all have probably complained at one time on another about having too much stress. It is a word used to cover a multitude of ills, but do we really know what it means? It refers to the effect on *you* of some particular event in your life. Some events are more stressful than others, and some people are more affected by stress than others. As science and technology made their presence felt in the world and began to affect human beings it became necessary to have a word like stress roughly covering the same sort of forces as in engineering. Noise, speed, pollution – all forces reminiscent of the external strains on metal – were now affecting us and we needed to be able to examine the power of such influences. Stress proved to be the right word, easy for everyone to use, short and concise; but of course the trouble is that we are not machines and do not lend ourselves to mathematical equations. As a result, although physical stresses such as noise can be measured to some extent, we cannot possibly predict at what point human fatigue will set in, because there is too much variation among individuals.

As homo sapiens we have immense variation in hair colour and facial features and our internal make-up is just as infinite. Psychological variety – personality, intellect and so on – is even more varied than the precise physical configuration of glands, organs and tissues. For instance, someone who sleeps very soundly whatever the circumstances is clearly in a better position to resist external noise than the very light sleeper would be. If on the other hand something happened in his life to disturb his slumbers he might suddenly become vulnerable to outside noise. And what factors distinguish the habitual insomniac from the lie-down, eyes-shut, straight-to-sleep individual? Indeed, no two people sleep in exactly the same way. If we take into consideration the whole range of activities that we regularly indulge in, the potential for being disrupted or not by stress is very enormous indeed.

Both physical and emotional stress are so variable, and produce such different reactions in different people, that any ambitious scientist who set out to measure them would flounder in a morass of conflicting evidence. We all have different *threshold* levels – the point at which an external event, physical or otherwise, begins to affect us, producing a response. Hence, each of us would have a different point at which that external event would produce stress. Many things impose strain and stress, and it is society's recognition of these factors which renders the word stress so useful to us. And when we talk about stress we should deal with aspects such as food shortage, poor housing and illness as well as the rather indefinable stresses caused by our expectations, our ambitions, our desire to live up to some image that may be totally inappropriate for us. Hunger and thirst for example are the most fundamental stresses known to mankind and they still affect many people in the developing world – and to some extent in the more prosperous Western nations. It is not possible to categorize hunger as solely physical, separating it from the complex emotional response to a stressful situation. Mind and body cannot be separated, although doctors and scientists have tended to promote this dichotomy during the past decades of scientific discovery. When medical science was in its infancy research workers had to separate mind from body in order to simplify their work and provide workable boundaries. Nowadays as we learn more we realize that this separation is quite artificial. And nowhere is this dawning realization of the interaction between mind and body more important than in the field and study of stress.

When studying the impact of stress we can see how the whole body reacts. Blood circulating the 'physical' part of the body also visits the brain and delivers 'messages' in the form of hormones and chemicals. From these the brain perceives what is happening and responds appropriately. The presence or absence of the right substances needed to keep the mind well oiled affects its mood. In response, the brain itself puts out chemicals in an attempt to make good the deficits and to compensate for the shortcomings in the rest of the system; or it might merely secrete its own chemicals in response to the 'directions' that it receives from the glands.

Stress is a very complex subject, as you can see. All we can say about it for certain is that it is the reaction to the stress that is important, not the stress itself. Pile on as many problems as you like, it is the way your body responds that is vital and signals that a dangerous level is being reached. Again, this reaction does not involve one section of the body, even though the symptoms may seem confined to one system, it is a whole body problem.

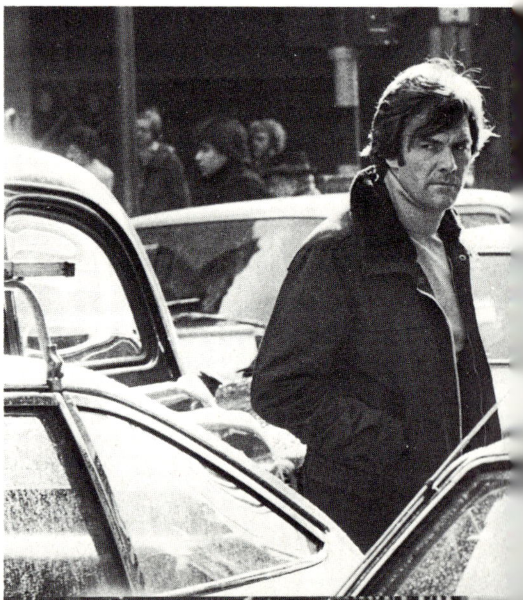

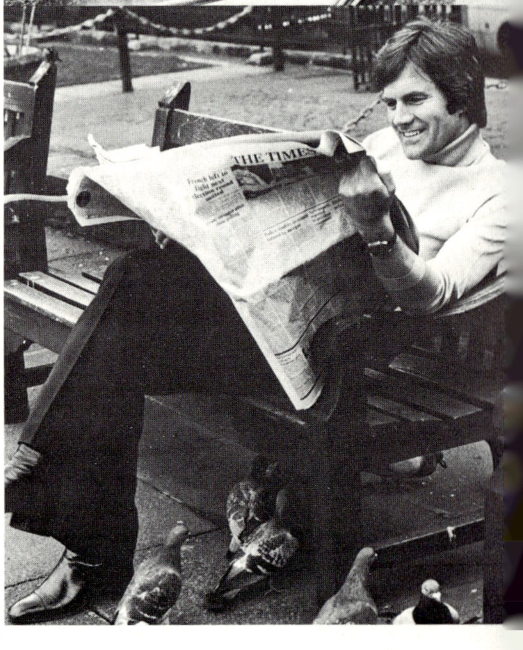

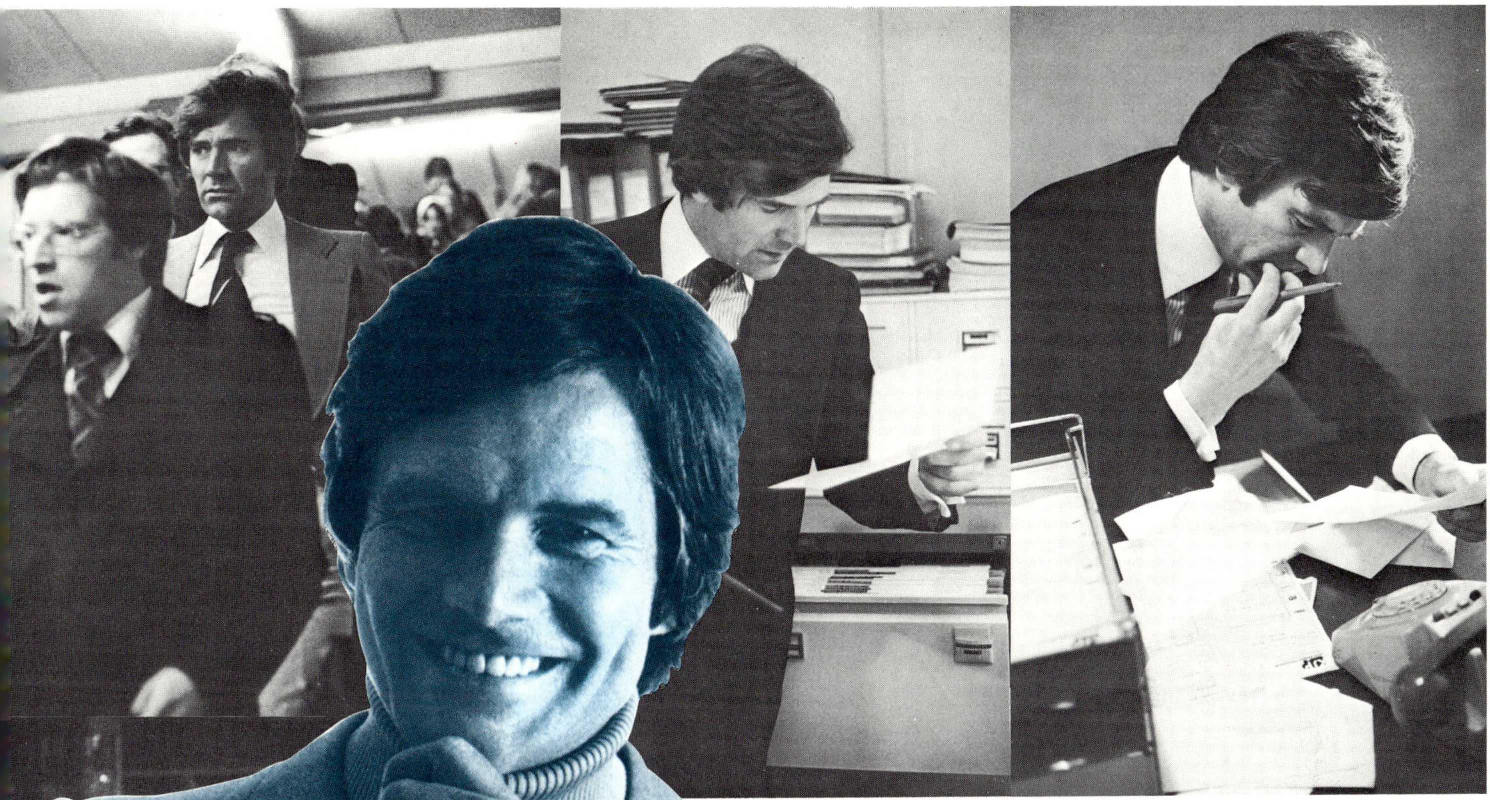

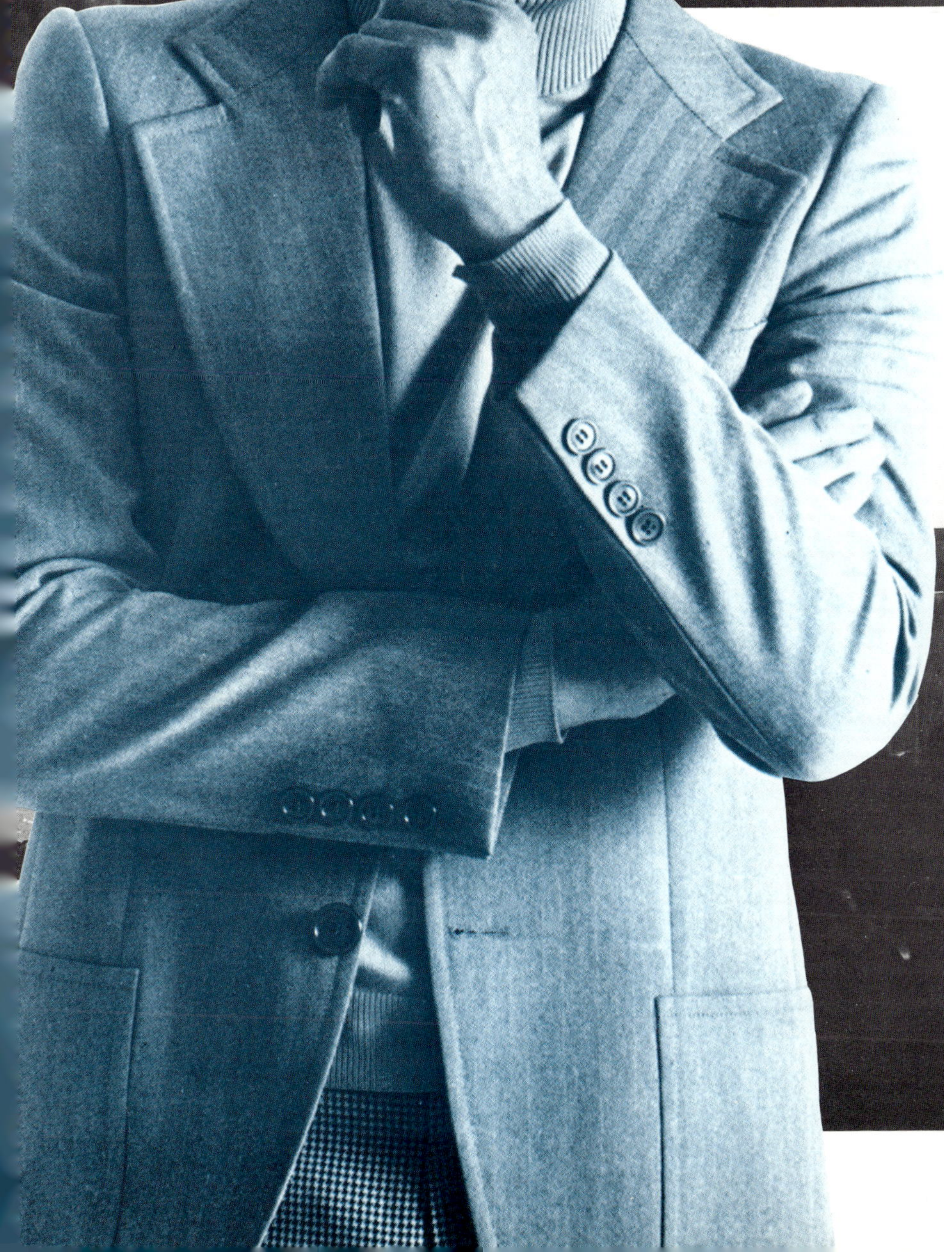

Many aspects of everyday life prove to be stressful. In the crowded city streets or on the subway there are traffic, noise and fumes. At work we experience pressure to make decisions and produce ideas, while at home there are bills to pay and perhaps an unpleasant atmosphere. Different people cope with the stresses in their lives in different ways. Some relax, for example, in the park, while others resort to more dangerous methods, such as secret drinking. When the problems mount, we all react with physical signs of tension and look for ways of release

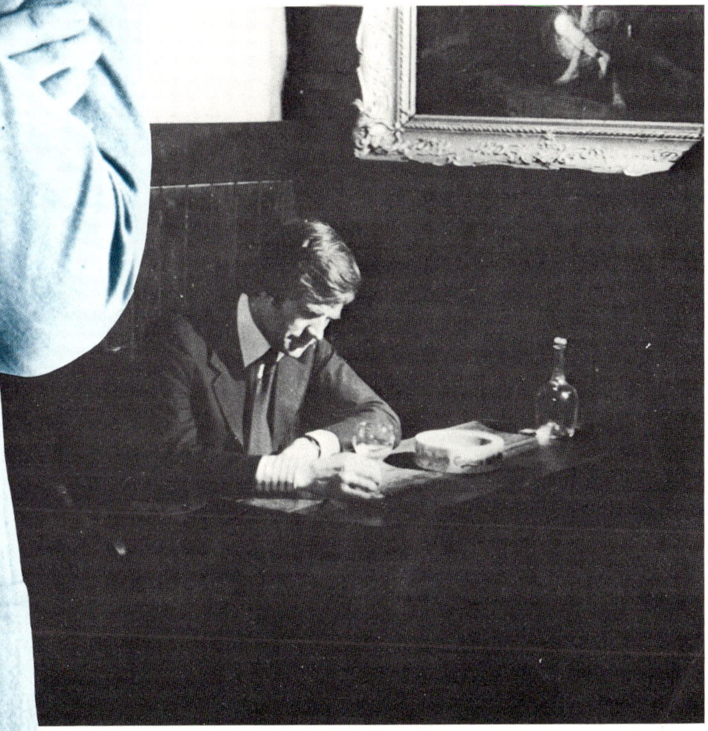

Is Stress Necessary?

Imagine a world without stress. What would we have to stimulate us into action, to change the course of our lives when things are going wrong? A world without the stress response – whether to physical danger or mental or emotional discomfort – would not only be duller, but certainly not as safe. We need stress – it is only when it exceeds a certain level that the problems begin. Where stress was once mainly a physical phenomenon, now it seems to have moved into a more psychological arena. But still it is adaptation to the circumstances that we find ourselves in that counts. It is still broadly survival of the fittest. But now we have to demonstrate our fitness in different ways. We are called upon to endure different kinds of stress today – and that is why we are so conscious about it. We are now concerned with overcrowding, violence and mugging, the need to keep up a certain material standard of living, the need to prove oneself in a social situation.

We must learn to adapt if we are going to survive. Some people are clearly more able to do this and ultimately the successful types will predominate as they tend to do better and pass their skills on to the next generation. For example, it was once advantageous if you could put on weight when food supplies were intermittent; now that food is plentiful such people tend to suffer ill-health because of obesity and the thin ectomorph is more likely to live longer. Theoretically, those individuals who are coronary-prone as a result of being overweight and the stresses they experience stand a lower chance of long-term survival and passing on the particular qualities which are responsible. In practice, however, they usually die *after* they have had children rather than before, thus potentiating the type of physique and personality which is at a disadvantage from the stress point of view. Also, evolution, which is what we are witnessing, works exceedingly slowly and it's likely that today's circumstances will have altered, thus changing the drift and putting other qualities at a premium, before appreciable alteration in the population has been made.

A small amount of stress is good for us, it is only when it becomes excessive as far as an individual is concerned that there is trouble. Environmental changes stimulate us, make us dynamic. If you are healthy, increasing the stress can increase the quality of your performance. For instance, a report must be completed by tomorrow morning and a great deal hangs on its completion. As a result, the strong motivation which this produces can drive you to levels previously undreamt of. The stress of an exam can bring out the best in you. Half-forgotten facts can suddenly be brought out of the recesses of the mind in response to a question from the examiner in a way that can take you completely by surprise.

Unfortunately, all too often the opposite can happen. The stress is so great and the individual's ability to cope with it so inadequate that the dominant sensation is one of anxiety. Instead of performing at his best, the candidate's mind goes blank and he completely fails to do himself justice. The causes of this type of anxiety are many and varied and sadly too many people in our society consider it natural to experience exam nerves of this magnitude. But examinations are part of our world, something to which an intelligent person must adapt if he wants to do well. If we can learn to reduce the anxiety with which we think of them and thereby reduce the total stress, we may be able to allow the natural low-level stress response to take over – i.e. stress bringing out a supremely good performance – if not every time then occasionally at least.

Some scientists describe this response to stress as the human function curve – a concept which plays a useful part in showing us how much stimulation any of us can take. Depending on the amount of stress (or arousal, as Dr Peter Nixon prefers to term it), the performance alters. The more the

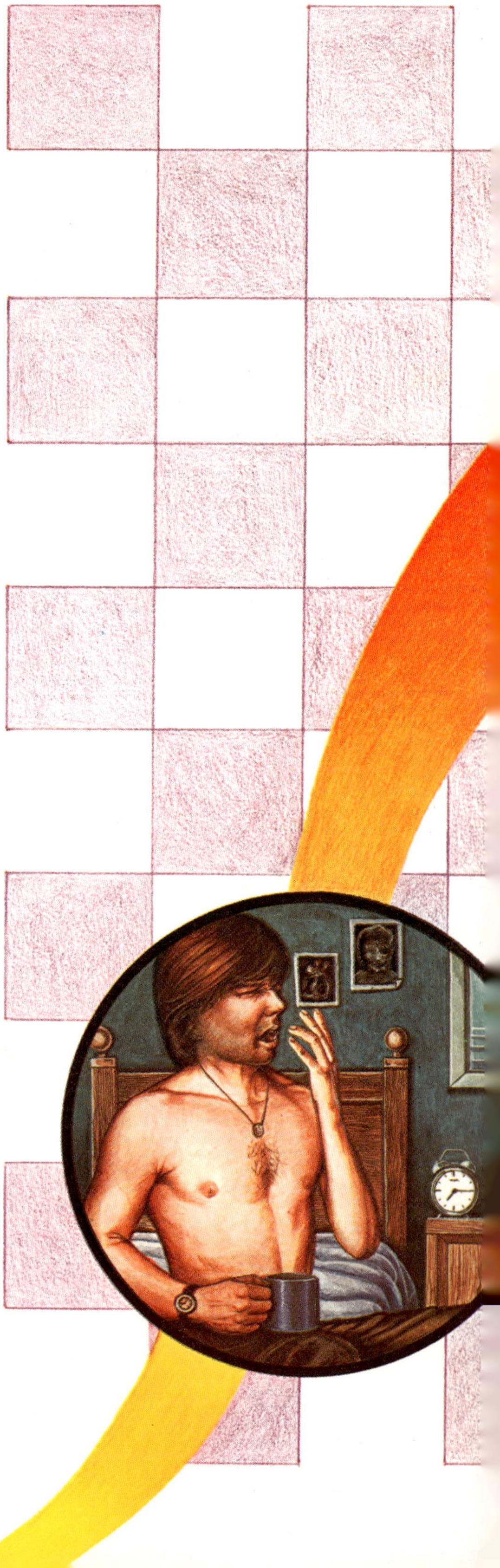

Our level of performance varies with our level or arousal. When waking up in the morning we are not likely to perform well as we are sleepy and distracted. In front of an audience, confident of our ability, adrenaline surges through out blood, so that we can give of our best. But if too nervous and under-rehearsed, we build up too much adrenalin, and whatever we do is likely to fail as we are over-aroused

arousal the better the performance – up to a point. This is the point when fatigue or excess anxiety creeps in. After that, an increase of arousal or an increase of stress leads to a marked deterioration. There is exhaustion, illness and possibly a breakdown. Again, the point at which the rising curve starts to tip downwards depends on individual factors: the point being reached progressively earlier with increasing age. In the early stages, the person is functioning well, like the person who thrives on examination conditions. Increase the demands and the person continues to respond with enthusiasm, with a capacity for original ideas and the ability to solve problems. When he reaches his limit and becomes fatigued or stressed he is aware of the fact and takes steps to recover his faculties. If he pushes beyond this and enters the stage of exhaustion or breakdown he may no longer be aware of what is happening and no longer be able to take corrective steps. This is increasingly a danger if he lacks insight into his own character and failings; also the problems are compounded if he has personality problems or insurmountable dilemmas of a personal nature that he cannot successfully resolve and come to terms with.

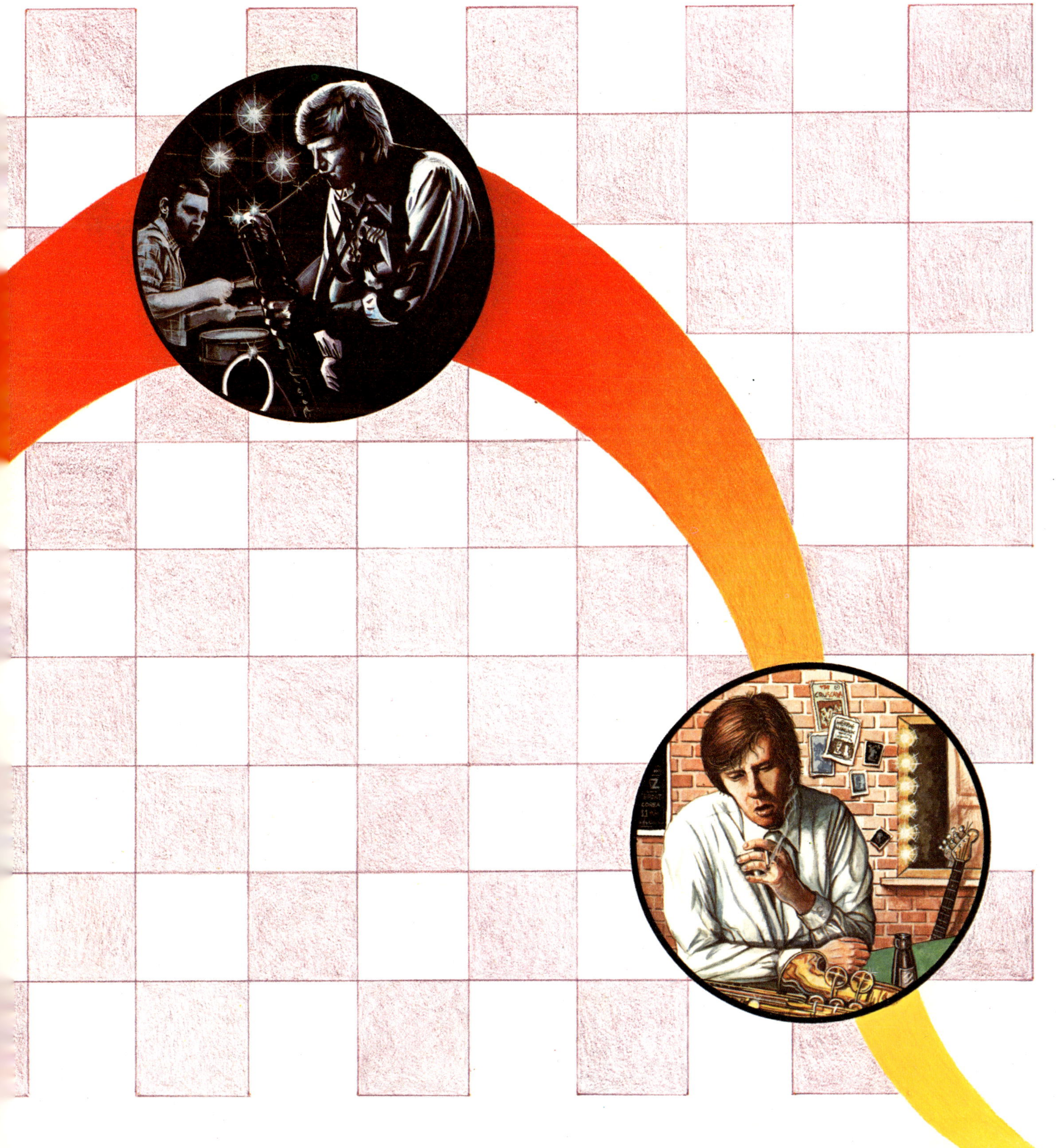

How the Body Reacts

Confronted with danger, our body immediately reacts, producing the energy with which we remove ourselves from the source of danger. This physiological reaction has helped man to survive. But the more subtle stresses of today are registered by the same physical reaction early man experienced when facing a wild boar or a forest fire. Whatever the situation, and however we have learned to express our stress, our *body* reacts in the same way.

If we imagine primitive man in the grasslands competing with wild animals for food, with only his wits, his fleetness of foot and rudimentary tools to help him, we can guess the sort of choices that were open to him in an emergency. If he was suddenly confronted by danger he could either stay and fight if the adversary seemed beatable or, if all hope of winning seemed impossible, he could run away. This is the well-known fight or flight phenomenon. Present-day man has a similar desire to act; to do something decisive: to either go in there and punch, or get away from the scene as rapidly as possible. But, instead of taking prompt action, today's man is only supposed to show his aggression through the use of expletives or body language. These are certainly a help, but nothing like the physical action that our bodies are prepared for. It is basically physical outlets that are necessary. Although this is still a fairly new line of research, evidence is accumulating to show that if the physical needs of the body are frustrated, be it a sexual impulse, the need to run away from a situation or maybe only to have a good stretch, the whole mechanism is somehow thwarted. The final outcome of the general disorder that results is anxiety to a greater or lesser degree, possibly leading on sometimes to mental or physical disease.

Faced with a threatening situation, the body pumps certain hormones into the blood. These are adrenaline and noradrenaline and they come from the adrenal glands, tiny pieces of tissue situated on both sides of the body, above the kidneys. They each have somewhat different effects, particularly on the heart rate, the dilation and

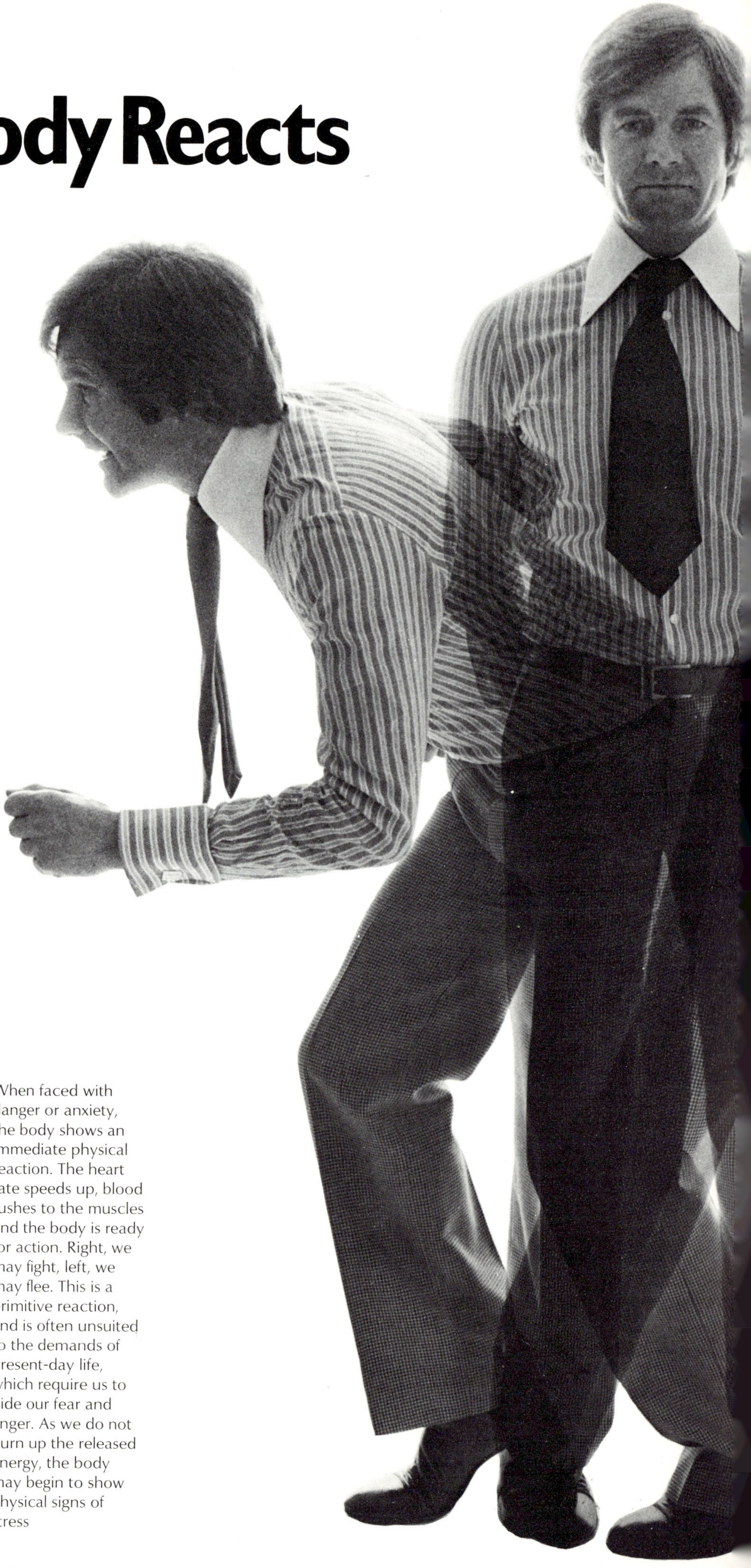

When faced with danger or anxiety, the body shows an immediate physical reaction. The heart rate speeds up, blood rushes to the muscles and the body is ready for action. Right, we may fight, left, we may flee. This is a primitive reaction, and is often unsuited to the demands of present-day life, which require us to hide our fear and anger. As we do not burn up the released energy, the body may begin to show physical signs of stress

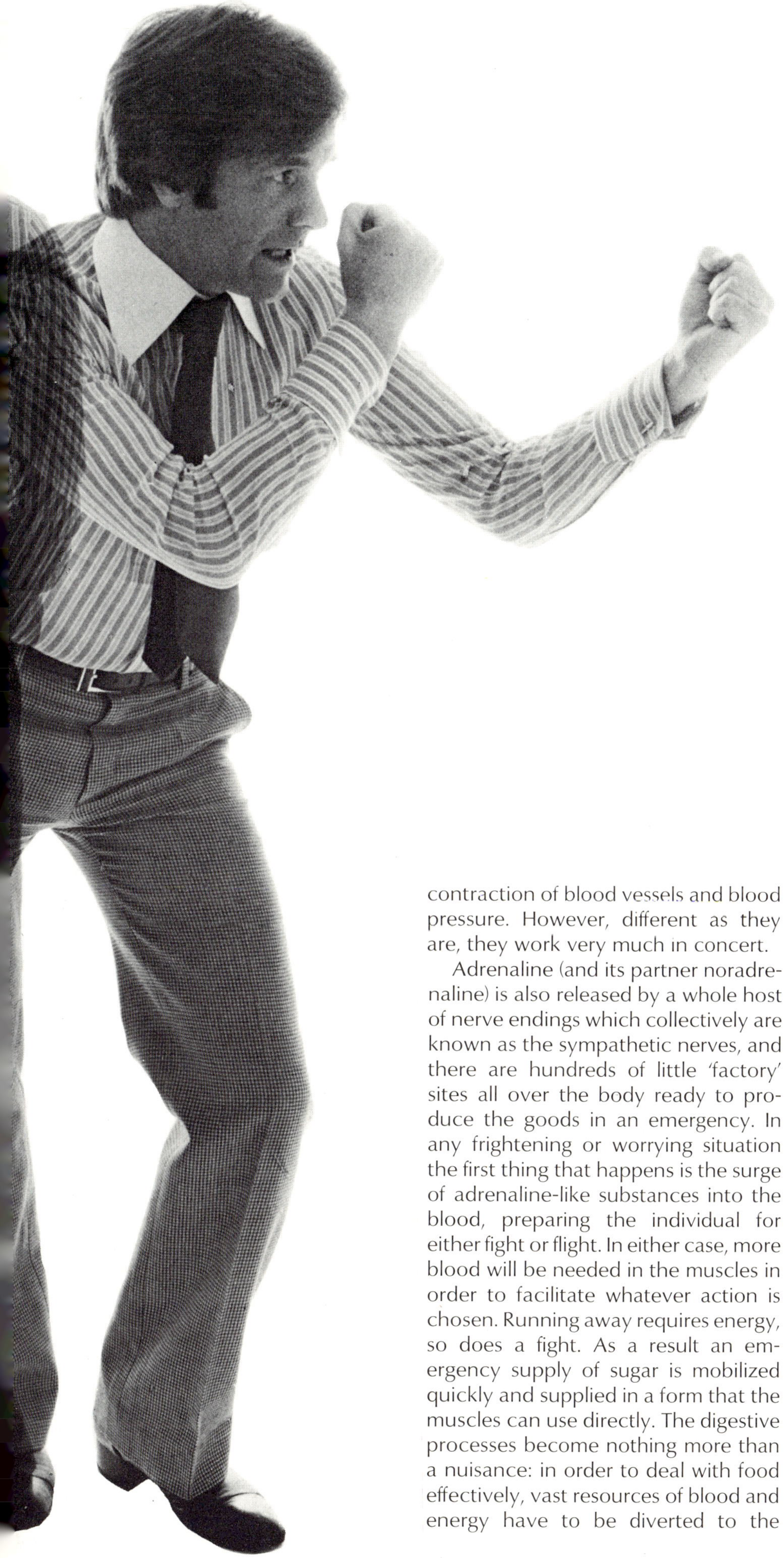

contraction of blood vessels and blood pressure. However, different as they are, they work very much in concert.

Adrenaline (and its partner noradrenaline) is also released by a whole host of nerve endings which collectively are known as the sympathetic nerves, and there are hundreds of little 'factory' sites all over the body ready to produce the goods in an emergency. In any frightening or worrying situation the first thing that happens is the surge of adrenaline-like substances into the blood, preparing the individual for either fight or flight. In either case, more blood will be needed in the muscles in order to facilitate whatever action is chosen. Running away requires energy, so does a fight. As a result an emergency supply of sugar is mobilized quickly and supplied in a form that the muscles can use directly. The digestive processes become nothing more than a nuisance: in order to deal with food effectively, vast resources of blood and energy have to be diverted to the stomach and intestines. This is wasteful at a time like this, so digestion has to slow down and the blood is pushed to the places where it is needed. The output of blood from the heart increases, resulting in a boost in pulse rate and a higher blood pressure.

If the reaction is particularly intense, the person's whole posture will change as he becomes alert, even rigid. His eyeballs move back a little into their sockets to improve the range of vision and his pupils dilate; this may also give him a wide-eyed appearance which may have originally served the purpose of frightening the enemy! The nostrils flare to make sure that the flow of oxygen into the lungs, and so via the blood to the muscles, is not impeded. Drops of sweat appear, the skin will change colour and the hair might stand on end – produced by extreme stimulation of the sympathetic hormones, adrenaline et al acting on the hair follicles in the skin so that again the enemy is intimidated!

Cortisone and hydrocortisone (often known as cortisol) form a different family of hormones, again produced by the adrenal gland, but by a part that is completely separate from the adrenaline production line, and are produced by stress. Cortisol helps the body cope with stress, and it sometimes provides a straightforward method of measuring just how taxing any activity has been. For instance, it has been used in cases of jet lag to analyze the disrupting effect of a certain flight pattern. In states of complete exhaustion, such as after a car crash, one of them might be adminstered in order to boost the body's ability to cope with all the demands that are being made on it. They are very useful and 'friendly' substances in any stressful encounter, whereas the body's production of adrenaline can prove to be a 'foe', as we shall see. However, overproduction of cortisone can have a weakening effect on the body's immunity system – so that the ability to fight off the invading organisms which cause infection is reduced. The exact role of cortisol in stress is not clear; but almost certainly the prolonged stimulation of the adrenal gland, forcing it to supply a constant flow of cortisone, may help to account for the stressed person's vulnerability to minor infections or illness of various kinds.

The Critical Balance

Some problems affect us more deeply than others, disrupt our lives more completely. If we know what these are, it may help us to deal with them. And do emotional stresses cause physical illness? Dr Holmes set up an experiment to answer this question.

Dr Thomas Holmes of Seattle, USA, has studied the factors in a person's general environment that contribute to illness. In order to find out what circumstances cause stress in human beings, Dr Holmes worked out a Life-Change Units Scale with psychologists. This is probably the nearest thing we have to an objective measurement of stress. Although every individual is different, assessing people on this scale does give an indication of what might happen to them. We can only talk in averages, of course, and there are some individuals whose make-up causes them to succumb earlier than others. Generally, if someone has just been through a whole collection of personal experiences which had great impact on him, he is more vulnerable than usual to accident and illness. The only way to categorize these emotional factors is to measure changes in life-style. This method doesn't pick everything up, of course – it cannot work out the rage you feel every day because your next-door neighbour burns rubbish in the garden, or because of the recent change in public morals. In any case, problems like these, though significant, are too personal to you to be meaningful in a questionnaire designed to be relevant for a wide number of people.

To obtain their measure, Holmes and his staff wrote down every conceivable event, happy or unhappy, that occurs during the lifetime of the average adult. Engagement, marriage, children, divorce, death of someone close, getting a good job, promotion, unemployment, dismissal, change in financial status, retirement, holidays, a new home. Changes in the life of children or grandchildren, major purchases such as car or house, were all included, so were quarrels with family or a significant tussle with a neighbour. The research workers allowed the public to make their own assessment of how important these various events were. As a result, people drew on their instinctive feelings regarding the seriousness of all the things that might possible happen to them, combined with their native commonsense.

Holmes worked out his scale based on the replies and he accorded a score to each event. The death of a spouse was seen to be the most traumatic stroke of fate by most people and its rating was set, for convenience, at 100. Marriage is much further down, rating 50 points. Marriage is certainly less of a complete change than death of a spouse, as the changes in the relationship that led to nuptials was presumably a gradual affair. Also, a happy event is universally perceived as less stressful, even if it does involve the same amount of change as bad ones.

Not only Americans were involved in the study; a group of ordinary Japanese people were also asked to scrutinize the same list of life events and evaluate their significance. Both Easterners and Westerners had the same basic attitude to the things that really mattered in life.

When the computer had finished adding up, it was found that those who had a high score on the life-event scale in one particular year were almost certain to be ill in the following year. Their medical records bore this out clearly. If too many significant events are crowded into a short period, such a big adjustment is called for that the person is ill-equipped to keep the normal bodily defences well oiled. Clearly, in terms of its resources, the body will not allow you to burn the candle at both ends, or even at several ends at the same time.

These findings have since been put to very good use. For instance, it is quite likely that a pilot might be kept on the ground for a period if a train of events have occurred in his private life to push him into the high-scoring category. If his life has been full of changes, so that every part of his system is being stretched in an attempt to come to terms with the new set of circumstances, the chances of his falling victim to a heart attack are theoretically increased: a risk that certainly cannot be taken in the air.

Dr Holmes used 3,000 men stationed on three US cruisers in San Diego, USA, in order to check just how true were his generalizations. Would it be possible to predict in advance which men would fall ill on the voyage ahead of them? The men all completed the relevant questions so that a score on the scale was allotted to each one. During the latter half of 1967 a careful check was kept on the health of each crew member. The computer came out with very definite results: those who fell within the top 10 per cent, as far as the life-change score was concerned, suffered twice as much sickness as those who comprised the bottom 10 per cent of the scale. And the higher on the scale – i.e. the most profound the alterations in their domestic circumstances – the more severely they were afflicted by ill-health later.

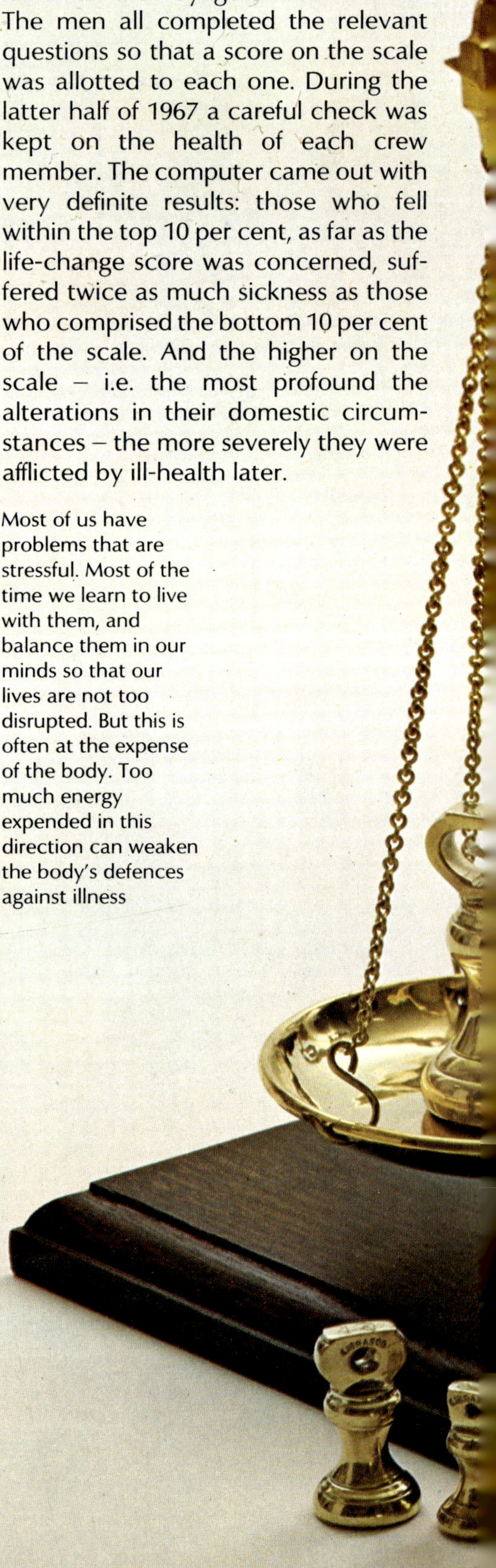

Most of us have problems that are stressful. Most of the time we learn to live with them, and balance them in our minds so that our lives are not too disrupted. But this is often at the expense of the body. Too much energy expended in this direction can weaken the body's defences against illness

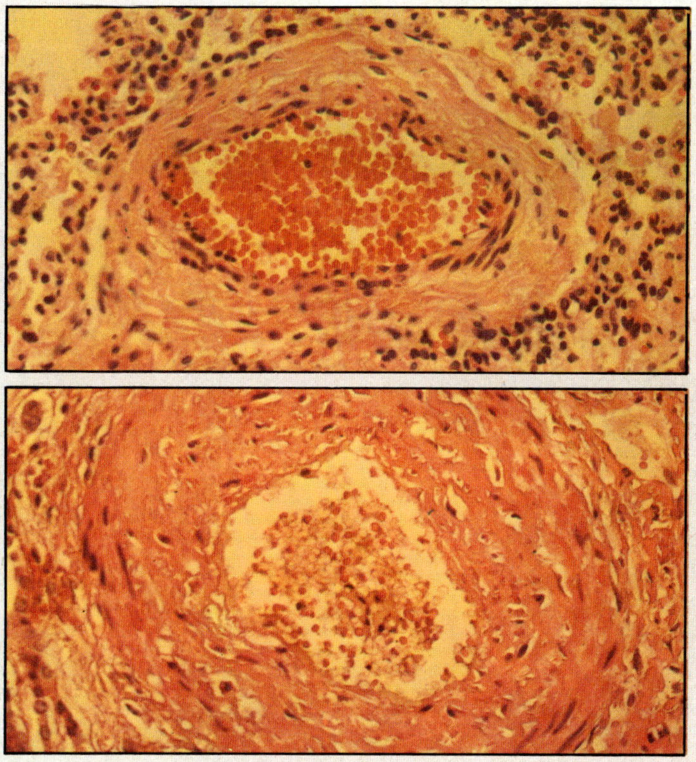

The artery of a baby (top) is wide and clear, allowing maximum passage for the flow of blood. As we grow older, though, the stress reaction releases cholesterol into the bloodstream and if we do not use this up through physical action, it may be deposited on the artery walls. The passage becomes narrower (above) and the heart has to work harder to push the blood along. People who experience a lot of stress in this way are more likely than others to suffer from heart disease

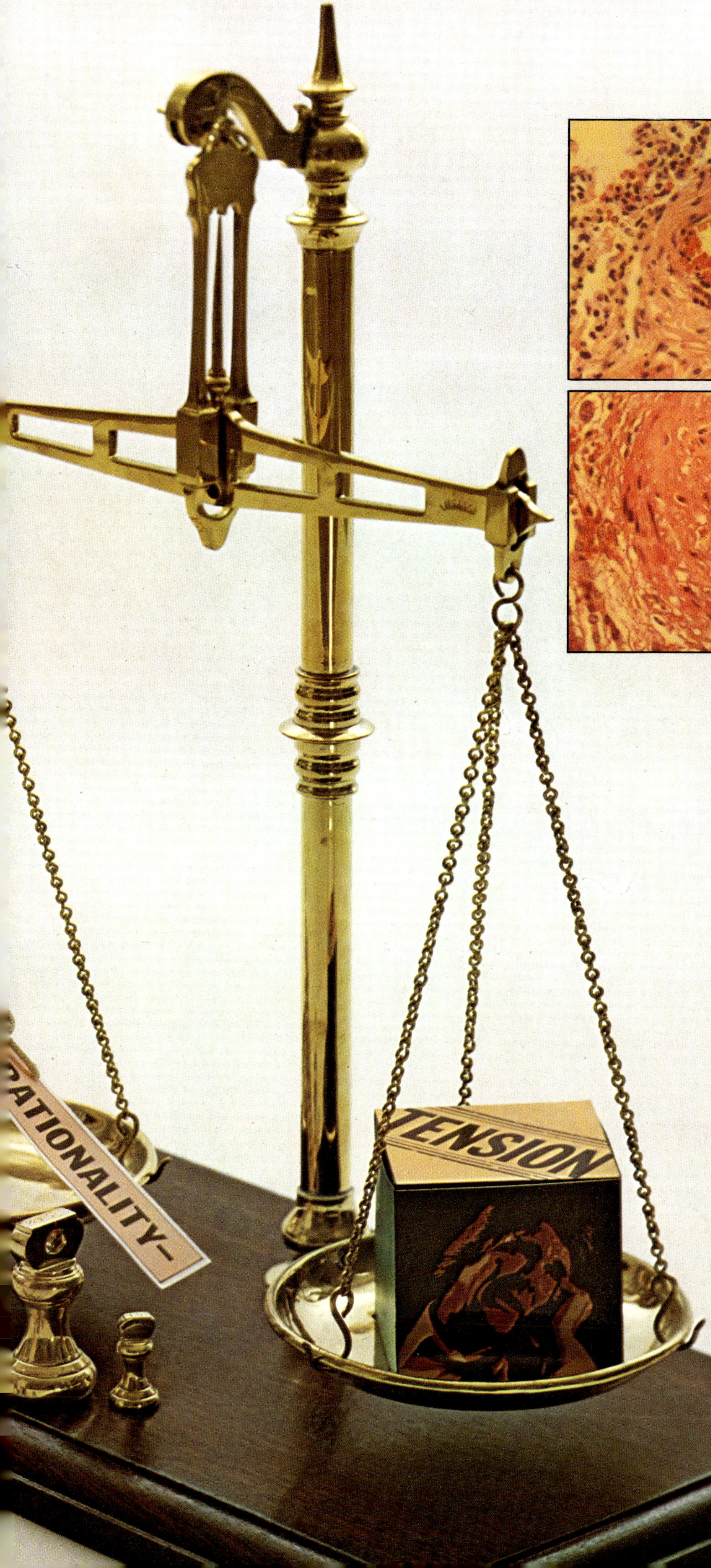

Breakdown

Sometimes life seems to move smoothly ahead. Other times, it seems that we are beset with problems, nothing is going right, and everything is conspiring against us. It is at these times of multiple problems that we try to cope, but if under a heavy load, or if something goes seriously wrong, we break down altogether. Dr Hans Selye has spent many years studying our reactions at these times, and he has given his findings the title of the 'General Adaptation Syndrome'.

The General Adaptation Syndrome is divided into three phases. The first and most dramatic is the one that we have already become familiar with – a general outpouring of hormones in response to some near-catastrophe. Crossing the road, we notice a car within a few yards of us. A swift jump, brought about by courtesy of the body's fight or flight mechanism, and we are out of harm's way. A situation that is soon resolved, except that the intense concentration of the body's resources for those vital instants leaves us feeling physically drained for a while afterwards. The withdrawal of hormones and the temporary exhaustion brings on a bout of trembling and a feeling of vulnerability once the worst is over. This also serves to help us learn something from the situation by assessing what went wrong.

If stress continues, even though it may come and go to some extent, the system is never free of it completely. A stage of long-term resistance is en-

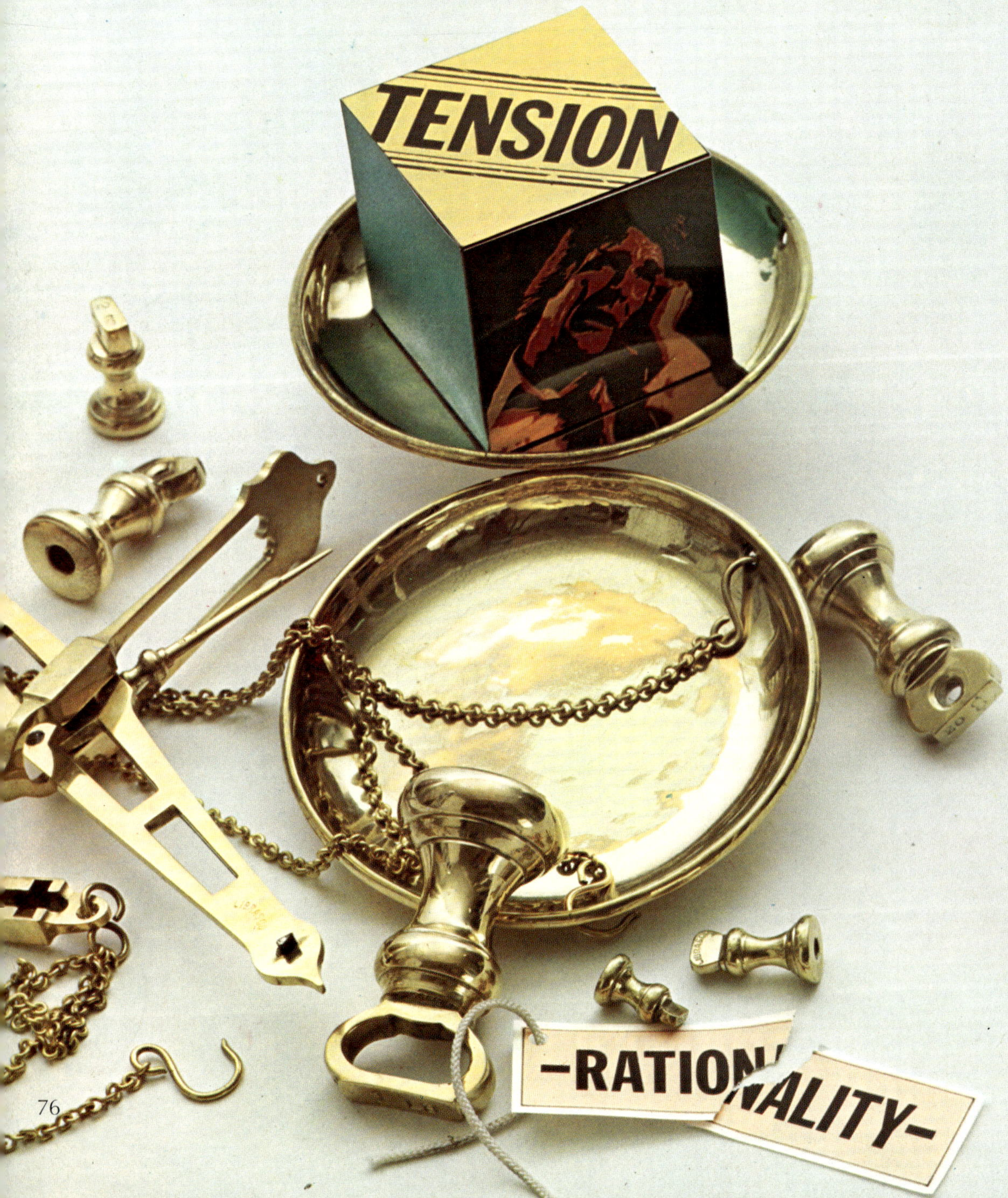

When that one problem too many is piled on top of all the others we carry, the critical balance is disturbed. The tensions become too great and we are then liable to break down. This often shows itself as a physical disease or very occasionally as mental illness

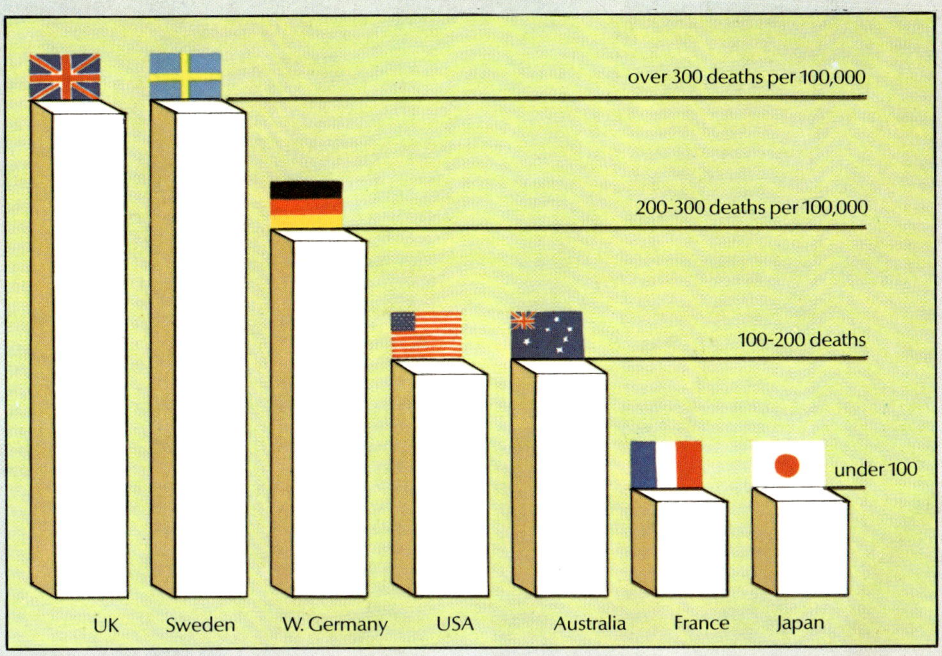

In the western world we have almost conquered infectious diseases. Instead, we are now killing ourselves by the kind of life we lead. Too much stress, especially if combined with drinking and smoking, weakens the heart. Heart disease is a major cause of death in the West. The UK and Sweden, two highly industrialized countries, have over 300 deaths per 100,000 due to heart disease. Germany follows closely behind, then the USA and Australia. The culture of France and Japan promotes a different outlook on life, and under 100 deaths per 100,000 is due to heart disease in these countries

tered. The system adjusts itself to the continual traumas that are encountered and a steady state is reached: equilibrium. Although this state of affairs can last for some considerable time, a state of exhaustion eventually sets in. At some point, something gives. The weakness may come in many different forms – it could be the result of an infection, or an emotional disorder, or it could be the physical strength to struggle declining.

Many of us are living permanently in this stage-two situation: we have jobs that bore us by their monotony which, in turn, causes its own stress. We may have to face an unsatisfactory marriage which bugs us continuously; it is a struggle even to tolerate it but other circumstances – children, perhaps – make any other way of life virtually impossible. Anxiety from whatever source is an especially important factor at this stage-two point, when equilibrium is the rule of the day, for any extra could tip the balance. Lack of security, the need to be loved, feelings of inferiority – all these are anxiety-producing situations. At stage-two, when a low level of stress has become a way of life, worries about the life situation form the major part of the burden. This helps to explain why some people love to involve themselves in dangerous sports; by risking their lives they lift themselves up into a state where the fight-flight reaction is acting as it was meant to operate, where the sensation is strong and clear-cut and in a way exhilarating. All the minor niggles of day to day worries are swept away. Not only during the moments of danger do they fade into insignificance, but even afterwards they are diminished by the magnitude of genuine feeling that has gone before.

Equilibrium cannot last for ever; sooner or later something has to give. The person may take himself in hand and change his way of life, so that he moves back towards a situation where only stage-one stress situations can operate. However, this is fairly unusual. As with any type of disease or abnormal process, the longer it has persisted the more difficult it is to treat. An acute episode has a good chance of being resolved quickly; the body responds with alacrity. Chronic conditions can take years of effort before they resolve themselves, although there is great individual variation. A decision to counter stress, after 30 years surviving in its clutches, will not be as easy as it would be for a very young person. But some people, unfortunately, progress inexorably towards the third stage, breakdown. This occurs when the body can no longer respond adequately to the constant demands upon it. The equilibrium between threat and response functions no more.

A person who is severely stressed, but in equilibrium, may find that his mechanisms would break down completely if he were to be involved in a car crash. The toll of the previous stresses makes it difficult for his body to cope as a result of the trauma, and possible loss of blood, he has to withstand. He will at this stage go into a state of shock. Hormones like cortisone, or occasionally adrenaline-type substances, will probably be administered in order to help revive him.

The third stage can occur in much more subtle ways, though. A whole host of illnesses could develop and the link is not always apparent; these are *psychosomatic*. The development of psoriasis or some other skin disease could occur. Intestinal problems such as indigestion or the development of an ulcer are not uncommon.

Breakdown is a complicated business that is different for everyone. It is possible that the body becomes just too weak to respond to any new addition to the 'brotherhood' of stresses that afflict you. In this case, the body is not able to produce any more adrenaline etc. Or the response may have been so powerful and inappropriate that an excessive concentration of these powerful chemicals and hormones backfires so that they are capable of attacking the body. As a result, the body's inability to cope with what is demanded of it brings total chaos to the system; the telephone lines get 'crossed' and a semi-blackout occurs. Resistance to disease is not at its best so the victim falls sick. Or the mind attempts to protect itself from overwhelming fear and anxiety and withdraws from the real world: the person becomes mentally ill.

Environmental Pressure

As well as the much-discussed psychological stresses that affect us, our surroundings can be equally stressful, and these conditions have been too long ignored. Continual physical hardship can gradually build up a lot of tension and lower the body's defences. Because it builds up slowly, the effects often go unnoticed until something seriously goes wrong.

Many jobs are carried out in conditions giving great physical stress; too much heat, cold, noise or humidity, and different people react differently to each of these situations. For example the speed and efficiency with which you sweat determines how well you would be able to adjust to the gruelling heat of a blast furnace. There is large variation, yet no checks are made on the men who push themselves to their limits in there. Most likely some of them are completely unsuited to the life. They may not become dizzy, but they may suffer from minor degrees of heat stroke, which reduces their effectiveness and their ability to work safely. In the executive world a lot of emphasis is laid on choosing the right man to do a job at the right level, so reducing stress. Far too little attention has been paid to the stress that the man on the shop floor experiences.

Of course, in the presence of excessive noise, virtually all the men suffer from the effects, although there is always a small variation. Persuading the men to wear ear-muffs is no answer, for the men are likely to see these as rather sissy; even if that can be circumvented they are a hindrance to a relaxed atmosphere. They cut out all normal communication. In everyone, the annoyance of continual sound causes irritability which, combined with other domestic worries, pushes people up the stress scale.

Humidity also affects both factory and office workers. A high humidity may be very uncomfortable and by making someone feel ill at ease with himself he may be less attentive, although from the point of view of health, high humidity is probably preferable to an atmosphere that is dry. Too little moisture in the air dries out the linings of the nose and throat; these are only effective if they are covered in a thin layer of damp, which helps to trap invading bacteria. Heating in houses and offices tends to produce an over-dry atmosphere. This can easily be tested by those who are interested (the relative humidity should not fall below 45) by a device rather like a thermometer. A humidifier which

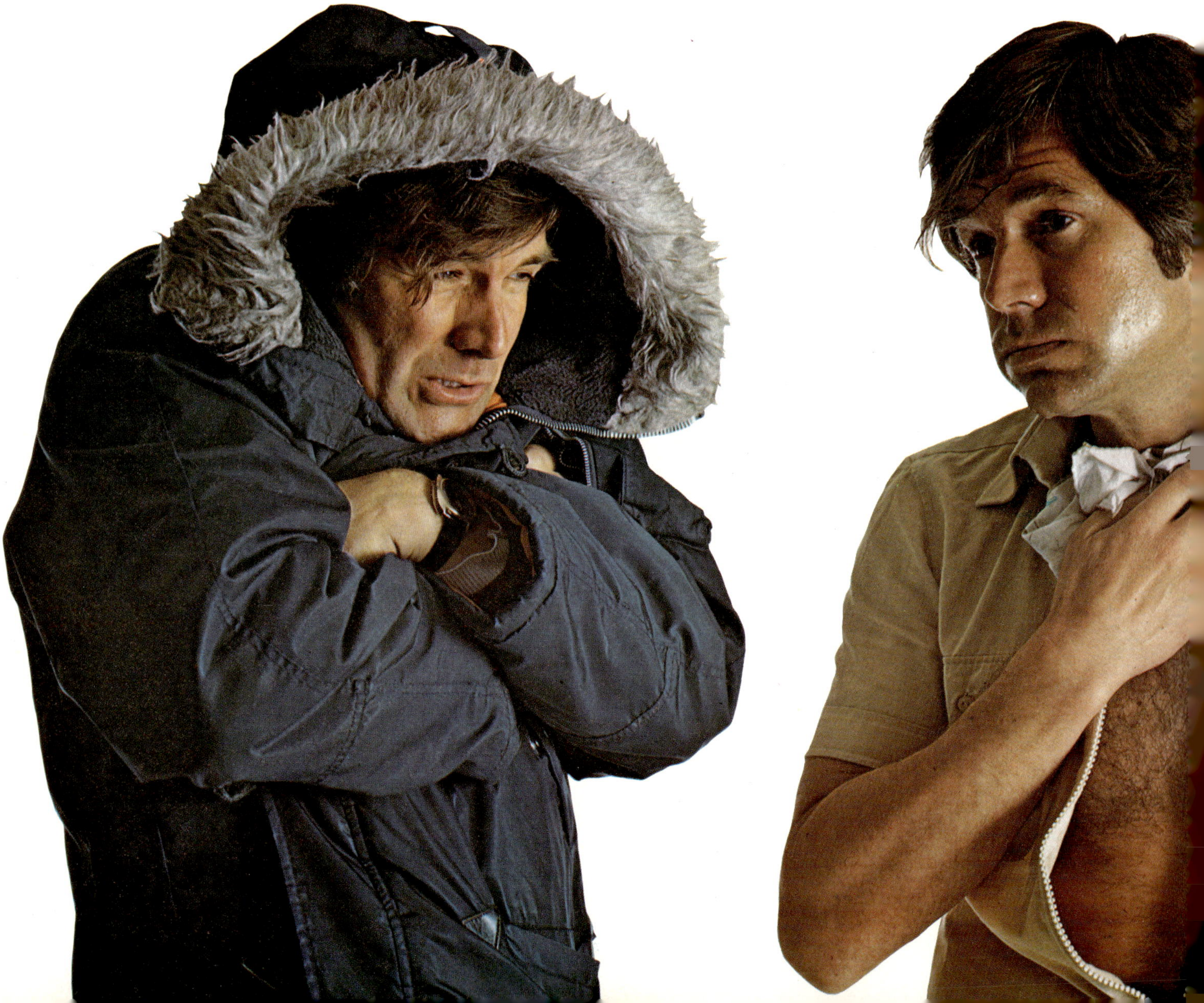

sprinkles droplets of water into the atmosphere can correct this defect which can cause coughs and colds.

The emotional environment is important too. The relationship between men to bosses, how those working next to each other on a production line get along. In factories men handle dangerous machines, with hundreds of lives and millions of pounds at stake. Yet management seems more concerned to iron out the stresses that push an executive towards a heart attack – a sad event, but an event which causes a limited number of ripples – whereas among working men a tragedy such as a heart attack could cost much more in human and financial terms.

Drugs form a large category of stressful agents. Tranquillizers and sedatives fall into this group and many people, quite rightly, are hesitant about their use, but there are times when their use actually diminishes the number of injurious agents in the body by stemming the flood of potentially harmful adrenaline, and similar substances, that the body is producing itself. All drugs, even though they are prescribed by the doctor for very good reasons, including the relatively innocuous antibiotics, put a strain on the system. However, a doctor weighs up the pluses and minuses before he puts pen to paper. But a warning should be provided about drugs like alcohol, smoking, marijuana, opium and others commonly known as addictive substances. They can undoubtedly cause great relaxation and have, over the centuries, been a great boon to mankind in its struggle to find a life-style that is tolerable. Alcohol has been of great help to millions in their attempts to evade some of the harrowing aspects of stress; but it can also be abused. The number of people in the West with an alcohol problem is growing steadily; they become emotionally if not physically dependent on the drug. It is easy to transform this cure for stress into an added burden.

Environmental as well as emotional factors can cause unwelcome stress. Cold, heat and excessive noise are just three conditions some people have to suffer at work. These place a strain on the body that builds up gradually, and may not be noticed till too late, when accidents have already happened. People should ensure that their working conditions are not stressful to the body

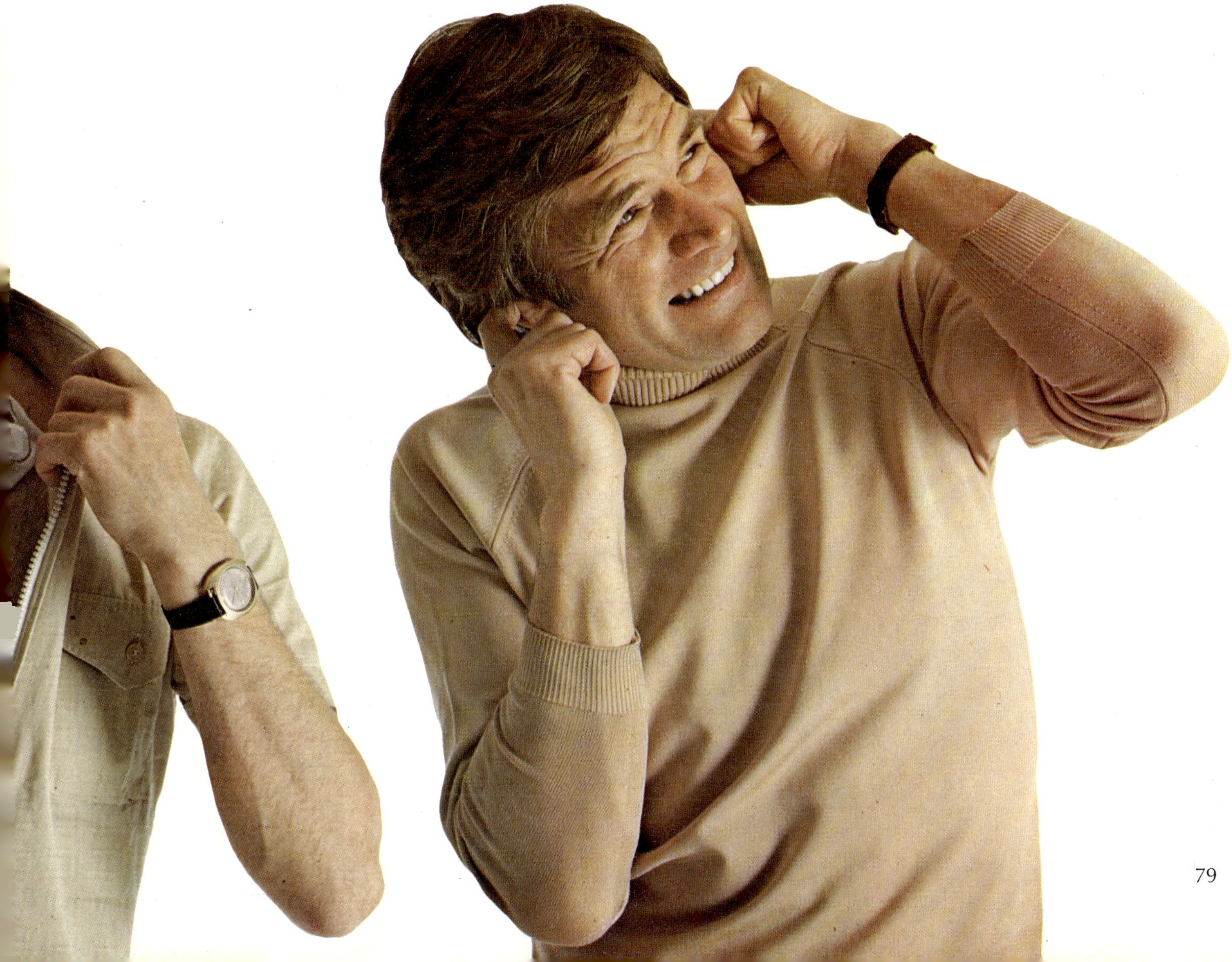

Executive Stress

The struggle for power in the boardroom, the difficulty of constantly making decisions, the responsibility of looking after other people's livelihoods, have long been suspected of causing a great deal of stress and stress illness. But is the executive more likely to succumb to these stresses, when in all probability he has the kind of personality that suits him for the job anyway? These stresses only begin to be felt when the man is no longer, or never was, competent – and they can be equally felt in many other jobs and walks of life too.

If a man knows he is competent at the job, then he is free from anxiety about it; he must of course recognize that mistakes can be made but that basically they are no more likely to occur to him than to anyone else on a similar level. He can have confidence in his abilities. If, on the other hand, he is promoted beyond his competency level, then he will become fearful; deep inside him he knows he's not quite up to it; he becomes sweaty, anxious, and the chance of mistakes in his work plus a breakdown of some kind are materially increased. The competent man or woman learns that there is no point in worrying about matters over which they have no effective control, but men who are promoted to the point where they cannot be effective often subsconsciously make themselves ill in order to remove themselves from a painful situation. Rarely do they have the insight to see their personal problem for what it is: they cannot admit to themselves that they are not as clever and competent as they and others would like them to be. Illness becomes a face-saver.

Being asked to make decisions that are beyond one's competency level occurs in every walk of life. For instance, consider the case of the man working in the greengrocer's shop who has suddenly been promoted. His new job involves grading oranges into small, medium and large sizes so that they can be priced accordingly. He found this constant weight of decision making very trying; after his breakdown the one word he kept repeating to his analyst was 'decisions, decisions, decisions'. He had been promoted beyond his natural level. The key comes, then, in finding the right level and sticking there. It involves having insight into one's own abilities and being realistic about them.

A great deal of the stress of the man who knows he is not quite up to his job is the fear of demotion or dismissal. The

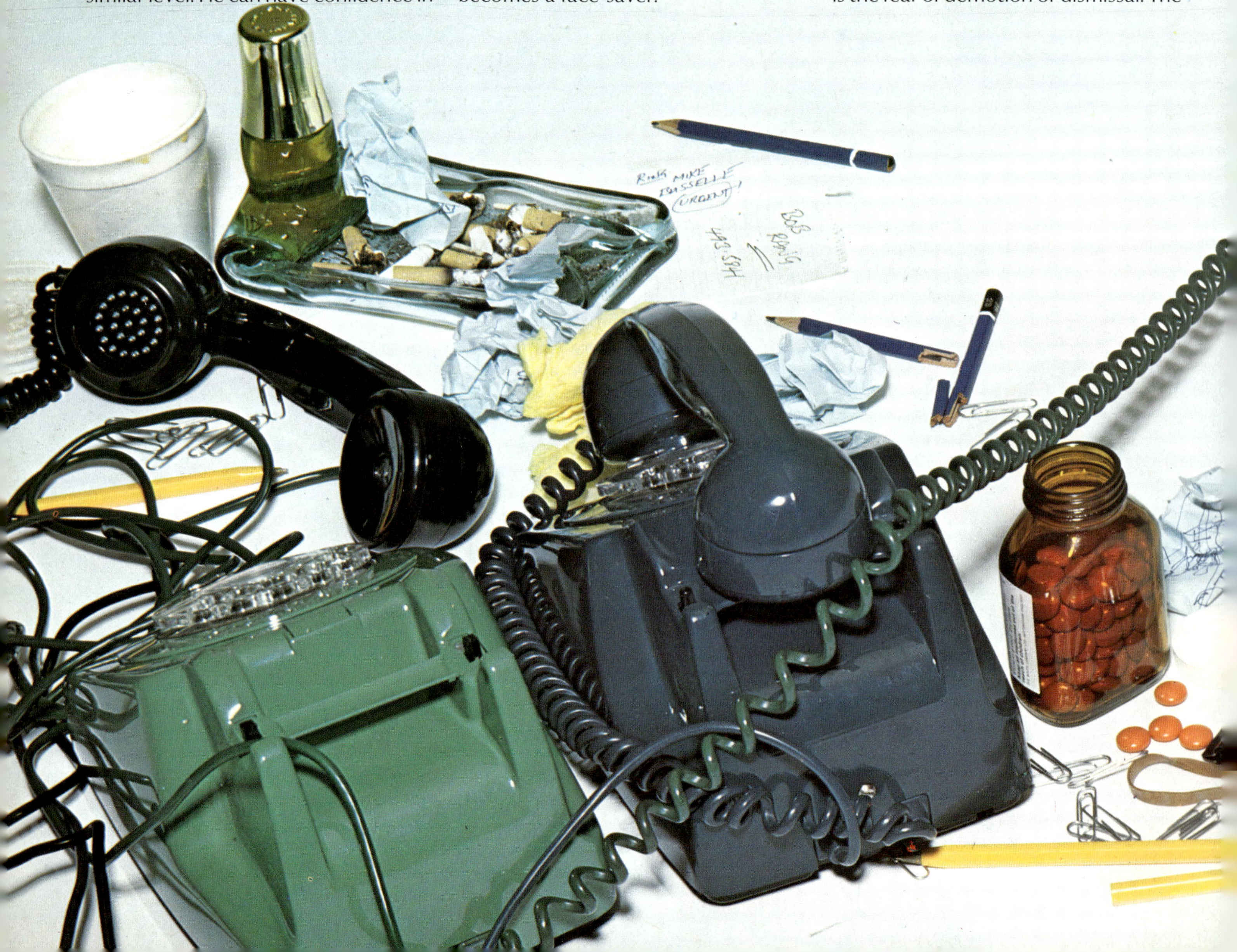

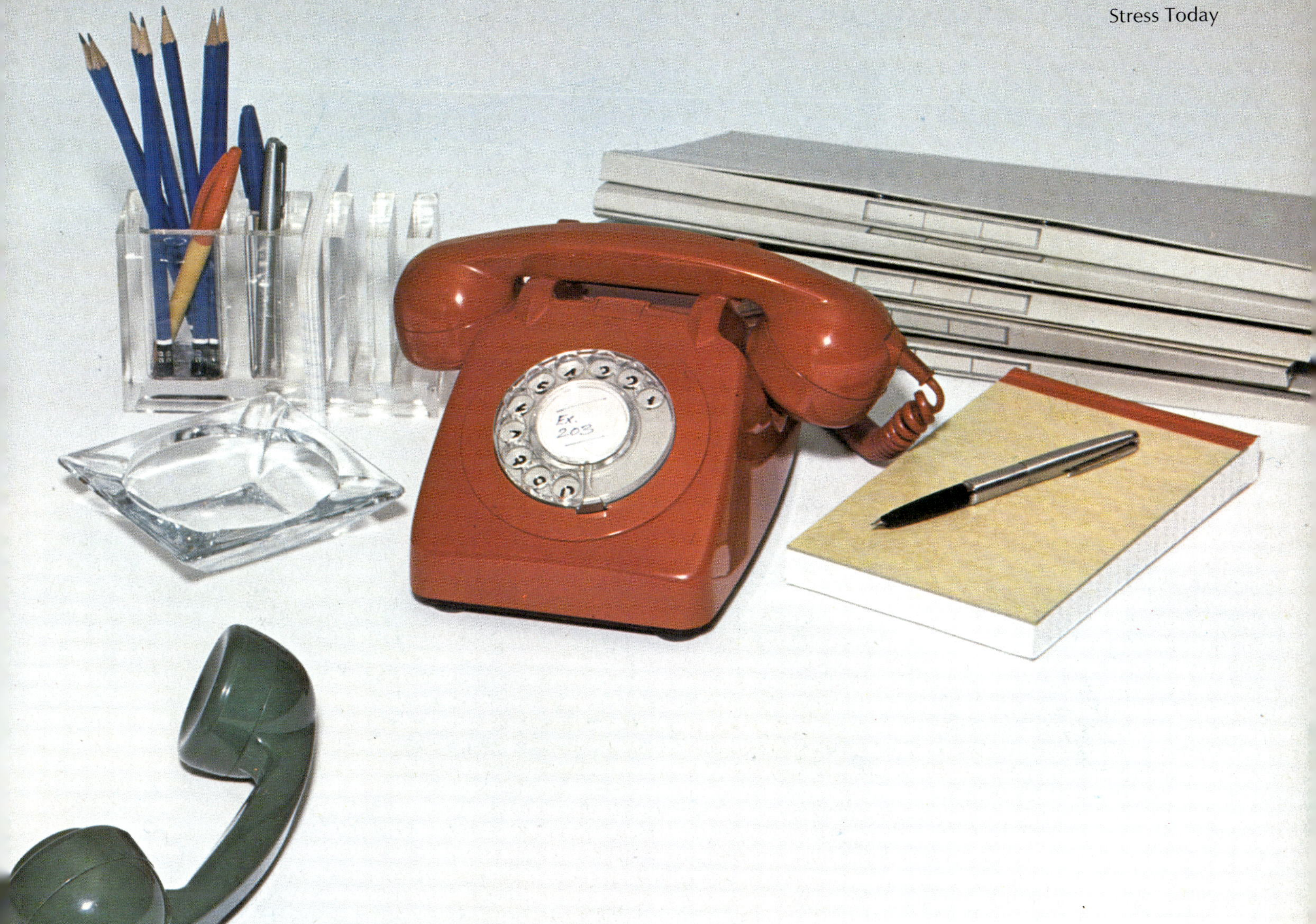

Ringing phones, the pressure to create and produce, the constant demand for decisions, are the hallmarks of executive stress. Of course any kind of job can apply this pressure. The person in the wrong job, or who has many other problems too, can succumb as his or her stress increases to an intolerable level. Pills, drink and cigarettes are often resorted to in excess, which only increase the physical discomfort. Removal of the problems alone can bring relief

disgrace and the financial difficulties either would impose make such prospects seem like veritable disasters. If the terrifying connotations of being down-graded could be whisked away, we might have more chance of helping everyone to find their proper level.

Those with weak or retiring (submissive) personalities sometimes find themselves at the top for various complicated reasons; and powerhouse characters are sometimes frustrated by being artificially kept back. These people suffer stress brought on by frustration, brought on by not being asked to do enough rather than too much, as in executive stress.

An experiment performed by the Bell telephone company in the USA in 1968 shows that stress doesn't just happen in the boardroom. All their outfits provide similar jobs so they were able to compare a tremendous total of employees from all over the country. The medical history, the educational background, job achievement, and other factors were scrutinized in approximately 270,000 men. As coronary thrombosis has been traditionally thought to be linked to executive stress, this was the disease that was of most interest. The men were divided into categories according to their function with the company. It turned out that the top executives were much less likely to suffer from coronaries than the workmen. The latter suffered coronaries at the rate of 4.33 per thousand per year. The men at the top had an equivalent rate of 1.85 per thousand per year. The foremen were worst off, it seemed, at 4.52. Supervisors and local area managers had a level of 3.91. The rate among general area managers dropped to 2.85. And, if anything, the top executives tended to be older, thus emphasizing the extra resistance to the scourge of heart disease they seemed to possess. And it is interesting that if education is taken into account, the highly educated who failed to 'make good' and rose no higher than foremen, seemed to be the worst off overall, whereas if an uneducated boy rose to the top he shared the invulnerability of his fellow executives. These findings must make us rethink some of the old clichés and look into the reasons behind them.

Body Rhythms

As day follows night, and the seasons follow each other, so our bodies have subtle rhythms that fit in with the world around us. We can be influenced by the phases of the moon, for example, and we react differently according to the time of day. Sometimes we have more energy, at certain times we feel hungry. But the kind of life we lead today can often upset these delicate mechanisms, whether it be too many late-night parties, jetting across time zones, or working at night.

But the rhythm which most concerns us is the 24-hour cycle, controlled by the progress of the sun. During the night temperature, pulse rate and blood pressure fall, and nervous activity – particularly the busy sympathetic – also decreases. In a deep sleep, your physical functions approach those of hibernation and if you are suddenly awoken from such sleep, you resemble someone in a state of shock which is a type of stress. The body immediately begins to pump out adrenal hormones.

In normal circumstances, the hydrocortisone in the blood starts to rise slowly just before your natural waking time and reaches a peak sometime during midmorning: at this point you are, from a physiological point of view, most able to do difficult work and withstand stressful situations provided something else hasn't gone wrong, such as a fall of blood sugar through lack of sensible eating habits. A lump of sugar in the mid-morning cup of tea or a biscuit could be enough to correct that discrepancy. The hydrocortisone, or cortisol, then falls off a little and reaches another peak in the early evening. From the point when you start naturally to feel tired until 2 or 3 in the morning there is a steady decline.

All our bodily functions show rhythmic fluctuations. Sleep, wakefulness, eating, digestion, elimination of waste products, sexual desires show a periodocity which depends largely on how the individual has adjusted to the overall 24-hour sun cycle that controls us. The simplest way to check your daily rhythms is to take your temperature at different times during the day. It is always slightly higher in the evening than the morning.

For top efficiency we probably ought to stay within the limits of our own body's adjustment to the day; although minor shifts are presumably very stimulating and therefore beneficial. A person who never deviated from the times of getting up, eating and sleeping through a lifetime is likely to stagnate – the odd healthy jolt to the system helps to keep it supple.

Although we have spent millenia adjusting to the 24-hour cycle the sun has inexorably forced upon us, we still have not made a perfect adjustment. When potholers and other adventurers volunteer to stay underground in self-imposed solitary confinement for long periods of, say, 100 days, they have electric light but no sun to guide them. They soon start to live a very regular day, but a day timed by their own clocks and not artifically imposed by the environment. A steady $24\frac{1}{2}$ hours, give or take 5 minutes or so, is almost invariably the rule in these cases. Blood tests on the 'guinea-pigs' at the end of the experiment show that their hormone levels followed their perception of day and night and not that of the surface. Of course, once back into physical contact with the surface world, their bodies soon made the necessary adjustments and the hormone levels fell in line with those of the people roundabout.

A pharmaceutical company devised an experiment to measure the change caused by crossing time zones. Several English students flew non-stop to San Francisco, where they stayed for ten days; whereupon they flew non-stop back to London. A sample of blood was taken from each volunteer approximately every four hours. It was found that hormone levels didn't settle down to normal for about five days after the outward trip; coming back, however, it took about twice as long.

Tests show that there is a deterioration in performance, impairment of concentration and a loss of the feeling of well-being, when the body stat has not been reset. The only cure for these ills is time and rest. As peaceful a journey as possible helps, plus as much sleep as possible, as soon as possible, at the other end. Take a sleeping draught unless you are God's own sleeper to make sure your confused body doesn't arouse you too soon. Attempts have been made to market a drug which will help speed up the adjustment process, but without success. The only safe way is to assume that at least 24 hours adjustment should be provided for every five hours of time-change. The main trouble is fatigue, which can be so severe as to cause attacks of trembling for days after a trip. Meanwhile, we can certainly say that interfering with your time clock, is stressful to some extent. Done repeatedly, this stress – by adding to all the others which may be weighing you down – could substantially add to the risk of a health catastrophe in your life!

Instinctively, people feel that shift work must be bad for the system. And to make matters worse, workers seem to prefer a few shifts on nights, followed by a few days off, when they immediately have to tune back into the habits of daytime people, instead of choosing two weeks on nights, two weeks on days, which would allow some period of adjustment. The mechanics of the shift-work system vary considerably and in each case the workers tend to get used to their own routine and are reluctant to change. Some studies have been made to see if permanent shift workers, or permanent night workers for that matter, were more prone to absenteeism – either for medical reasons or because of psychological distress, the latter percentage being a good indication of whether people are unhappy at their work. To their astonishment, scientists have found so far that, if anything, shift workers and night workers seemed to be happier than average with their lot. The record of actual, i.e. medical, sickness seemed the same in the various groups but emotional absenteeism was, if anything, reduced. From this the researchers assumed that shift workers are more satisfied because of the extra pay they receive and the easier pace. Also they are a self-selected group. Those who don't like it and find the shift system stressful soon opt out.

Our lives follow the 24-hour cycle of the sun. All our body systems fluctuate during the day and at night, so that we feel hungry or sexy, sleepy or energetic at particular times, each 24 hours. During the night the amount of hormones released into the blood falls, as does our temperature – often by as much as 2°C – and around 2-4 am our energy level is at its lowest. Towards dawn both begin to rise again, and this process continues throughout the day till early evening. We are at our fittest for physical work during the morning, for mental work in the afternoon, and in the evening we wind down, becoming naturally tired. Disrupting these natural rhythms can unsettle our bodies

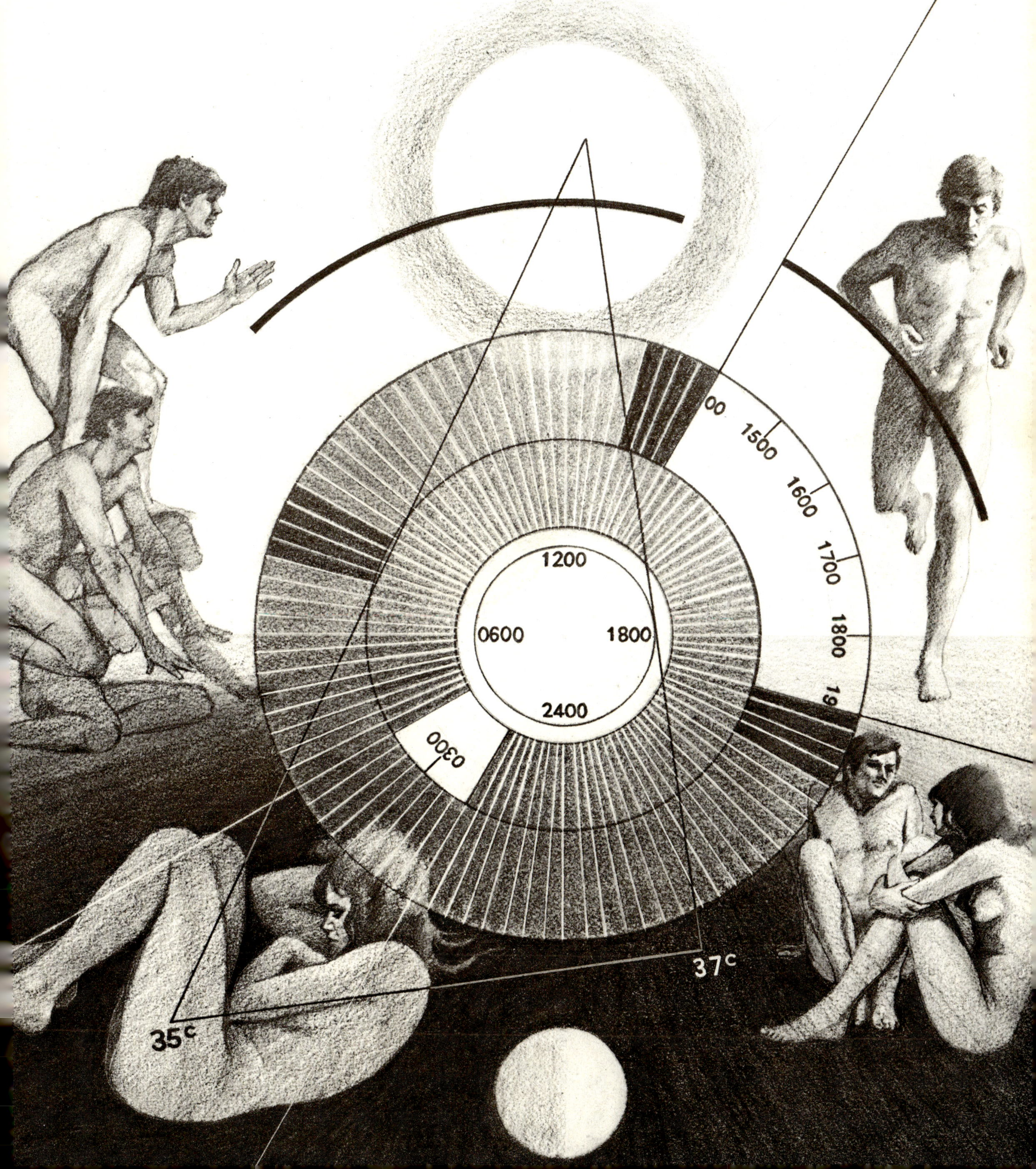

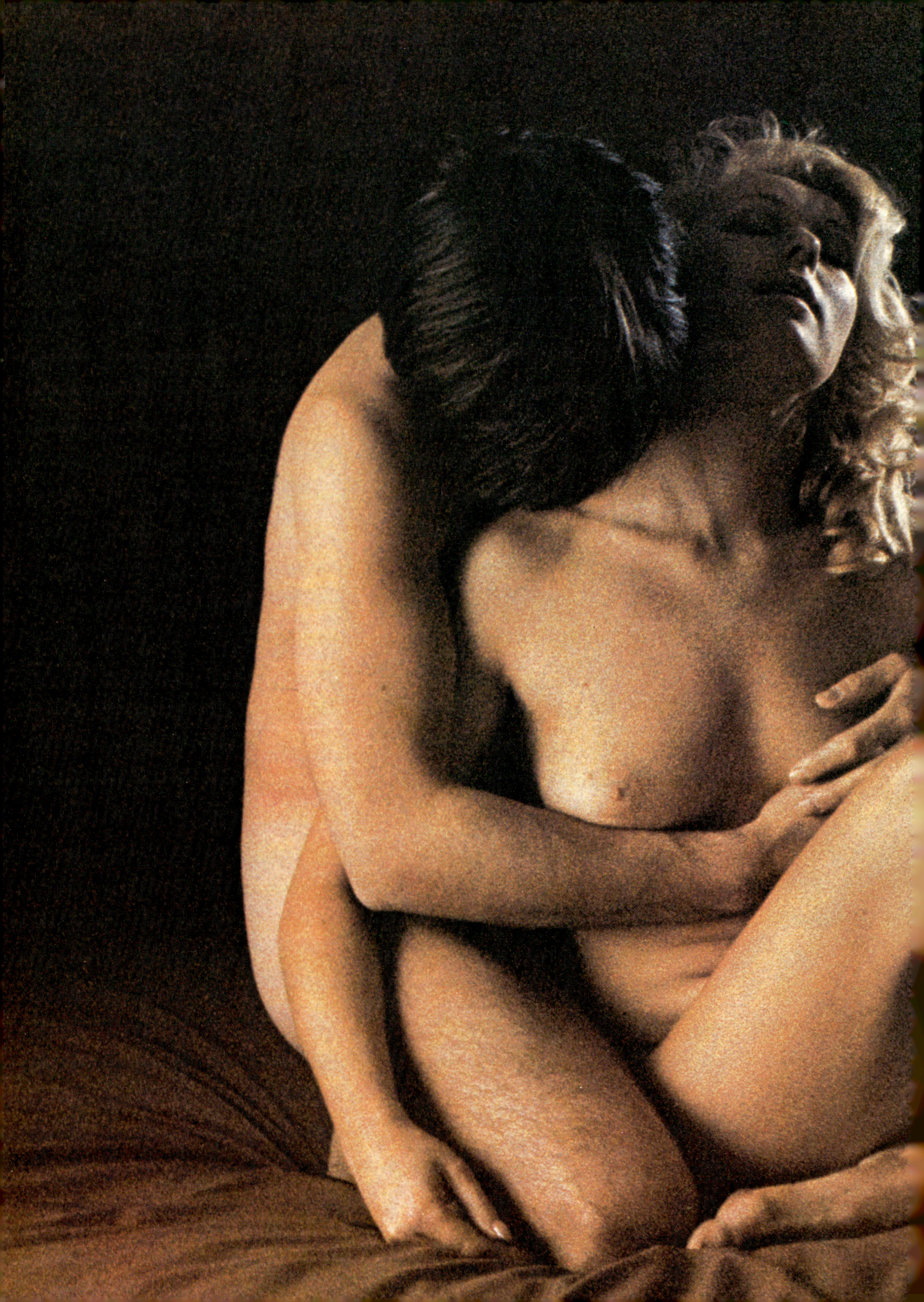

YOUR SEX LIFE

Sex stimulates our imagination far beyond the normal boundaries. It brings out the elements of curiosity and excitement in each one of us and cuts through sexist barriers. Sex expresses our deepest feelings as well as being a biological necessity for our own survival. Each generation imposes its own limits on this exhilarating experience, at present we judge ourselves to be in a permissive age. But the fundamental drives of sexuality, sensuality, lust and capacity are still treated with caution. Our knowledge and understanding has vastly improved and in this section we illustrate the advances that now enable us to increase our sexual fulfilment.

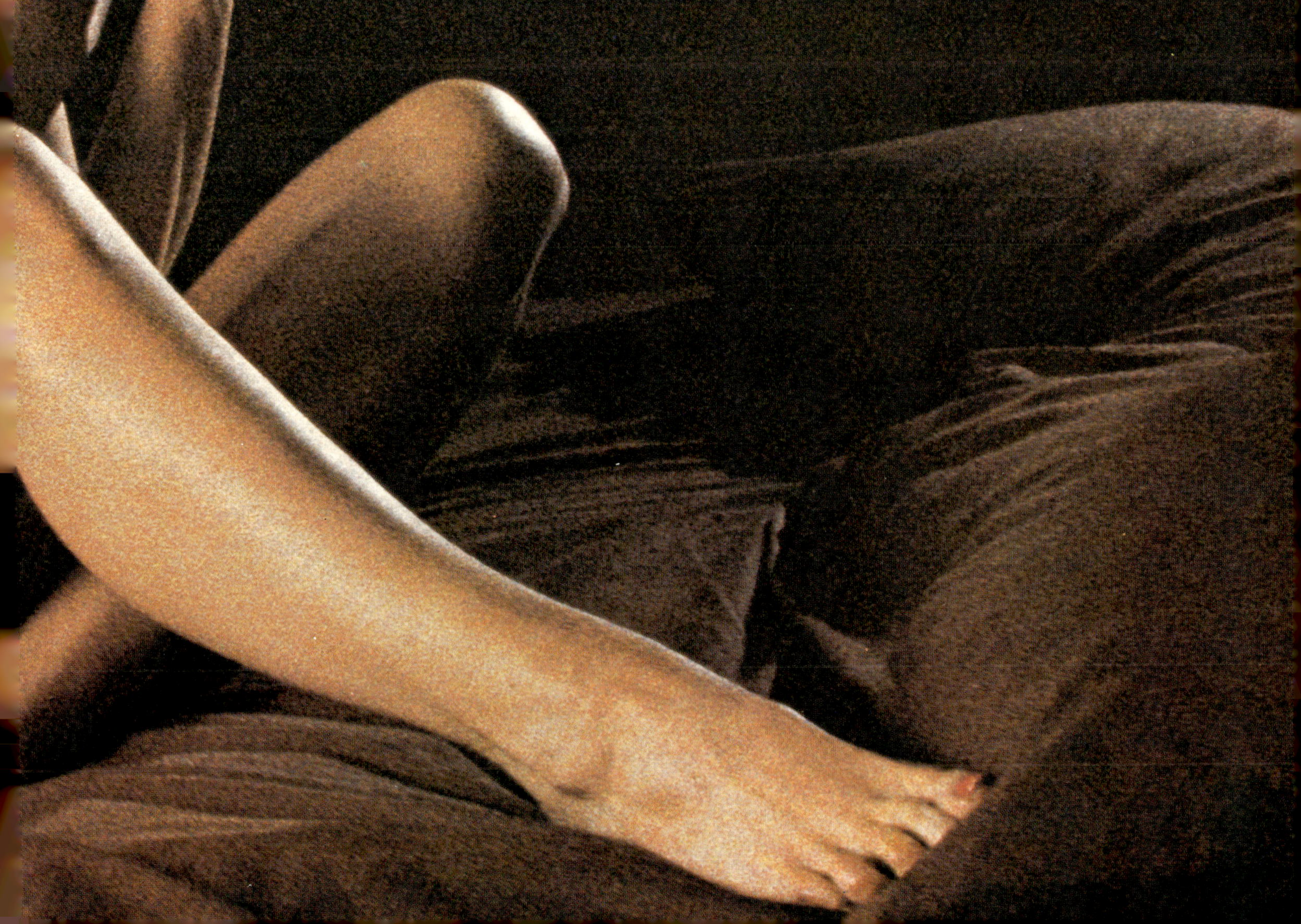

Sex in a Perspective

The survival of the human race as a species depends on the fundamental sexual attraction of the male to the female which drives a man to desire intercourse with a woman. Or, to put it biologically, his penis responds to sexual signals by erection which causes him to insert it in her vagina and ejaculate.

Although this act is vital and often pleasurable, procreation is not the sole reason for its existence as on most occasions no pregnancy results. A woman can only conceive about one tenth of the time, that is, at or around ovulation, even at the most fertile period of her life which is from the early twenties to the mid-thirties. In the ten years or so before and after this period the chances of conception are lowered and, of course, before menstruation and after the menopause, or 'change of life', a woman is sterile, although exceptions do occur.

The idea that sexual intercourse exists solely for the purpose of reproduction was introduced into the western world by the Christians and still holds a wide currency, although usually at an unconscious level in the mind where it has remained since childhood. Its effect can be seen in women who are intolerant of all forms of contraception and for whom a risk of pregnancy has to be present if they are to enjoy intercourse. Such women are usually unaware of the true nature of their difficulty and needless to say, they do not necessarily have to hold Christian beliefs.

Another view, namely that sex is a pleasurable recreation, is opposed by two attitudes which, at first sight, appear to be totally opposed to each other. The first is again that of the Church, which has been preoccupied with sex throughout its history. It says, or has said in the past, that sex is a very special act of which God will take particular note and the congregation is threatened with burning in hell for sexual indulgence. This notion of the sinfulness of sex is deeply ingrained in all of those with Christian upbringings and probably no one is altogether free of it, although it is more unconscious than conscious in many people. Such extremism has called into existence an equally strong reaction in the opposite direction which, in its most extreme form, acknowledges neither reasonable restraint nor sense in its devotion to sexual practice more or less as a way of life. Intercourse can become an activity where elaborate technique is a substitute for simple pleasure. Neither attitude can be a guide to the rational man or woman who wishes to love, to be loved and to make love.

Man, it is supposed, evolved from aquatic origins, in which reproduction is usually achieved by the female laying large numbers of eggs in the water and the male releasing millions of sperms over them. The water acts as the transport medium facilitating fertilization. When animals began to live on dry land a means of internal fertilization became necessary and the penis and vagina system resulted. Live birth from within the mother, care of the young after birth, and breast suckling also evolved. The number of eggs released by the female has been progressively reduced until now, in humans, it is usually only one at a time. The woman has no voluntary control over the event. Men continue to produce millions of sperms per ejaculate but their release is under the man's control – he does not have to discharge any if he does not wish to do so. For men, releasing the ejaculate is associated with the pleasure of orgasm but there is no comparable link between the release of the egg, or ovum, and orgasm in women. Ovulation, or release of the ovum, usually occurs 14 days before the next period is due to start. If semen is deposited in the woman's vagina a day or so before or after an ovum is released from the ovary into the outer end of the adjacent Fallopian tube, then it may encounter an ovum after travelling up

In women the ovaries, which release one egg roughly every 28 days, are sited deep within the body. The egg, if fertilized in the Fallopian tube, embeds itself in the wall of the uterus. If not, it passes out of the body through the cervix and vagina. In men, the testes, which produce millions of spermatozoa each ejaculation, are held outside the body in the scrotal sacs

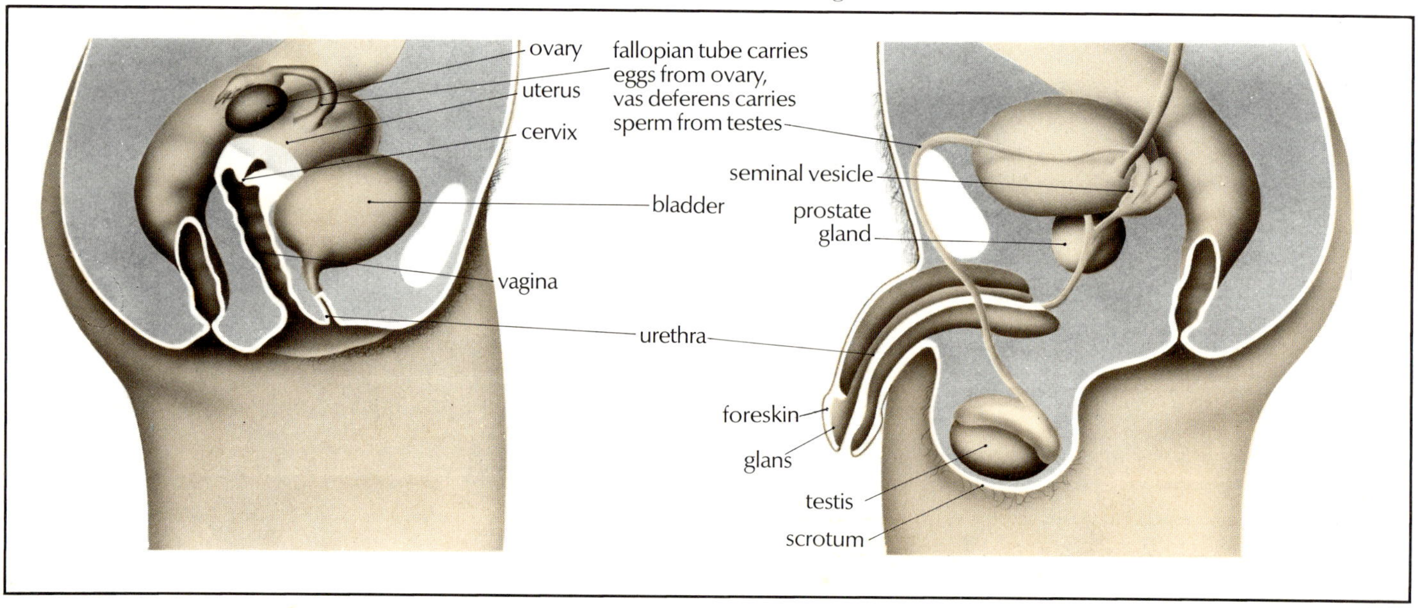

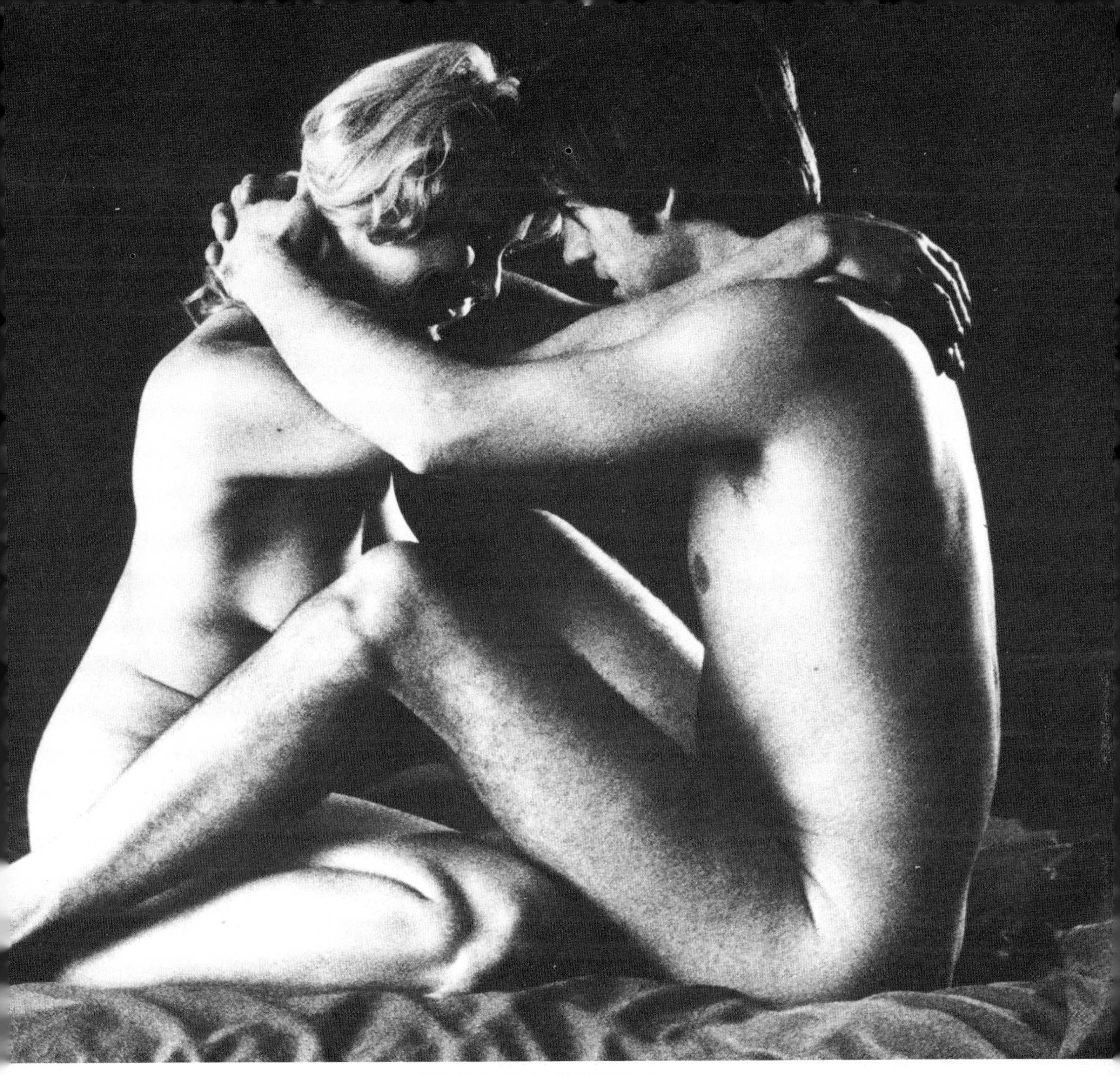

Human beings feel sexual arousal whether or not the woman is ready to conceive. This, coupled with modern contraceptives, means that sex is not purely an adjunct to reproduction. Nor is it purely seeking after pleasure with slick techniques. The bed is not a battleground, but somewhere that love, affection and acceptance can flourish. The shared intimacy of physical contact is an important form of emotional expression. Exploring your own and someone else's body is not only enjoyable but gives confidence

the tube and fertilize it. Then the fertilized ovum or conceptus, after passing along the Fallopian tube for a number of days, implants itself on the wall of the womb or uterus and the pregnancy begins. If the woman does become pregnant she may produce a baby some 280 days after the first day of her last period but, especially in the very early stages, perhaps a half or more conceptuses do not thrive and are aborted without the woman necessarily even realizing she was pregnant. This happens perhaps because the conceptus was defective in some way and, if the pregnancy had continued, an abnormal baby would have resulted. Even so, about one baby in 50 has some imperfection but it is usually of a minor character.

Thus, it could be argued that since we are social animals leading a complicated social life, scarcely to be compared with that of the wild animals, it is reasonable to take a woman's social situation into account and if this is also defective in some way, from the point of view of rearing a baby, it is justifiable to copy nature and induce an abortion if a woman so wishes.

Some people see such an act as selfish and in a sense they are right. Having and rearing a baby may gratify wishes in the parents but it is basically an altruistic function based on love. Although the personal pleasure of sex receives much emphasis, its reproductive aspect is altruistic because another individual, or generation, is the vital beneficiary. It is the pleasure which tempts us to the act and this is vital for the survival of the species just as indulging the pleasures of eating and drinking are essential to the survival of the individual.

Affection and Desire

Sexual intercourse, in the true sense, is impossible without a mutual feeling of affection and desire between two people. Copulation, however, is possible with or between anyone. Physically, almost any man who is capable of an erection is able to insert it in the vagina of almost any woman. Both men and women experience promiscuous thoughts and dreams, although some disguise the fact from themselves, and both sexes are almost equally liable to undertake sexual activity on brief acquaintance. However, many people cannot break down the mental barriers that prevent them from doing so. This is one reason why there is a need for prostitutes.

Nevertheless, there is a fundamental difference between the sexes, in that a man can force intercourse on a woman whether she is asleep, unconscious or even dead, a woman cannot force a man to feel aroused and maintain an erection. It is possible for a woman to have intercourse with any man whether she likes him or not, but the vast majority of men would be unable to have sex with at least some women although any woman is attractive for at least some men. If both partners are to enjoy sexual contact there has to be some attraction between them although some individuals appear to respond less to the actual partner than to a stimulus which that person can supply, such as those who are only capable of full response if the partner beats them before intercourse. Indeed, in some, the associated activity, such as being beaten, is the end in itself and penetration and intercourse is neither welcome nor desired.

For the majority of people, the sexual attraction which has to exist for sex to become really pleasurable, is sometimes called lust. The evidence from fantasy and dreams as well as from behaviour, shows that most individuals can lust after a large number of the opposite sex. Some people make the fulfillment of these desires their main work in life but this is a form of personality defect based on fear of the opposite sex. In most people it emerges as a social drive which promotes social activity and as a general liking for the opposite sex expressed as a tendency to flirt with and fantasize about them. Some men and, probably, more women are likely to exaggerate these feelings into love, especially when they are young, often in order to justify sex.

The capacity to be sexual with the opposite sex and to love a member of that sex develops at different stages in adolescence. At puberty, or shortly after it, the interest in sex increases rapidly, as does masturbation. Although commonly afraid, most members of both sexes begin to experiment with the opposite sex. Progress tends to be slow for most and is carried out over several partners. Thus a girl may first kiss a boy at 13 years and gradually proceed to first intercourse at 18 or 19 years. Boys are more variable. For boys particularly at this stage almost anyone who is willing and available will serve. Their interest is in sex itself more than relationships whereas girls are more interested in the romantic side of sex. Gradually experience should be acquired which does eventually allow partner choices to be made more on grounds of general suitability.

Although we start to learn to love probably from the minute we are born, the capacity to love a member of the

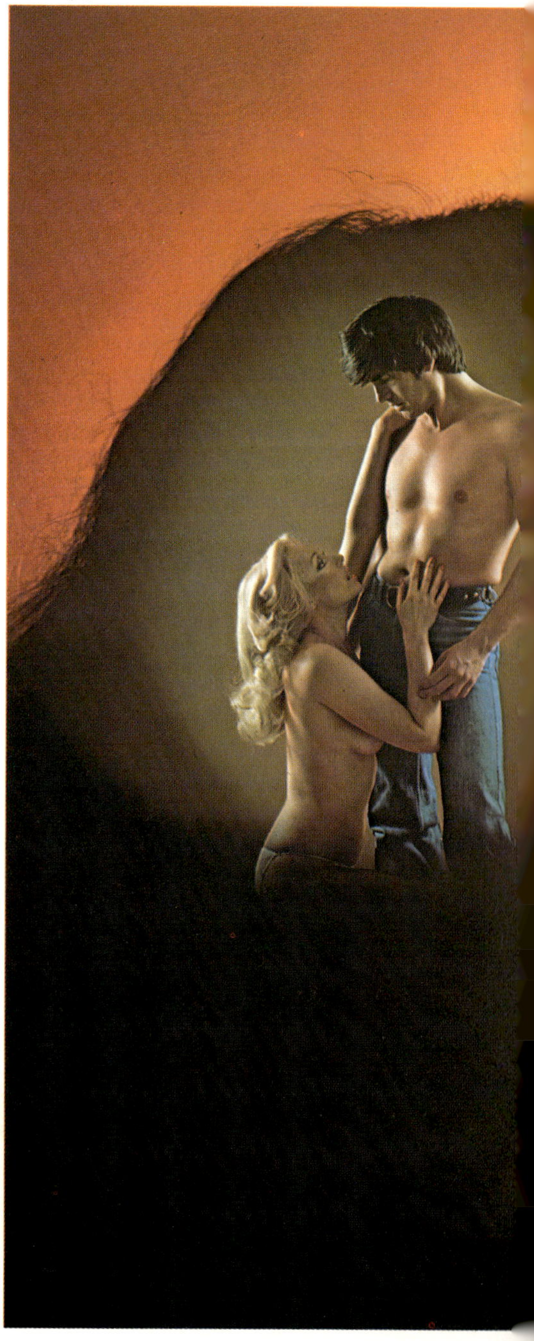

Discussing fantasies can often enrich a couple's sex life. The man (centre) wants a sexually aggressive woman, the woman wants to be submissive. If they don't talk about their different needs, difficulties may occur

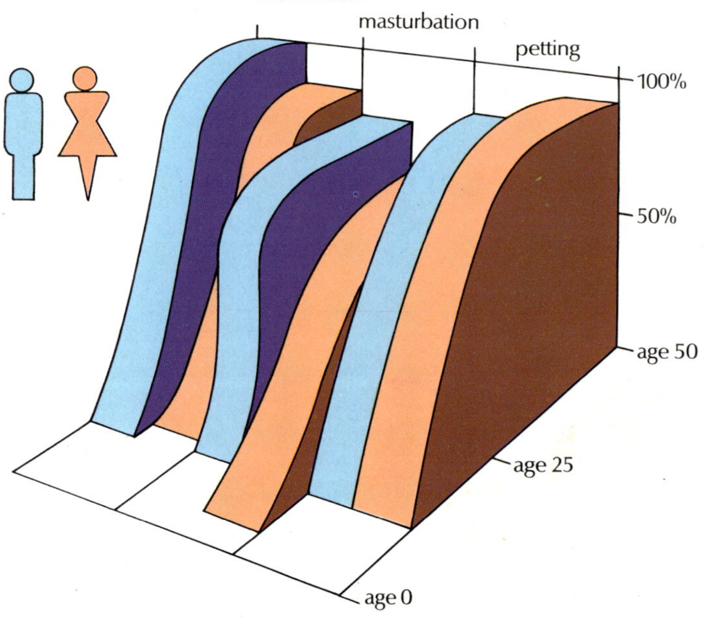

Throughout life the pattern of source of orgasm changes for both sexes. Petting is a more important source for women. Women begin to masturbate later and to a lesser extent than men

opposite sex who is also sexually preferred to the others does not fully emerge until late adolescence or early adulthood. Choices made before then, no matter how much the couple feel they love each other, tend not to endure. Some individuals never develop the capacity to love someone else fully while others cannot simultaneously regard the person who is loved as a sex partner. Such people have either never learned to love or are arrested at some earlier stage of emotional development and unconsciously still love, for example, their opposite sex parent or themselves.

So, both the development of sexual and loving capacities can go wrong but where it does not, the possibility of

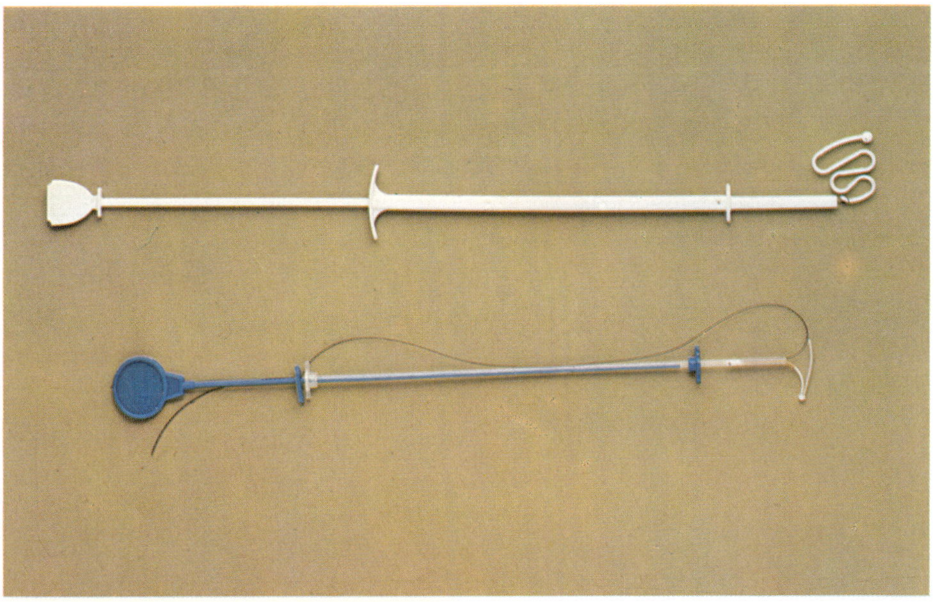

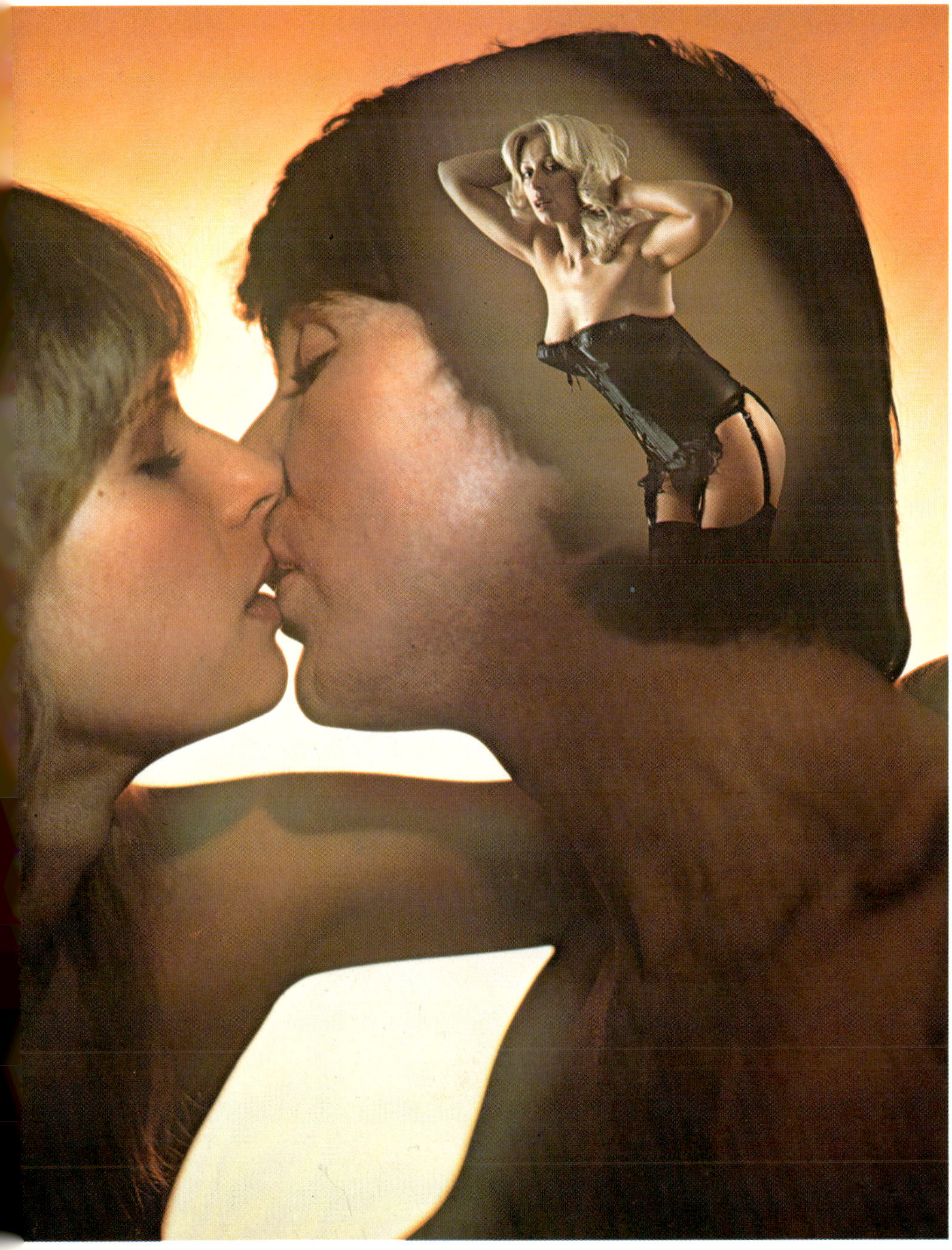

Planning a family is an integral part of any stable relationship today. Above are two intra-uterine devices (IUDs) with applicators, two popular and widely used contraceptives. Together, a man and woman can decide when and how often they would like to have children

combining the expression of both with one member of the opposite sex comes into existence. In this condition, the individual is neither loving simply for the sake of being in love and is not undertaking intercourse simply because it is a relief from sexual tension. The basis of choice mainly centres on personality and on the capacity to understand and communicate with the partner. This is most likely to be harmonious where the personalities and the backgrounds are similar. Thus, the foundation of a satisfying man-woman relationship for most people is friendship. The individuals are then able to give expression to their feelings in loving and in accepting love as well as in physical sex.

Since men and women probably innately possess complementary rather than conflicting qualities, they can cooperate when suitably matched and afford each other mutual support. Although it is possible to dispute the point, it seems that this is the ideal context for a man and a woman to find self-expression, satisfaction, security and a sense of purpose, which for most also involves the production and rearing of children. Within such a framework copulation, which is really the use of the genitals of the opposite sex for masturbatory purposes, gives way to intercourse.

Attitudes and Society

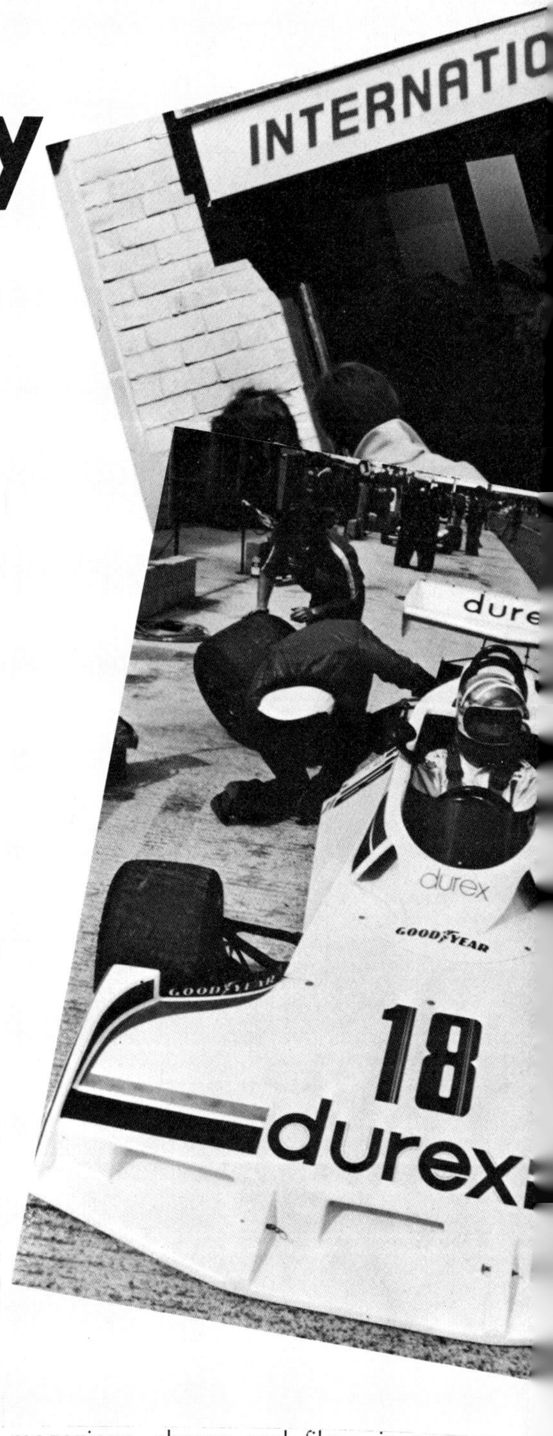

Sex and sexual behaviour is affected by society in at least three ways. The first is the manner in which individual parents consciously and unconsciously teach their children about sex. The second is through legislation and the third is through general public opinion.

The task of the family is to socialize the child to fit into society but, as far as sex is concerned, this is almost always in the direction of excessive suppression of sexuality in our society. Thus the influence exerted by the parents tends to modify and, perhaps, inhibit the spontaneous and rather formless sexuality of the child.

Society legislates to control both the sexual interests and sexual behaviour of its members. When it is considered that a society is enriched by change and by the creation of an environment in which each can fully express himself or herself, it might be thought that in sexual matters as in all else, a free society would have established laws that, in effect, are mainly variations of the rule that you can do as you like provided only that you never harm anyone else or their free interests. Again, children are a particular case and should be protected against both excessive suppression or excessive stimulation of their sexual interests in order that they can develop in a balanced manner suitable to their own personality and free of distortion.

Sadly, almost none of this is the case and the situation current at any particular time reflects the progress in the battle between the suppressors of sexuality and the militant pro-sex extremists who react against them. In the western world, and in much of the rest of it, the second faction are increasingly asserting themselves, assisted, to some extent, by the entirely just and welcome Women's Liberation Movement and, perhaps, efficient contraception and legalized abortion. However, the case for a rational approach to sex is probably gaining ground, although slowly because the largely unconscious anti-sexual attitudes induced in childhood, and reactions against them, change only slowly through the generations. Most parents, who may have acquired some sexual wisdom themselves, still tend to rear their children more in accordance with their own early sexual rearing and its restrictions, than in accordance with their own actual practices.

The third way in which society controls sexual interest and behaviour is by what might be termed the expression of opinion and expectation. Thus marriage is encouraged to a point where it occurs too early for many people in contemporary society which powerfully contributes to later divorce. Extramarital and homosexual relations are condemned so that an individual whether he has any reputation to lose or not can be successfully blackmailed in an attempt to conceal it. Revelations about sexual behaviours of which a particular society disapproves can bring a political career to an end in many parts of the world. In the not too distant past British Cabinet Ministers had photographs of their genitals taken in order to prove they were not the male performer in a series of pornographic pictures which had come to light. Most women keep the fact they have had an abortion secret and many men are afraid to buy openly explicit pornographic magazines in areas where they are known. Prostitutes claim that all sections of society, such as doctors, teachers and clergymen, use their services although their clients rarely proclaim the fact publicly. Most VD and Sex Clinics have to be discreet or they would lack for patrons and it is quite uncommon for say, syphilitics, to tell anyone they have the disease.

The fragility of sexual control by the expression of opinion is shown by the fact that most people are capable of considerable lack of inhibition when away from their home territory and people who know them.

Although it is commonly said that recently society is more 'permissive' and although it is true that, due to the extremists, harder pornography and indulgences of other kinds are available, on any overall view, western society, as experienced by most people, is still very restrictive to a person's capacity to express himself sexually. I would suggest that the rise in substitute sexual gratification, such as magazines, shows and films, is probably an outcome of the frustration this implies. If everyone was enjoying such a marvellous and free sex life, as is suggested by many commentators on the contemporary scene, it would be unnecessary for these types of activity to be widely sought and hard to find.

Different societies establish different sexual attitudes which influence both child rearing and sexual practices. Many of these societies are much more sexually permissive than our own and they are also less technically advanced. It has been argued that the two circumstances are linked and that a society which restricts sexual expression by its members frustrates them to such an extent that sex energy

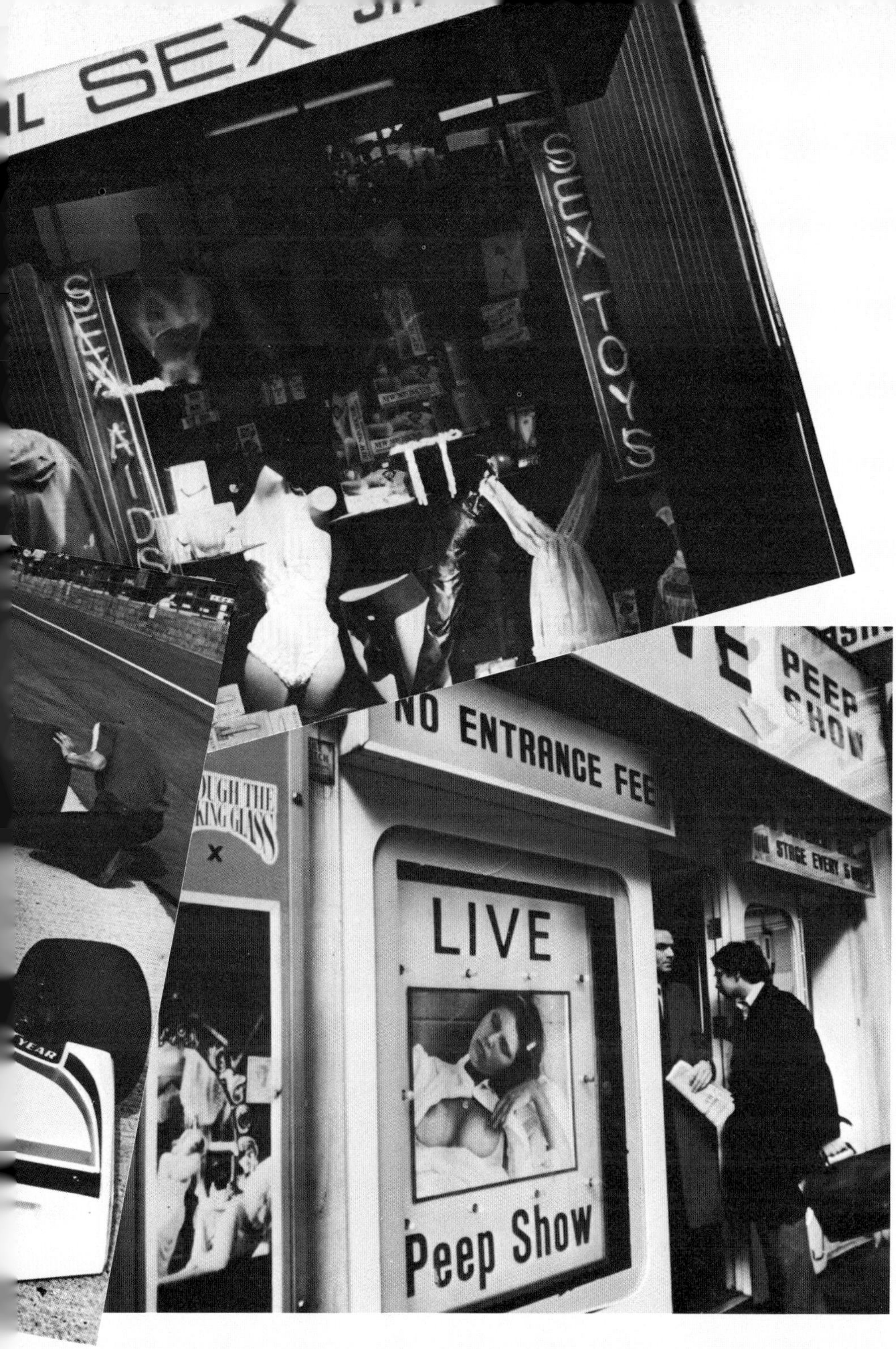

Different societies have different attitudes towards sex. Unfortunately, in the West, a hangover of repression means that much sexual activity is secret and has also become big business for sex shops and strip clubs. The promotion of racing cars by companies producing contraceptives is a healthy sign

is released in other ways which are of benefit to society economically. It has also been argued that if society places restrictions on sexual behaviour then sex becomes more enjoyable as a result of the opposition it has to overcome.

Both arguments are probably false for if they were true they would amount to a neurotic misuse of sex by society. There is no real evidence that enjoyment of a happy sex life weakens a society in any way and neither is there any indication that members of more sexually enlightened societies than, for example, our own enjoy intercourse any less than we do. In fact the evidence appears to suggest the opposite since members of sexually free societies encounter few sexual difficulties whereas ours suffers many.

In an ideal society we would rear our young to take pride in the development of their sexual and other talents, setting as wide limits as possible on what is regarded as acceptable. Children should not be unduly screened from sex and neither should their interests be severely repressed. However, they should be shielded from seductive behaviour and 'abnormal' sexuality. Undue emphasis on sex, whether by way of stimulation or restraint, should be removed and more balanced views about the importance of sex should be instilled. Although much debate is possible on the point, the aim in an ideal world should be to rear children to their adult tasks of loving and making love to a member of the opposite sex in a natural way that is free of embarrassment, shame or inhibition. Adolescent sexual experimentation should be accepted but those who engaged in experimentation should be made aware of all the possible dangers and of its purpose; that it is a way of learning not only about sex but about the opposite sex and relationships with them. Masturbation should be accepted as normal and, perhaps, encouraged to a degree since its suppression, apart from causing psychological problems, can lead to intercourse before maturity as an escape from the 'sin' or 'dirtiness' of masturbation. However, parental involvement in child and adolescent sexuality should probably be best kept to a minimum and parents should avoid sexual provocation.

The anti-sexual elements in society should be prevented from endeavouring to reduce everyone to a sexually infantile level by seeking to restrict sexual material on the grounds that it will harm children. As in the ancient world, the human body and its genitals should be permitted reasonable display and be accepted as unexceptional. Excessive emphasis on the privacy of the body and sex, or the denial of the attractiveness of the body to the opposite sex, especially that of the female to the male, as insisted upon by the radical feminists, is a form of prudery which can produce its own inhibitions later and should be avoided.

Men and women should be a source of joy and pleasure to each other and anything which diminishes this is hostile to the man-woman relationship. Since a stable society of the type preferred by most individuals can only be based on the man-woman relationship, society's opposition to sex runs the risk of undermining itself. It may be that societies which preach sexual repression also diminish the capacities of individuals to love and to make love and thereby make them more prone to aggression.

Sexual Capacity

Sexual capacity is one of the most discussed aspects of sex as everyone has their own ideas about what their personal capacity should or should not be and it rarely agrees with what experts report. The rates of intercourse from one individual to another can vary enormously from twice a day to once a month to once a year. It also fluctuates with age, rising to its peak in men during adolescence and declining thereafter towards old age, while for women it achieves its full potential only in the middle years.

Although there is no direct way to measure it, it seems likely that, to a certain extent, most people possess roughly similar sexual drives with perhaps the average woman's being stronger than that of the average man. This is not to say, however, that everyone undertakes the same amount of sexual activity. Inhibition, personality, experience and relationship to partner can affect the translation of basic capacity into actual acitivity.

Although newborn children may show signs of sexual arousal and children of a few months of age have been observed to masturbate to orgasm, the mouth is their principal source of body pleasure. At a later stage in childhood, around three or four years or even earlier, the genitals become a more important pleasure centre and it is usually at this stage that the child is very strongly attached to the opposite sex parent. This does not mean that the child wants intercourse but simply that it recognises its own sex and responds to sex difference. Later still, the child is thought to become anxious about the attachment and surrenders, for a while, both its interest in the genitals and its special attachment. Thereafter it tends to become more interested in the same sex parent and his or her interests.

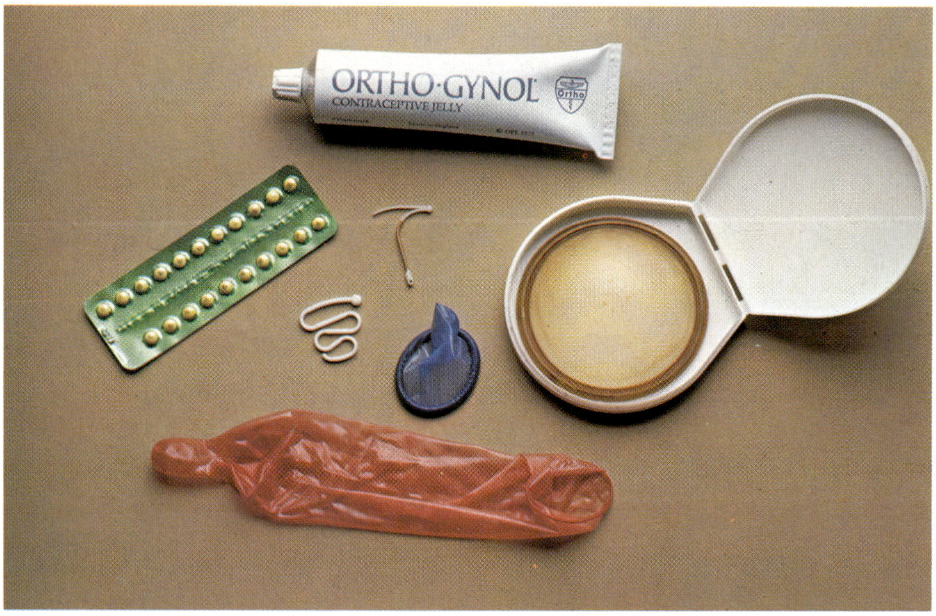

The sheath can inhibit sexual capacity, as it reduces sensation in the penis, and inserting the cap may destroy spontaneity

The pill and IUD are safe, unobtrusive contraceptive methods

If the child does not negotiate these stages successfully he or she may subsequently have an inhibited capacity to respond properly and fully during heterosexual activity, even to the extent that sexual activity is prevented. Fearful attitudes towards the genitals of the opposite sex or disgust at one's own can sometimes also be the result of mishaps during the child's sexual development.

Inhibitions of sexual capacity also come about through one's parents' attitude to sex. The small child readily learns the rules and regulations of the society and family into which it is born and thereafter it conforms most of the time to these rules, many of which are implanted so early in life that the child has no recollection of learning them. These are the hardest to overcome subsequently. Although most parents claim to possess reasonable and sensible attitudes towards sexual interests displayed by their child, the actual evidence is much to the contrary. Some families never mention or appear to see anything sexual and this is a form of denial of sex. Adults who have been

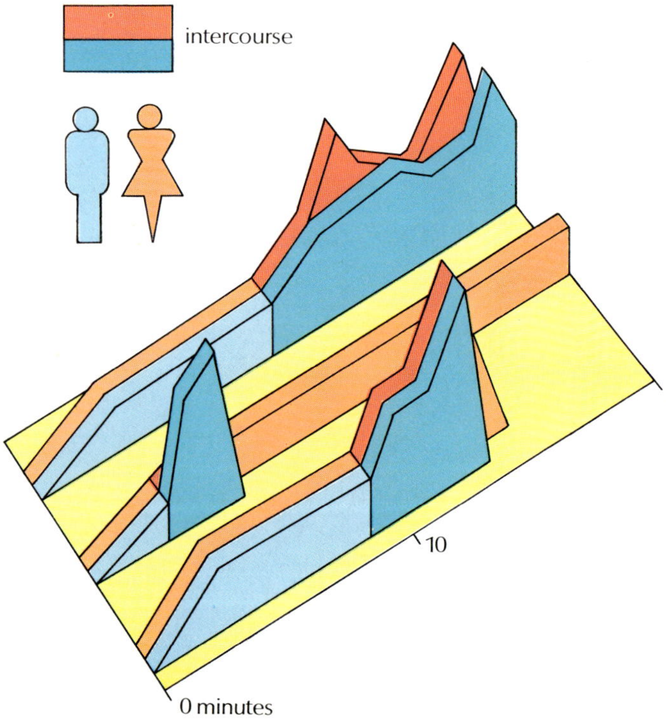

Men and women differ from each other in the pace with which they reach orgasm. Men can climax very quickly, whereas women usually take longer. The man and woman move together through the first stages of arousal. The woman starts to climax first and the man follows (top). Sometimes (centre) the man climaxes very quickly when the woman is nowhere near orgasm. The man and woman (below) move together towards simultaneous orgasm, a fairly rare occurrence

reared in this way will deny sex with statements such as 'Sex isn't everything', or 'I can't see what is so special about sex' or 'Sex is a beautiful mystery that should not be talked about'. Some may unconsciously behave in ways that deny the existence of sex and sex pleasure, causing impotence or vaginismus, that is, painful intercourse from spasm of the muscles surrounding the entrance to the vagina.

Other families seek to suppress sexual interests on the grounds that they are 'dirty' in the same way that any interest in the body's excretions is seen as dirty. For many in our society, dirty is synonymous with sexual and children who have been given this attitude grow up with notions that to be sexual is something akin to having leprosy – everyone will avoid you. When knowledge of the venereal diseases is acquired later in life fear of VD may become a way of expressing this fear providing a restraint on sexual activity or a depressing and self-punitive belief that he or she has caught VD after some sexual adventure. Another inhibiting belief is to equate semen and vaginal fluids with excretion which makes oral sex impossible for them to undertake due to this unconscious association. Some men regard the vulva as horrifyingly repulsive to look at, touch or smell because of its association with excretion and dirtiness in their minds. Others appear to perceive it, unconsciously, as being contemptible or distasteful simply because it is not like their own genitals.

Religious families often emphasize the sinfulness of sex and how offensive it is to God who will dole out punishment for any interest in it. Many patients with sexual problems feel that they have, or might, commit some awful sin. Adolescents will often swear to God that they will not masturbate again because of guilty feelings.

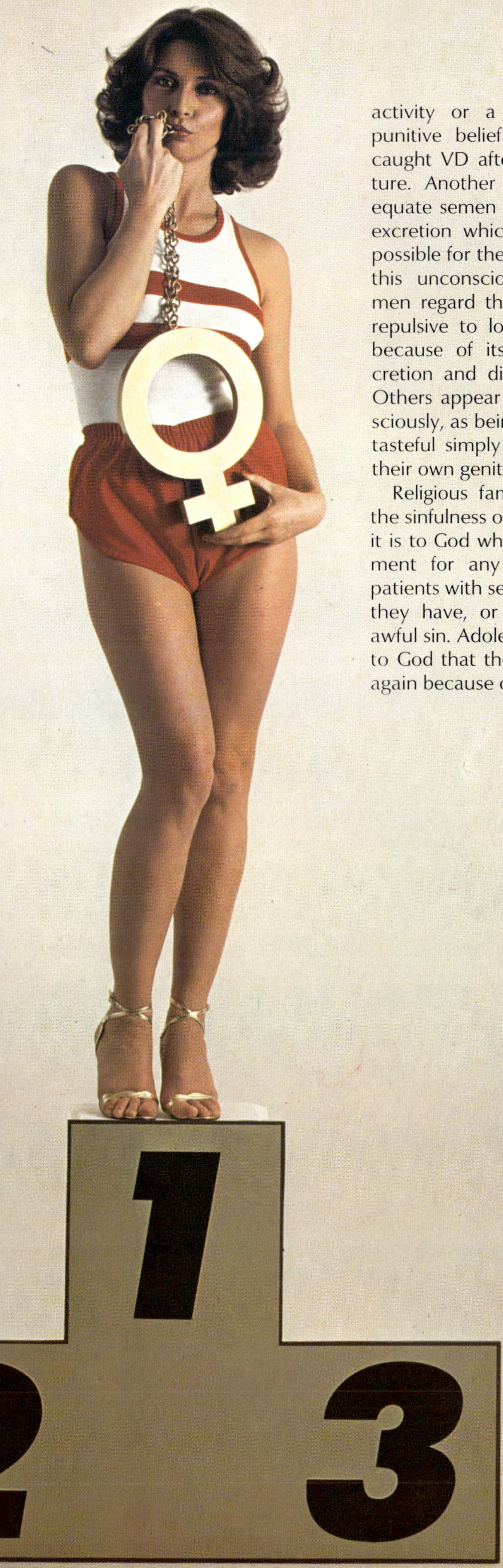

Because of their different physical structure, men are usually capable of only one orgasm during intercourse. Some men, after a short rest, are then able to achieve erection again. Women, however, can theoretically achieve many orgasms during love-making

Some parents rear children to believe that sex and sexual expression are shameful. Girls are probably more vulnerable than boys to this type of suppression because they are more dependent on their parents' affections, and it is often combined with threats that the parents will not love them if they persist. As adults such women can be so ashamed that they cannot admit to ever having touched or looked at the vulva, to having sexual thoughts, ever being sexually aroused or ever wanting to have intercourse. Boys are affected in a different way. Often women are represented to them as being pure and sexless, undertaking sex only for the male's benefit, whereas he is sexual and should be ashamed.

Direct punishment, whether physical or not, creates the attitude of fearful sex. Some people show signs of fear as they become sexually aroused and may become so agitated and tense as orgasm approaches that they cannot attain it. In our culture girls are more suppressed than boys and have standards of 'nice-girl' behaviour drilled into them. Although they may subsequently believe that they are free of such nonsense, the vast majority of women do modify their sexual behaviour in order to conform to these standards and so are inhibited, in varying degree, even within the context of marriage, over such matters as displaying their bodies freely, making advances, uninhibited foreplay and masturbation.

Punishment can also distort the form of sexual development and the problems of many adults with sexual disabilities seem to date back to such episodes. For example, boys who have been caught and seriously blamed for 'looking and showing' games with a girl are later often sexually unadventurous even with their own wives. Girls rebuked excessively for masturbation may thereafter undertake it in deceitful ways, such as lying prone, through knickers, or even by non-touch methods all of which are poor training for subsequent intercourse.

Parents can also bring about subsequent inhibitions by hammering home one particular theme such as that erections are 'bad', or that sex is only for 'making babies'.

All such inhibitions exist within one's sexuality and are often in striking contrast with the rest of the personality. Thus a man who is outgoing, resourceful and self-confident in dealing with all other aspects of life may be found to be timid, cringing and submissive in sex; he may even be impotent. A woman who is lively, imaginative and self-assured in all else may be found to be excessively self-conscious and inefficient at sex due to inhibitions implanted in her during childhood.

More usually, sexuality is an aspect of one's personality as, for example, those who are generally energetic will be energetic in sex, while those who are lethargic by nature will be lethargic sexually. It follows then that people with similar personalities are likely to display very similar sexual needs and characteristics. There is evidence that we unconsciously assess the sexuality of members of the opposite sex we meet and in whom we are interested. This assessment could be behind the judgments we make about personality.

In spite of frequently made statements that the sexuality is in fixed form by the middle of adolescence this is only true for abnormal states; more usually a person's sexuality is not fully delineated until the personality is completely and finally established in young adulthood, which enables adjustments to be made to accommodate the future partner.

Inhibitions could be said to be the product of experience imposed by the parents but really it is more a matter of the child being 'planned and programmed' by the parents. Purely fortuitous experience is random and yet it can also exert an effect on sex. A child walking in on parents having intercourse is usually not planned and some children react very badly to it, perhaps perceiving it as an assault on the mother or, by older girls, as hypocritical self-indulgence on the mother's part. Boys may become jealous of the father. Parents' reactions of horror or embarrassment to such an intrusion on the child's part may also create a strong effect. Similarly, the experience of being interfered with by an adult, of seeing a male exhibitionist, of being forced into sex games by older children and of being told by a teacher that he or she is 'diseased' when caught playing sex games during the homosexual stage of sexual development, and many other similar misfortunes can all exert profound effects on subsequent sexual capacity. Being seduced into homo or heterosexual activities by much older individuals during childhood or the earlier part of adolescence can also do damage. Although it is difficult to substantiate, it is also said that the first person with whom a man or a woman has intercourse markedly influences future choices and sexual practices. One of the reasons sometimes advanced for premature ejac-

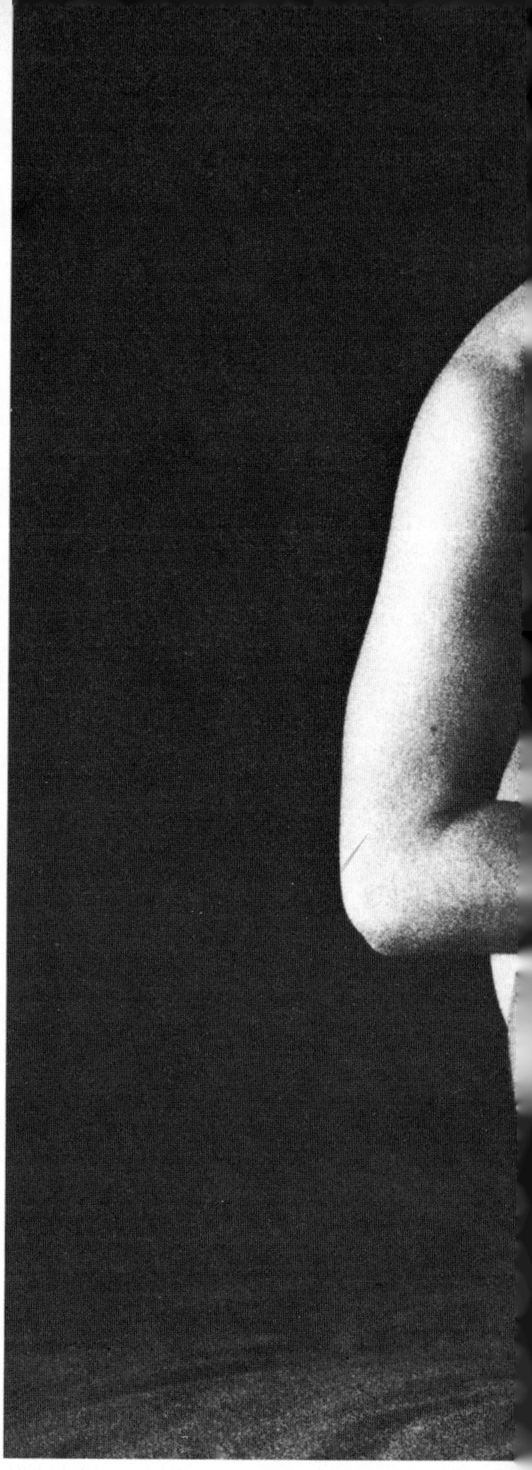

Apart from coitus itself, foreplay provides the most intensely pleasureable stimuli there are and an opportunity for men and women to completely explore all the levels of their mutual sensuality and love

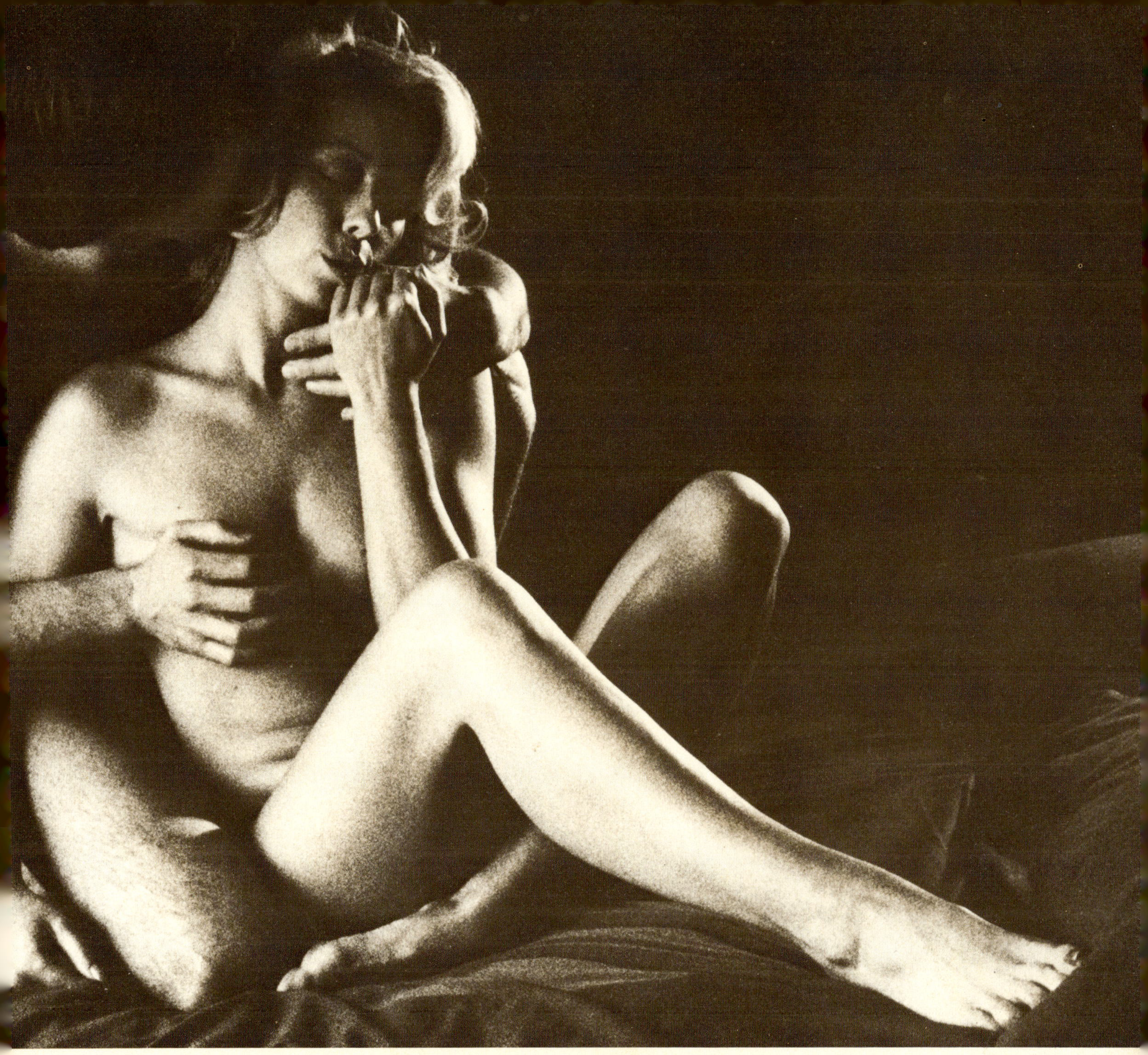

ulation, in at least some cases, is that the man's first experiences were with prostitutes who made him hurry. Certainly, the reactions of the first or early partners towards the body and genitals can undermine or promote confidence and therefore capacity. Thus many kinds of experience can affect later sexual activities.

Theoretically, a woman can have intercourse almost endlessly whereas a man is limited by biological considerations to, say, six times in 24 hours. Although some can manage more very few reach this level, except, perhaps, over short periods. The frequency of intercourse in a relationship is probably most governed by the man's rates of masturbation as an adolescent since this indicates his potential sexual energy. This in turn is an aspect of his personality unless he has been affected by experiences and inhibitions. If either partner is not inclined to frequent intercourse he or she may eventually deter the partner whereas if he or she is appreciative and keen it may provide encouragement.

Most usually rates of intercourse decline along with the man's physical powers although this is more gradual than many suppose. Within the relationship, disharmonies, discrepancies, disappointments and desires for revenge can reduce both rates and capacities below this line. For all couples who are not mutually inhibited it is probably wisest for the partners to encourage each other to keep up a good rate of intercourse and to make it as interesting and exciting for each other as possible. Refusal should be rare or non-existent and gaps should be kept, as for example in pregnancy, illness or absences from home, as brief as possible in order to prevent the loss of habit. In both young and especially in older couples, the loss of habit can lead to a more or less permanent loss of capacity.

Although many individuals may secretly regard themselves as being oversexed, due to their sexual thoughts and wishes yet it is a fact that the vast majority of people in our culture do settle for a low rate of expression – in fact the minimum necessary to ensure the lowest state of satisfaction. Nevertheless, the sexual capacity of most people does tend to vary from time to time and in the inhibited it is often very variable, with bouts of sexual activity followed by long periods of abstinence.

Female Sexuality

Women are physically and physiologically equipped for the major role in the reproduction of the species. Although they certainly could not do without men's contribution, it is women who must give their entire bodies over to an almost parasitical being for three quarters of a year; who, unless they can afford not to, must give up any other social commitments to care for the child; and who, in the best interests of the children, must do so more than once. Luckily, few women feel this way about childbirth or we would be a doomed species. Basically, women are highly adapted to their role.

Apart from the obvious anatomical differences, behavioural differences between the sexes do exist at birth and probably before. These small differences possibly form the basis for the different patterns of development later pursued by the sexes. These may be reinforced by society but it is almost certainly incorrect to assert that femininity and the female role are forced onto girls. Convincing evidence to the contrary is to be found in colonies of infant chimpanzees reared away from the example of adults. Under these conditions males and females show markedly different patterns of behaviour and interest. It is not so much that the two sexes are totally dissimilar but that each undertakes certain behaviour in different ways or with varying degrees of interest. Other research into animal behaviour has revealed that if the sex hormones are altered before or soon after birth then the animal's behaviour becomes more like that of the opposite sex.

However, having said all this it must be admitted that rearing powerfully affects subsequent behaviour and, due to the special capacity of young children to learn, it would probably be possible to rear boys to behave like girls and vice versa. Therefore it is partly as a result of genetic factors and partly through rearing and social expectation, that patterns of behaviour appropriate to the sex of the individual emerge. It would seem, then, that psychosexual growth and development proceed in accordance with an inner blueprint which is universal in basic structure, but which varies in detail between every individual in response to personality factors, while the whole is subject to modification, as required by the general attitudes of society and the particular attitudes of the family. Eventually a sexuality as unique as the personality emerges and yet, like the personality, all members of the same sex have much in common with each other and for that matter, with the opposite one as well. On this basis a number of generalizations can be made, some of which apply to all members of the sex and others only to the majority but none can safely be regarded as being beyond dispute.

In sex, as in all else, girls develop more rapidly than boys. The astute conclusion has recently been made that this may be another reason why girls seem to be more vulnerable to suppression than boys.

Perhaps because it is more obvious in boys, it used to be thought that genital excitement, handling and masturbation were commoner in boys than girls. More careful observation, taking account of the greater variety of less obvious modes of stimulation available to girls, reveals that the honours should go to them. A far greater proportion of women than men assert that masturbation was a continuous activity from childhood onwards. However, the majority seem either not to have realized or to have forgotten auto-stimulation in childhood. Of these most say that masturbation commenced at some age between about eight and twelve years. More women are prepared to admit that they masturbate, probably because the activity is spoken of fairly openly and is no longer regarded as shameful. Until this process of deshaming female sexuality is complete no statistics are likely to be utterly reliable.

There is no 'right' pattern of sexual response, only what is pleasurable for you. The woman's response (left) may peak to one orgasm; she may experience two or three, or she may remain in the plateau phase. The typical male response (below) is to climax once, and occasionally twice

Understanding your body (right) and the way it responds and feels is an important part of sexuality. We should not be afraid of our bodies; this can lead to inhibitions which may make a couple's sex life suffer

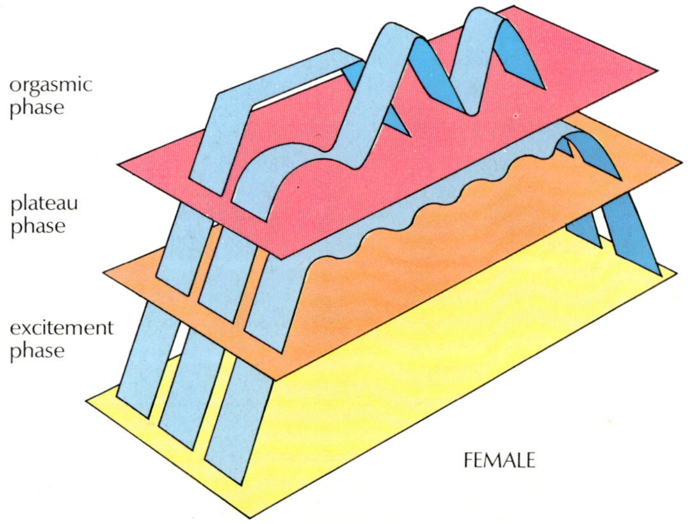

FEMALE

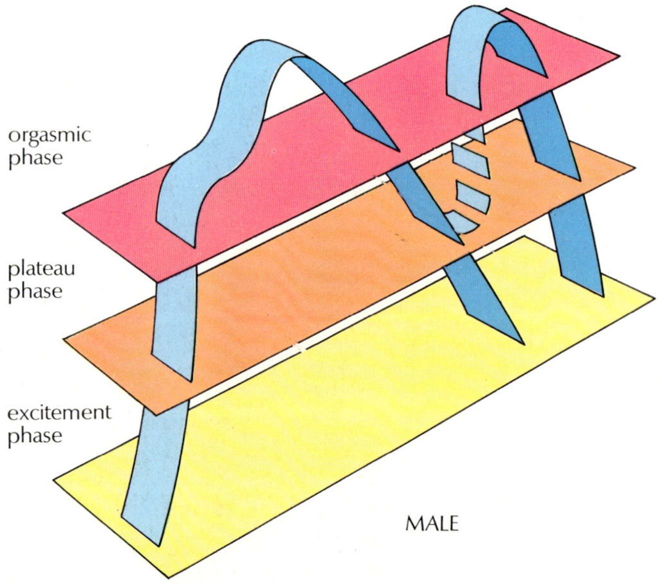

MALE

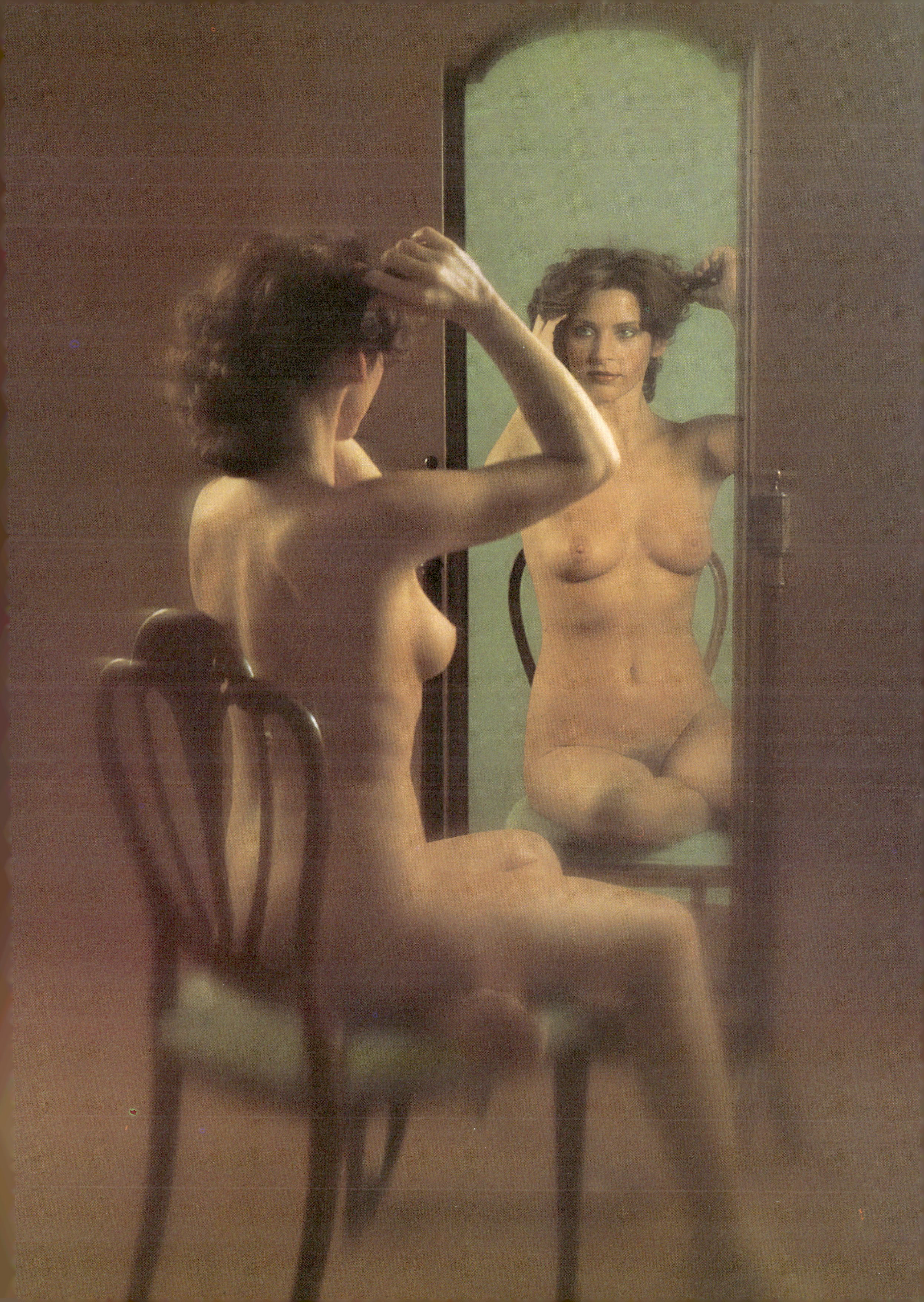

A number of characteristics of masturbation in women illustrate some aspects of their sexuality. The activity is an important source of information about the woman's own sexuality because it is a self-activity which, curiously as it may seem, tells more about her than her behaviour in connection with intercourse which she may well modify in accordance with her belief as to what is 'nice' and 'normal' and acceptable to her partner. Few girls seem to learn of masturbation from books or from other girls, that is, for most, it is a self-learned or instinctive act. Secondly, women can masturbate in many ways. This does not mean that an individual woman has a great repertoire but simply that a group of women display many different forms of the same act. This capacity is based on the fact that in both mind and body, women possess a greater potential for arousal than men. A few women can masturbate, that is to say obtain orgasms, simply by thinking erotic thoughts, or by listening to certain music or to a particular man's voice or even by a man sitting or standing next to them on a bus. There is scarcely a part of the body from which some woman has not obtained an orgasm when she, or more usually a man, has stimulated it. Pre-pubertal boys are probably similar but later lose the capacity. This observation seems to make sense since the general excitability of women, even to orgasm, when touched is more conducive to frequent sex. However, if men erected and ejaculated on having an ear nibbled we would scarcely get reproduced.

As well as being reflected in different modes of masturbation, this excitability means that granted the woman likes the man, he can probably achieve intercourse if he attempts it properly. This is important and husbands should be advised not to be too easily discouraged but rather to regard a rebuff not as a matter to sulk over but as a hint to vary their approach and technique. If this is the case, and it seems to be, then the starting point of a lot of unnecessary marital discord, which may eventually lead to divorce, could be avoided. Alternatively, it may also be concluded that in a relationship which is proclaimed to be loving but in which the woman often refuses sex and this state of affairs is accepted by the man then the man may not really wish to succeed and is inhibited, although it may look at first sight as if the woman is to blame.

Men should try to really understand the sexuality of their partners so that they can encourage them to express themselves fully and unselfconsciously. This involves trying to discover the method or methods of masturbation and the associated fantasies, in order to incorporate what most excites her into foreplay. Women who masturbate by stimulating the vulva do so in their own way which the man should learn. This helps to establish intercourse as a true inter-personal activity and is probably one basis of sexual loyalty since only copulation, but not intercourse, is possible with a new, casual or unknown partner.

Many women, although a minority, masturbate by methods which avoid direct genital touching, due to maternal prohibitions in childhood. Common forms include pressing the vulva against objects, contracting muscles, retaining urine, thigh rolling and pelvic rotation or thrusting. This group can often be encouraged towards better habits by the use of some indirect method such as use of an object like a vibrator before finally establishing the normal method, from which she was distracted in childhood, that is, the use of the hand.

Most women can obtain several orgasms, perhaps five or even more. Orgasms are pleasant feelings for women and not the exhausting business they are for men. There is scarcely any limit to female capacity, except, perhaps, loss of interest with satiation, soreness or tiredness. Contrary to what is said in most books on sex, most women say that both in masturbation and in intercourse orgasm can arrive with great rapidity if they feel very aroused before they start. Also, whereas men say they masturbate to relieve sexual tension or because they are bored, women will also often claim that

At orgasm there are profound and noticeable anatomical (as well as physiological) changes (right) in the uterus, cervix and vagina, compared with the resting state (left)

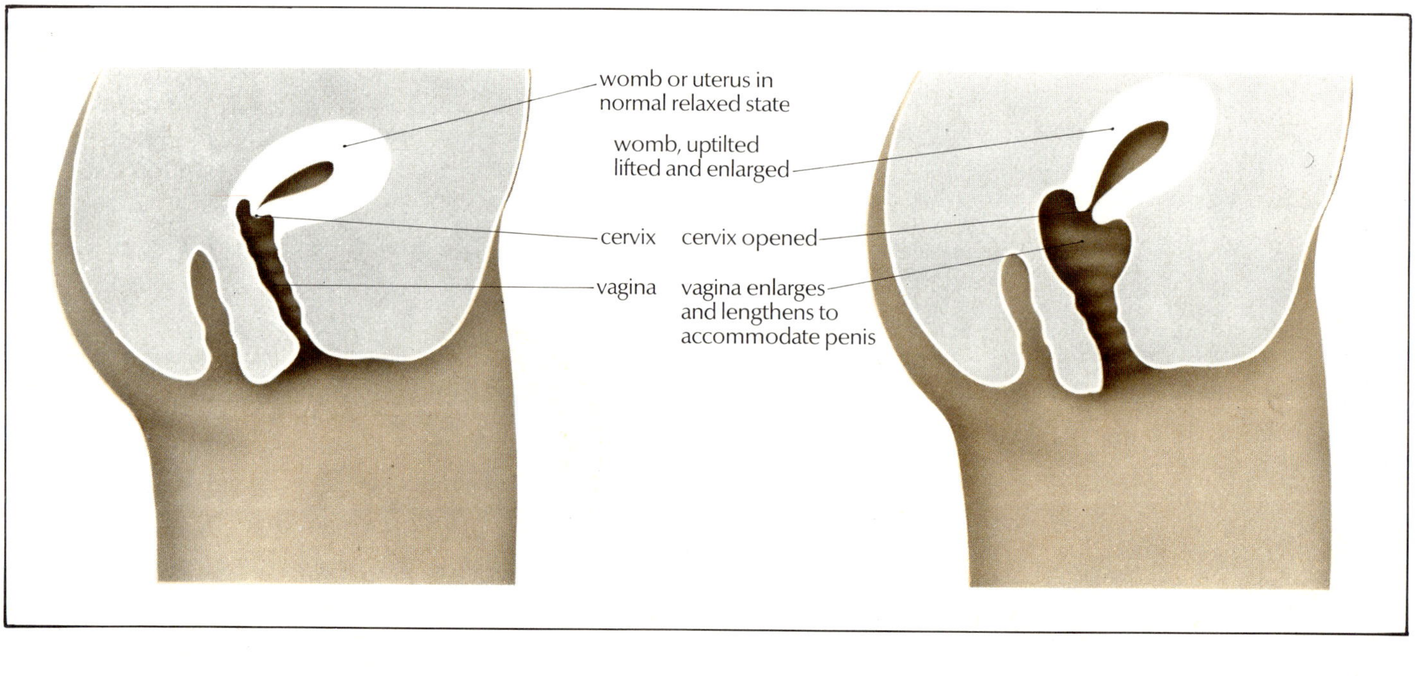

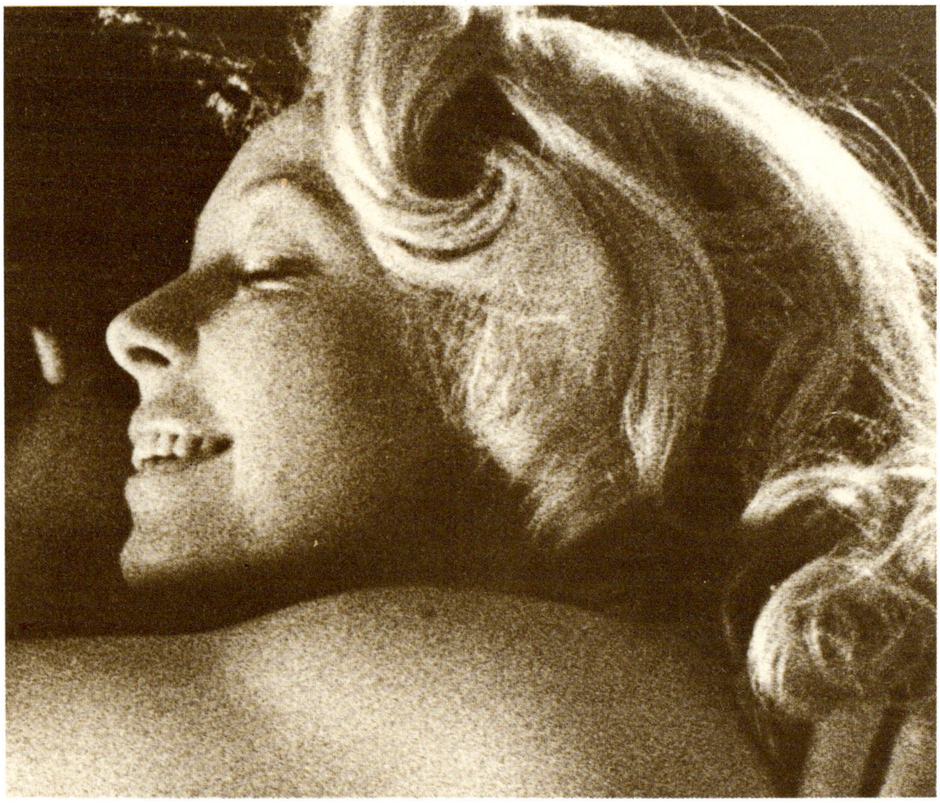

Following orgasm, both partners experience pleasantly lazy feelings of post-coital tenderness, satisfaction and complete physical and mental relaxation

in addition they will masturbate if they feel anxious, depressed, over-excited or to induce sleep.

Women often display a feature of enforced submission to men in their fantasies. Sometimes the men in them are repulsive or faceless. This may be a true aspect of female sexuality or it may be derived from the shame women are reared to feel about their sexuality. If so it is extraordinary that even in their fantasies they have to placate the self-criticism induced in them in childhood by placing the total responsibility for the act on the man. Although such fantasies may provide a basis for a number of sex games with her partner, as a part of foreplay, they are not likely to lead to total sexual cooperation with a partner.

In some women, this capacity for a form of self-deception about their sexuality, extends more seriously into their behaviour and they may happily think one thing, say another and do a third. A woman may be genuinely unaware of her sexual motivations at a conscious level and this explains how some women take the risk of becoming unwantedly pregnant and how they can sometimes unfairly accuse a man of having used force. It is interesting though, that most women only too readily take the blame themselves for any untoward consequences of casual intercourse and in cases of adultery the wife is prone to blame the other woman rather than her husband. In fact, it is women more than men who hold double standards of morality and are much more prepared to overlook sexual misbehaviour in men than they are in women based on the notion that men cannot help it since it is their nature whereas women can help it and are therefore at fault if they indulge. To some women, men who do not show signs of sexual interest in them are likely to be regarded as homosexual.

Although disputed by women's liberationists, even from girlhood women do seem to be aware of their exhibitionistic role. Unless it has been suppressed or her self-confidence undermined, even small girls can display a degree of attention-seeking behaviour towards males which can only be regarded as womanly. If the relationship with her father is good she develops these capacities and experiments in the exertion of influence. Many mothers of small daughters say the child is more effective in obtaining her own way with the father than is she herself. It has been suggested that the father is more influential on the establishment of sex roles in children of both sexes than the mother.

Perhaps the most fundamental aspect of female sexuality is its relationship to emotional feelings. From the time a woman is small she seems to use body contact, cuddling and service to express her loving feelings towards the things and people she loves. When her sexual capacities and her body begin to develop rapidly at puberty, the effect is intensified. It is perhaps the underlying feeling which women identify and label as 'spiritual', or in some similar way, in distinction to the physical demands of the body for gratification. Nevertheless, being a woman is a very physical business and there is perhaps a progression in the subjects of her love and care starting with her dolls, passing, perhaps, to the dog and then daddy and from there to the man she eventually loves and finally her baby. Her capacities to care for the people she loves, to understand them and empathize with them is truly remarkable. The pleasureable, sexual and in some cases orgasmic sensations she can obtain from her breasts and the rest of her body surface encourage maximum skin contact between her and the baby she loves. This is of enormous importance to the future welfare of the child, since it induces a sense of security and of being loved. Sexual care for the man she loves and maternal care of the baby she loves are not very different.

In fact everything about female sexuality, far from being pornographic, and the word literally means the writings of prostitutes, is at least as beautiful as the flowers and blossoms which, of course, are all part of the same story. This is not to deny that women are capable of making all manner of other contributions to society and can achieve distinction in any field of endeavour. However, one aspect of liberation for women is the acknowledgement of their own sexuality and the admission of its right to expression. For many women sex is still something done to them by the man rather than a fully cooperative effort. One way of ensuring a happier world may be to encourage women to claim their full sexual heritage.

Male Sexuality

Compared with the average woman, the average man is larger, heavier, stronger, fleeter, darker, hairier, less fat, more aggressive, less inhibited by novelty, more interested in things, less interested in people, more voyeuristic, more sadistic, more active, less verbally skillful and less prone to depression. Society permits him to express his sexuality more openly than it does the woman but insists that he conceals his emotions more. His true nature may be the opposite of these last two restrictions and although he may be less affected by emotional feelings and mood changes than women, he may be more adversely affected by emotional deprivation. For example, unlike girls, unloved boys may cease growing. Generally, however, boys are less likely to modify their behaviour to gain or retain love. Married men fare better in almost every aspect of general health than those who are unmarried.

Men may be more romantic than women, although this could be the result of emotional suppression, and the word may signify something different to each of the sexes. For women it seems to mean the environmental and emotional circumstances surrounding the association at a given time whereas for men the term seems to mean long enduring mutual love and total mutual support. It is difficult to gain access to the romantic fantasies of the average man but they probably consist of ideas of total dedication to a woman he loves who turns all her efforts, affection and sexuality towards him alone amongst men. When he feels this is lacking because of her irritations with him and criticisms of him, her sexual refusals and the attention she pays to other men, he rarely says anything directly but may punish her in other ways. Gradually this leads to deterioration in the relationship as he withdraws his emotional warmth and even his sexual interest. In a way this sort of reaction is immature and may be a price the man-woman relationship pays for society inhibiting the emotional development of males.

The greater proportion of fat in the woman's body is largely arranged to make her soft to touch and the man's psyche is organized so as to be exquisitely sensitive to her curves which probably accounts for the greater arousal value visual stimuli have for him compared with her. In this sense she is certainly the seducer and he responds with erection and nearly irresistible desires to look at her, stroke and cuddle her, and make love to her. He wants her to enjoy his attentions, reciprocate them and respond to them because this is flattering to him. In a culture which gives to boys, during adolescence, the idea that a real man is one who is attractive to women, can seduce many of them and sexually satisfy all of them, the consequence is anxiety about performance added to the other anxieties boys already possess about sex. These are derived from earlier suppression and also from the phase of intense attraction to the mother in childhood. They can so overburden a proportion of men that they never subsequently make any determined move towards heterosexuality. In one sense the culture is right, however, since only women can affirm the masculinity of a man just as only men can affirm the femininity and attractiveness of a woman. What is most valuable to the sexes is the gift of the opposite one.

Around the age of five or six, boys do seem to give up most of their interest in the penis and also their special interest in the mother, provided she allows him to do so by avoiding being over close or over hostile to him. Thereafter they tend to avoid and denigrate girls whilst

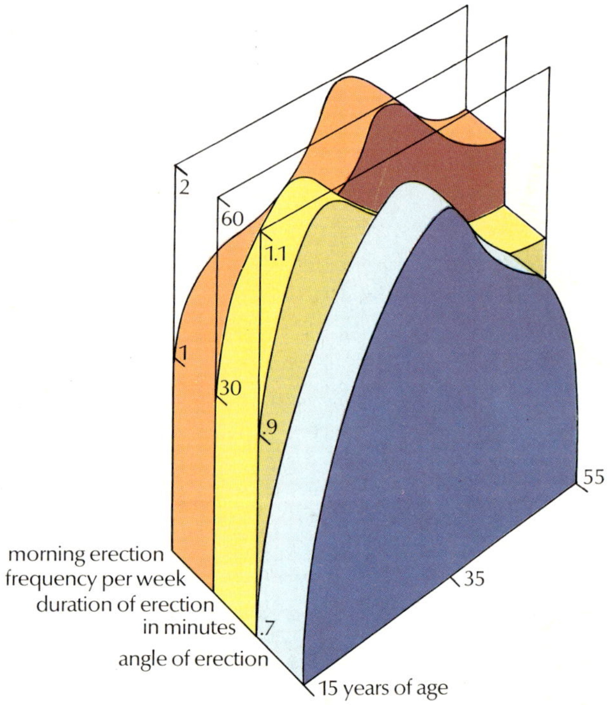

Throughout life the male's sexual response continually changes. The frequency of intercourse per week (left) peaks at about 35 years, although the duration of erection is longer at about 25. The angle of the penis to the body is at a maximum at about 30 and then declines

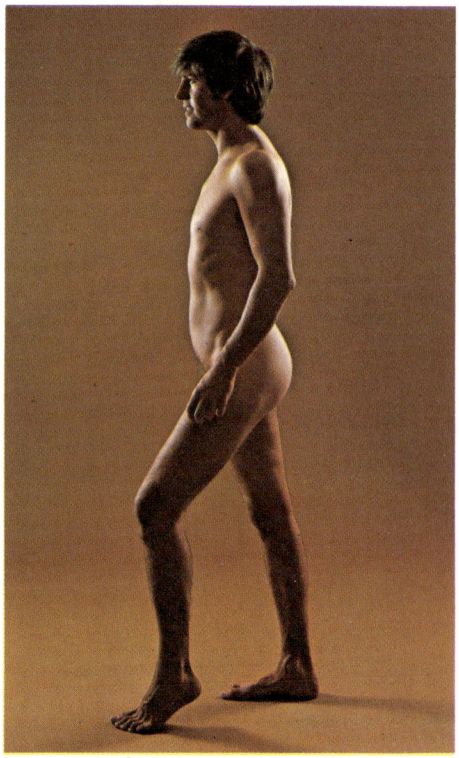

From adolescence the male becomes stronger, darker, hairier, more aggressive and less prone to depression

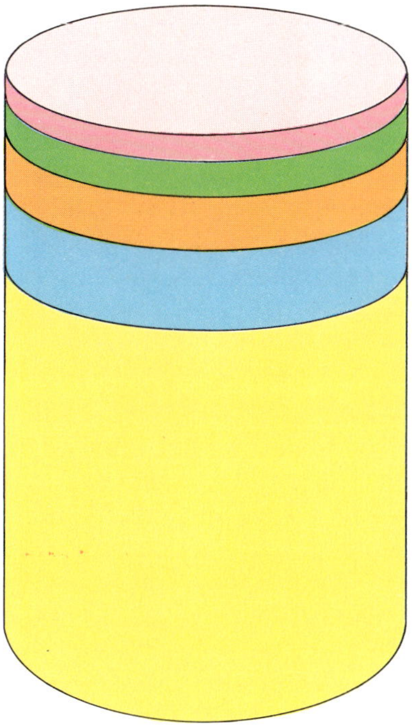
3% others
5% petting
11% intercourse
13% nocturnal emission
68% masturbation

This diagram depicts the various cases of the male's first experience of ejaculation

acquiring interest in matters evidently considered important by the father such as sports, cars or whatever else. Sometimes the father is absent, disinterested, uninteresting or frightening and the boy may turn back towards the mother if no other adult male is available in whom he can take an interest. Boys may join gangs or groups of boys in the stage before puberty and although there may be a certain amount of sex talk and sex play, such as mutual exhibitionism, the stage is more one of social rather than actual homosexuality. Boys generally are more able than girls to let their friendships cross group boundaries. This social homosexuality may be important in later permitting men to cooperate in large groups for purposes of communal defence, and other large enterprises for social, commercial, industrial and similar purposes.

The pre-pubertal stage in boys is different to that of girls in which for many it is one of physical homosexuality in which they may play explicit sex games such as 'mothers and fathers' with their best girl-friend. They may show the vulva to each other, smack bottoms and even explore the vagina of the other but mutual masturbation is rare. When puberty is reached girls usually take an emphatic turn towards heterosexuality and begin to test the effect of their body changes in attracting male attention. Some girls become frightened of their increase in sexuality and may retreat into work, obesity, anorexia nervosa or even religion.

In boys the true homosexual stage arrives after puberty and there is much talk about and comparison of pubic hair development, penis enlargement, ejaculation and masturbation. The slightly older boys seem to serve the function of drawing the attention of the slightly younger boys to masturbation and they most promptly become ardent practitioners. Thoughts of the mother or of a mother substitute such as an aunt or a friend's mother may come to mind during fantasy at first but these rapidly give way to thoughts about girls and desires to look at pictures of them naked or near naked. At this stage the boy is learning to put a real value on girls but if he is caught masturbating or if his masturbation material is discovered he is likely to be labelled 'dirty' by parents or teachers.

A boy with a previously over-close mother or with one who preoccupies herself with his masturbation, as some do, may be unable to rid himself of fantasies about her and may either try to give up masturbation or turn towards boys in a more permanent way for sexual relief. Boys who have been led to believe by parents that they are ill-favoured or ones with poor prior experience of women such as a dominant mother or a very jealous older

Man's image of the sexually stimulating woman, provocatively and 'dangerously' semi-clothed in black underwear, stockings and suspenders, can be an ideal fantasy figure

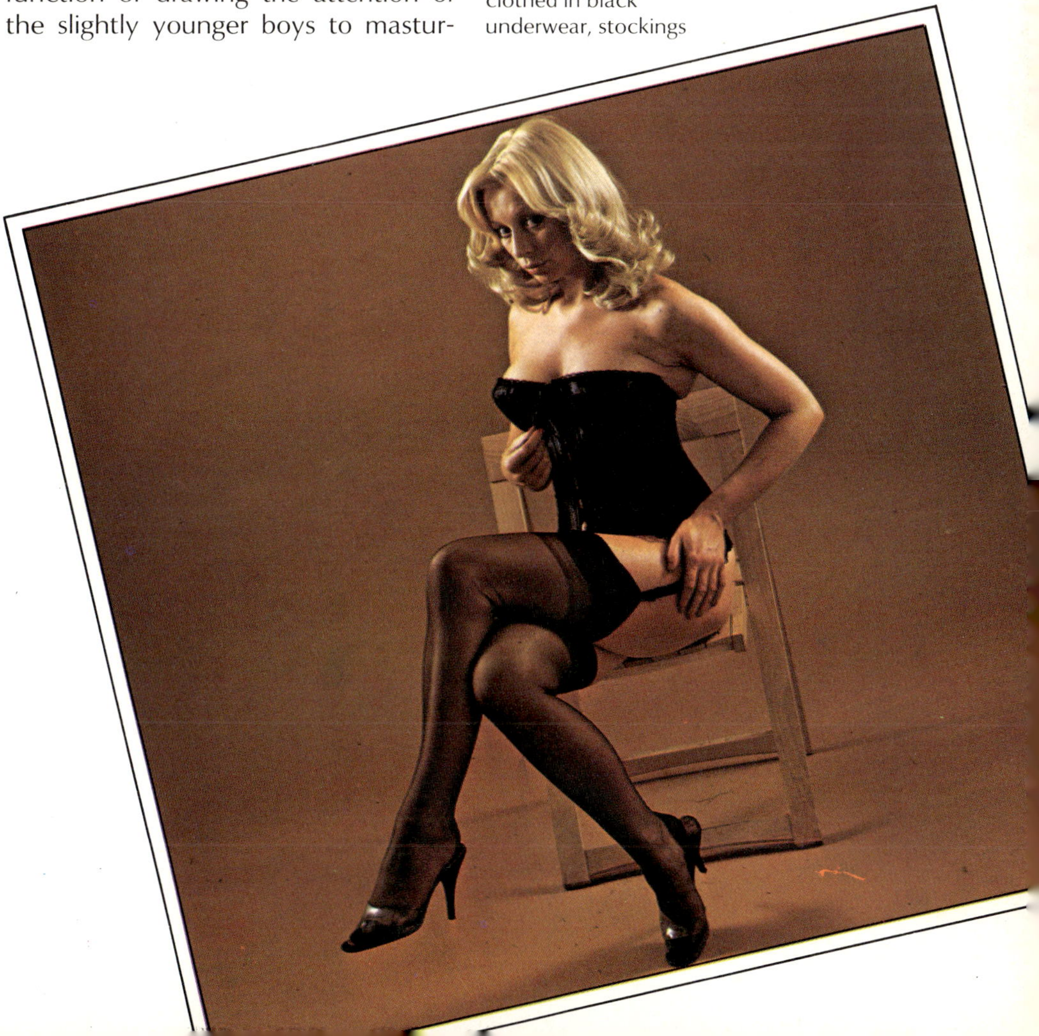

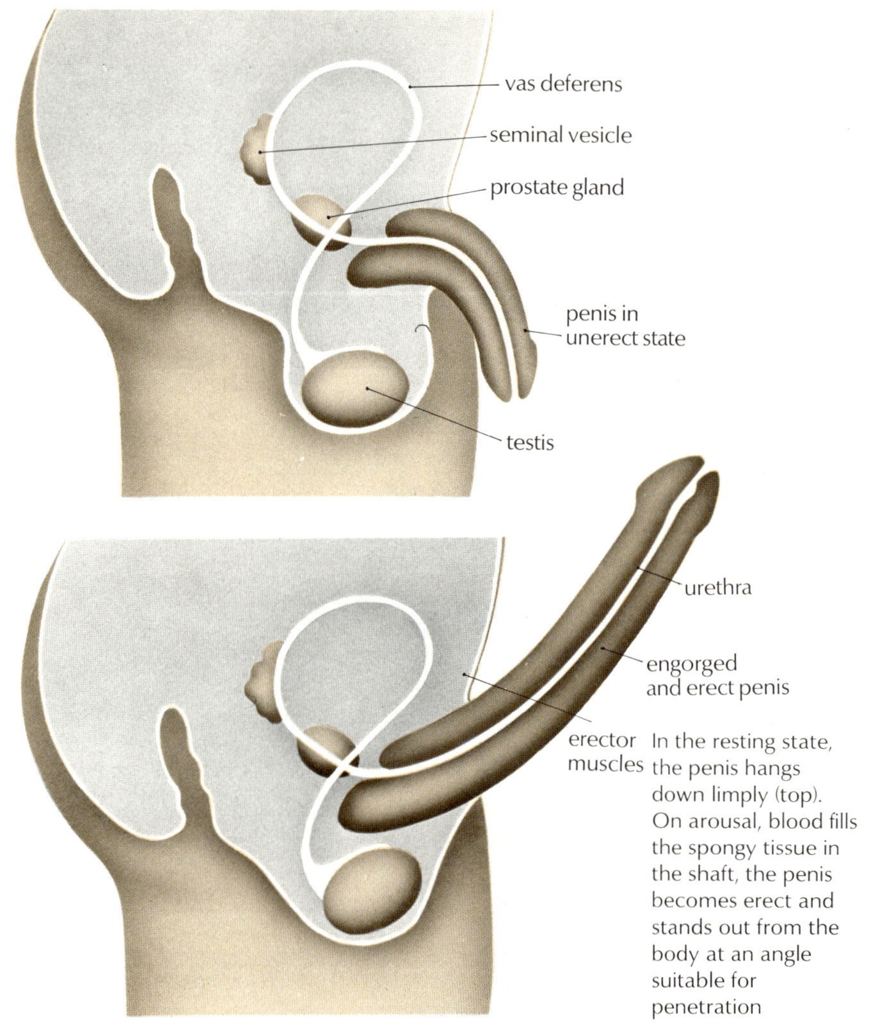

In the resting state, the penis hangs down limply (top). On arousal, blood fills the spongy tissue in the shaft, the penis becomes erect and stands out from the body at an angle suitable for penetration

sister, may show considerable anxiety about contact with girls or even thoughts of them. They may have difficulty in leaving the homosexual stage for the heterosexual one but are not truly homosexual.

Adolescent boys who have been suppressed and inhibited earlier in life may have difficulty in establishing satisfactory masturbation and may be excessively guilty after doing it. Girls at the same stage are prone to excessive handwashing or the washing of any object used in masturbation and some boys become equally if not more involved in self-cleansing or even self-punitive rituals and obsessions after masturbation. Guilty boys and girls may confine masturbation to sleep or when dropping off to sleep or waking from it. Some boys make no attempt to conceal the evidence of nocturnal emissions, or even normal masturbation, from the mother and in some the unconscious aim is seductive. Some boys and men learn to reduce levels of consciousness in order to remove inhibition and promote pleasure during masturbation and this may be achieved by 'sniffing' various substances, by taking certain drugs, by over-breathing or by partial suffocation or strangulation. All are very dangerous and it is a matter for indignation that the boy should have had such a degree of inhibition imposed on him in the first place.

As well as affecting the frequency and also activities associated with or after masturbation, earlier imposed inhibitions can also effect the mode of masturbation, as also occurs in girls. Although most adolescent boys may experiment with alternative forms of masturbation some concentrate on them and a high proportion of these encounter sexual difficulties later. In fact, it seems that the persistent adoption of any method except the encompassment of the shaft of the penis with the dominant hand, with the thumb and index finger encircling the lower rim of the glans or head of the penis, is a poor form of training for boys. The grasp is not too tight and the hand is moved to and fro so as to stimulate not so much the shaft as the rim of the glans. The shaft is not particularly sensitive and may well be the sensory equivalent of the vagina, which is also relatively insensitive. Some boys move the hand in quick movements and some more slowly. Some, like some girls, perhaps the guilty ones, masturbate direct to orgasm presumably to get it over quickly whereas most pause occasionally to allow the mounting tension to dissipate a little and so prolong the act. Such pauses may be important since they may teach a degree of self-control which is of value in intercourse subsequently. It is during such pauses many girls, during mid-adolescence, begin to incorporate the insertion of the fingers into the vagina during masturbation. Since they associate this with fantasies of penetration by the penis it has a high preparatory value for intercourse. Masturbation trains both sexes to be competent sexually.

Orgasm commences as semen enters the portion of the urethra, or water-pipe, which is closest to the body and is a sort of intensely pleasurable spasm. From this point ejaculation is inevitable and with a few more rubs, or thrusts if the penis is within the vagina, the man brings on the again intensely pleasurable throbbing sensation which accompanies the first few spurts of the ejaculation. During orgasm the muscles contract, the face may be contorted and the man wishes to push hard with the penis. Thereafter, unlike the woman, he does not want any more stimulation to the penis since it is experienced as pain. With this last exception, and also the lack of ejaculation in women, the sensations and body reactions at orgasm are very similar in both sexes although orgasm in the woman may last longer than in the man. Very experienced women, who have watched many men have an orgasm, comment on the differing intensity of orgasm between men and on their differing bodily reactions to it.

Although members of both sexes who are incapable of coping adequately with the stresses of life may masturbate to comfort themselves, quite un-neurotic boys may masturbate up to six times a day in adolescence. Once a day is a fairly common frequency during adolescence and perhaps once every two days thereafter. However, just as in women, there is considerable variation. Most boys eventually find masturbation unsatisfactory and this combined with desires for the company of a girl eventually overcomes their fears and they begin to make substantial advances towards girls in the hope of achieving copulation. Other things being equal, the vast majority of men would agree that a vagina is more satisfactory than the hand. Thus, most men would have intercourse in preference to masturbation but because the two are not mutually exclusive in women, as they are in men, women do not have to make such a choice and can and do undertake both even at the same time. Nevertheless, the vast majority of men do occasionally masturbate no matter how attractive to them and available their sex partner may be. Such masturbation may not go as far as orgasm. Often they are very ashamed and admit to it only with reluctance. Masturbation after marriage in both sexes may serve the purpose of assisting sexual loyalty by permitting promiscuous thoughts to be discharged in fantasy rather than fact. It may also have an innovatory purpose in that new sexual techniques, or elaborations of old ones, may be worked out in fantasy. Incorporating them into intercourse may help to retain the quality of excitement in the sex life.

Although men like to receive general body stimulation from women, just as women do from men, to be really sexually arousing it has to occur in the area covered by the underpants, but some men also find the nipples exciting. Within the pelvic area stimulation of the scrotum and testes is usually enjoyed and some men even like a woman to squeeze the testicles hard. The anus is pleasurable and for some, the buttocks. Prostitutes who specialize in such services say that for some men, being beaten or whipped on the bottom is so exciting that erection, orgasm and ejaculation may occur with no genital stimulation. The theory usually put forward to account for it is that either the mother smacked the boy on the bottom during his phase of special attachment to her or that the man is a masochist and wishes the woman to assume responsibility for his sexuality. Unless she really enjoys her work he is unlikely to obtain the maximum benefit. Most masturbation fantasies in most men are of them doing things to the woman but most men occasionally have fantasies of their own submission to the sexual wishes of the woman. In the fantasy, at least, she may make him do all manner of things to her and she may do all manner of things to him before permitting him to reach orgasm. This strain of passive fantasy seems to parallel a corresponding feature in female sexuality in which most women at least occasionally fantasize about being in charge of the man and working him up into a tremendous passion before she allows intercourse. Properly used in the man-woman relationship this can lead on to occasional role reversal and so doubles the repertoire of the couple.

Just as a woman, especially a young and inexperienced one, may criticize her body, and particularly her breasts, as being less than perfect, so many men believe their penis to be unacceptably small. During early adolescence when their own penis is still less than fully developed, boys are given the notion that all women desire a huge organ. The sex jokes which convey this information to the boy often also assert that a coloured man is likely to have huge genitals and the preference that this is supposed to grant him with women is one source of colour discrimination. Since an average implies that half will be more than the average and half less than the average, a number of men will have a relatively smaller penis just as some women will have smaller breasts. However, most breasts and most penes are very adequate and in any case one of the features of our heterosexual system is that virtually everyone is included. Thus, some women prefer a smaller penis and some men detest even average sized breasts. There is no universal agreement in either sex as to what is ideal in the other. Beyond this, personality factors tend to be more important than physical ones.

Foreplay is immensely important, specially to the woman, enabling her to experience the fullest possible satisfaction from sexual intercourse

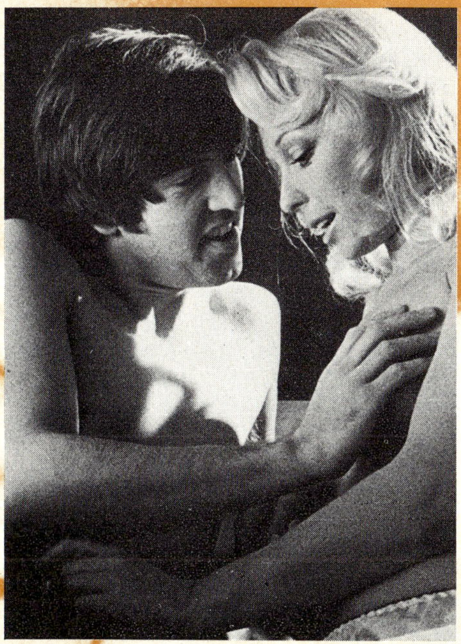

The size of the flaccid penis is no indication of its erect size but in some men there is little difference in the two states. A man with a small flaccid penis may assume that a man with a large one will still enlarge in the same proportion as his own and thereby attain huge proportions. In public lavatories, a homosexual may be so excited as to be half erect and may be careless about showing it in the hope of thereby obtaining a partner. This may make the unexcited heterosexual creep off feeling inferior. Again, when a man is being prepared for a male photograph for a sex magazine, a girl usually stimulates his penis to half erection beforehand. Even photographs of an erect penis can be misleading due to the skill of the photographer in making it appear larger than it is. Such photographs expose men to the same inferiority-inducing pressures that our women have endured from advertizers to promote the sale of their beauty enhancing goods. However, long before advertizers existed, men in some eras, and most women in all, have used artifice to enhance their attractiveness to the opposite sex.

Really it is a measure of the enormous values we place, and rightly, on the other sex. This has survived two millenia of opposition. The old Adam and the old Eve are present in everyone. If they are wise, partners flatter each other both in words and behaviour about the bodily characteristics of the other.

Living Together

Almost everyone yearns for the ideal one-to-one relationship which can be all things to both partners; one which is romantic, sexy, fun and that has deep mutual understanding, lots of common interests and no annoying habits. Unfortunately, this storybook relationship is extremely difficult, if not impossible, to achieve for most people as so many things conspire against it. Judging a real relationship against idealistic fantasies perhaps nurtured in adolescence tends to cause eternal disappointment. Poor rearing and training for the relationship, due to the opposition to sex and sexual interest by parents, adds a further difficulty, as does the perpetuation of myths about, particularly, female sexuality. Too early marriage before the personality is mature and having children before the parental relationship is sufficiently secure to withstand the stresses of pregnancy and child-rearing, are both seriously likely to harm an apparently good relationship.

Another threat is our own tendency to promiscuity. It is true that society imposes barriers against such indulgence but this is probably of no real benefit to the man-woman relationship since it may lead to resentment. Some marriages are greatly improved by some extramarital involvement since they enable a fresh assessment of the value of the existing partner to be made. One difficulty is the need that some men and women impose on themselves to love a partner before they are sexual with them. When this is combined with the notion that he or she can only love one person at a time it means preparing for extramarital adventure by 'deloving' the existing partner before progress can be made elsewhere. In this way, again, unnecessary divorce may be occur.

Communication, friendship and mutual acceptance by a similar personality are probably the basis for a happy and fulfilled man-woman relationship. Earlier misrearing might cause either partner to have unreal expectations of the other and resent deficiency. For example, some women by their behaviour rear a son to believe that a woman who loves him will more or less wait on him hand and foot but, unless carefully chosen, his wife may be less than willing to continue the practice. One partner's insecurity may cause him to become over-excited and prone to unreasonable behaviour when certain topics are mentioned and this then establishes a communication blockage.

The participants in the man-woman relationship usually fulfill a series of roles in relation to each other which answer to a need in oneself or one's partner. Thus, on different occasions a man may be the protecting and providing loving father towards the woman, and at other times be her best friend, her lover or her son. These are not games but are states of total intimacy. In a particular relationship one particular role may be the most common adopted by that relationship. Possibly the father-daughter one meets the needs of most people most of the time but it is easily switched and changed. In 'abnormal' relationships one role exists to the exclusion of others and both partners may, for example, wish to be the perpetual child or the man may want the woman to be an eternal, and sexless, mother. The happiest situation of all is where the couple unconditionally love each other regardless of the role being filled.

Although both sexes benefit from a good man-woman relationship it is possible that women are more easily upset and depressed when it goes wrong. Because of their special relationship to any children, especially

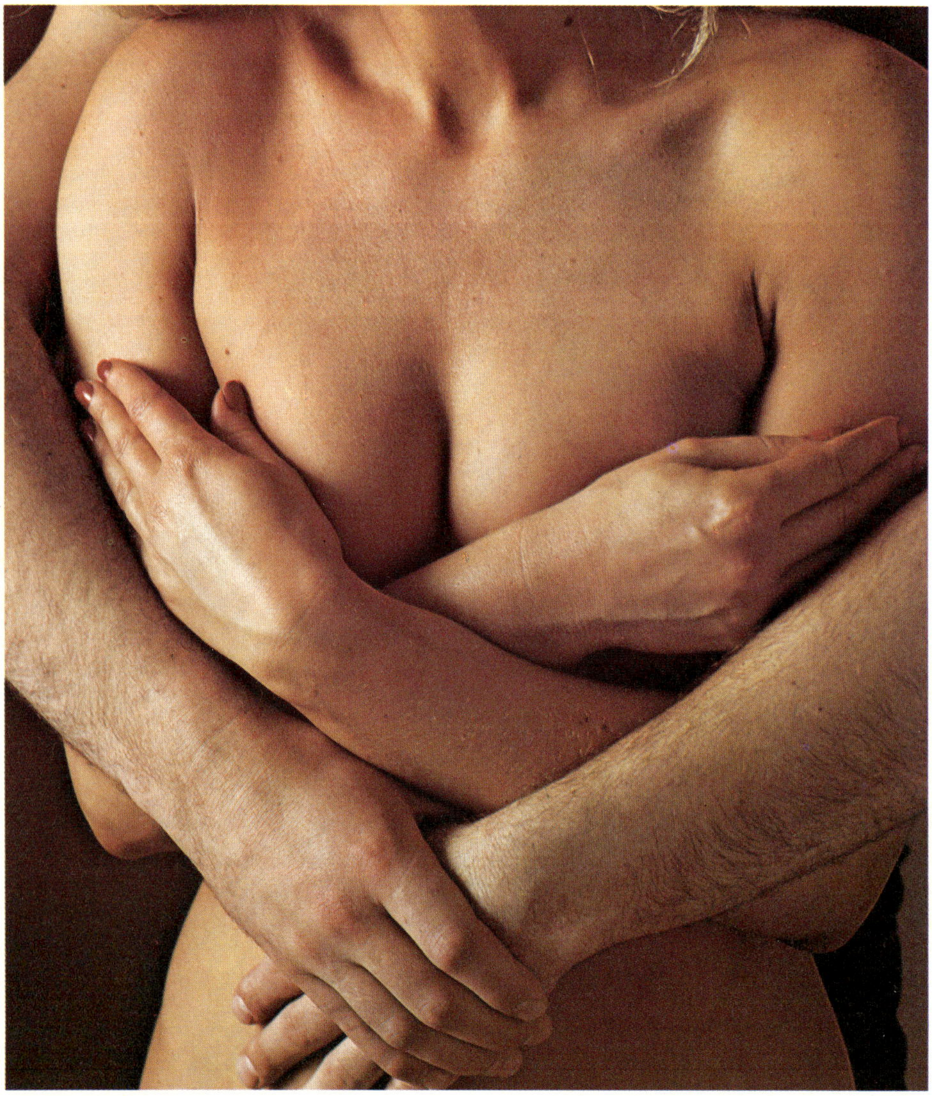

Loving physical contact – not necessarily of an overtly sexual nature – is a vital part of the man-woman relationship

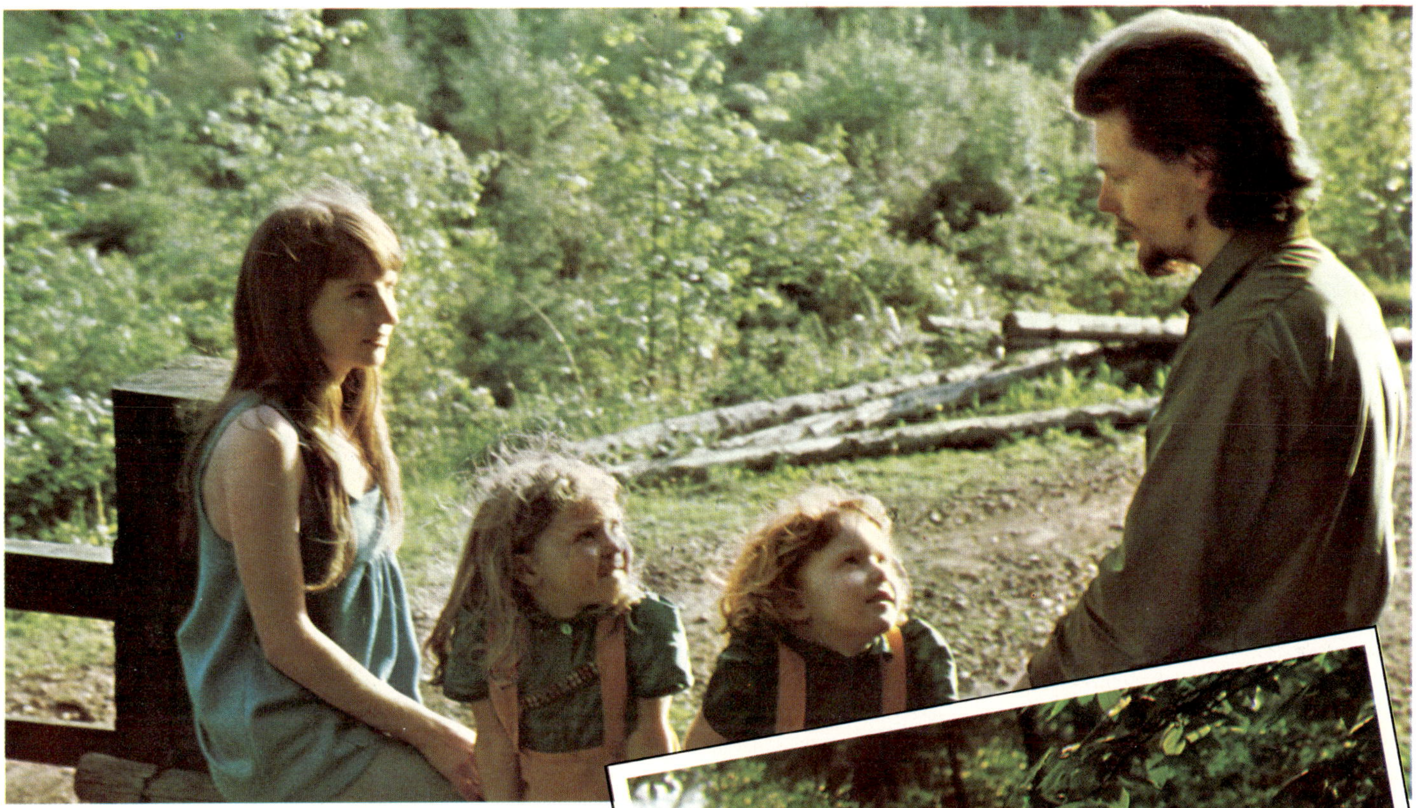

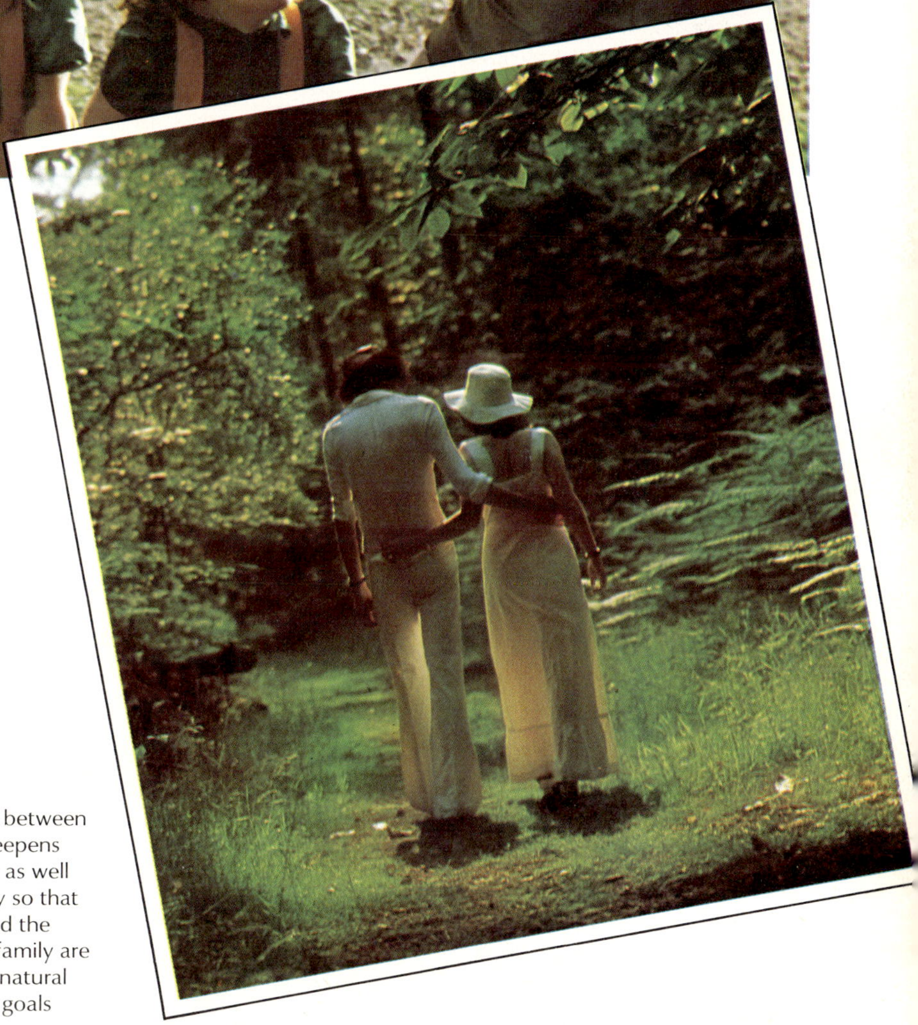

Ideally, the relationship between the sexes deepens emotionally as well as physically so that marriage and the raising of a family are seen as the natural and mutual goals

young ones, it could probably be said that it is more important to the family and society that its women are happy. For most this probably implies that the man will also be happy but it must be admitted that some women seem happiest when they are testing, challenging or frustrating the man. This is not quite the same as the more frequent complaint made by women that their male will not have a row with them and so 'clear the air'. This probably means that a number of doubts or misunderstandings have arisen and that these are hurting her feelings; she therefore wishes to resolve them and discharge the negative emotion at the same time. She may also wish to draw attention to some distress for which she would like some husband therapy. An occasional woman may seek to indulge masochistic and rape fantasies by provoking her partner to rage in the hope he will force her to have intercourse. This may be one of the reasons why the partners of many battered wives are not brought to justice; the woman knows she is responsible for it. Shame, of course, is another. When a woman is really and severely upset it is almost invariably found that in some way or another she is perceiving herself as being the woman scorned. Although it may be easy to label her as hysterical she is severely distressed and the matter should receive proper attention. Men may feel the same but are less allowed to show it.

It has become fashionable to advise divorce in some marriage guidance circles when there is much difficulty in a relationship, with the idea that a bad marriage is best ended. Not much effort may be made to save the marriage and yet in many of these the partners are found to only differ on trivial grounds which have become magnified. Society would perhaps do better to emphasize later marriage rather than early divorce. Marriage seems to be a good cure for love which is an indictment of our moral religious, educational and social values.

Sexual Intercourse

Achieving mutally satisfying intercourse is not as easy as most books and magazines would have us believe and the young receive very little real preparation for it in our culture. It can take a number of years for a couple to learn to make it work for both of them and if they do not realize this, early disenchantment and divorce may result. The tendency we have to settle for minimal satisfaction often prevents much progress being made and couples of long standing may be incompetent at sex to a point which would be a disgrace in any other aspect of their lives. Both may eventually become involved extra-maritally not so much because of real promiscuous desires to do so but simply to relieve the tedium of their sexual existence before they become too old to attract another partner. The tragedy is that they may both fantasize about doing with each other what they do with others but be too ashamed or embarrassed to say so.

The central act both in copulation and intercourse is the insertion of the penis into the vagina, the only function of the latter being to stimulate the penis sufficiently to bring about ejaculation. The sensitive entrance to the vagina is 'H' shaped so it offers sensations to a penis of almost any size and the area engorges in sexual excitment thereby increasing the effect. In side view the vagina is 'S' shaped and this again affords the tip of the penis more stimulation than if it were a simple straight tube. Although the vulva and vagina are always damp, a clear lubricative fluid exudes from the vaginal walls as the woman becomes excited, by a process which is similar to that which causes erection in the man, and the resultant wetness reduces friction but increases the sensitivity of the glans by facilitating gliding movement. It is interesting in passing to note that when in masturbation women rub their equivalent of the penis, the clitoris, or the area around it, they will first wet the fingers with saliva or with fluid from the vagina.

Another feature of the vagina is its acidity which helps to prevent germs which may be introduced into it from gaining a hold and perhaps spreading upwards leading to inflammation of the uterus, tubes and peritoneal cavity. It is also quite short being, in most women, no longer than three or four inches. In any position where the penis can be fully inserted it is almost always a good deal longer than the vagina and may cause pain to the woman by stretching it and pushing on the organs above. However, about nine out of ten women say they enjoy deep penetration, perhaps because of the low level of sensation they otherwise obtain from the barrel of the vagina, and this is just as well in view of the man's desire to push at orgasm.

Although the penis may seem to be moving inwards and outwards easily in the vagina during intercourse, the vulva moves a lot, the inner lips clinging to the penis and being pulled outwards and then being folded inwards on the return stroke. Many women pull, rub, stroke, compress or roll the inner lips as a part of their own masturbation and in addition to being a source of pleasure in their own right, the lips transmit mechanical forces to the sensitive clitoris which is thereby stimulated. The inner lips divide over the clitoris and form a little foreskin similar to that in the male. It has been suggested that in both intercourse and masturbation, the very sensitive tip of the clitoris more or less has intercourse with its own foreskin and this is the main way in which the woman is brought to orgasm. Certainly many women, especially young ones, need either to additionally stimulate the clitoris during intercourse, or to have it stimulated, if they are to reach orgasm.

Variety, experimentation and exploration in foreplay is an essential part of a full and enjoyable sex life. The act of intercourse marks the culmination of arousal which begins with foreplay and sexual caressing

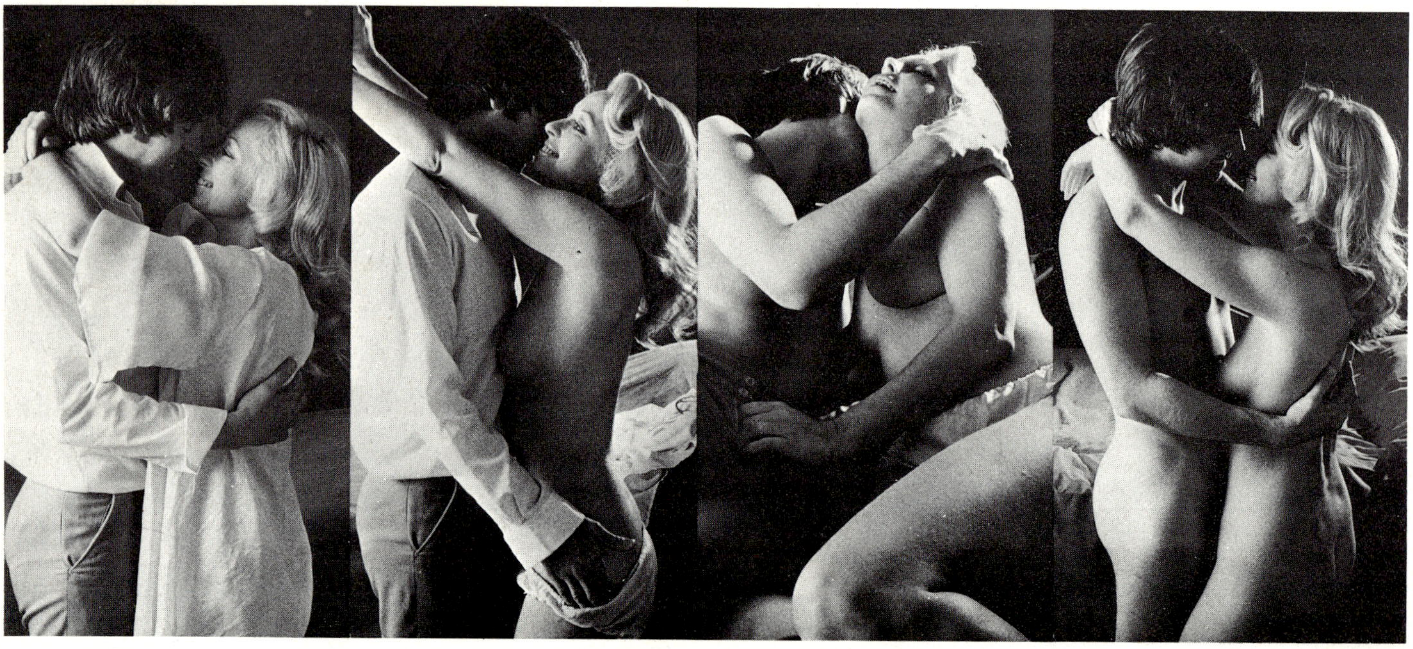

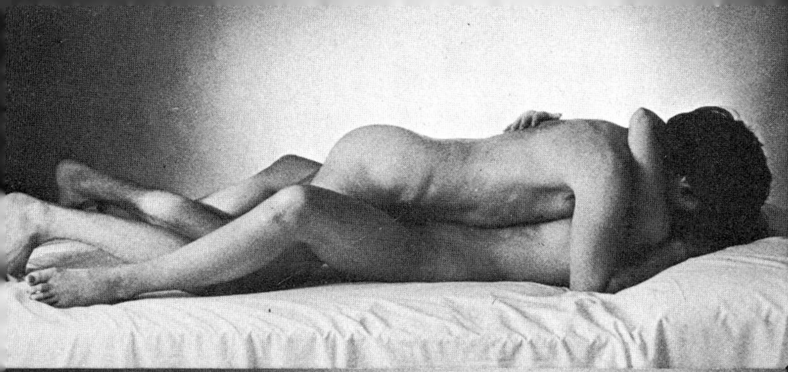
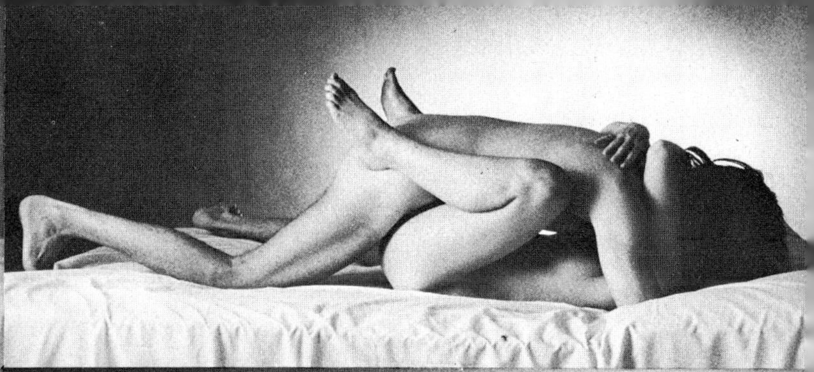
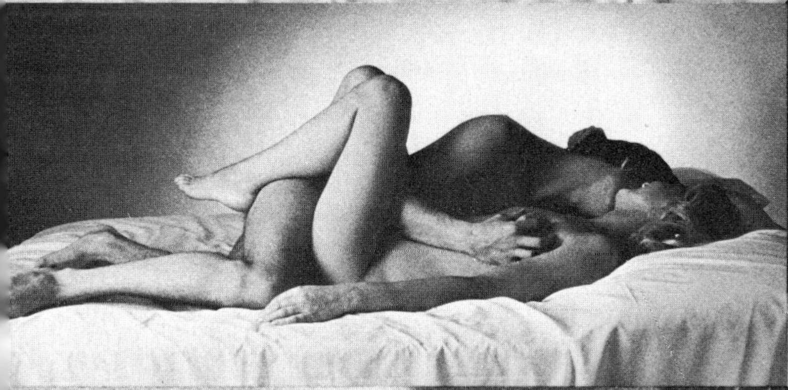
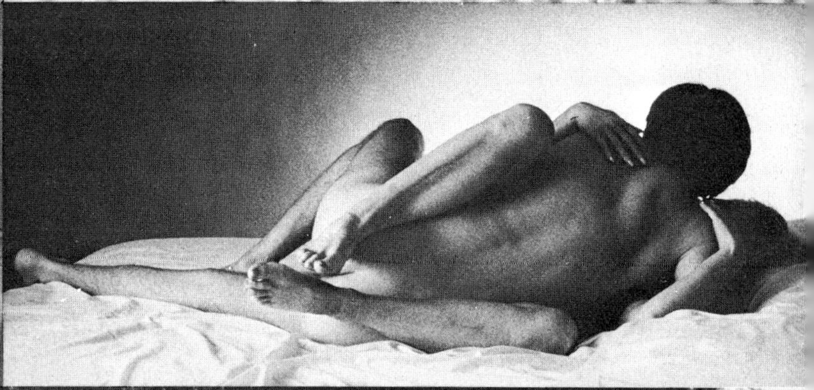
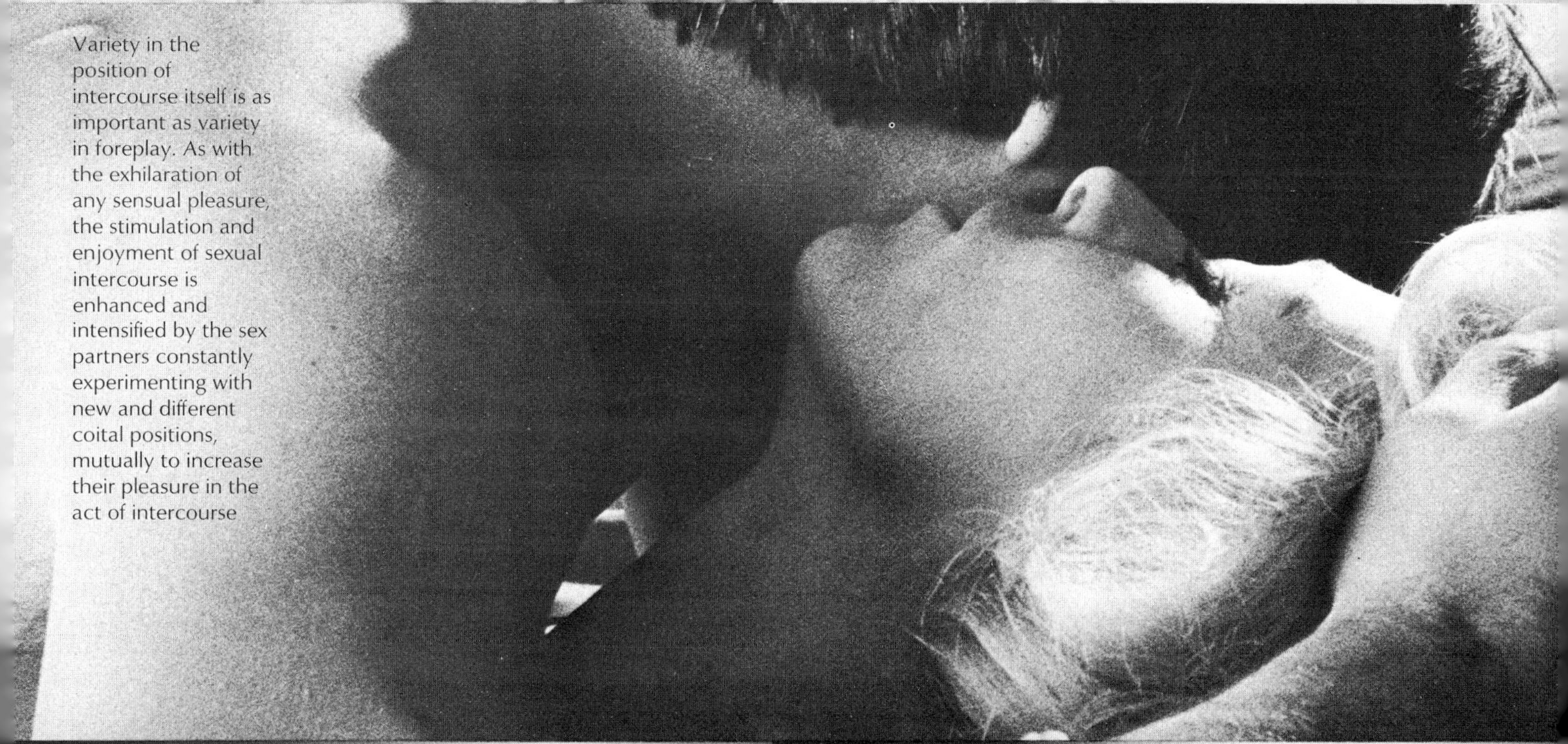

Variety in the position of intercourse itself is as important as variety in foreplay. As with the exhilaration of any sensual pleasure, the stimulation and enjoyment of sexual intercourse is enhanced and intensified by the sex partners constantly experimenting with new and different coital positions, mutually to increase their pleasure in the act of intercourse

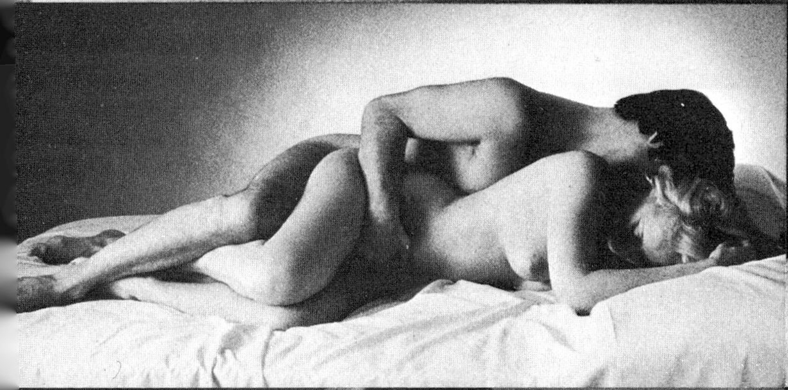
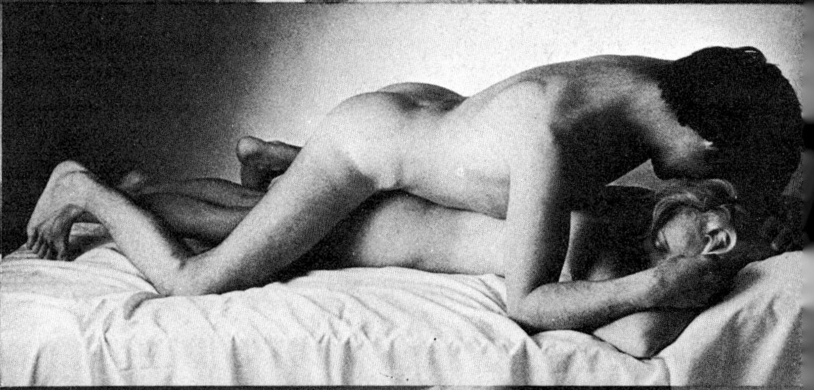
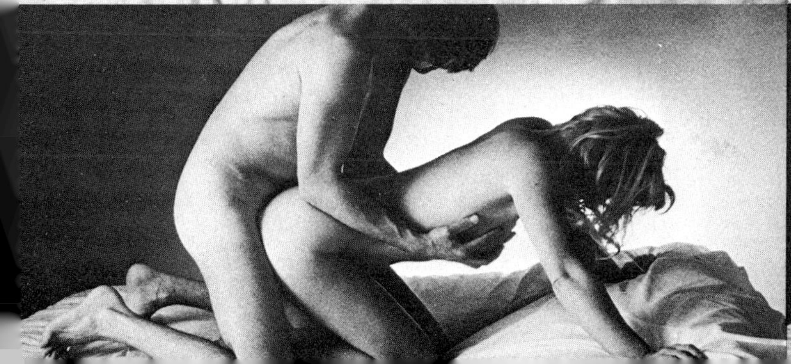
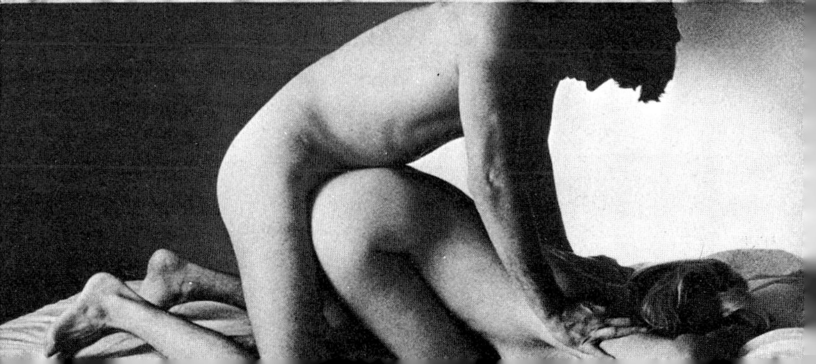

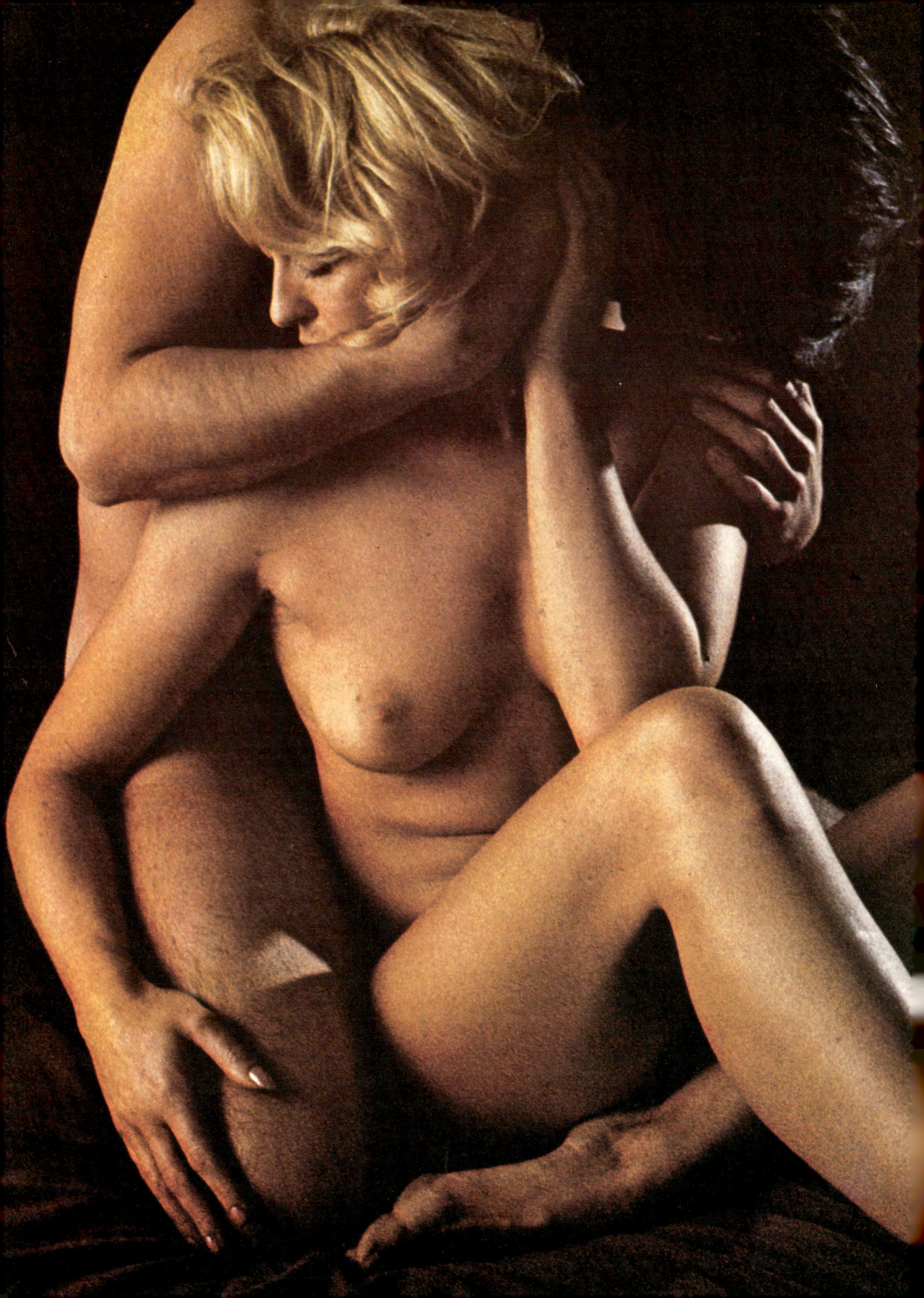

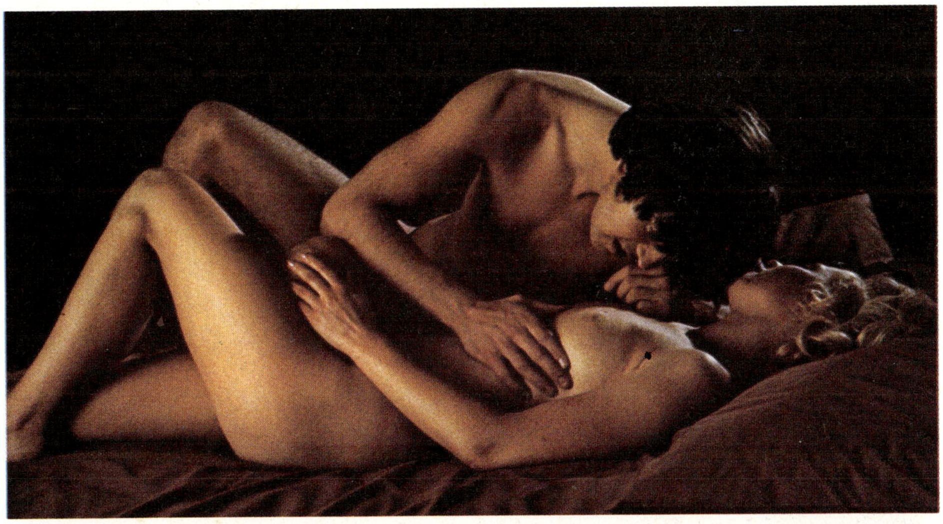

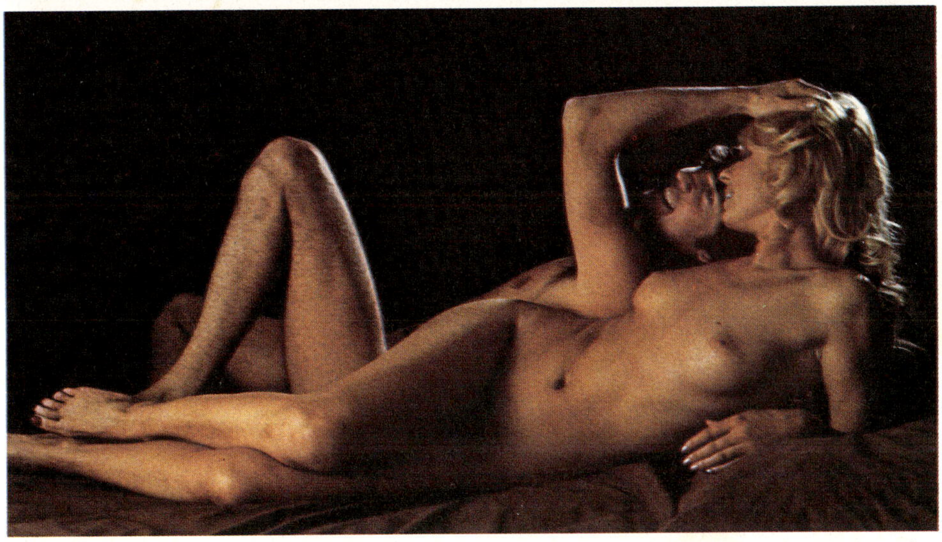

Foreplay provides both partners with the opportunity to achieve maximum erotic and sensual pleasure prior to the actual penetration and coitus. No social or cultural 'taboos' should be allowed to restrict this acutely stimulating and enjoyable phase of intercourse

One good way of assisting a woman to overcome her inhibitions regarding intercourse is to persuade her to masturbate in the normal position and manner she usually adopts and then to try to combine it with vaginal penetration by the penis. A good position in which the man can masturbate her during intercourse is to have her lying on her back with her knees up and apart whilst if he is right handed he lies at her right side more or less folded round her, lying on his left side, so that the penis is lying at the vaginal entrance. She can rest her right leg on the hollow of his waist. The vulva is widely exposed in this position and can be easily masturbated with the right hand. Not being overlaid, the woman can easily move her pelvis and if she does this in a rotary fashion, as if she were drawing a circle with her hips it has the effect of sweeping the penis round the vaginal walls. When some women insert fingers into the vagina during masturbation they rotate them round the walls rather than simply move them in and out. The vagina is sensitive to movement and perhaps, for some, this is a way in which maximum stimulation can be obtained. In this position too, the woman can easily play with the scrotum and testes with her left hand and she may even be able to reach the anus. As in any position, the woman can add to the man's pleasure and her own by learning to contract the muscles around the vagina in order to grip the penis on the inward strokes and relaxing on the outward ones.

When asked what are the sources of pleasure during intercourse, most women mention in addition to the obvious ones, the thought of the pleasurable sensations she is inducing in the penis and the excitement she feels as the man's orgasm approaches. If he is pleased with the act, and says so rather than asking her whether she had an orgasm, it adds to the pleasure and increases her self-esteem.

The evidence from studies of chimpanzees and other animals, indicates that there is a greater learned component in the conduct of intercourse for the male and a greater instinctive component in the female. If this is so, mislearning is a greater threat to men than to women. Judging from the greater number of men than women who avoid intercourse, or who are incompetent at it or who need all manner of special circumstances to be present in order to achieve it, the observation could be correct. The average man is far from being the bull at the gate envisaged in the fantasies of many inexperienced young women.

Self-confidence is necessary for a man to commence intercourse and for a woman to obtain orgasms. Most sexual problems in men are connected with performance and in women with sensation. Due to rearing influences, fear of criticism, distracting worries, anxiety and so on, the pleasure for both sexes can be lost and intercourse may be impossible either to undertake or to complete satisfactorily. With a stranger who will not be seen again and whose opinion, therefore, is of little consequence, a fuller response may be possible than with a known partner whose opinions or criticisms matter. Ideally, the partners should be so self-accepting and other-accepting that total trust and confidence exists thereby permitting the loss of all self-consciousness. Good intercourse should be something like eating good food in that the mechanics underlying it should be only at the edge of consciousness. In a way, really good intercourse is something akin to the pleasure the baby shows and feels during breast-feeding and our behaviour and the noises we tend to make as orgasm approaches are very baby-like. Some women may urinate and some men may expel wind, vomit or even defaecate at orgasm – just like a baby!

For many couples, the best way to conduct intercourse is for the man to

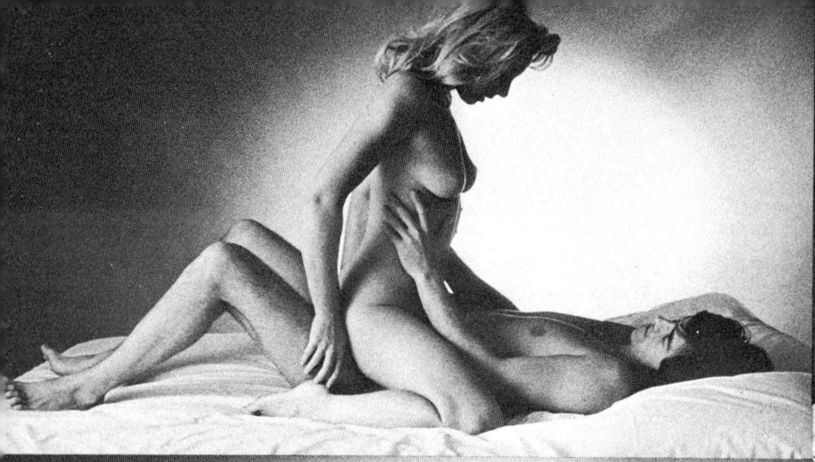

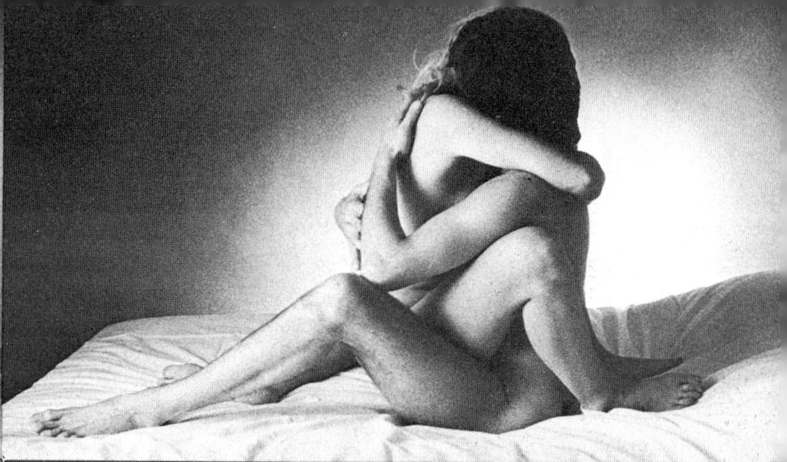

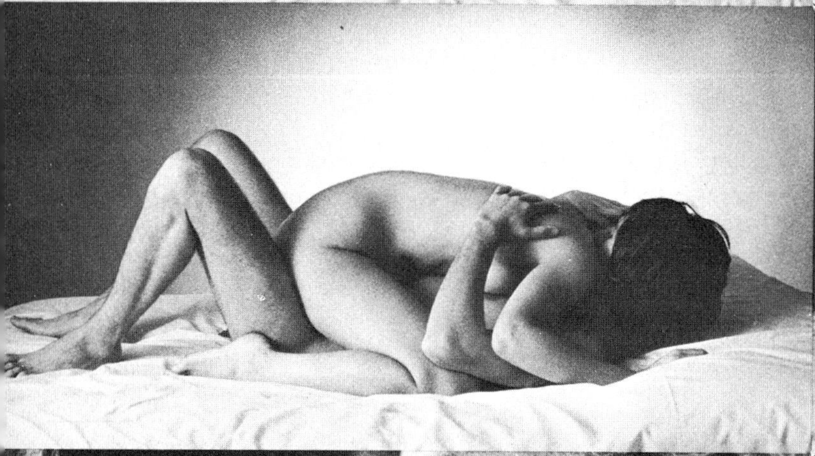

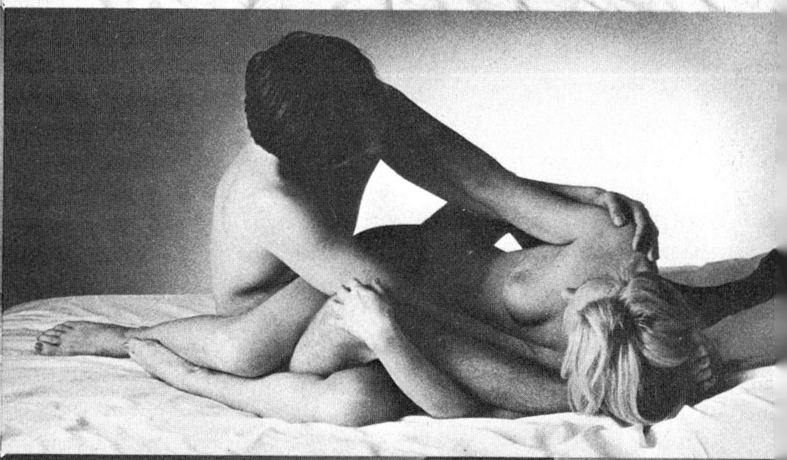

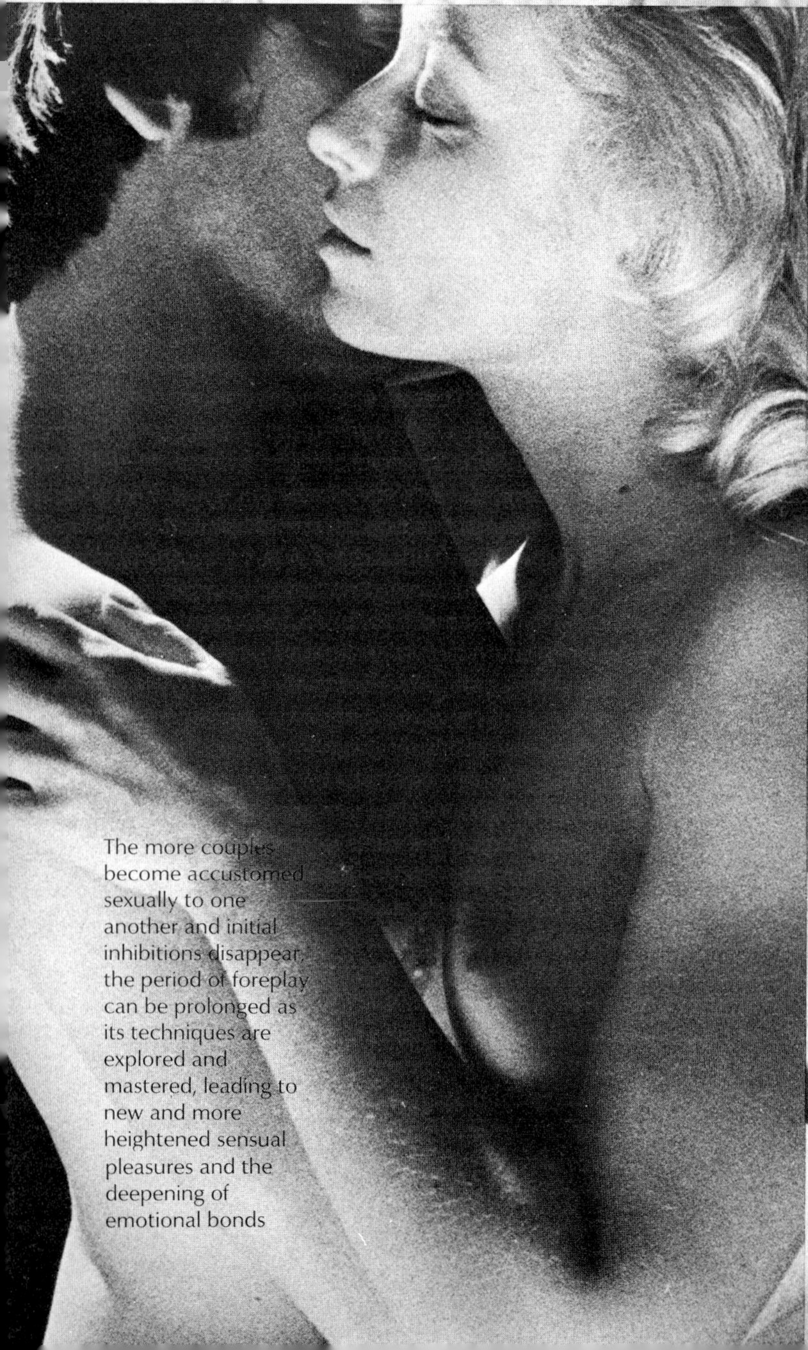

The more couples become accustomed sexually to one another and initial inhibitions disappear, the period of foreplay can be prolonged as its techniques are explored and mastered, leading to new and more heightened sensual pleasures and the deepening of emotional bonds

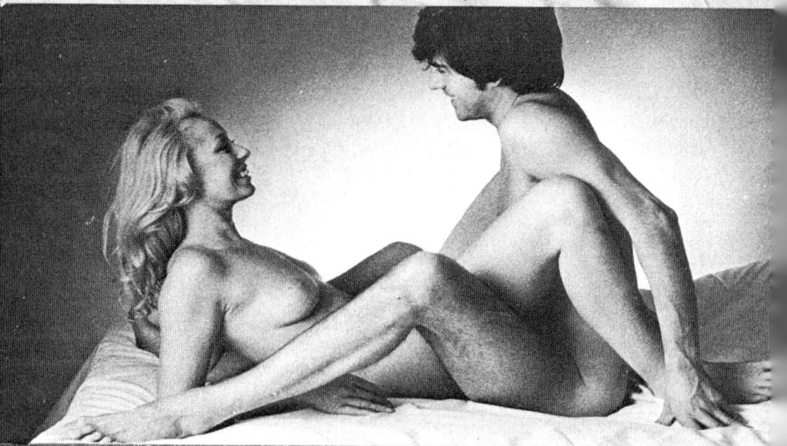

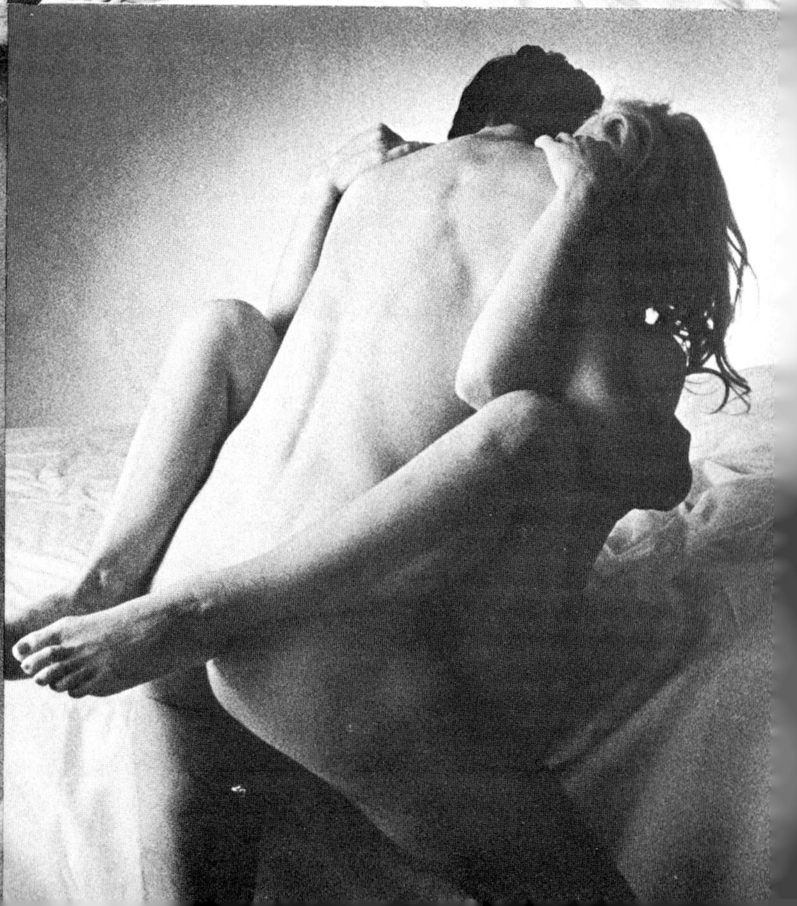

regard the first portion of penetration as a part of foreplay. The aim should be to try to induce one, or more if she is capable of it, orgasms in the woman and then for the man to fully let go of conscious control and really enjoy himself. His abandon and passion may induce further orgasms in the woman. If one coincides with his own so much the better but it is probably counter-productive to strive for simultaneous orgasm. If a woman has a series of orgasms any one, and not just the first, may be the best.

Foreplay, which receives much attention in sex manuals, is a more personal and variable activity than is actual penetration of the vagina. Some men who tend to become over-excited and ejaculate early may wish to avoid or minimize foreplay. Some women dislike foreplay, either because of inhibitions induced about the dirtiness of touching and being touched for pleasure, whereas the penis in the vagina is a necessary duty, or because they wish to reach the stage of penetration quickly or because their partner is so unskillful that the stage may as well be omitted.

Almost any activity preceeding penetration which increases the pleasure the couple derive from the act is of value and constitutes foreplay. Where the two find similar or complementary activities exciting the situation is ideal. Oral elements, such as kissing, sucking, nibbling and licking any area including the genitals, are a component of foreplay for most but not all people. Looking, showing and touching are also components of foreplay and intercourse itself is only an elaborate form of touching. Romantic, in the woman's sense, and loving talk and play are essential for many people, especially at the commencement of the relationship. Their continued incorporation not only into foreplay but into the general life of the couple assist in the creation of more occasions on which intercourse is mutually desired. Intercourse should emerge from a general and continuous background of affection, touching and feeling which can be given and accepted without necessarily implying an instant commitment to intercourse. Many women claim that their men scarcely notice them or show affection except when intercourse is desired. It is understandable that such women may be less than enthusiastic.

Individuals who require something additional to intercourse in order to undertake or enjoy it sometimes cause concern in the partner. Really they want to use tricks to overcome inhibition and these may involve the use of special rituals, the presence of special objects, the woman wearing special clothes or saying or doing special things. In some cases an object such as a glove or a shoe may come to stand for the whole woman and the response is entirely to that object. Women fetishists also exist but the condition is not so noticeable. In a similar way some people require partners of a special type or group activities in order to obtain a full release. Such people are often regarded as being over-sexed but in reality they are inhibited and need an addition to ordinary sex in order to function. Some men and fewer women prefer anal intercourse but this is far from being an invariable sign that the man is really homosexual.

Some men and women have a dread of actual intercourse and become more preoccupied with foreplay activities such as oral sex or mutual masturbation which may come to replace intercourse. Although the term immature is frequently bandied about, such individuals could be reasonably regarded as being immature sexually as are all avoiders of intercourse. Some men are inordinately jealous in a sexual sense of their woman and yet may obtain little value from them sexually. Often such men are found to masturbate to fantasies of watching another man have intercourse with their women whilst they masturbate. This is also the product of an inhibitory fear of intercourse.

Men who wish, no matter how unconsciously, to avoid intercourse in general or with just a particular woman, may respond to the situation with failure to erect, loss of erection as penetration approaches, ejaculation prior to penetration or soon after. Various techniques exist to overcome the anxiety which underlies most such cases, the most famous of which consists of re-education about the acceptability of sex followed by the partner training the man to last longer by recurrently masturbating him almost to the point of orgasm and then enforcing a pause in which the tip of the penis may be pinched between the thumb and first two fingers placed at the level of the rim. In this way, the man is taught to control himself. Many men with premature ejaculation experience the reverse condition, that is difficulty or inability, to ejaculate in the vagina when successfully treated for the original condition. This is not the product of any desire to avoid inducing pregnancy but is probably something to do with guilt about earlier wishes to possess the mother.

Some women encounter difficulties of a similar nature. They may not lubricate or lubrication may cease as soon as penetration approaches or soon after it commences. Others involuntarily contract the muscles around the vaginal entrance making penetration painful or impossible. A part of the changes in growing up is to amend the image that exists in the mind as to what the body is like. The task requires some effort at puberty, especially in girls, since the body is rapidly changing. Due to earlier inhibitions, which may or may not be connected with the father, the girl may not, as it were, be able to admit to the existence of the vagina and a man trying to insert his penis is perceived more as trying to push a knife through an intact body surface. Such women may be sexually competent in all other ways and may freely masturbate, but only by using the vulva and not the vagina.

Considering the immense pleasures associated with intercourse, in order to ensure its occurrence, and the value it has for the man-woman relationship, it is regrettable that it evokes so much secrecy and is surrounded with so many anxieties of various types in our society. Some of the justifications which have been advanced for the massive suppression of sexuality over the last two thousand years are that it has prevented women from becoming unwantedly pregnant and has attempted to ensure that every child has two parents to care for it. Such problems do not seem to have been any more common in the ancient world, which did not require so much restraint, than in the present one and yet the price which has been paid is to make sexual incompetence and lack of sexual enjoyment widespread.

WHAT IS NUTRITION?

Too much over-refined food and too little nutritious food is rapidly finding a way into all our diets. This is causing a major health problem throughout the western world. We seem unaware of and disinterested in what constitutes a properly balanced diet. But it is not too late to learn. There is no need to give up our favourite foods but it is necessary to recognize the ill effects of refining, processing, overcooking and the convenience packaging of many staple foodstuffs. Food is exciting as well as essential but care and thought must be applied to choosing your diet.

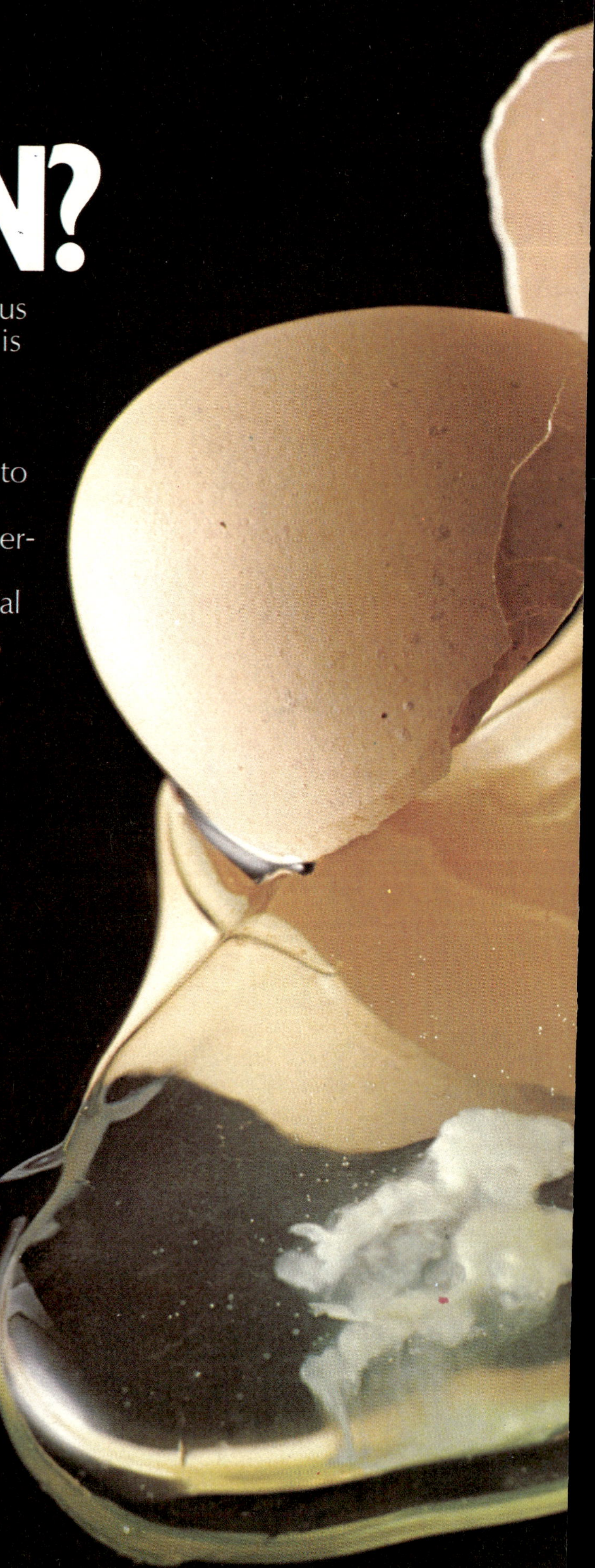

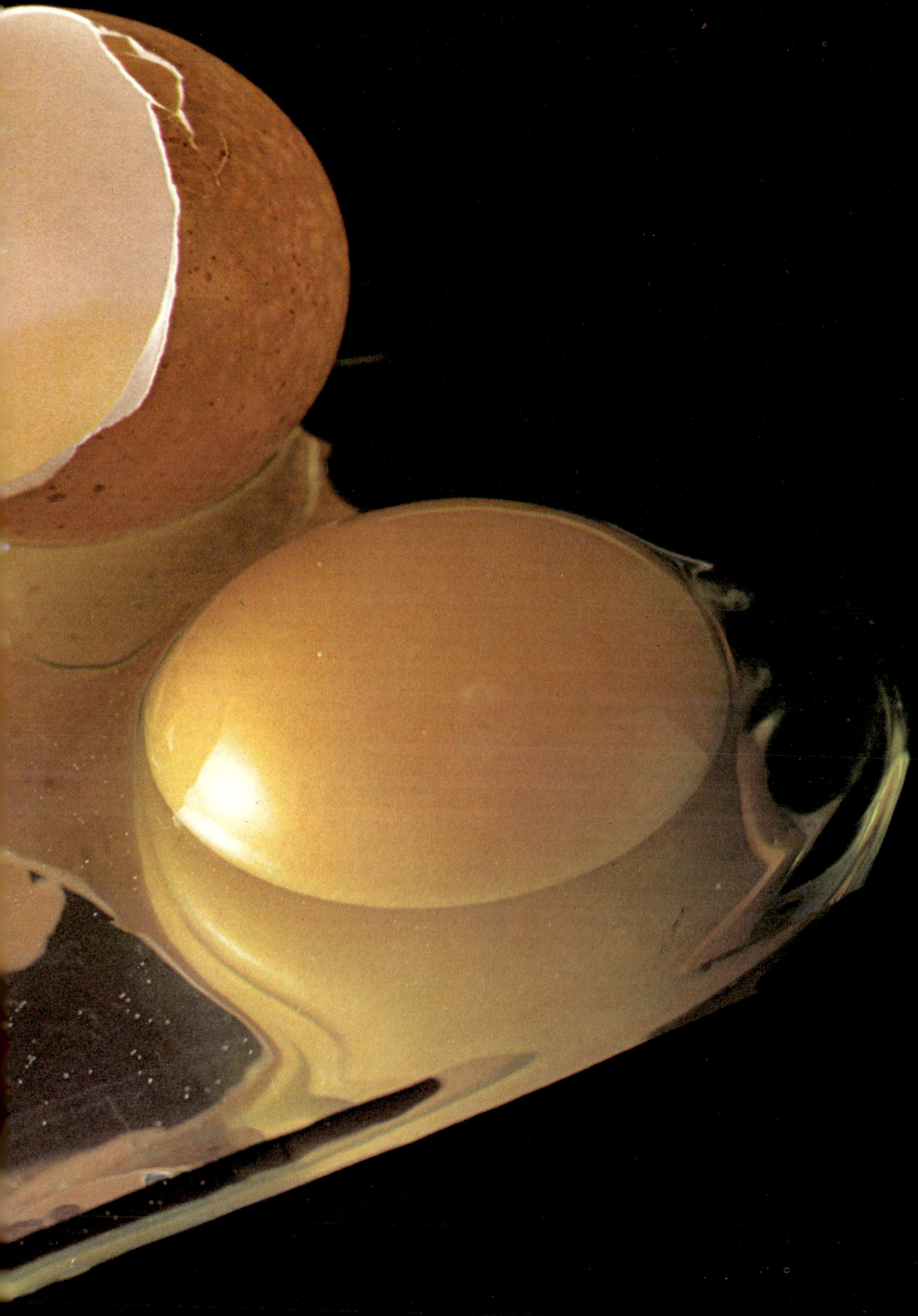

Eating Habits

We too often think of diets as the restrictive menus that slimmers mean when they say 'I'm on a diet'. Actually we are all on a diet, because diet means the type and pattern of food eaten. Centuries ago, diet referred to the whole way of life. Now it is restricted to our way of eating although this is influenced by our way of life. Whatever combinations go to make up our diet, it should be adequate for good health, be pleasing and palatable, and serve the social and psychological roles food has in our particular life and culture.

There is a great variety of different diets in the world, based on different staple foods, such as rice, corn, wheat or potatoes. Many factors influence the type of diet adopted, but three are particularly important: availability, wealth and tradition. Availability of foods is determined by what can be grown or imported: the former is still important for most people in the world, but is less so for the rich countries which can provide any kind of food, for a price. This introduces the question of wealth: a food may be physically available, but is it economically available, can people afford to buy it? The poorer the person, the more restricted are both the type and amount of food available. Tradition and belief also play an important role in what we regard as food. The British tend to avoid horses, Hindus do not eat beef, the Jews eschew pork, and so on. Tradition also affects the way we deal with staples. Wheat, for example, can be made into breads or pastas.

A wide range of different foods can be combined to give a nutritionally adequate diet. For most people in the world, that is inhabitants of poor countries, the choice is limited to what will grow where they live. For most people in the industrialized countries there is a great variety of fresh and processed food to choose from, particularly over the last 20 years as the amount of processed foods has mushroomed. Paradoxical as it may seem this great abundance has led to problems. With so many processed foods, it is possible to pass over the basic food groups and have an unbalanced diet. There is also the problem of overconsumption of food which leads many to be overweight. Our ability to buy food and satisfy our desire has increased while our capacity to absorb it has not. In most wealthy countries the actual need for food has fallen as work becomes less strenuous, often involving little physical activity.

Increased affluence has been accompanied by an increased consumption of meat, fat, eggs and dairy products. Partly this is a learned response: we were taught by our parents that these were good foods to eat; it

In different countries and among differing cultures there exist a wide range of foods which can be satisfactorily combined in order to provide the appropriate diet – diets that combine nutritional value with appetisingness. These dishes do not transgress ethical lores

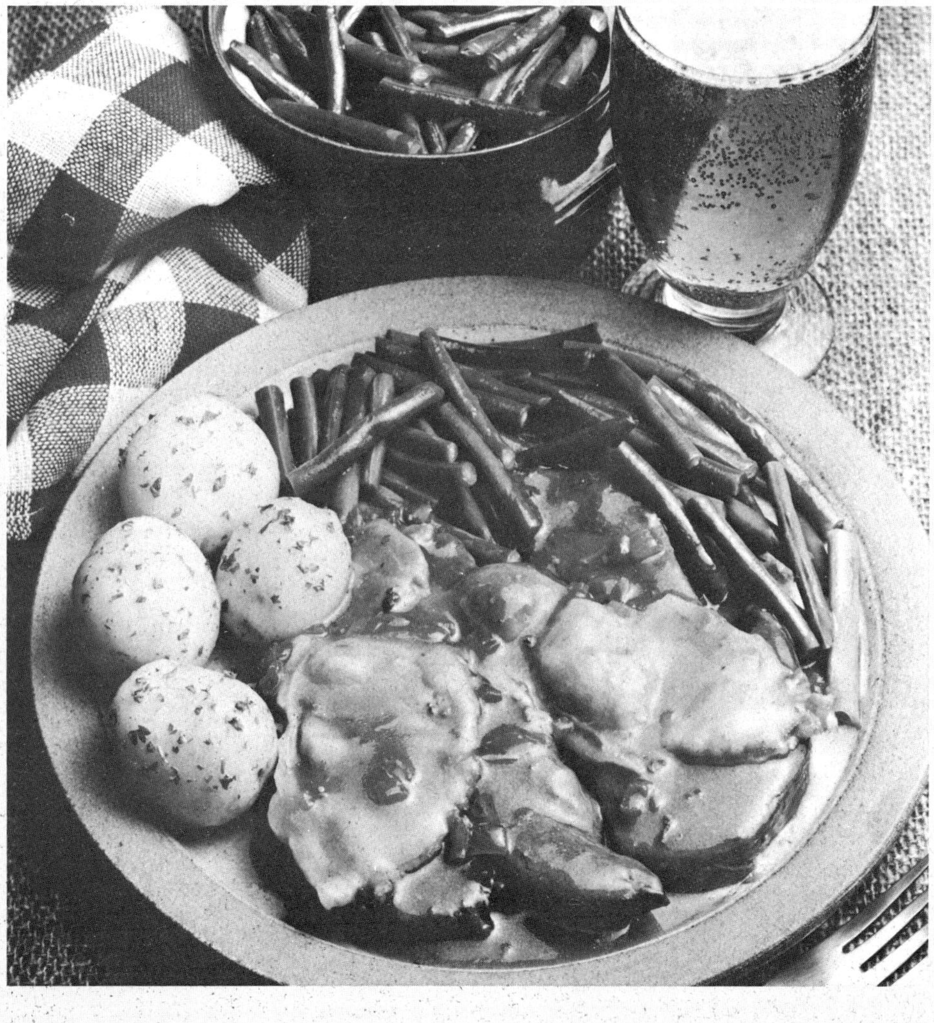

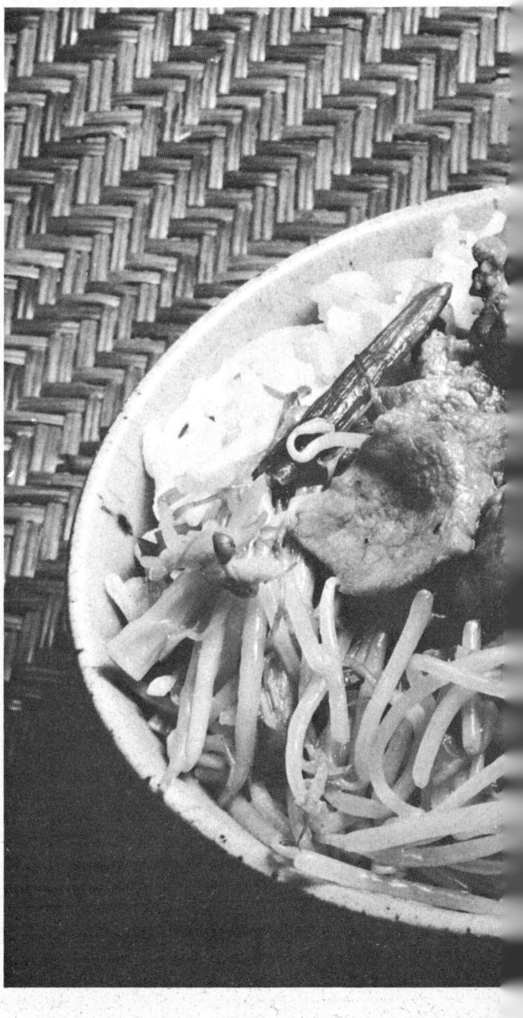

has also been well supplemented by advertizing. In the past when these foods were relatively more expensive and diets were built around large quantities of staple foods like bread, potatoes and vegetables, most people could only afford a little of the expensive meat, butter, eggs etc. With increased affluence many can afford them and with both a liking for them and the feeling that if a little is good for you, more is better, consumption has increased. Some authorities are now saying that this is not a good thing. The modern diet in industrialized countries, as found in America and Europe, may be partly responsible for the prevailing types of diseases like cancer, heart-disease, diabetes and many others which people in these countries increasingly suffer from.

Many people have become concerned about additives in food. The need for additives, which are being used on a growing scale, has increased as the nature of the food system has changed, from a locally-based farmer/market/consumer nexus to a highly mechanized industry, with different crops increasingly concentrated in certain areas. As the length of the chain from agricultural supply industry, through the farmer to the food processor and manufacturer, distributor, supermarket and finally customer has increased, so has the need to package food, make it look appetizing and ensure that it keeps for longer. The food that the farmer produces is turned into an increasing number of products, which often bear little resemblance to the original, some being made entirely in the factory. All this processing means that different chemicals have to be added during production. Sometimes the chemicals are needed to preserve the food so it will keep until it reaches the consumer, others to enable the technology to work, and others to give it a particular colour, flavour, texture and so on. Consequently there are about 1,000 chemicals which can be added to food during processing, the exact number depending upon the particular country's food laws. You can avoid most additives, but not the chemicals used in agriculture, if you do not eat processed foods. However, there is unlikely to be a general reduction in their use without a drastic change in the food production system.

Leaving additives aside, how do we tell if the food we eat will provide an adequate healthy diet? There is no one perfect diet but any diet should contain enough of the nutrients our bodies need for growth and maintenance. A good diet will contain a mixture of foods, drawn from the four food groups which contain the nutrients we require. Our precise diets will vary depending upon where we are, the beliefs we hold and what our circumstances are and what kind of work we do. The right balance of energy intake varies, favouring either side of the needs of the mythical 'average' person. If no particular element is missing, our diet will give us the basis of a healthy life.

Thus an English meal may consist of liver, bacon and potatoes, the nutritional requirements of the Chinese may be satisfied with fried pork and bean shoots, while the Italians are able to get what they want primarily from pasta dishes such as spaghetti

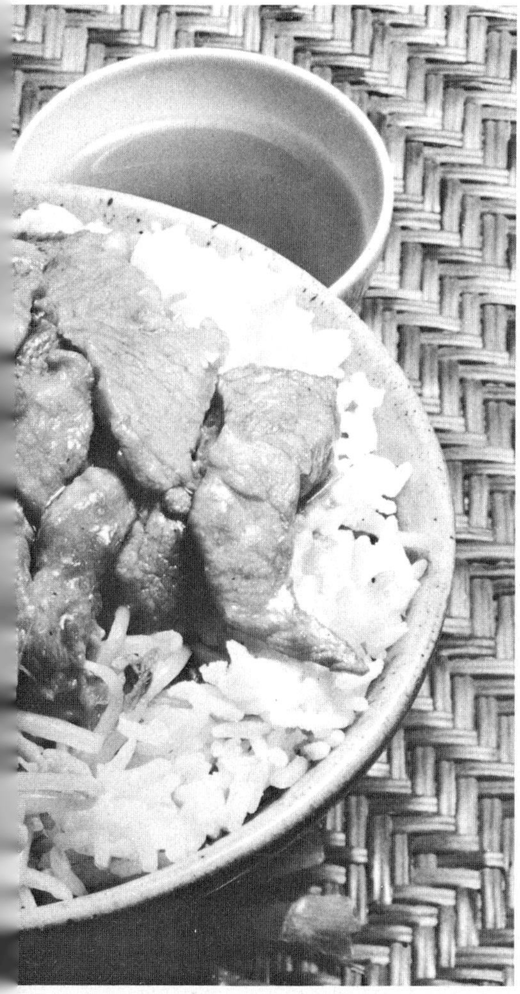

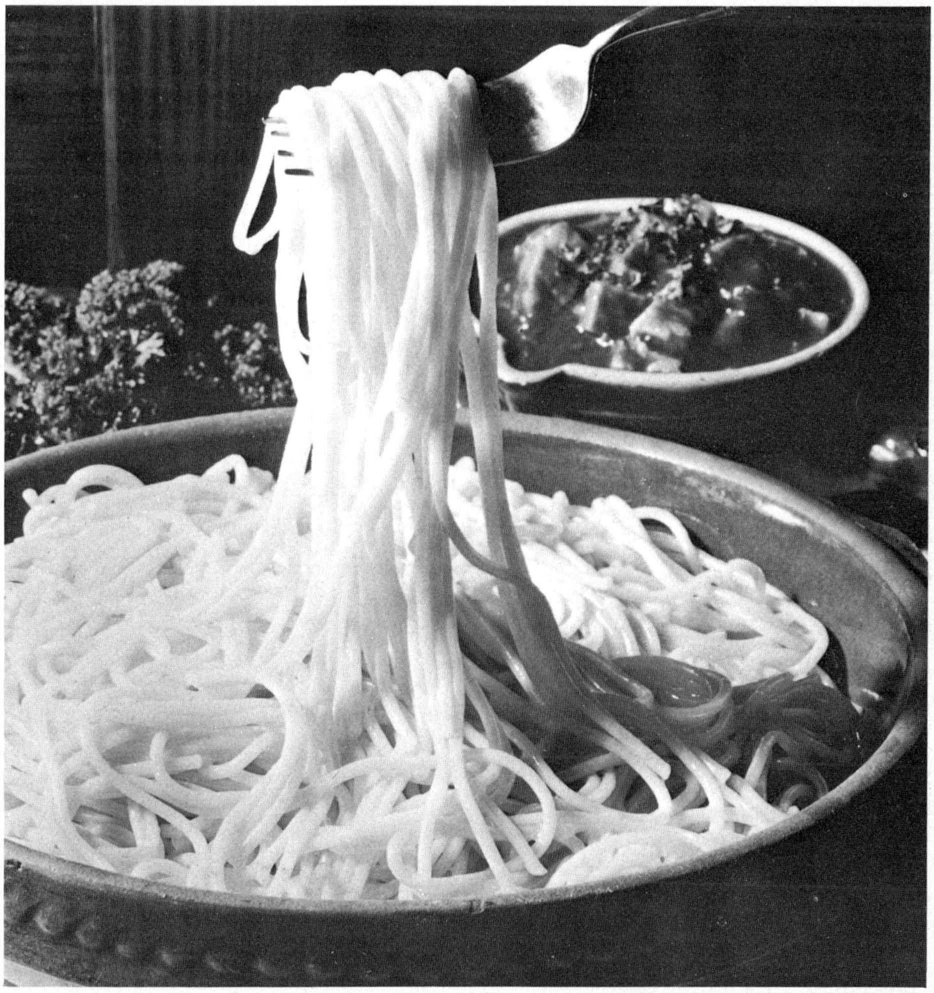

Energy

We need food to stay alive but what does food do? Food gives the body the energy it needs to keep functioning. Energy enables all the different processes to go on in the body – from breathing to running to repairing to repelling infections. Food also provides the many building materials that are needed for growth and repair.

The energy a food provides is usually described in terms of the calories it provides. A calorie is a measure of energy: the amount of energy required to raise the temperature of one gram of water 1°C. Although in most popular literature the word calorie is used to describe the energy value of food it should really be called the kilocalorie or kcal as it is 1000 calories, that is, it will raise the temperature of one kilogram of water 1°C. We can get some idea of what this means if we consider what just one American teaspoon of butter can do. It contains 33kcal, enough energy to raise the temperature of one kilogram of 1 litre of water 33°C. Metrically, this energy value is expressed in kilojoules (kJ). A kilojoule is 4.18kcal.

Whatever the measure, the energy in food is released in the body to enable the thousands of different biochemical reactions to take place and to keep us warm. The various components of food contain different amounts of energy. One gram of pure carbohydrate or protein provides about 4kcal; one gram of fat, however, contains about 9kcal. If we know how much of these food components we are eating we can calculate the amount of energy the body is supplied with. For example, if a day's food contained 50g of protein, 100g of fat and 300g of carbohydrate we would get 4×50 kcals from the protein, 9×100 from the fat and 4×300 from the carbohydrate, i.e. a total of 2300kcal.

Average energy requirements for males and females at different ages can be found from tables, but they only give an approximate guide. This is because the recommended energy intakes represent an average and like and any average there is a whole range of values on either side. For example, experiments have shown that energy intake in women can range from 1900 to 4400kcal, with the woman remaining healthy and maintaining their correct body weight. There can, then, be very considerable individual variation in energy requirements. For the other nutrients the recommended intakes are based on a value which meets the needs of over 90 per cent of the population.

Energy requirement depends upon what we do, our activity, and how our bodies function when we are at rest. The resting energy requirement varies from person to person. It is the amount of energy the body needs to maintain body functions while we are at rest.

The amount of energy that can be provided by a food source will vary greatly from one type of food to another so that, in this case, the calorific value of the piece of steak is equivalent to the value of all the apples surrounding it

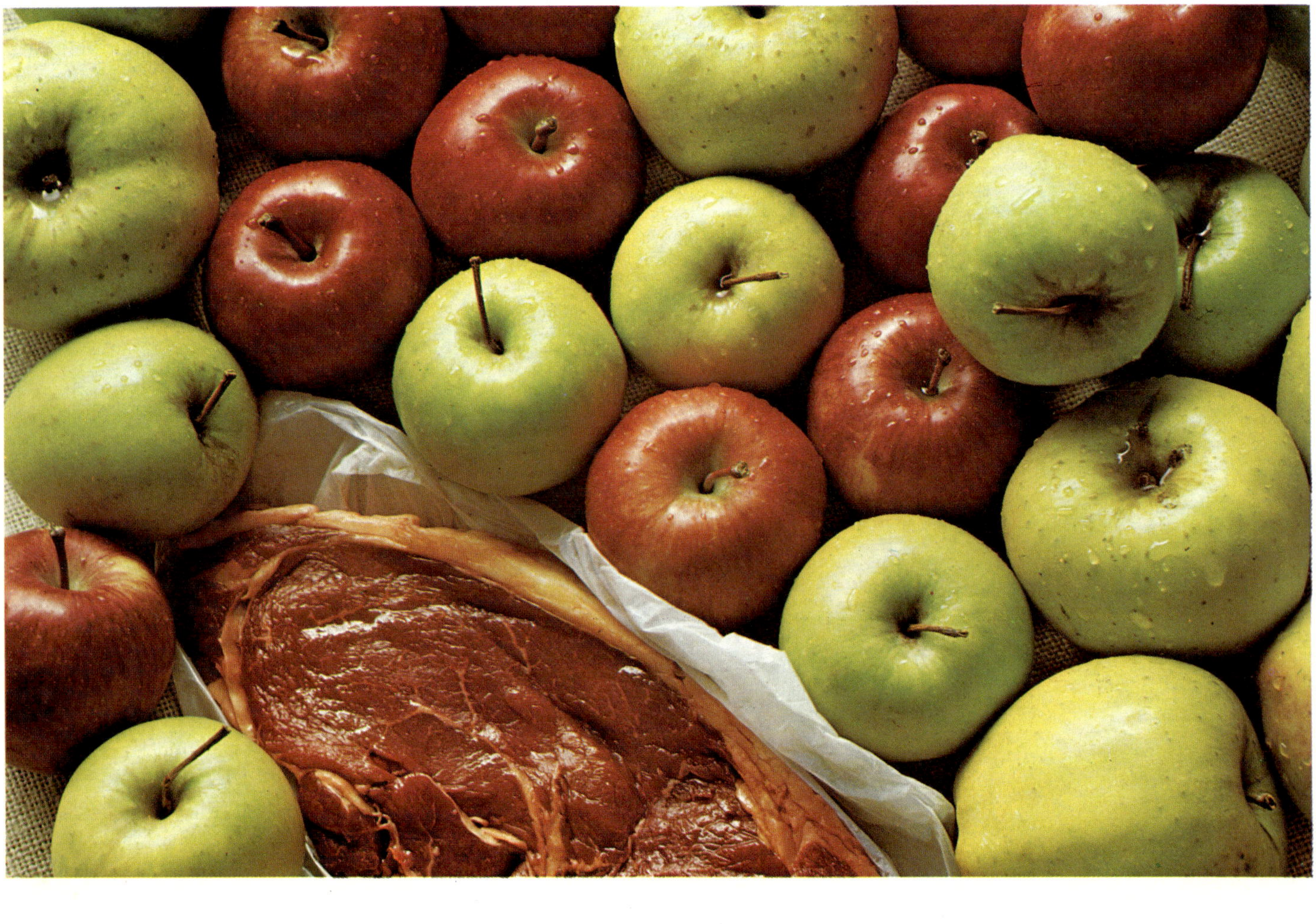

This includes breathing, blood circulation, cell functioning, body temperature maintenance, and the functioning of vital organs and glands. The speed at which the body operates and requires energy to maintain itself is called the metabolic rate.

The activities we pursue also affect the amount of energy we require. If we are sitting at a desk all day, doing little walking, sport or other exercise, our requirements will be much less than if we were doing heavy manual work. Typing rapidly on a manual typewriter uses up about 1kcal per hour for every kilogramme of body weight, that is 60kcal per hour for a 60kg man, whereas playing table tennis takes up 4.4kcal, boxing 11.4, driving 0.9 and walking at 3mph 2kcal. The amount of food we eat also affects the metabolic rate. It has been shown that if food intake is increased on a regular basis then the metabolic rate increases both at rest and in activity. This increase in energy expenditure means that people who eat a lot of food do not necessarily become fat. Conversely, when people regularly consume small amounts of food, energy expenditure is lowered. However, there are limits to the body's ability to increase or decrease the metabolic rate.

Generally speaking, if the energy used over a period of time equals what has been taken in then body weight is maintained. If more is eaten than the body can adapt to using we gain weight; if less we lose weight.

As an example let us look at an 18 year old woman, 5′3″ tall. Her average resting metabolism might require 1475kcal. If she were a student, her activities could be divided up between dressing, eating, driving, studying, walking, watching TV and sleeping. Her activity requirement would be about 550kcal, giving her a total energy requirement of 2025kcal per day. But, even if she did these same things for the next 50 years her energy requirement would not remain the same. This is because the energy required for body functions decrease with age. As we get older we need less food to maintain the same weight. Unless we realize this then weight gain is almost inevitable if we keep eating as much as we did at the age of twenty five.

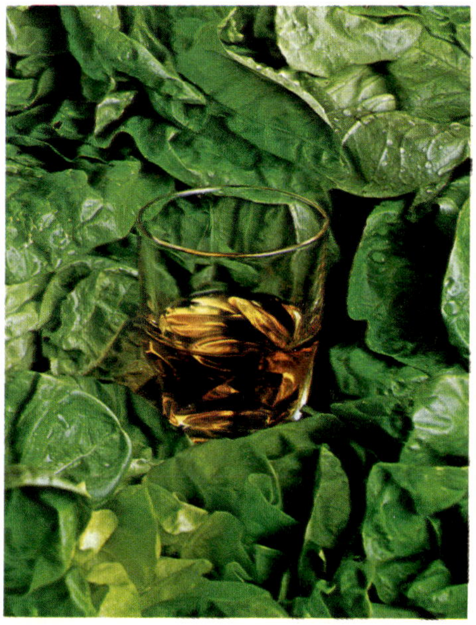

This is an extreme example of the amount of energy supplied by different foods, the calorific value of many lettuces is equalled by one glass of spirits

Fish is a source of food that is high in the amount of energy it provides, but a few chocolate biscuits can have the same calorific value. The essential difference is in the nutritional value, the benefit lies with those who chose fish

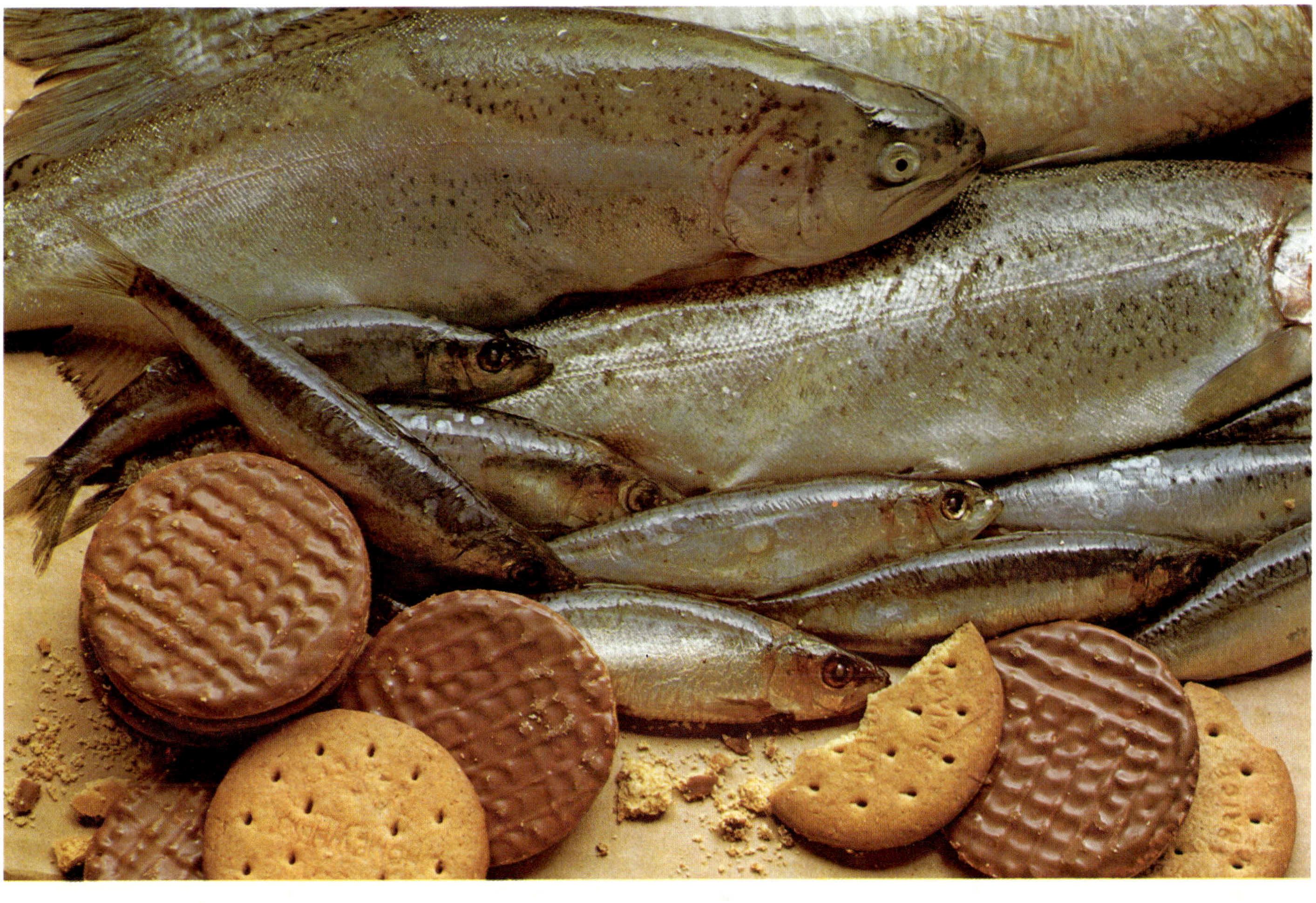

Diets

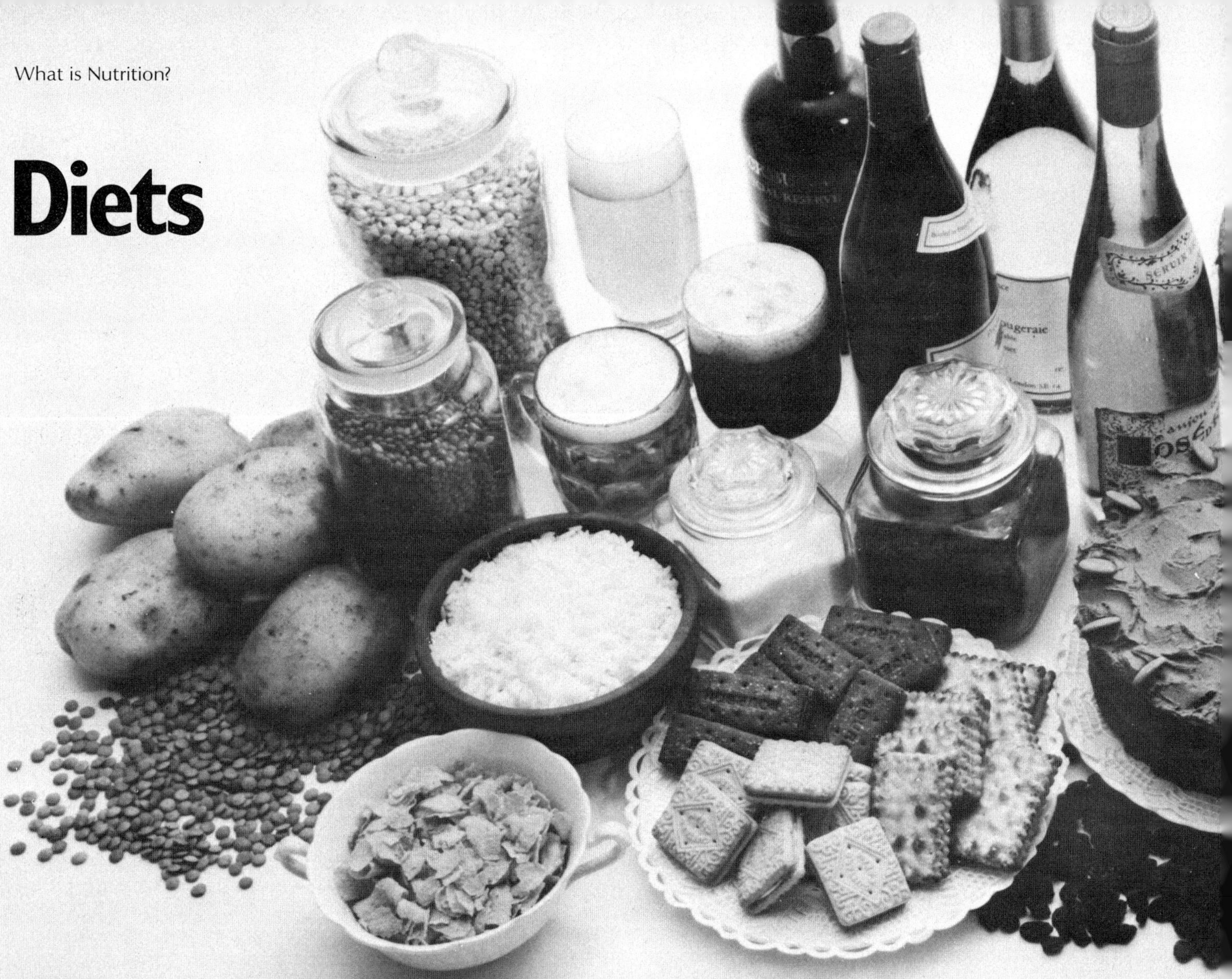

Nothing is simpler for anyone to understand than the external differences between people. From our earliest moments we learn to make assessments according to external characteristics such as facial features and shape; up to a point we judge the attractiveness of people in this way. It is not surprising therefore that we are anxious to have as attractive an outside form as possible and we try to project our inner feelings onto the image that confronts those around us. This means that if we are dissatisfied with something in ourselves we might think this can be cured by changing our external image—by fitting our figures into a fashionable mold we will also become more acceptable as personalities! It also explains why sometimes psychology and feelings are so intimately bound up with patterns of eating.

This emotional component to dieting makes the subject very complicated and means that hard and fast rules cannot really be laid down. However, for the moment let us stick to the purely physical aspects of the affair. As already stated, bodies differ tremendously in shape—some human beings are tall and thin, others rounded and dumpy and nothing science has yet devised appears able to change these parameters. It is certain that these different physical types use food differently and that, as a result, fat people do not necessarily consume more than thin individuals. But, it is still true that the overweight eat more than they need. The plump had an evolutionary advantage at one time—they put on weight as fat whereas the lean types put on any excess (and to a much smaller extent) as muscle—this gives the spare tyre individuals greater efficiency when they suddenly need extra supplies ie. in times of great physical activity when there is a deficient food supply.

Thin individuals are able to double their intake of calories over many months and they merely put on a little and then maintain their weight at a steady – somewhat higher – level. They seem to lose the excess fairly naturally once the food intake approaches a usual level. This has been shown conclusively in various clinical studies. The overweight types, however, enjoy no such luck. Their weight might also rise to a certain level and then climb no higher but it seems to creep to a much more unacceptable point before it levels off. The reasons behind this difference are not clear—but almost certainly they are many and varied and as individual as people themselves. In some cases it could be that only a certain amount of food is absorbed from the intestines, the rest passing straight through. Or else, only the required amount is metabolised inside the system, the rest being discarded again. Other possibilities are the increased activity that is noted among thin individuals—so that they use up surplus energy by a myriad of little movements, such as waving their arms about in conversation. Then there is the whole question of heat production and metabolic rate; almost certainly these play a considerable part in the whole story.

Eating in itself puts our temperature up ie. the sheer calorific value of the food produces heat as a by-product

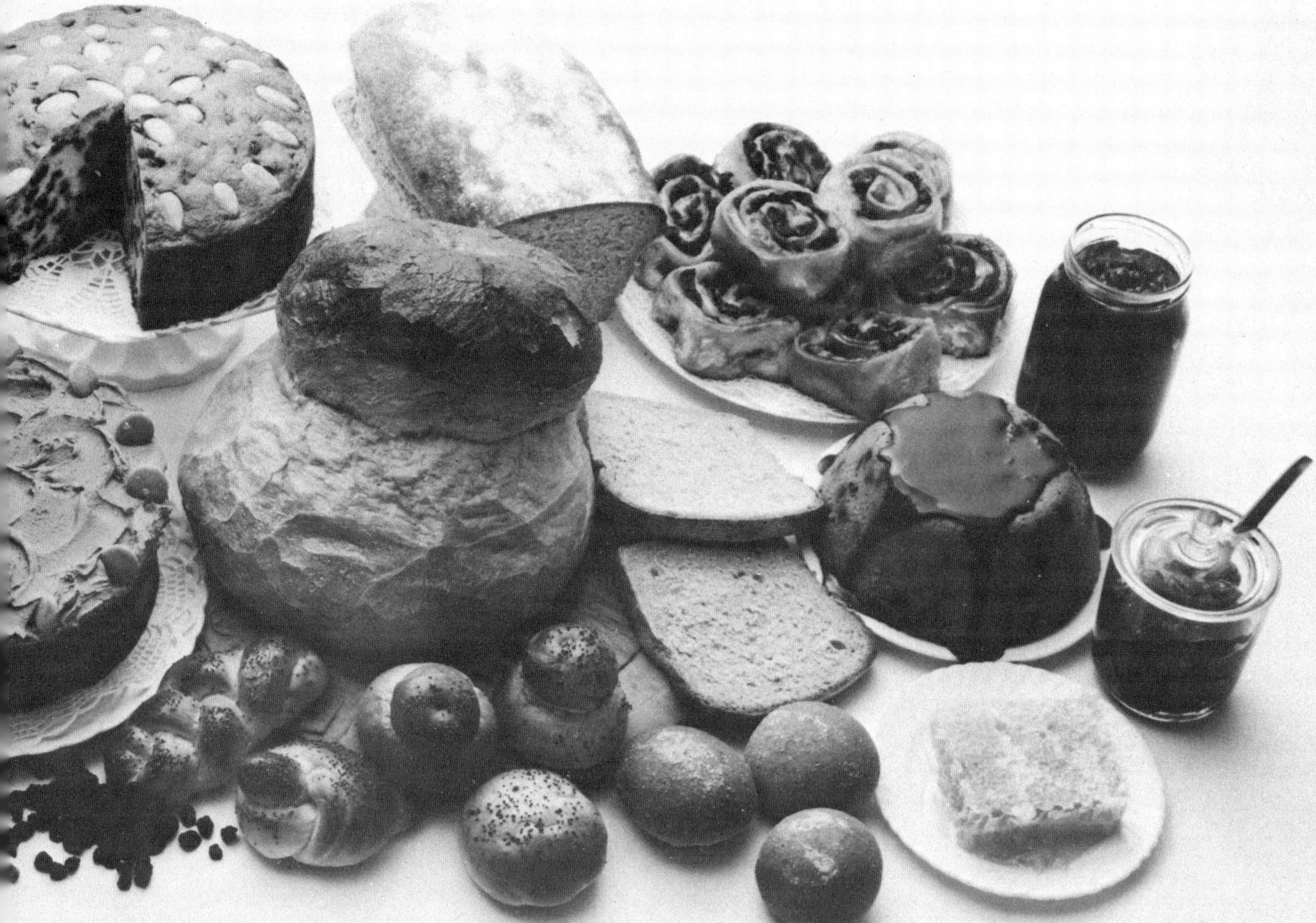

Here are a selection of foodstuffs in which we constantly indulge but are, by and large, superfluous to our dietary requirements. Eating too much potato, rice, bread, cream, biscuits, cake, and currants is inadvisable. The very high carbohydrate content of these foods means that a large amount of energy would have to be burnt off to balance the body; so unless strenuous exercise is taken a weight problem will result. Alcohol in the form of beer, lager and wine, is an extremely pleasant and useful addition to any meal. But, again, the carbohydrate content is high so these drinks should be taken in moderation.

and often makes us feel more comfortable in cool surroundings—this also explains a relative lack of appetite in warm weather. Exercise also, by mobilising all our chemical production capabilities and getting the bodily systems moving, puts up the body's temperature—as a result, exercise can reduce appetite by warming us up. Some people always produce more heat than others even when they are asleep, this is known as basal metabolic rate and it has considerable value as a crude measure of the differences between various individuals in energy production.

Metabolic rate can be conceived as amount of energy turn over—rather like the performance of an engine is measured; and we work it out by determining the amount of heat produced by the person's body during a certain time span. Obviously every bit of work done requires an appropriate amount of energy which must come, ultimately, from food; just as the car needs a certain amount of petrol for every mile travelled; however, in the human beings there is great variability, just as there is with cars and number of miles per gallon. Efficiency varies enormously and cannot easily be correlated accordint to the size of the person and the amount of labour undertaken. When reducing diets are considered exercise generally tends to be undervalued: comments are made suggesting that it takes so many miles to walk off the calories resulting from a glass of beer, or it is said that activity increases the appetite and thus results in a greater intake of calories than ever. These comments may be true as far as they go but they ignore other facets of the question which are now thought to be important. For instance, exercise makes you feel warmer thus eliminating one of the reasons for eating; it also puts up the basal metabolic rate for many hours, possibly days afterwards, thereby increasing your ability to dispose of any excess calories for a prolonged period. Exercise stimulates the whole metabolism making it more efficient and allows the appetite-regulating mechanisms to become more efficient along with the other 'production lines'. It is as if the appetite control device situated in the brain, known as the appestat, along with other parts of the machinery, had been well oiled.

It is still true in every single case that if you are overweight you have—at some stage of your life—eaten too much. If your weight is static, then at this point you are eating merely enough to keep things steady. And this does not have to be an enormous amount.

Protein

In any discussion of nutrition, protein is usually the dominant theme. Certainly it is essential in the diet, but so too are all the other nutrients. What is so special about protein? It is the very stuff of life: protein provides the essential amino acids the body needs to build and maintain itself. We must ensure a balanced intake of all the essential amino acids from the food we eat, as the body cannot originate them itself. Some proteins only contain six or seven essential acids and must be supplemented by other protein containing the missing material, or there will be a protein deficiency. Even if only one essential amino acid is missing, the body will not be able to make the proteins it requires.

Proteins are large complex organic molecules containing carbon, hydrogen and oxygen, nitrogen and sometimes sulphur. There are a wide variety of proteins, each with a specific function to fulfil, but they are all made up of different combinations of 22 amino acids, the body's basic building blocks. Eight of these are essential in the adult diet, nine for children. Proteins are described as simple, in which case they only contain amino acids, or conjugated, where a simple protein is joined to one or more other molecules to make a complex. These conjugated proteins are vital to life and include those that contain the genetic code, DNA (deoxyribonucleic acid) and the haemoglobin in the blood. Proteins are also sometimes referred to as native or denatured. Native means they are as found in their natural state, whereas denatured means they have been altered. For example, the white of a raw egg is a native protein but when it is cooked it becomes solid and opaque and is denatured. The protein still contains the number of amino acids but its molecular shape has changed and this gives it different properties.

Unlike carbohydrate or fat, protein digestion begins in the stomach. The large molecules are broken down into their constituents by enzymes. Enzymes are themselves proteins which the body has made from the amino acids derived from food. Each enzyme operates in a very specific manner and will only split up a particular part of the protein molecule. Splitting up protein is a long job and is not completed until the protein reaches the small intestine, where the amino acids are absorbed into the bloodstream and distributed around the body.

When they reach the cells the amino acids can be recombined in different ways to make the kind of protein the cell needs. Some proteins are used to form the nails and hair, others become part of haemoglobin, some act as hormones which regulate the body functions, others build the flesh, and yet others make the en-

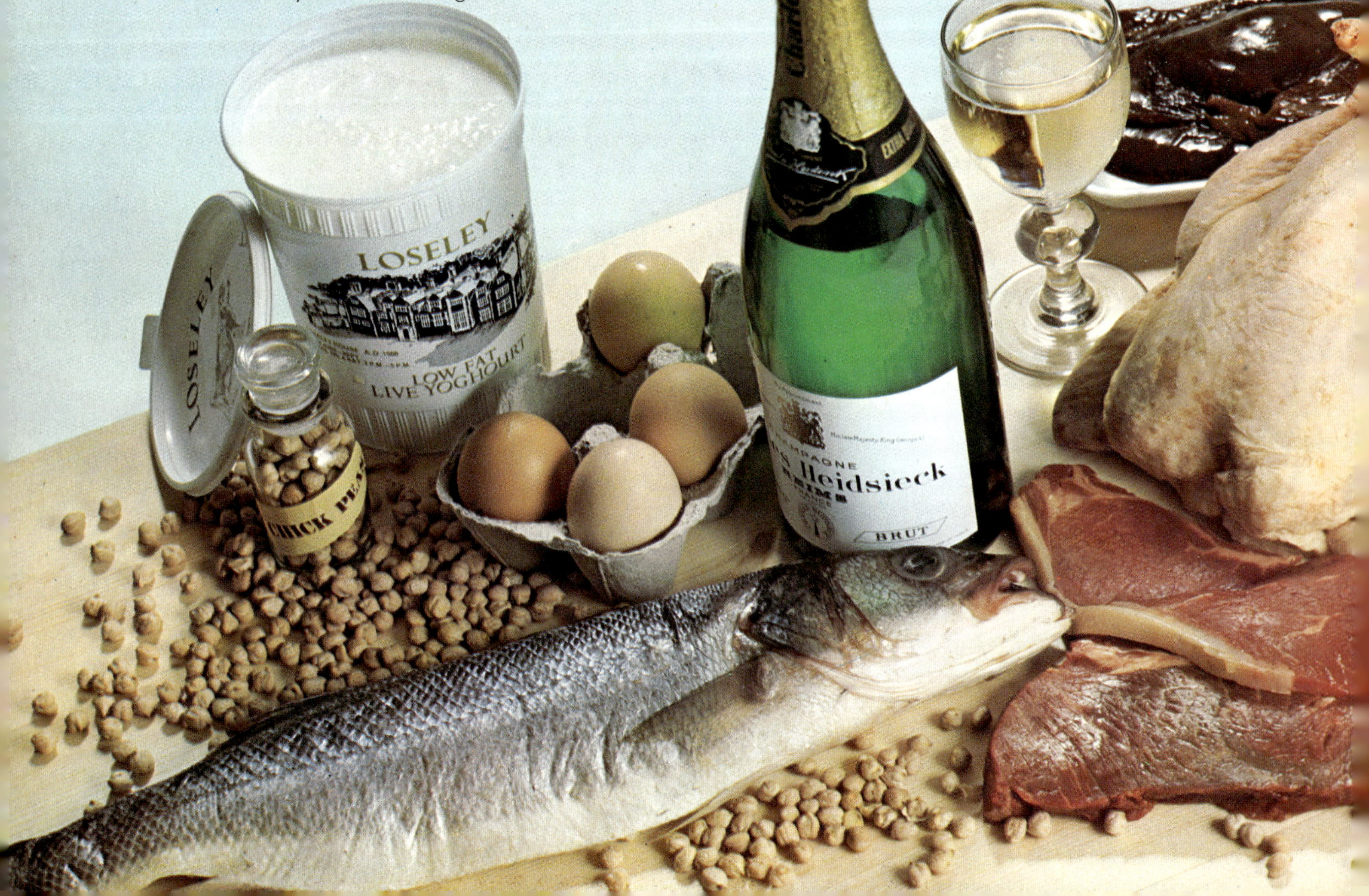

Water

Water is a nutrient but perhaps because it is so obvious and easily obtainable we tend to forget about it. Actually we can do without food for weeks and still live but if we are deprived of water for more than a few days we will die. Over half of our body weight is water. Some 40 per cent is the water that is in the cells and another 15 per cent is water in the bone, connective tissues and bloodstream.

Water is essential to most of the body's functions: nearly all activity in the body takes place in a solution; water makes the bloodstream and the lymphatic system efficient transport systems; it lubricates the joints; it plays a part in the reactions needed for digestion and elimination; it helps to regulate body temperature through sweating, and it is important in maintaining the structure of the cells. Excess water is lost through perspiration, breathing, and in the urine and faeces. As water passes out of the body in the urine it takes with it other waste products which if left in the body would build up to toxic levels. How much water we take in varies greatly from person to person although a rough guide is 1 litre of water for every 1000kcal eaten. Much of the water is consumed in beverages like tea, coffee, beer and soup, but most food contains surprisingly large amounts of water. Bread, for instance, is over one third water, most apparently dry foods contain 25-50 per cent and fruits and vegetables may be over 90 per cent water. It is safe to say that you can never have too much water, but too little may lead to all kinds of disease.

zymes, which regulate the body's biochemistry. Proteins help in maintaining the fluid balance in the cells and in keeping the body slightly alkaline, and are intimately involved in tissue production and maintenance, which is one reason why growing children and pregnant and lactating women need extra protein.

Body protein must be replaced all the time: some is lost in the nails, hair and skin; old body protein is broken down and new material substituted; nitrogen is made into urea and excreted in the urine; and carbon, hydrogen and oxygen are burnt off to produce energy and warmth. In the end, the protein we eat is used to provide energy. If insufficient energy is provided by the diet, any protein that is eaten will not be used to make tissue and other vital substances, but will immediately be transformed into energy.

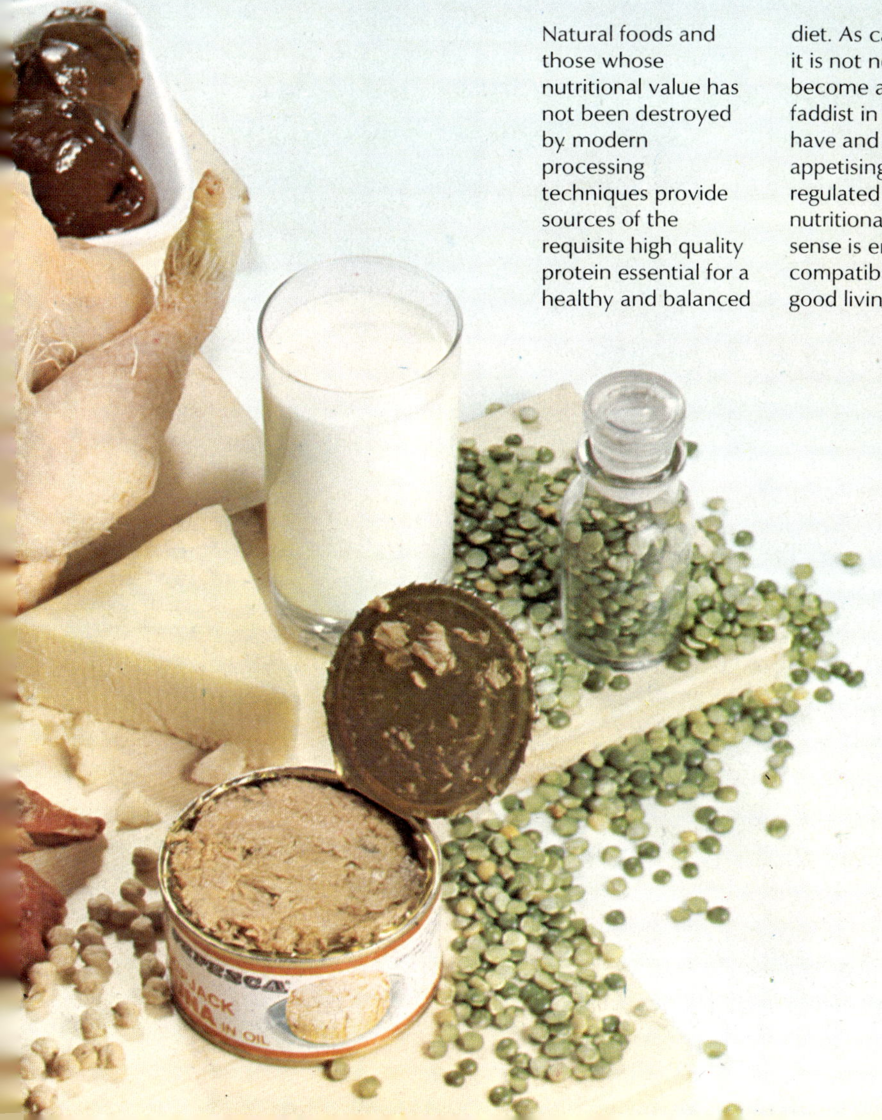

Natural foods and those whose nutritional value has not been destroyed by modern processing techniques provide sources of the requisite high quality protein essential for a healthy and balanced diet. As can be seen, it is not necessary to become a food faddist in order to have and enjoy a full, appetising and regulated diet – nutritional good sense is eminently compatible with good living

Fortunately, there are many sources of protein and a complete intake of amino acids can be obtained from both animal and plant foods. Animal foods – meat, eggs, milk and milk products, fish – are sometimes said to provide complete protein because they contain all the essential amino acids. Plant sources are sometimes called incomplete because one or two amino acids are missing. However, a complete range of amino acids can easily be obtained from a vegetarian diet. Different plants have different amino acids missing from their protein, so if properly selected they can be mixed to complement each other. Thus if grains are mixed with pulses such as rice with lentils, all the amino acids will be provided. No foods, except sugar and salt, are single substances. They are complex compounds containing varying proportions of protein, fat and carbohydrates. Most carbohydrate foods, especially those containing starch, supply certain amounts of protein. Legumes (peas, beans, pulses) and nuts are rich in protein and there is a significant amount found in the various grains. Measured as a percentage of the dry weight, rice contains 7-8 per cent protein, maize 9-10 per cent and wheat 10-12 per cent. Potatoes, usually thought of as a source of carbohydrate, are also a source of protein, a raw potato containing about 2 per cent protein. In fact, a daily diet for a woman which contained about 3kg of potatoes, a cabbage, water and sunshine would be quite adequate nutritionally, but not a very exciting prospect.

Carbohydrates

As every dieter knows, carbohydrates are sugars and starches. Most of the sugars consumed in the industrialized countries are refined from sugar beet or cane. The sugar we eat comes in the form of sucrose, the pure white substance used to sweeten drinks and cakes. This is the only pure compound in the diet that is eaten in quantity, either on its own or in other foodstuffs such as jams, candy, and biscuits. Many vegetables and fruits contain small amounts of various sugars, and honey is mainly a mixture of glucose and fructose. The major part of the starch in the diet comes from cereal grains, both from the grains themselves, notably rice, corn and oats, and the flour derived from them and subsequently used for baking. Potatoes and other tubers, seeds, legumes and other vegetables all contain varying quantities of starch and the non-digestable fibrous form of carbohydrate, cellulose, which is essential for healthy digestion.

Why do we need carbohydrate? Primarily carbohydrate is a source of energy but it also plays other roles in the running of the body, such as fat metabolism. The chemical story of carbohydrates is complex. All sugars and starches contain only carbon, hydrogen and oxygen in the ratio of 1:2:1. The type found in our food are usually based on compounds containing six carbon atoms. The simplest sugars, the monosaccharides, contain only six carbon, twelve hydrogen and six oxygen atoms and are not joined to any other molecules. Glucose, fructose and galactose are monosaccharides. Sucrose the best known sugar is a disaccharide, that is it has two basic six carbon units in a molecule. Another disaccharide is lactose, the milk sugar. When hundreds of the basic units join together, they form large molecules called polysaccharides. Starch, for example, consists of over 2,000 glucose units, the precise number and way these are joined depending upon the source of the starch. The size and shape of the carbohydrate molecules influence their properties. Monosaccharides such as glucose and sucrose are sweet and will dissolve in water; polysaccharides like starch are not sweet and will not dissolve in water, but turn it into a thin paste.

The digestion of sugar and starch begins in the mouth, where enzymes in the saliva start to break them down. However, most of the starch and sugars are digested in the small intestine, where enzymes help to split up the large starch molecules and complex sugars into simple monosaccharides so that they can be absorbed through the intestine wall into the bloodstream. Once in the blood, gluc-

An enormous variety of cereal products act as a primary source of carbohydrate. Cereals are refined to flour and then, with added ingredients, baked into a multitude of breads and derivatives. The greater the refining process, as for white flour, the less the nutritional benefits. Brown or wholemeal bread retains the roughage which in turn increases the dietary advantages of bread as a carbohydrate source

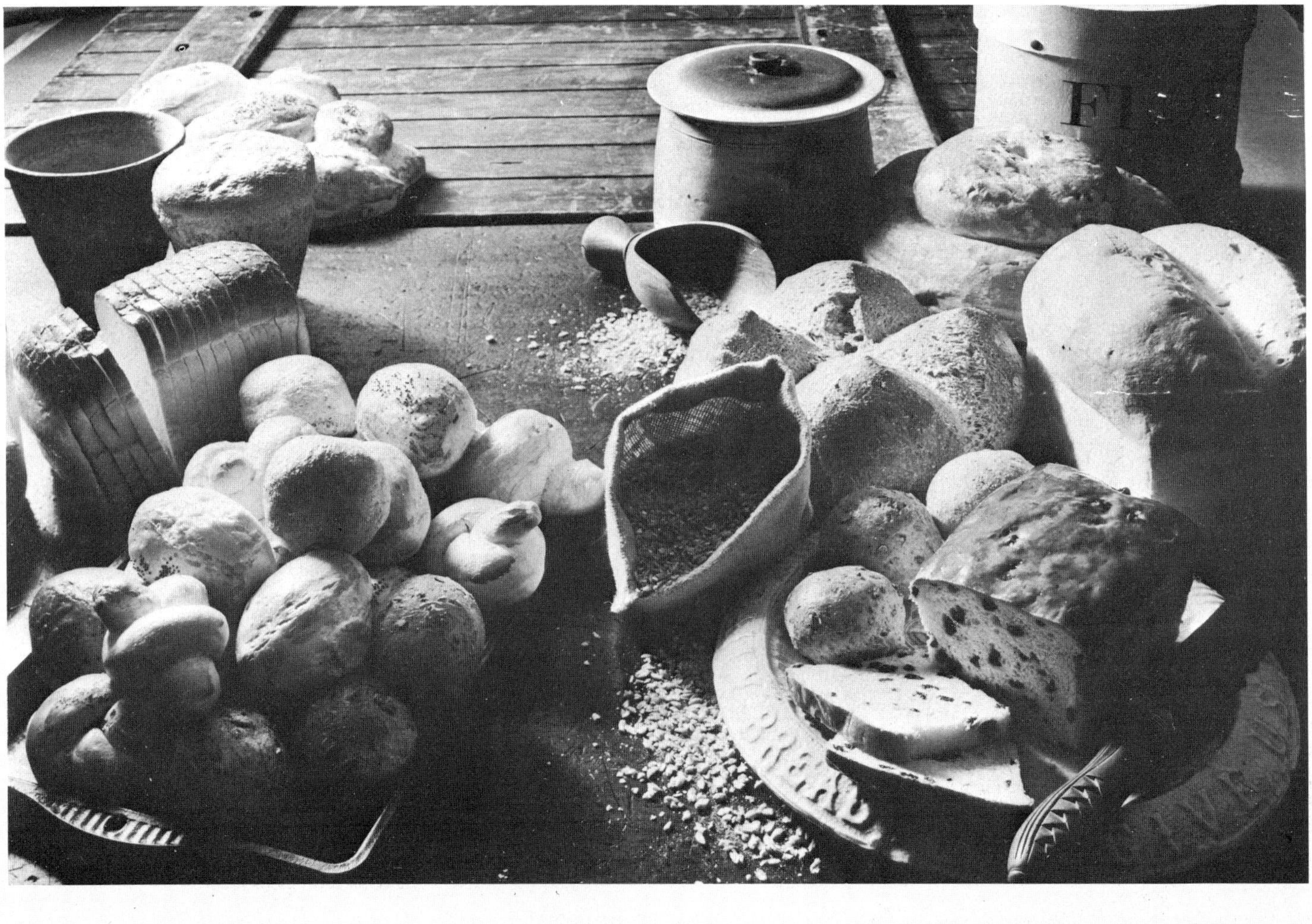

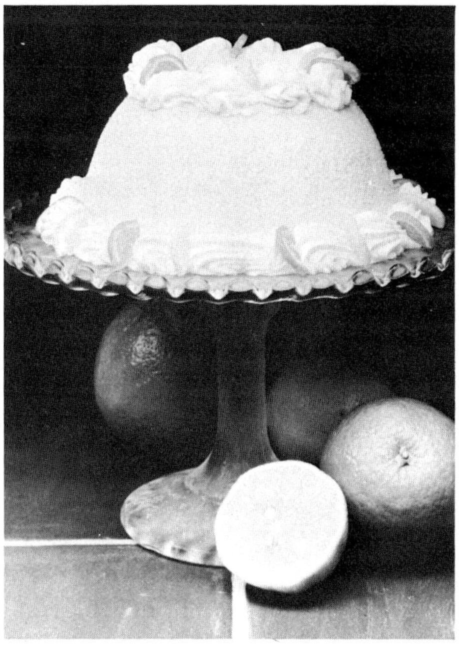

There is evidence to indicate that foods made from refined sugar, such as ice cream (above) are not only inherently less nutritious than foods prepared using natural sugar but the refined product may actually tend to hasten arterial disease. Foods which contain a lot of refined sugar or which are sticky and sweet pose risks not only to the arteries but to the teeth where such food helps to promote dental decay (below)

ose can be used by any of the cells and tissues, but non-glucose monosaccharides must be modified by the liver first. The glucose which carbohydrates ultimately provide can be used in three ways: it can be stored in the liver where it is transformed into another compound called glycogen; it can be carried to the cells where it is burnt up immediately as energy; or it can be converted into fatty acids and eventually laid down as fat.

When glucose enters the cell it is broken down, in a series of steps, into simpler chemical substances, releasing water, carbon dioxide and a considerable amount of energy. About half of the energy released goes in heat and the rest is stored in complex molecules called adenosine triphosphate (ATP) in 'energy rich bonds'. This compound and others like it are very important: they take part in various biochemical reactions in the body and release the stored energy to allow cells to function properly. Energy rich bonds can be replaced by the breakdown of more glucose.

The carbohydrates in food are important in ultimately providing some of the energy that the body needs to function, but they can also give problems. Not only carbohydrate digestion begins in the mouth; so does tooth decay. Carbohydrates are prone to stick to the teeth and this allows bacteria to act on them. Weak organic acids are produced by the bacteria, which form a plaque on the tooth, and the acid can eat holes into the teeth. Although both starch and sugar can lead to this reaction, sugar is particularly guilty. Individual susceptibility to tooth decay varies and is influenced by how our teeth developed. If flouride is present in drinking water in small quantities this is incorporated in the teeth during growth and increases resistance to tooth decay. Sticky, sweet foods, especially eaten between meals, helps to promote tooth decay. Sugar consumption, which is between about 100-200 lbs per person each year in the industrialized countries, should be curtailed if we want healthy teeth. It may also be desirable to reduce sugar consumption for other reasons as it has been suggested, but not proved, that sugar is implicated in other diseases of the affluent society.

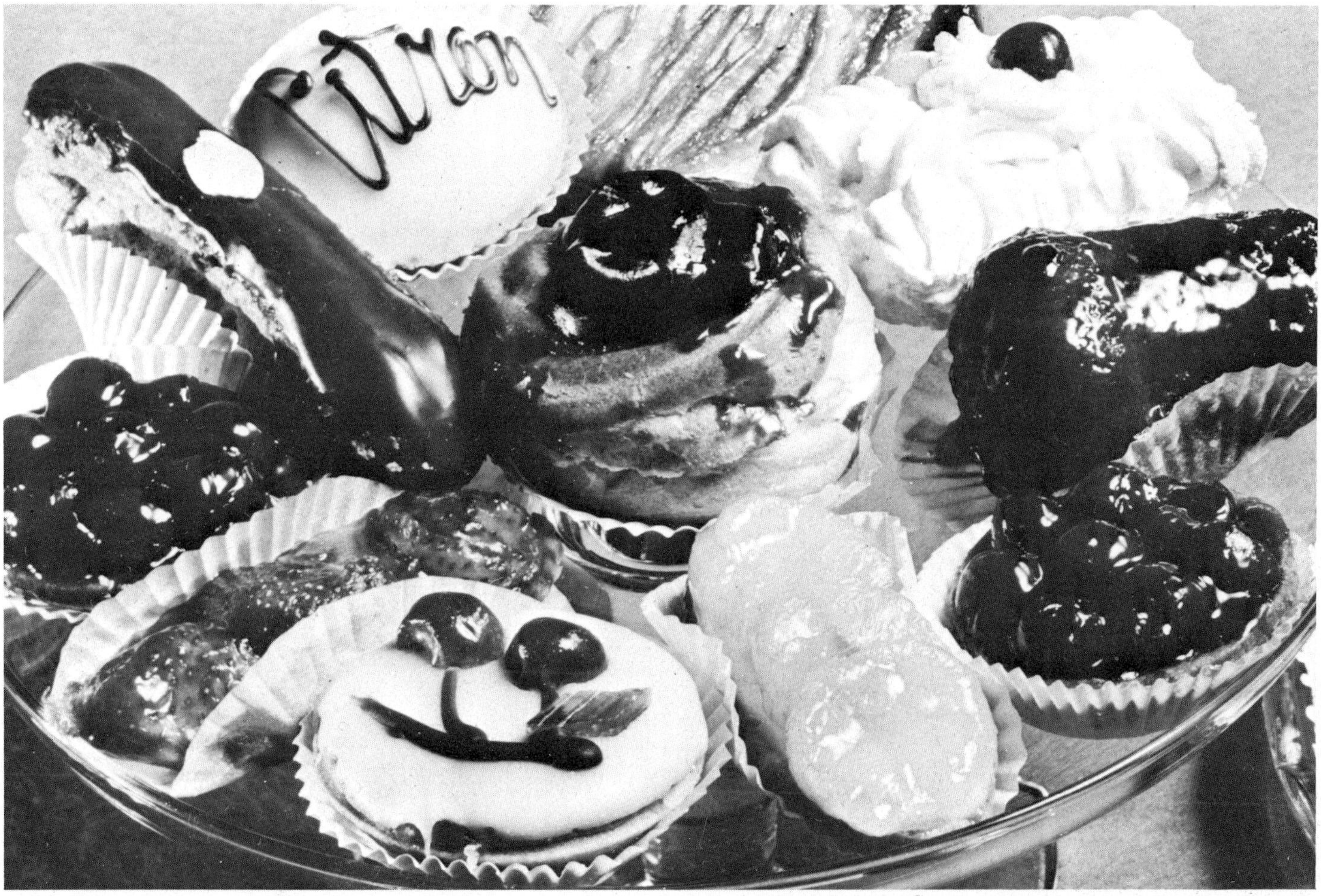

Fibre

One of the most important components of our diet for a healthy life is one that we get virtually no nutrients from but which passes out of the body as faeces. This component of food is dietary fibre. Fibre used to be thought of as unimportant since it did not seem to contribute anything to the body but now this view is changing.

The clues that fibre plays an important role in body function and maintaining health came from the rural areas in the developing countries, not from the sophisticated laboratories of the affluent countries. The disease patterns in the rich industrialized countries has changed so that now it is not contagious epidemics but degenerative diseases like coronary heart disease and cancer that are responsible for most deaths in the rich world. Some doctors noticed that many of these ailments did not occur or were generally very rare amongst people in the rural areas in the developing countries.

A major difference which seems to be linked to the changed disease patterns is the greatly altered diet in rich affluent nations and in the cities of the developing countries when compared to that of the rural population in the poor countries, or to that of our ancestors only a few generations ago. The rural people, by and large, have a diet based on whole unrefined foods whereas that of the rich is much more highly refined and high in processed foods. In the refining process generally and in that of cereals and sugar in particular it is the fibre that is lost, a loss that has led to a ten fold decline in the fibre intake of the rich this century despite an increase in food consumption.

Fibre is the material that forms plant cell walls – paper and cotton, for example, are both plant fibre. Dietary fibre is the part of the plant cell walls that is not broken down by the enzymes in the stomach and intestines during digestion and which passes out of the body. It consists of polysaccharides such as cellulose, pectin and hemicelluloses, and lignin, a complex organic polymer. Fibre helps to give plants their shape and strength but it is not necessarily fibrous or rough.

Dietary fibre is not the same as

Fibre is now believed to be of prime importance in a healthy and balanced diet but much of civilized living depends on foodstuffs which have been processed to exclude the natural fibre. Shown below are various pulses, lentils, cereals and breads which provide excellent sources of dietary fibre

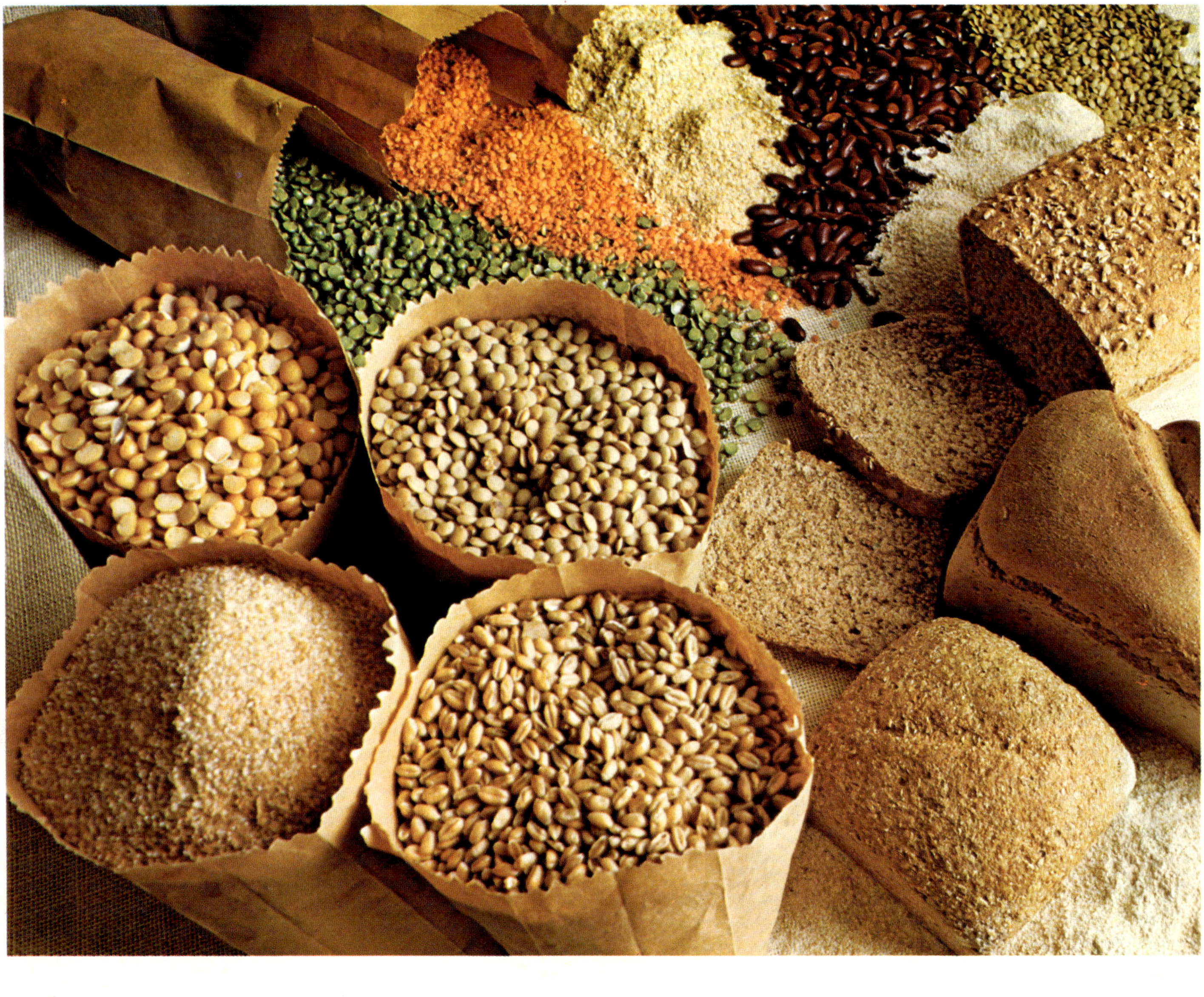

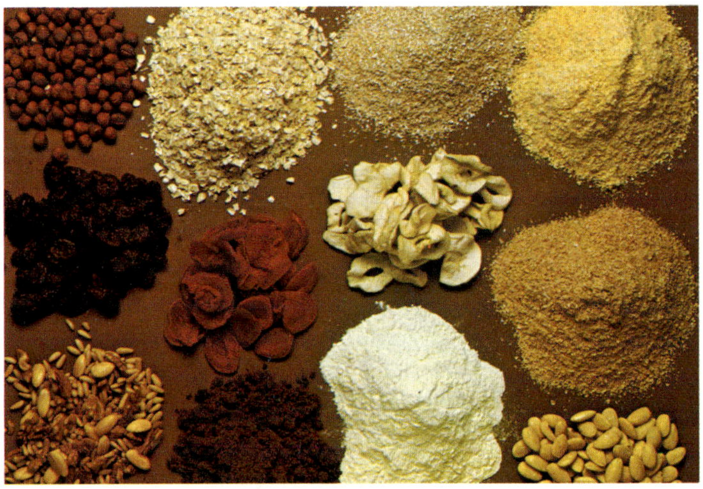

A most effective and enjoyable way of ensuring that your diet contains a sufficient quantity of natural fibre is to begin each day with a bowl of *muesli*, a high source of the fibre and one which is no way out of the range of the normal diet

roughage or crude fibre. Both of these terms are used to describe the material left after food has been boiled with dilute acid and then alkali. This is a harsh treatment which destroys certain kinds of fibre and in cereals, for example, the amount of dietary fibre may be five times greater than the amount of crude fibre.

Only plant foods contain dietary fibre and the richest sources are leguminous seeds like peas, beans and lentils and cereals which may provide up to 81g of fibre for every 1000 kcal of energy they supply. Most of the fibre intake in the affluent countries used to come from cereals and potatoes but consumption of these has declined and the cereals eaten are more highly refined than in the past. The loss of fibre this entails has been offset to some extent by an increase in the consumption of fruit and vegetables which also contain fibre. The nature of some of these has changed as breeders have produced varieties suited to mass production for freezing and canning which usually contain less fibre than older ones. Cereal fibre seems to be more active physiologically than that from other sources and the refining of cereals removes virtually all of this fibre. Two other foods derived from plants have also had all the fibre removed – sugar and vegetable oils, and the margarine made from the oils. Animal products contain little or no fibre.

When fibre enters the body it does, by definition, pass through the stomach and small intestine unaltered. However, it is now becoming clear that it does play a role in the digestive system, and that a low fibre diet is implicated in development of a wide range of diseases – dental caries, obesity, diabetes, gallstones, coronary heart disease, various bowel diseases and bowel cancer.

One of the major properties of fibre is its ability to absorb water which is important in the bowel or colon as a high level of fibre helps to produce soft bulky stools which are easy to pass. The amount of fibre present in the colon also affects the type of bacteria present which may affect our vulnerability to some diseases. Fibre is also able to act as an ion exchanger, rather like a water softener, and may help to keep the right balance of salts in the body. If we look briefly at how it is thought a lack of fibre makes us more susceptable to the seemingly diverse range of diseases, the value of these properties is revealed.

When we refine foods and remove the fibre from cereals – to produce white flour – and from sugar cane and beet to produce sugar we produce foods which can be absorbed quickly by the body. They do not fill us easily or make us feel full for long. In fact removing the fibre has carried out part of the digestion process for us but because it takes longer to feel full on low-fibre diets we are more likely to eat more than if all the fibre was there. If we eat a high-fibre diet it makes us feel full longer and we eat less. The prevelance of low fibre diets seems to be one of the main reasons for the occurence of obesity in the affluent countries. A diet including one pound of potatoes, which are relatively high in fibre, a day has helped people to lose weight over a period because the bulk of the potatoes meant other intake was reduced.

The processes of refining and concentration, such as the preparation of the aerated fruit juice may appear to concentrate the food value of its fruit equivalent of four fresh apples: in fact, dietary requirements would be much better served by eating the apples

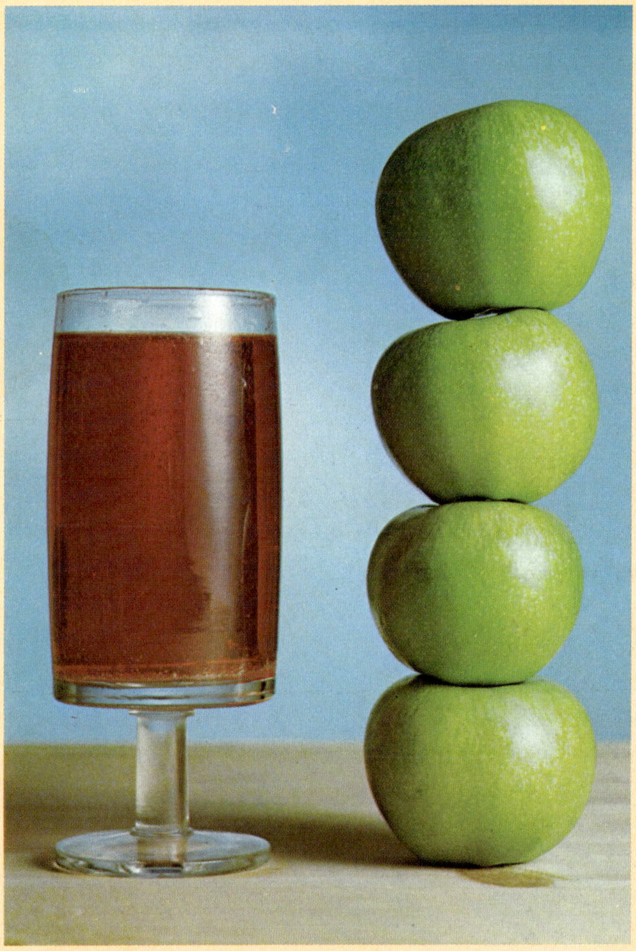

The refining process has also helped us to eat large quantities of sugar which causes tooth decay (dental caries). Refined sugar or sucrose is the most vigorous agent in promoting decay although all carbohydrates do to some extent. Fruit and vegetables do contain various kinds of sugars but they are much more dilute than sucrose. Also associated with a generally high intake of sugar is diabetes, in particular that kind which begins in maturity. Obesity increases the risk of becoming diabetic and fat consumption may also play a part.

Another illness which eating a refined diet increases the liklihood of contracting is gallstones. The precise cause of these is not known but evidence suggests that a combination of an increased cholesterol production coupled with the type of bacteria found in the colon of people with low fibre intakes increases susceptibility to the condition which is very rare in the rural areas of the developing countries.

Coronary heart disease is another disease where a high fibre diet may offer some degree of protection. What causes the disease is not yet known and what is known presents a confusing picture. One thing which is clear is that sufferers from obesity or diabetes are more likely to have coronary trouble than average. If a high fibre diet helps to reduce these conditions then it will also help to reduce coronary heart disease.

There may also be a more direct link between fibre and heart disease, however, as the type of bacteria found in the bowel of those on low fibre diets, seems to be linked to the degree of fat absorption and blood triglyceride levels which in turn increase the possibility of heart disease.

A much more clear cut and direct link is to be found between the amount of fibre in the diet and the prevelance of bowel diseases such as constipation, appendicitis, varicose veins and piles. A high-fibre diet makes for an easier passage of the remains of the digestive process. The fibre absorbs water and produces a soft stool which can be moved along the colon easily. Low-fibre diets produce small hard stools which require considerable pressures to be exerted by the colon wall to force them out. This is perhaps one of the most common strains felt by those on low fibre affluent diets. The pressure takes its toll over the years and the colon wall may blow out like a tyre. These blow outs give rise to the diverticular disease of the colon. Many blow outs may occur during life and leave rather vague but annoying symptoms like nausea, a bloated feeling and some discomfort in the gut. If a blow out becomes blocked off and the contents become infected it may burst causing peritonitis which can be fatal.

A similar blocking of the appendix can cause appendicitis which is generally only found amongst those on a low fibre diet. The pressures caused by straining at stool are also linked to the occurrence of varicose veins and piles. A low fibre diet means too that any substances in food that are not absorbed by the body may be left in the colon for days or even weeks if they get stuck to the sides. If any of these

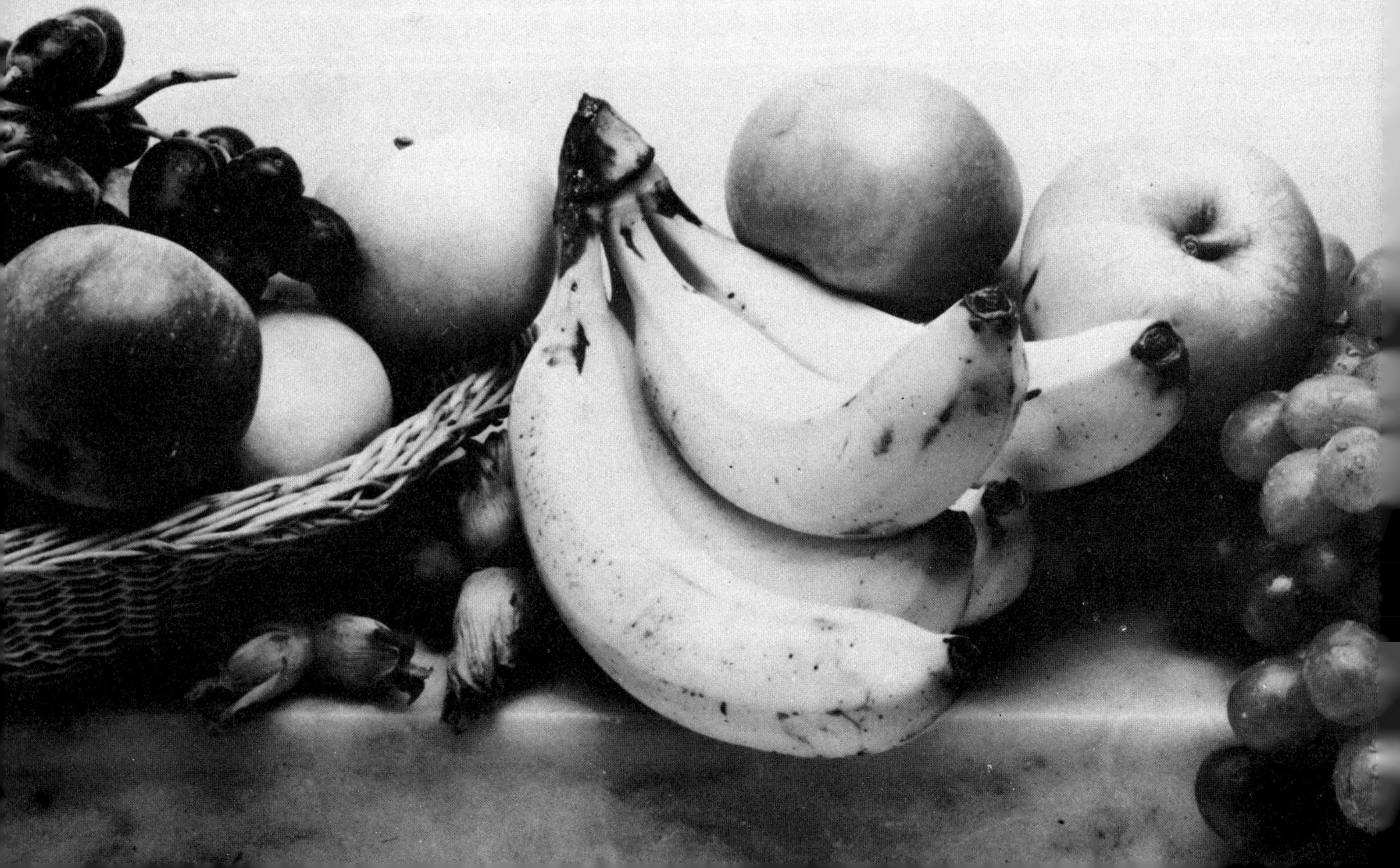

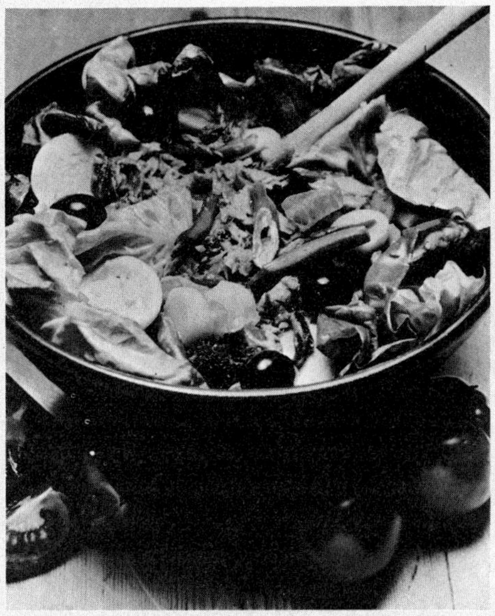

When fresh fruits are processed – whether by cooking, canning or preserving them by another method – much of their nutritional value, particularly their fibre content, is destroyed. The same applies to the processing and cooking of vegetables and so, ideally, a well balanced and healthy diet should contain adequate quantities of fresh fruit and vegetables

substances are carcinogenic they will have close intimate contact with the colon wall for considerable periods of time when they may do some damage. If there is a lot of bulky fibre present these substances are diluted and pass through more quickly. The different types of bacteria present in a low and high fibre regime in the colon may also influence the effects of the substances.

Just eating a high fibre diet, or adding bran to food, will not necessarily prevent us from contracting any of the diseases mentioned. It seems clear, however, that these diseases are linked to the widespread adoption of a low fibre diet containing much refined food. The adoption of a diet higher in fibre content may well help to reduce the incidence of these diseases. Even if there is no guarantee that it means we will avoid them at least the problem of constipation and the strain and out of sorts feeling that it engenders would be reduced. So what does following a high fibre diet entail?

Generally it is a way of approaching food and means that we would avoid white flour and products made from it and replace it with wholemeal. We would eat as little sugar as possible – indeed it may come as a surprise to discover how sweet many fruits and vegetables are once the palate ceases to be deadened by consumption of large amounts of sugar. We would also eat more fruit and vegetables, eat less fat and fewer processed and synthetic foods. In the process of changing to such a diet it may be that bran should be added to food to achieve the benefits of overcoming constipation early on in the change. Obviously if the adoption of such a diet became widespread considerable changes would be needed in the food and agricultural industry.

Eating a high-fibre diet will lead to some flatulance at first but this goes after a few weeks as the body becomes used to it. It is also advisable to increase the amount of water drunk as more water will be needed than before so that the fibre can absorb it and produce the soft stools which pass easily from the body.

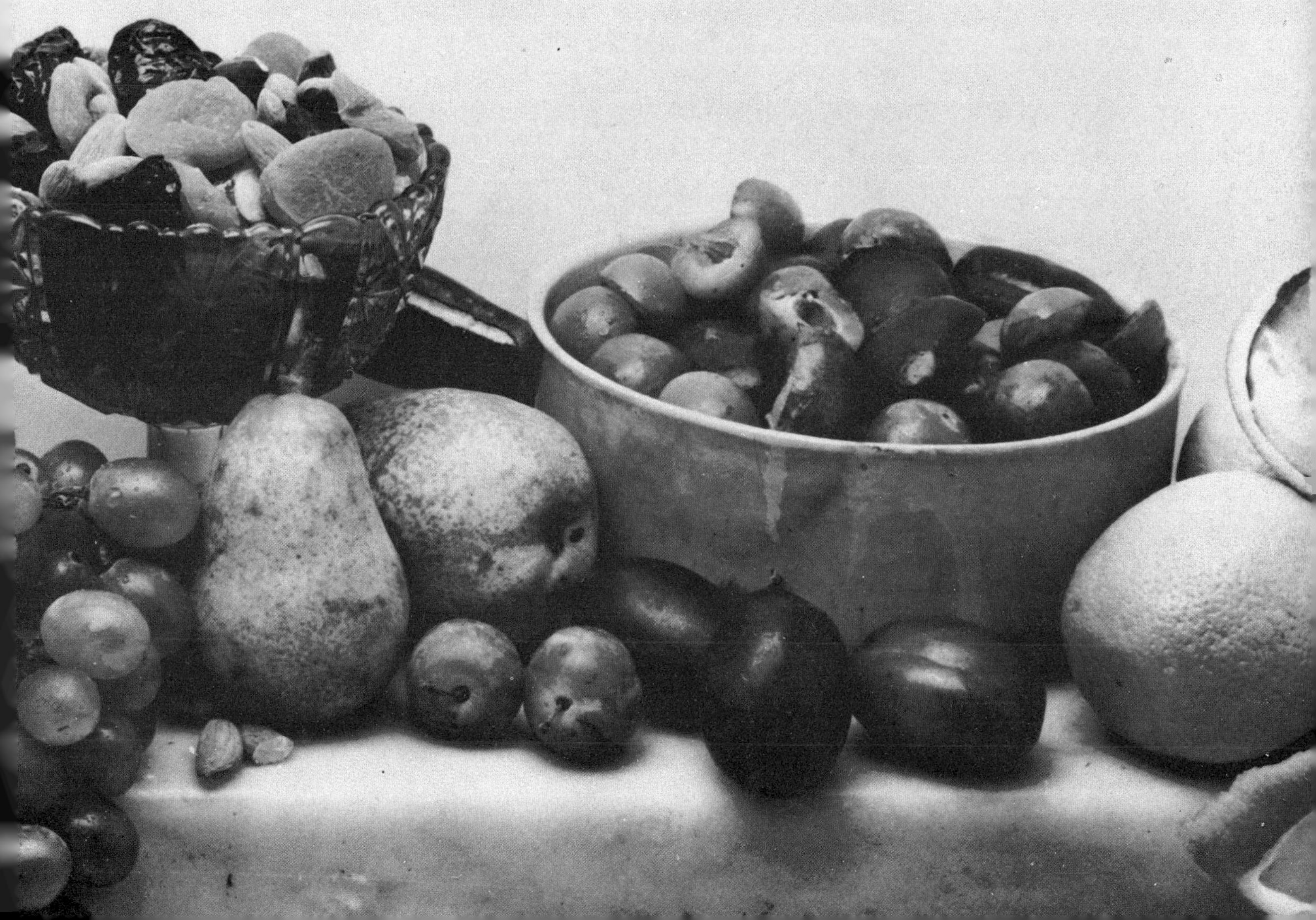

Fats

Fats are a concentrated source of energy; one gram of fat provides more energy than one gram of protein and one of carbohydrate put together. They also contain the fat soluble vitamins and polyunsaturated essential fatty acids, such as linoleic acid – which is vital for the promotion of growth. Gastronomically speaking, one of the joys of fats is their ability to give or hold flavour. Many of the complex compounds that produce flavour are soluble in fat and food derives much of its palatability from the fat component wherein the flavours are dissolved. Most of the best tasting foods contain a high degree of fat. We get fats from visible sources like cream, butter, margarine and the fat round meat but also from invisible or hidden sources like the fat in meat, milk, cheese, egg yolks, avocados, nuts, chocolate, and in baked goods such as cakes, pies and biscuits.

Like carbohydrates, fats are made up of carbon, hydrogen and oxygen but the proportion of oxygen to carbon is lower, and the three elements are combined in such a way as to give fats very different properties. Most of the fats found in food are called triglycerides. These consist of three fatty acids joined to a molecule of glycerol (glycerine) which is an alcohol. If only one or two fatty acids are joined to glycerol the fats are called mono- or diglycerides. A fatty acid consists of a chain of carbon atoms with an acidic group on the end. The chain of carbon atoms can be from four to over twenty carbons long but is usually in the 16-18 range in dietary fats. The nature of the fats depends on the number of carbon atoms in the chain and how they are linked. If the chain is short, the fat is softer than if it is long. (If the fat is liquid at room temperature it is called an oil).

The way the carbons are linked also affects the properties of the fat. This linkage that determines whether a fat is saturated or unsaturated. Normally, each carbon atom is linked to four or five other atoms – one carbon on either side and two hydrogen atoms, or three at the end of the chain. When all the hydrogen links are filled, the fat is said to be *saturated*. Sometimes, only one hydrogen atom is linked to a carbon atom in the chain and instead of there being a single bond between two carbon atoms there is a double bond. The molecule is no longer completely filled with hydrogen, but has space for some, it is *unsaturated*. If there is one double bond in the fatty acid chain it is said to be monounsaturated, if two or more double bonds, polyunsaturated. Unsaturated fats tend to melt at a lower temperature than saturated fats.

Animal fat is high in saturated fats; polysaturated fatty acids are found largely in vegetable fat (oil). Many margarines boast of their vegetable oil origin but this can be misleading as not all vegetable oils are high in polyunsa-

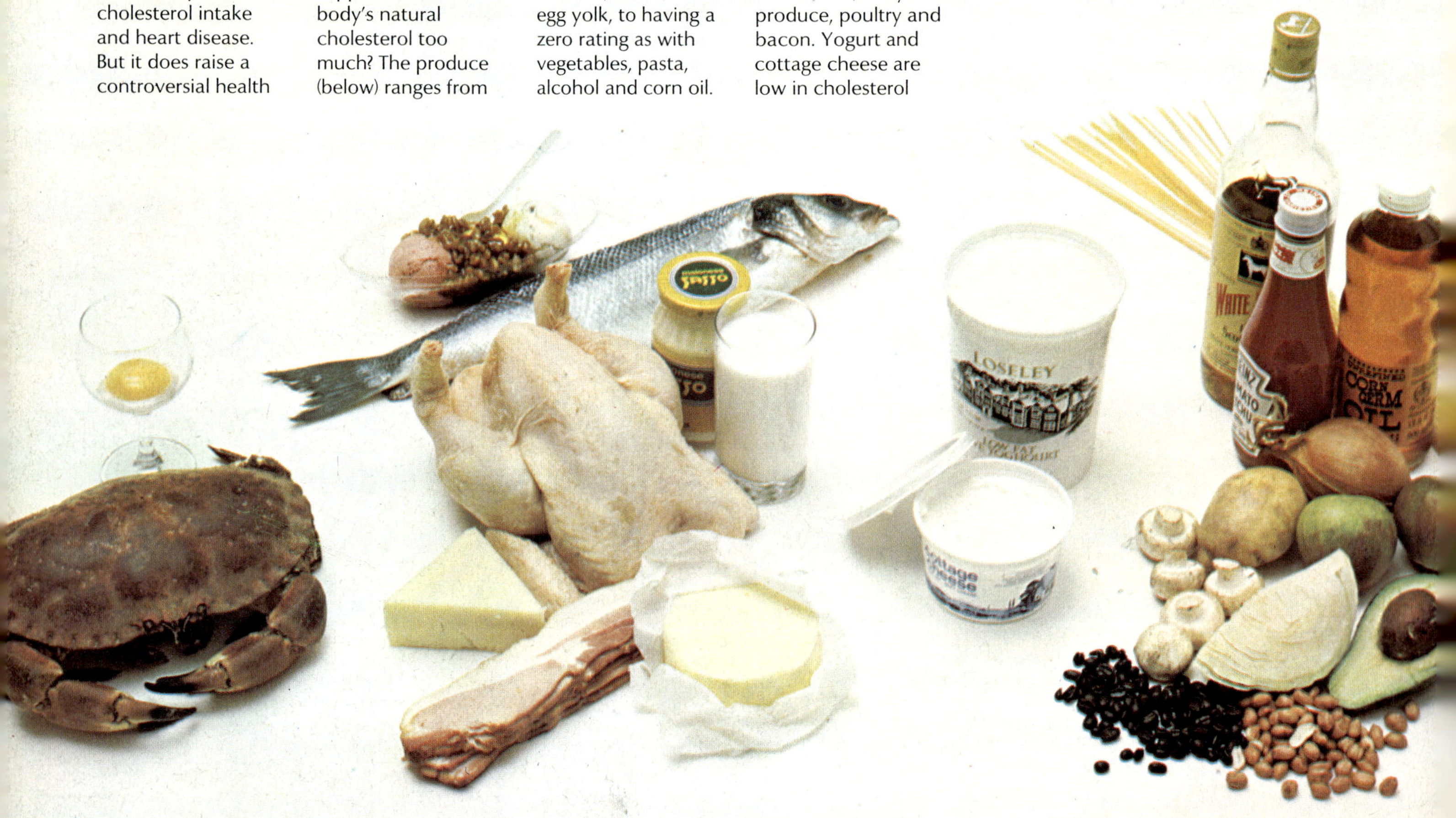

There is no simple relationship between cholesterol intake and heart disease. But it does raise a controversial health question – do we supplement our body's natural cholesterol too much? The produce (below) ranges from having a very high content, crab and egg yolk, to having a zero rating as with vegetables, pasta, alcohol and corn oil. In the medium range we find fish, dairy produce, poultry and bacon. Yogurt and cottage cheese are low in cholesterol

turated fats, eg olive oil. Of those which are the amount remaining in the margarine will depend upon how it was processed. Some of the polyunsaturated fats have to be hardened, or made into saturated fats by the addition of hydrogen, in order to produce a margarine that is solid at room temperature.

Fat digestion begins in the mouth as the food is warmed up and swallowed. In the stomach the fats liquify and any eaten in the form of an emulsion – a fine suspension of fats in water, such as salad dressing – begin to be broken down. Fats stay in the stomach longer than sugars and starches and help us to feel full longer. Most of the digestion of them takes place in the small intestine where they are emulsified by bile secreted from the gall bladder. Emulsion contains very small particles, giving the fat a very large surface area. This makes it easier for the fat-splitting enzymes to break down the fat molecules into their constituent fatty acids and glycerol, which then pass through the intestinal wall during digestion.

About a third of the fatty acids and glycerol are directly distributed around the body in the blood after being absorbed. Glycerol provides energy in much the same way as carbohydrate. The long chains of the fatty acids are split up to provide substances which make such important compounds as cholesterol and sex hormones. Energy is a by-product of this process. The rest of the fatty acids and glycerol recombine, once they permeate the intestinal wall, to form mono-, di- and triglycerides. These team up with protein to form a complex molecule called lipoprotein, which is soluble in water. The lipoproteins do not enter the blood supply immediately but go into a special fat transport system, the lymphatic system, and are taken to the neck. Here they enter the bloodstream and are taken to the tissues where the fat in them can be stored or used immediately for energy.

Fat intake seems to be a wealthy pastime, as a large amount of fat is eaten in the rich countries while the poor, developing countries have a low intake. Fats of all kinds provide a large percentage – 40-45 per cent in American diets – of total energy intake in the diets of rich countries. It is generally recommended that this level should be reduced to 30-35 per cent. It seems that the amount and type of fat in the diet may influence the prevalence of heart disease. The type of fat, saturated or unsaturated, may also effect the liklihood of heart disease and some authorities suggest that the bulk of the fat intake should be of polyunsaturated fats. It would be simple if we could point to one factor as the cause of any particular degenerative disease, but the body is not that simple. Certainly fat consumption plays a role in increasing susceptibility to heart disease and arteriosclerosis, but so too do other dietary factors as well as environmental and genetic considerations. The story of fats and heart disease is by no means clear yet but it would almost certainly be wise for most people in the rich countries of the world to reduce their fat intake as this may well benefit their health. However many of the apparently sophisticated low-fat diets have no scientific foundation but do reduce butter and cream intake.

The volume of saturated fat (below) in our diet is usually thought to be too high to be healthy for us. Dairy produce and meat have a very high content; peanuts, with little animal fat fall into the medium range and fish, chicken, pasta, egg yolk, corn oil and yogurt have a low content. Alcohol, vegetables and sugar derivatives have no animal fat and are therefore free of saturated fat

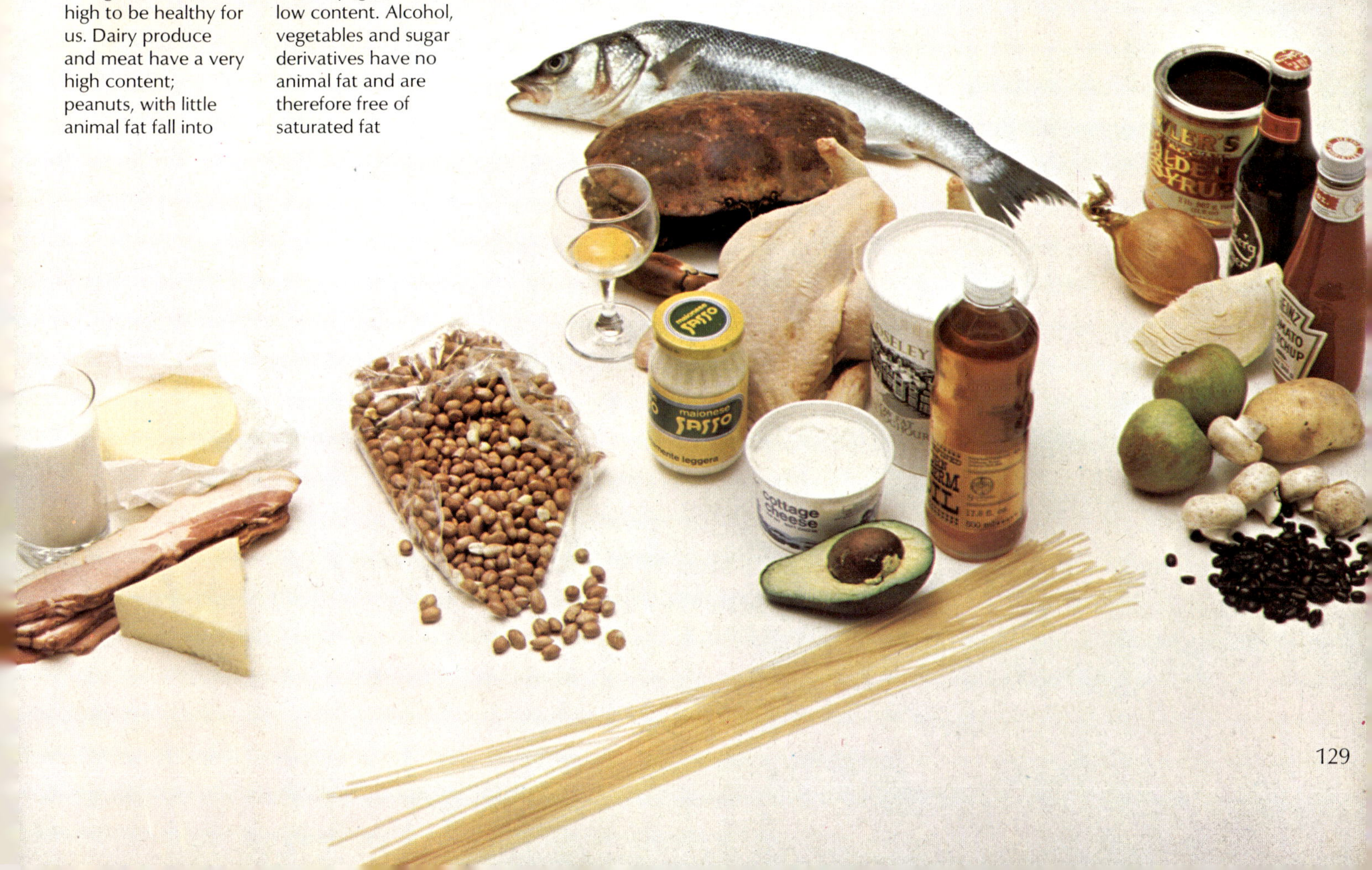

Vegetarianism

There is a surprising amount of disagreement about whether or not the vegetarian is adequately nourished by his chosen diet even among people who profess to have some expert knowledge. There are those who claim that some animal protein, however little, is essential for the proper maintenance of health and yet others who say that the vegetarian attains longer life relatively free from scourges like heart disease. Actually, both points of view are correct to some extent and reflect a certain amount of confusion regarding terminology.

It is also interesting to note that research scientists themselves have not reached a consensus until recent years—partly because information about the relative values of different foodstuffs used to be rather scanty. In 1935 the report of the Mixed Commission of the League of Nations stated categorically that some quantity of animal protein was essential. More recent knowledge suggests that this oft-quoted statement is almost certainly not correct. Over the last thirty years we have learnt a lot about the way proteins can be mixed together to provide a wellbalanced whole and there is no doubt that a mixture of vegetables can provide sufficient of the various 'building blocks' needed for our complex metabolism to maintain full efficiency. However, that is the story only as far as protein is concerned, as one of three basic groups of foodstuffs, absolutely essential in fairly large quantities for the maintenance of health. But the minor substances can become significant too if they are in really short supply in the diet. And, although our present state of knowledge makes us confident that every vegetarian can, with a little attention to what he eats, get a more than adequate supply of protein for his needs he may be short of one of the vital vitamins. Some of the advantages of animal protein are derived from the presence of non-protein material such as minerals and vitamins.

One of these substances, vitamin B12, is completely missing from plants and yet it is essential for life. Without it the individual suffers from pernicious anaemia. Most vegetarians do eat some animal protein—quite enough for them to get adequate supplies of B12—they merely avoid the flesh of the animal meat. They have no objections to the consumption of milk, eggs and cheese and all of these are rich in animal protein and all the other vital substances that are included.

However, there is a group of vegetarians who eschew all animal products and make it a point of honour never to let these substances pass their lips. Known as vegans, they form a very small group and they have to work very hard in order to maintain full health. Nowadays they are able to obtain sufficient supplies of B12 which, as we have seen, is the crucial substance which plants cannot supply, from the by-products of moulds that are grown to produce antibiotics such as penicillin. Of course, they could take B12 supplements but this would probably not fit in with their notions of what constitutes a natural diet. Fortunately incredibly small amounts are sufficient, provided your body has a normal ability to cope with the vitamin. An ounce is sufficient, on a daily basis, for more than ten million people!

Many people think that vegetarianism is more natural than eating meat; this is a quite erroneous view as agriculture and the cultivation of cereals that form the mainstay of such a diet are relatively recent inventions in the history of Man. He was eating meat long before he discovered how to tame crops. In fact, his ability to get sufficient nourishment for his needs quickly from meat left a lot of time over for development and the creation of civilization. All exclusively plant eaters among the animal world spend a massive proportion of their time just eating because so much more bulk is required in order to get the same amounts of useable nutrients. A possible advan-

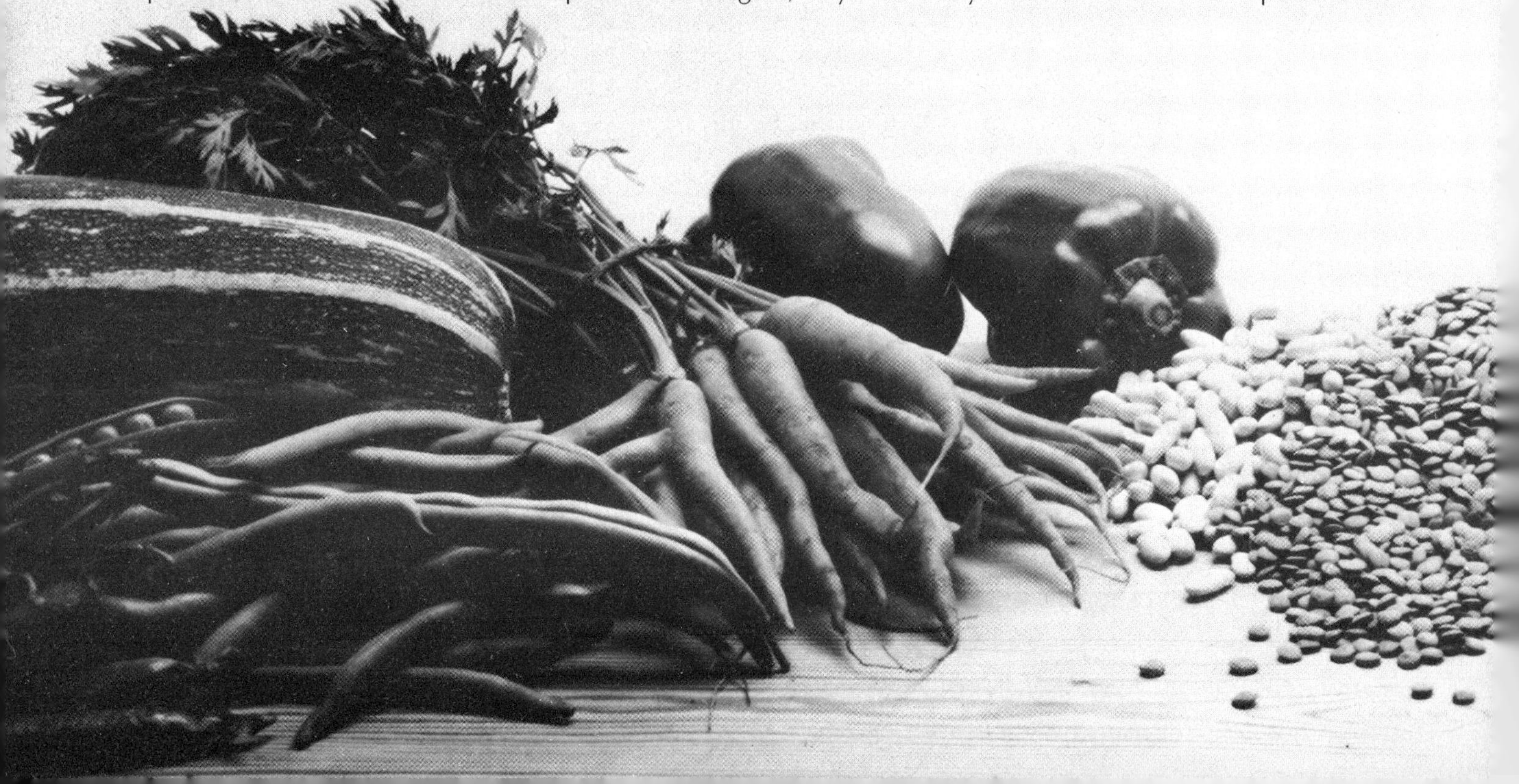

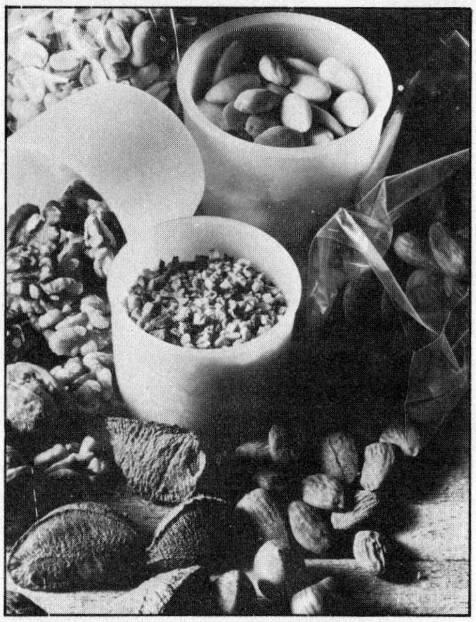

The vast array of vegetables (below) available to the vegetarian invariably means there is no shortage of invention in the dishes they prepare. A skilled cook will produce nourishing, stimulating and appetizing meals

Nuts (above) are typical ingredients in a vegetarian diet. They are a wholefood and are usually eaten in their natural state. Walnuts, hazel and brazil nuts are a few of the nutritious and readily available kinds

tage in today's world, of course, and this tendency not to overeat may be the reason why vegetarians do seem to do well from a health point of view, certainly as far as diseases like heart disease are concerned—although there have not been enough studies for us to be sure of these facts.

One of the misconceptions that vegetarians are prey to is the idea that some vegetables contain as much protein although with a different composition weight for weight, as meat. It is true that the pulses such as peas, beans or lentils do have as much protein as beef—but only when the pulse is in its dried state. Water must be added before the peas or beans can be eaten and they automatically swell and absorb a large quantity of liquid. This often results in the reconstituted food having only a quarter of protein by weight.

There are certain essential amino-acids which must be eaten and obtained from food, as they cannot be produced by our bodies: meat closely resembles our own flesh and thereby gives a good ready-made mix which is not far removed from our own. As plant metabolism is so different from our own, they do not contain the essential amino-acids in the combination that is appropriate for us. And in many plants one or other of the essential amino-acids may be completely absent. It is for this reason that earlier pronouncements were made, such as that from the League of Nations, suggesting that a vegetable diet could never be adequate. But now we know that whereas one plant may be insufficient to sustain life on its own, a mixture works out well—because the plants all differ in their make-up and what is missing from one will be found in another. There is no doubt that provided several vegetables are mixed in the diet no trouble will occur. Even small amounts of another product will be enough to ensure adequate nutrition even if one particular legume forms the staple. Some plants are obviously better than others from the human point of view: wheat is much better than rice; the potato too is a well balanced food. But do avoid refined or processed vegetables.

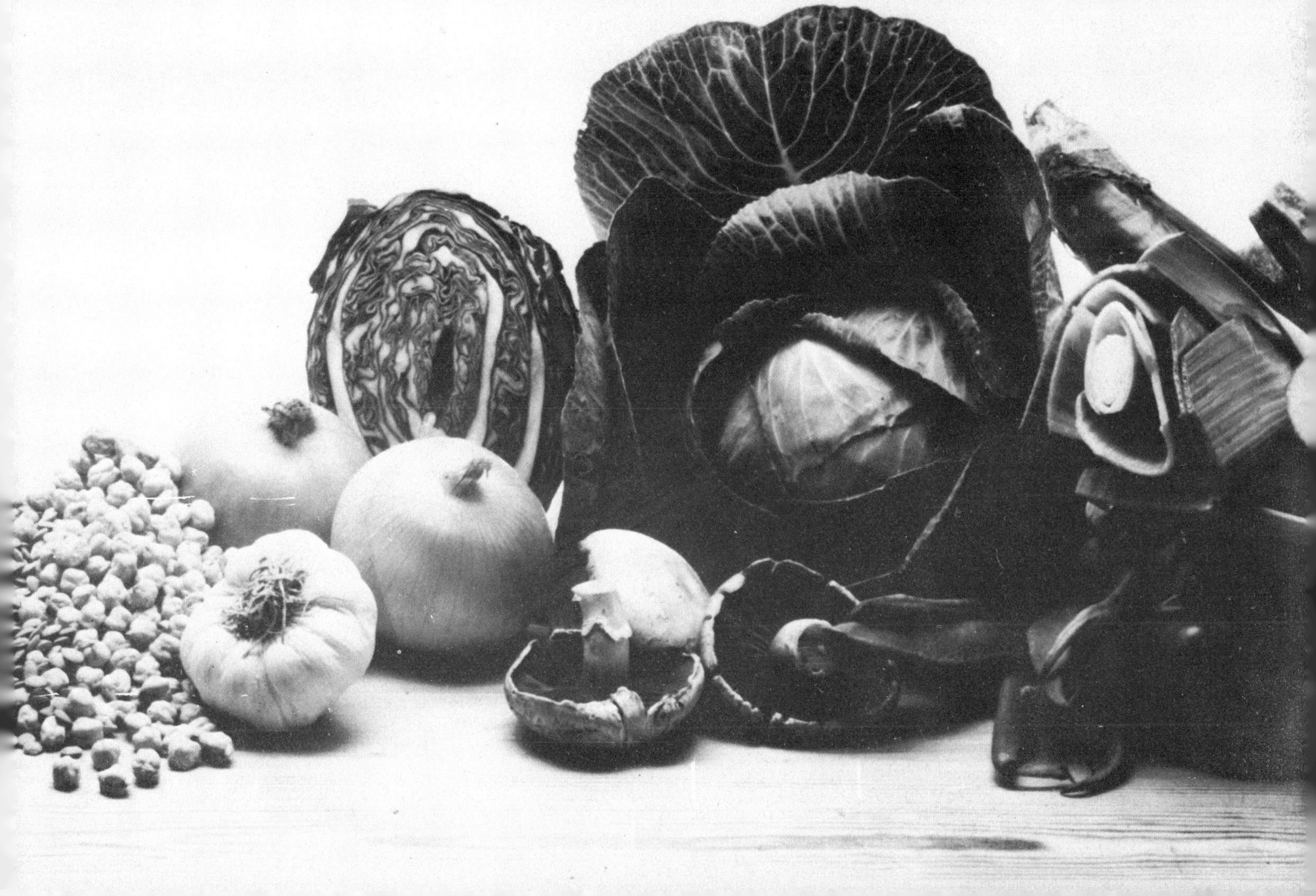

Minerals and Vitamins

Although we need large daily supplies of fats, carbohydrates, water and protein, there are many necessary elements which are only required in small quantities – ranging from about one gram a day to a few thousandths or even millionths of a gram a day. Small though these quantities are, their absence can lead to illness and, if prolonged, even death. Minerals are inorganic compounds and are found in small quantities in food, animals and people. If a food is burnt completely a little ash is left and this is the mineral content of the food: only about 4 per cent of the human body is ash. The minerals needed by the body are often divided into two groups, macronutrients and micronutrients, depending upon how much of them is found in the body. The macronutrients are calcium, chlorine, magnesium, phosphorus, potassium, sodium and sulphur, and the micronutrients are chromium, cobalt, copper, fluorine, iodine, iron, manganese, molybdenum, selenium and zinc. Other minerals such as gold, lead and mercury are present in the body but are thought to play no role in its growth or functioning and may be harmful if present in any quantity.

Minerals have many and varied functions. Calcium helps to build bones and teeth, as does fluorine; iron is an important constituent of haemoglobin in the blood; and sodium and potassium help to maintain the balance between the fluid inside and outside the cells.

Vitamins are also needed in very small quantities, but unlike minerals they are complex organic compounds. They are needed to promote growth and maintain life, and are divided into two groups: those soluble in fat – vitamins A, D, E and K – and those soluble in water – all the B vitamins and vitamin C. Of major importance is the part vitamins play in the construction of enzymes or of substances which enable enzymes to be made: enzymes enable the reactions which keep the body going to take place.

All the vitamins we need are available in our food, and adequate vitamin D can also be obtained through the action of the sun on skin. The whole collection of B vitamins, each now usually given a name as well as a subnumber, arose because when it was first discovered vitamin B was thought to be one substance. Vitamin C is now often called ascorbic acid.

A lack of vitamins can cause illness, but so can an excess of certain vitamins, A and D in particular. Illness due to excess is known as hypervitaminosis. Self administration of these vitamins is not recommended and may be fatal if prolonged high intakes are taken or even if one massive dose is administered.

With vitamins and minerals we again see the principles of balance and limiting factors. A good diet should provide the right mix of fats, carbohydrates, proteins, water, minerals and vitamins but it can do this within fairly wide tolerance limits. Meat for example is an important source of vitamins and minerals and in many affluent diets it is for these that it is important rather than its protein potential. If meat is replaced by textured vegetable protein, or single cell protein made to look like meat, which lacks the minerals and vitamins in meat, deficiencies could arise. For those who do not eat meat, a careful balancing of other foods is needed to ensure deficiences do not occur. This is perfectly possible and there are many healthy vegetarians and vegans walking around.

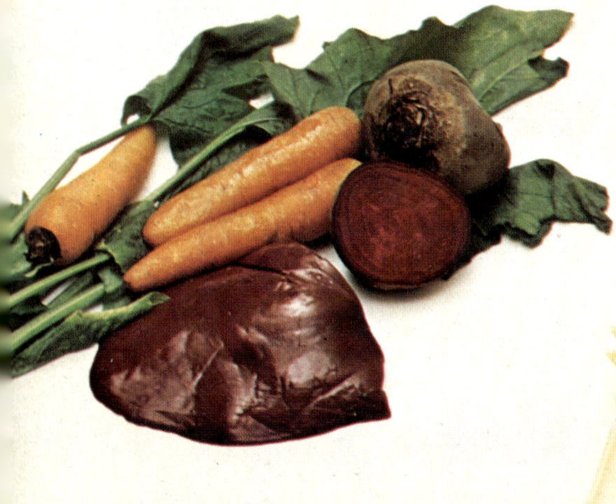

Vitamin A is essential for good vision in poor light and some of its major sources – which include carrots, spinach and beets – are shown here

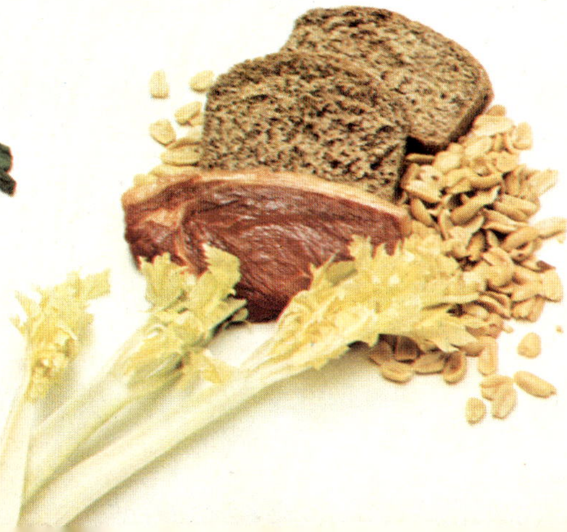

Vitamin B is, in fact, a genetic term for a number of quite dissimilar substances which, because of the effects of their deficiency from a diet – including beri beri and pellagra – have been grouped together. Major sources of the B vitamins, shown here, are bread, nuts and celery

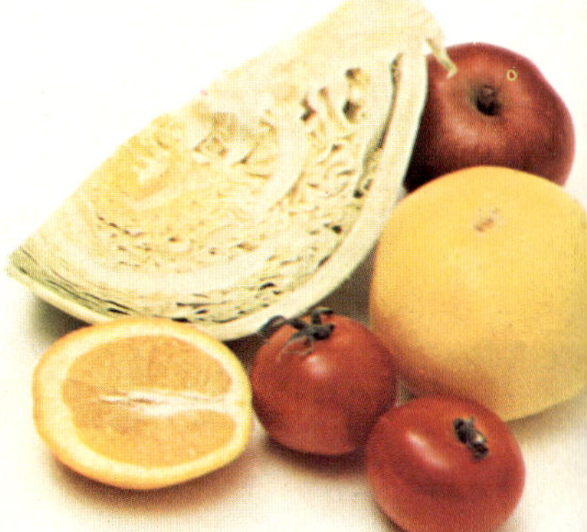

Vitamin C was the first whose lack was noted in the form of the deficiency disease scurvy which was known to be susceptible to treatment with fresh fruit or lime juice. Major sources are fresh fruit and vegetables – cooking destroys most of the vitamin C content

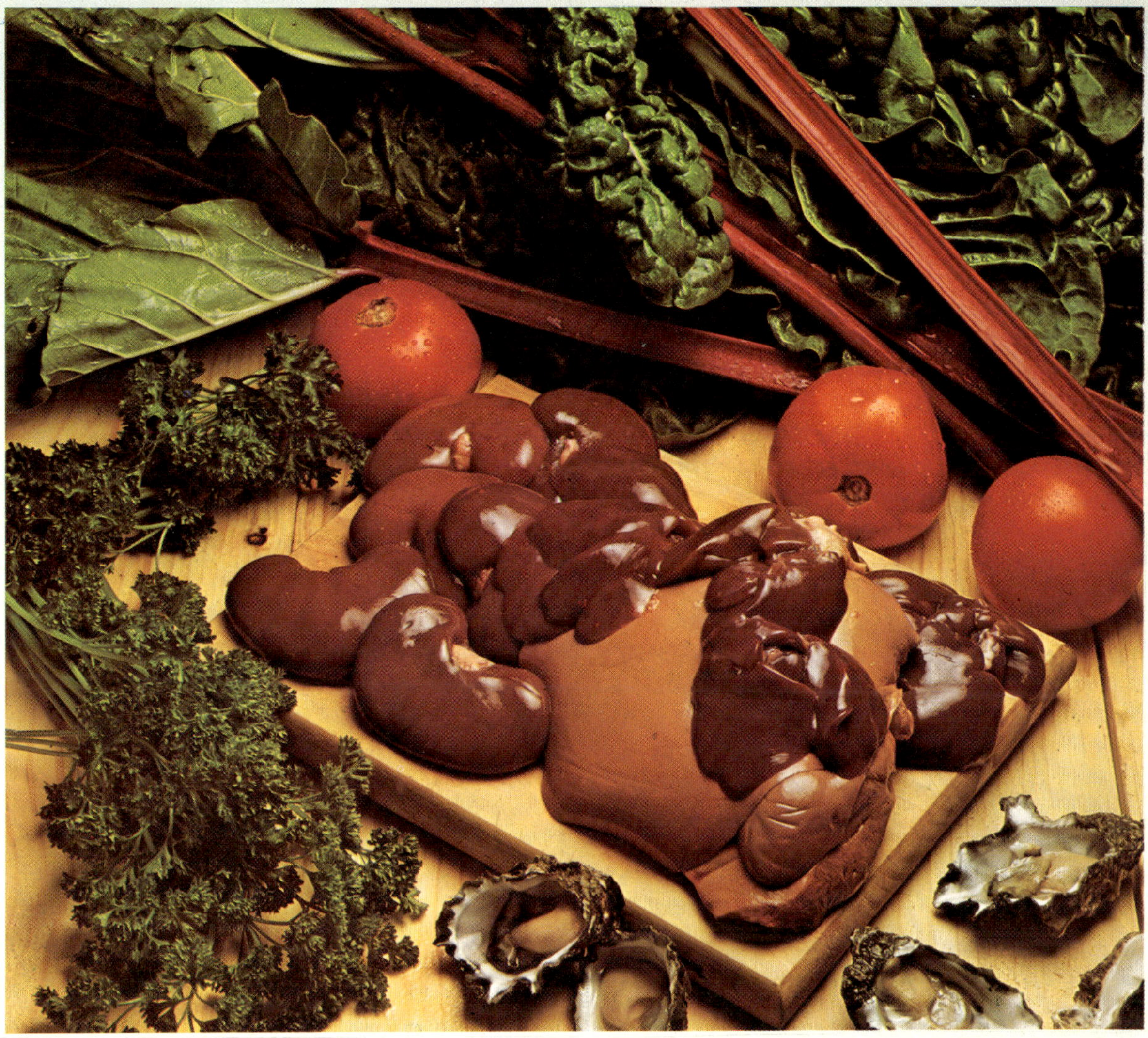

Iron is an essential mineral in human metabolism, its main use being in combination with protein to form haemoglobin, the oxygen-carrying component of the blood. It is also involved in enzyme action where oxygen is used throughout the body. The adult absorbs some 10 to 20 mg of iron daily and shown here are some foods – liver, kidneys, shellfish and tomatoes – that are particularly rich in this element

Vitamin D is essential for the formation of healthy teeth and bones. It can be formed naturally in the body as the result of the effect of sunlight on the skin but its main nutritional sources, shown here, include milk, cheese and eggs

There is little evidence to suggest that man is ever short of Vitamin E but it is found mainly, as shown here, in fish, bean sprouts and olives

Vitamin K is required for the synthesis of the enzyme thrombin, without which the blood would fail to clot. One form of this vitamin is formed by the action of bacteria in the intestines but natural sources include fish and green vegetables, especially spinach

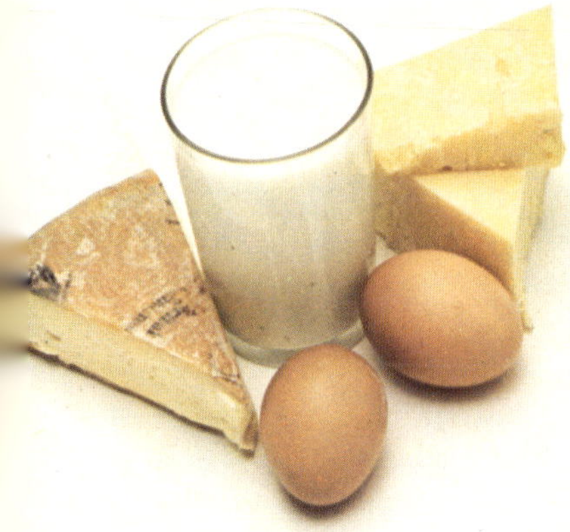

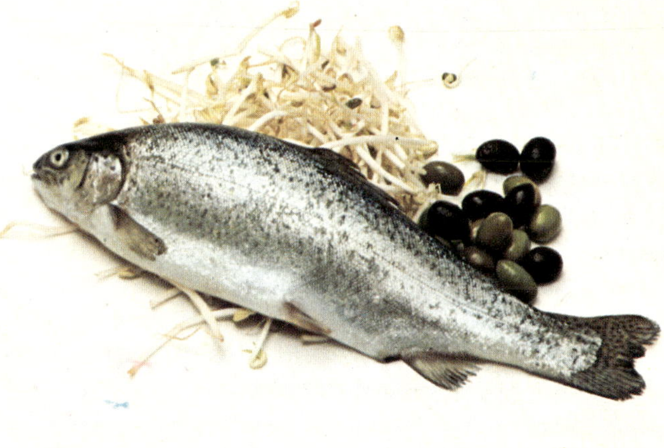

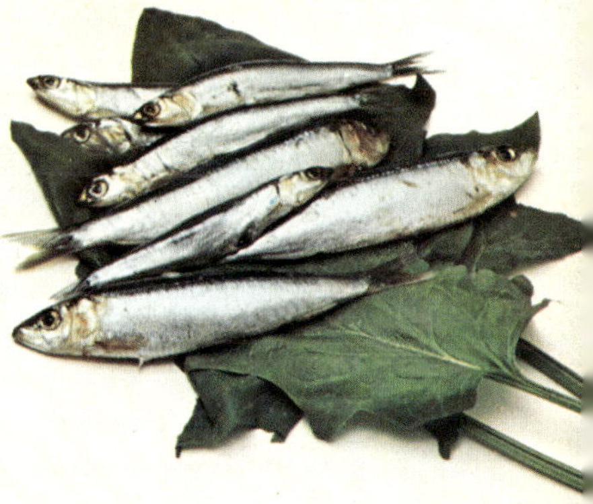

Reducing

Fasting is one way of losing weight: this is used in health farms and in hospital. Though very effective this drastic method should never be used over any extended period unless there is adequate supervision—because medical problems can occur. Also it can produce a strange state of euphoria so that the person concerned may begin to think he or she can live indefinately without food—and there is a danger that they might be tempted to try. Some forms of anorexia nervosa seem to fall into this category—girls can be so successful at cutting out food that they often lose all sense of reality and are transformed into an emaciated shadow of their former self, a downward slide that can go much too far to be attractive. Anorexia nervosa is a very difficult condition to treat because of all the psychological implications. In practice most of them do not fast, but alternate between hardly eating at all and then indulging excessively. Sometimes they feel remorse, as a result of all this overeating, and make themselves sick and rid themselves of all those excess calories. When they reach this stage their appetite has got out of control and no longer shows any relation to the actual needs of the body: part of the time they deprive their system, then they treat it equally cruelly by overwhelming it with foodstuffs. They can no longer trust their instincts regarding appropriate food intake and instead of being welcomed as a life-sustaining and pleasureable substance food becomes an obsession, victim of a love-hate relationship; food is an object of fear.

This fear of food is by no means confined to this group—who in practice nearly all become excessively thin; a lot of fat people fall into this category. They are the food addicts, the compulsive eaters. They love their addiction but hate it also—they despise their lack of control. They may starve themselves all day by eating nothing but cottage cheese and a wafer only to overindulge at night. Members of this group might consume as much as 5,000 calories at one sitting—enough for two women for a whole day.

It is then possible that their horror at this brutal act of self-destruction will assert itself and they will also artificially induce vomiting, after which their physical aches tend to be satisfied—until the next time. Once a person has got into this state they lose faith in their ability to resist food, particularly things like chocolates, but, in actual fact, it doesn't matter much what they eat once they are in full swing, they no longer appreciate the subtleties of taste, it is only the physical act of

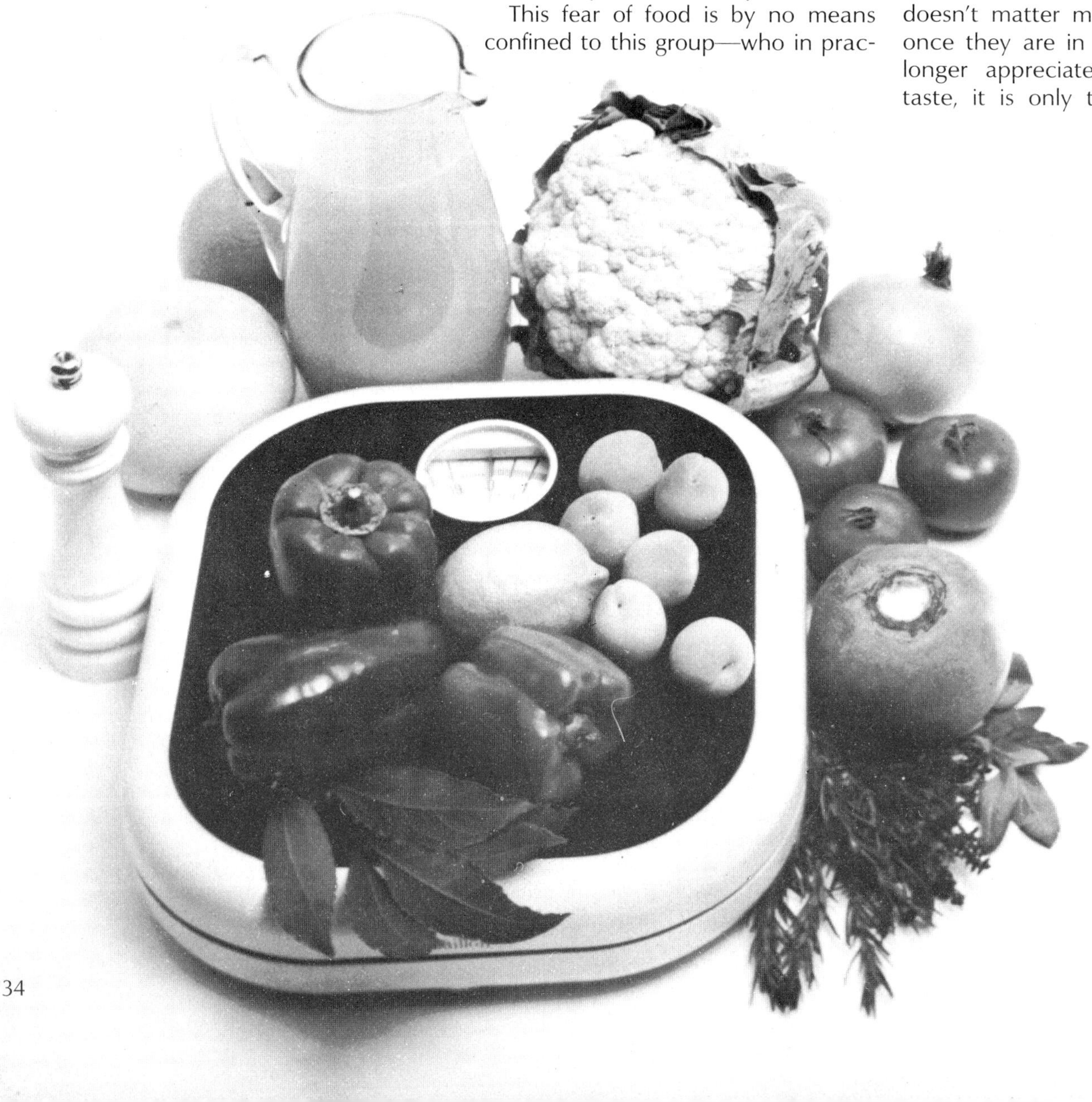

Successful reducing requires discipline, organization and enlightenment. Loss of faith or an apparent irrational inability to control your appetite is often the downfall of many a slimmer's regime. Fruit, fruit juices and selected fresh vegetables form an intricate part of a planned diet

eating that counts. In a case like this, the pyschological factors have become paramount, whatever the original cause for the overeating, and it is generally not very helpful to give lots of advice about a balanced diet.

Despite all the best intentions, it is because slimming diets tend to ignore the sweet tooth that so many diets fail. The afflicted person thinks he must avoid anything sweet like the plague and at the slightest lapse he is in despair—failed again.

Of course, the compulsive eater is in a different category from someone who genuinely does not need much in the way of calories to survive and each individual is very different in this regard. The compulsive eater is fortunate in one respect because he really does consume far too many calories and so there really is something to cut down—however he has many other anxieties linked with this cut down—and one of the most difficult things is the maintenance of a steady weight once it has fallen. It is only by paying great attention to the maintenance of weight loss that a steady slimmer state is achieved and it is for this reason that a diet that includes some sweet things, if the person craves it, should be included, if possible, right from the start.

It is not possible to devise the perfect diet—and the number of different possibilities and variations on a theme constantly presented in magazines and slimming publications bears ample testimony to the truth of this fact. It can only be arranged on an individual basis—because of individual needs, metabolism and also varying reactions to the foods available. For instance, some people tolerate very well a high fat diet, others feel sickly if their menu is too rich. People must make up their own minds. The first essential is to work out, completely honestly, exactly what is eaten on the average day. The best way to do this is to write everything down, each detail included. That way it is easier to remember the bits you'd like to forget like that mid-morning snack. It is the inbetweens which go uncounted that are responsible probably, for a majority of failed diets. There is absolutely no point attempting to slim unless you know exactly what you are consuming. You can then work out something realistic that you can live with and is a considerable reduction in calories as well. Fads diets work well for a time, mainly because they are so tedious but sooner or later you are bound to get tired of them—the milk and banana diet is one example, the apple and yogurt is another—also they are not well balanced; but this is unimportant for a few days. In hospital it has been found that fasting individuals do better if they are given a little protein and glucose mixture—the pure sugar and protein cope with all the body's basic needs for the fasting period and reduce side effects besides ensuring enough energy to allow normal living.

It is impossible to make firm recommendations regarding the foods that should be cut out—for scientific opinions are still somewhat conflicting. A low-protein diet is advocated by some people, as it reduces appetite, but that is not a good idea in the long run as the diet may become deficient in this substance. High fat diets are not to be recommended either: the relative lack of carbohydrate causes a metabolic imbalance causing bad breath and the kidneys have difficulty getting rid of all the waste products, known as ketones, also the brain needs sugars in order to work efficiently so that the person often feels sluggish. A diet that is very high in protein can be subject to the same disadvantages. Carbohydrates cannot be cut out completely, and too little fat reduces satiation; the key to a good diet is to keep an even balance.

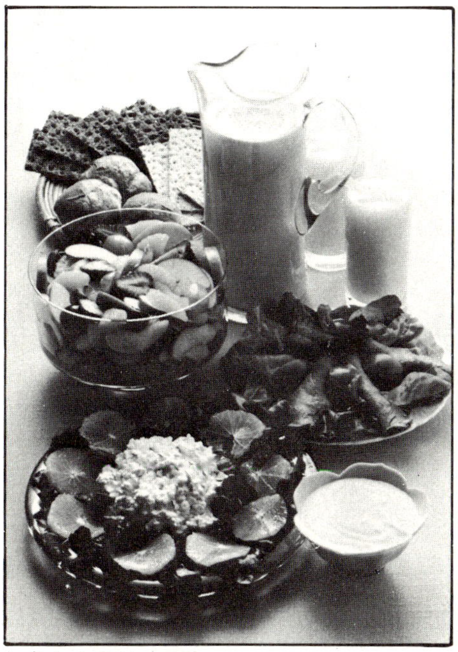

A dieter's light meal of crispbread, fruit, salad, orange juice, cottage cheese and a beef salad can be augmented by more solid food such as a jacket potato, as shown here

A beautiful body (below) is the ultimate goal to the slimmer. Attaining a well-proportioned, attractive physique is often the incentive for reducing.

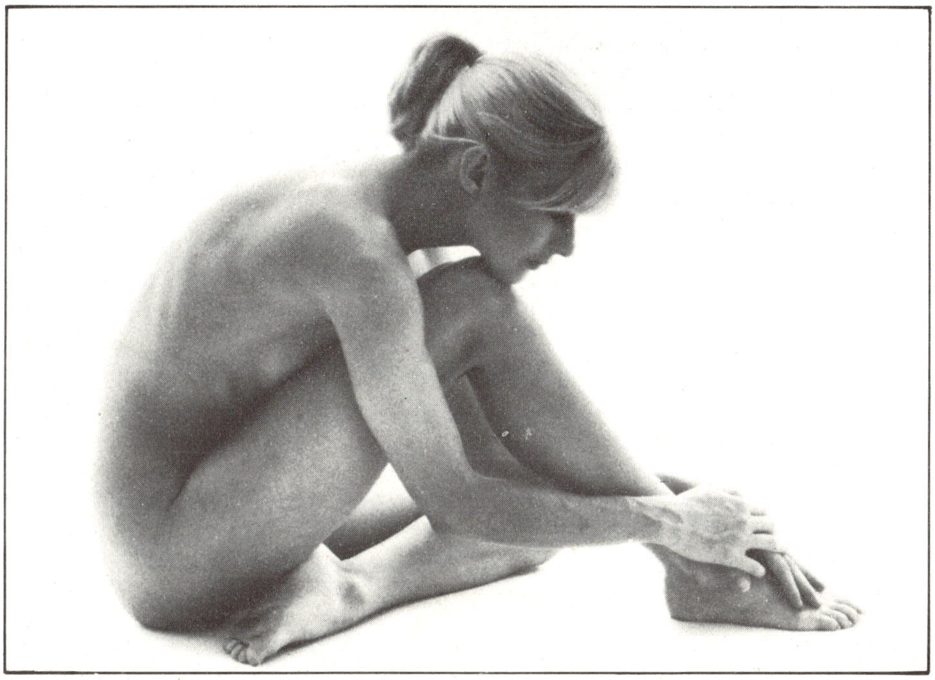

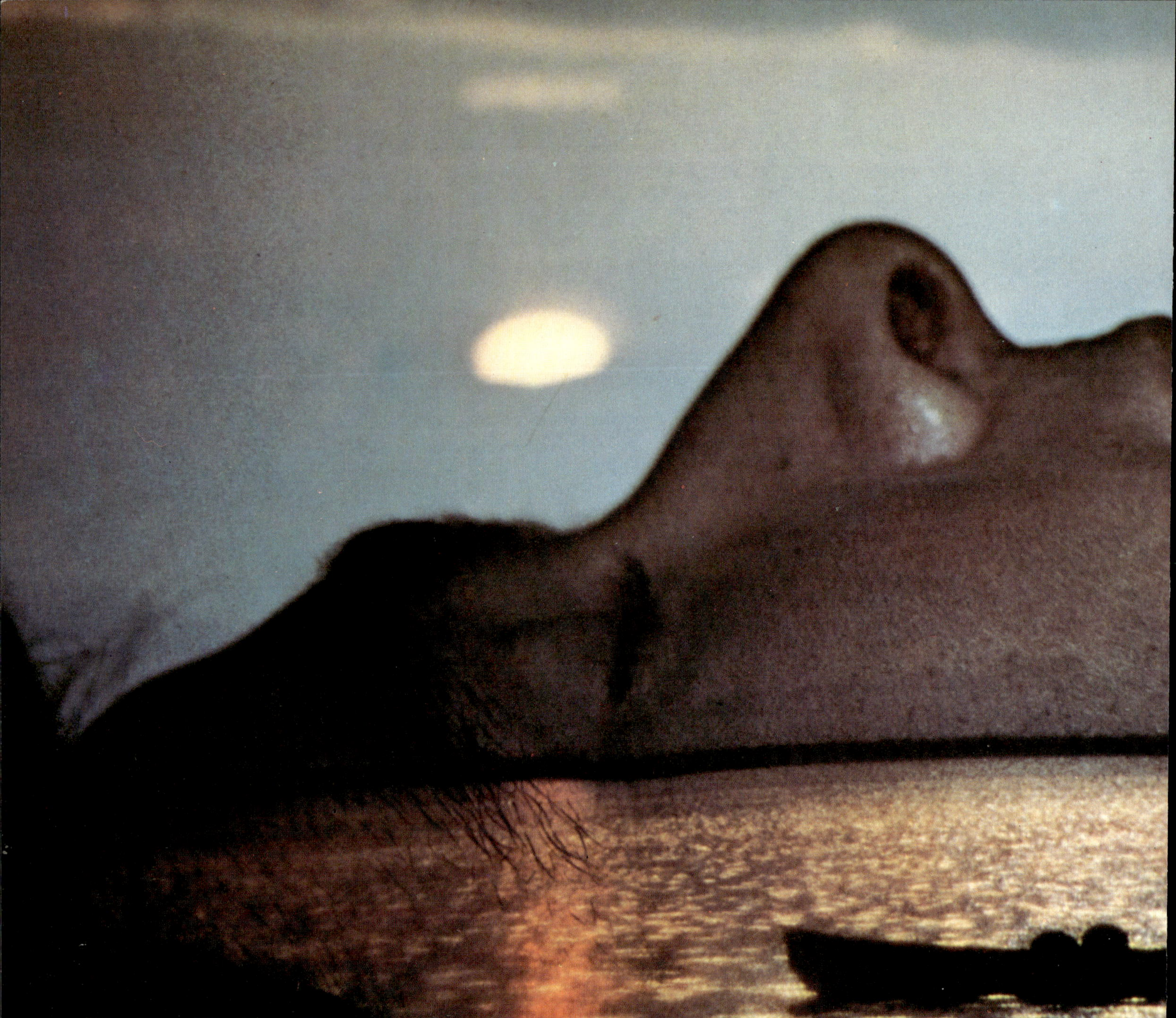

HOW TO RELAX

Learning to relax is important to health and happiness, even if we do not feel that our lives are particularly stressful or tense. Usually we relax by indulging ourselves in food or drink. More positive methods, though, include Yoga, meditation and massage. Whatever you feel choose a method which is suitable to your needs and personality. Learning to relax correctly should help you lead a fuller life, with mind and body able to harmonize in complete comfort.

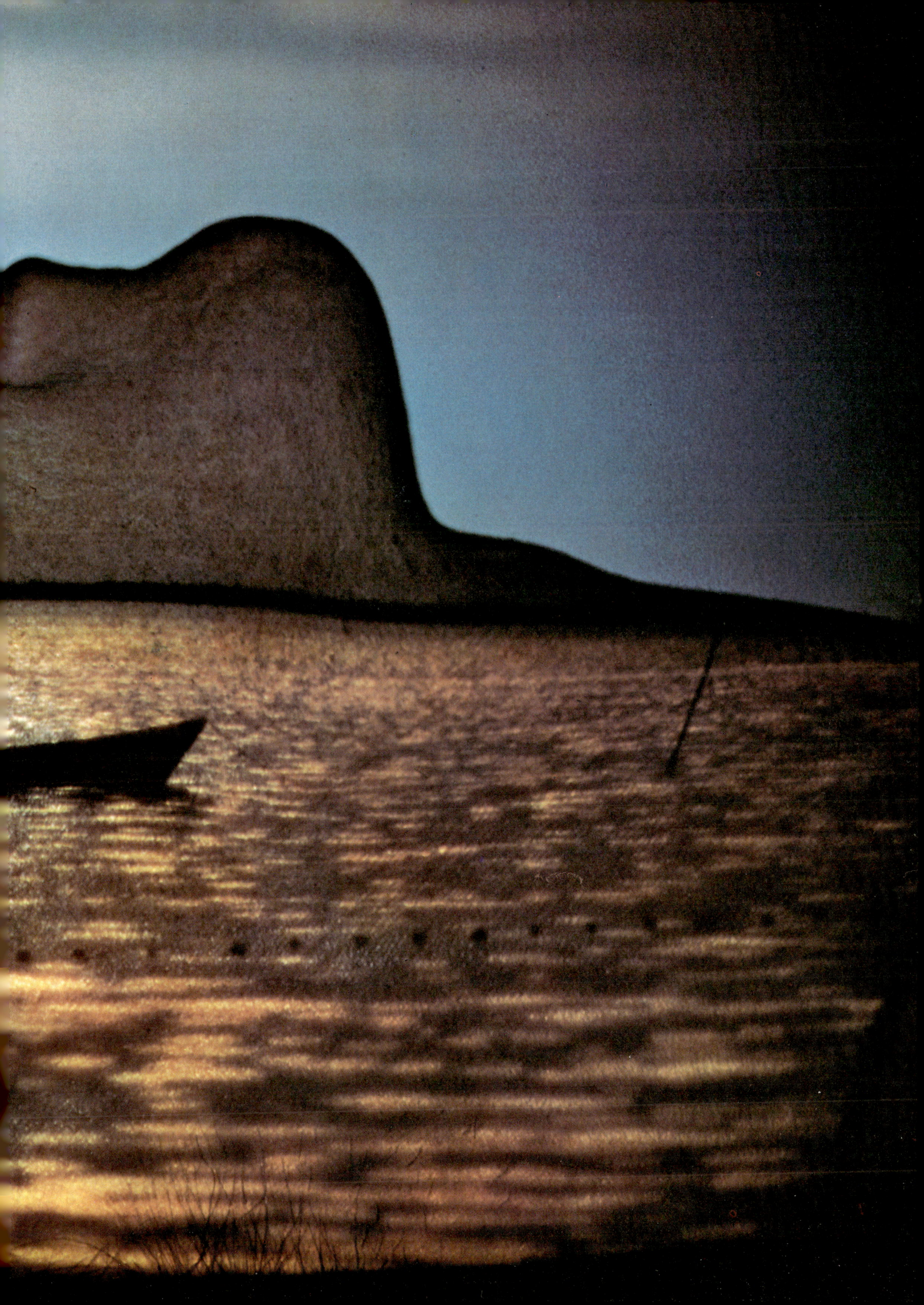

Why we need to Relax

Modern life, especially in the western hemisphere, is a nasty, brutish tense business. In the achieving society, the need to be always at peak alertness takes a heavy toll. Look at the rush-hour crowds in any major western city: their faces are stamped with unmistakeable signs of strain and anxiety.

Many of these people do not realize the state they are in. They go home and rest, they sleep what they consider a reasonable number of hours. They gradually get used to feeling a little bit less alive. Most of their problems could be completely blown away overnight if they learnt how to relax properly.

In this section we will examine various methods, both new and old, for helping modern man and woman to relax. Some of them are a little unusual as far as 20th century Western Man is concerned, but considering the acuteness of his problem, drastic methods need to be considered. In many cases, methods like meditation – which to many will sound more like hocus pocus – is not as alien to our culture as you might assume. It was practiced by the early Christians and was most likely the original purpose of prayer.

Relaxation is very difficult to define and impossible to measure accurately, although there are a number of guidelines that can be laid down. Basically it means freedom from mental anxiety and its corollary, bodily tension. Anxiety can take many forms: worrying about the mortgage, about the need to get up early in the morning to get to the office, about whether or not to wear a tie. These are not very serious concerns, compared with some of the life and death struggles that our ancestors had to face as part of their daily routine, but they can eat into our substance just the same. Our modern lives are constantly full of minor worries. We hardly ever have major crises, but lots of little ones that are never fully resolved. These prove to be much more difficult for the body to deal with than a few major problems.

We want to concentrate on the absence of anxiety and anger. Anger is a basic emotion, and complete relaxation means absence of anger as well. We all have some anger, some bitterness stored up and only we ourselves understand what it would mean if we could eliminate this thorn in our flesh. The opposite side of the coin is pleasure, a positive attitude. It is on this aspect that we need to concentrate.

Animals feel fear or anger when it is relevant to their lives, but these sensations are fully worked out and disappear once the crisis is over. They return to their resting state, one of contentment provided they are healthy. Children tend to be the same, manifesting their emotions immediately. Then it is over. As a result, animals and the vast majority of children do not suffer from tension. Adults, however, submit to a slow process of socialization which encourages them to hide their real feelings. It becomes an addictive habit, one that we often carry to ridiculous extremes. Tension builds up. This tension is socialized fear or strong feelings turned inwards, instead of outwards and therefore never released. The muscles which have been prepared for action never achieve release – they are kept in a perpetual state of readiness, akin to the battle fatigue that soldiers experience when they are in a constant state of readiness for action, and possibly death. The muscles never quite lose all their tension – so that even when we are resting we are still not completely relaxed. For the sake of argument let us assume that 0.1 per cent of the tension remains in the muscles after each crisis which prompts them to readiness has passed. The muscles become used to being tightened – in time the tension accumulates and a permanent tautness, even shortening of the muscles can result. Look at the back of the neck in the typical office worker and see how taut these muscle fibres are. Over the whole body this spasm-like condition of the muscles is bound to accelerate the pressure on the spine, encouraging it to shorten: the wear on the spinal discs is increased, leading to premature ageing, stooping and potential disc problems. Similarly the tight muscles, acting like a vice, lead to decreased flexibility of the joints and possible osteo-arthritis. There might be pressure on nerves where they leave the spinal column, causing sciatica-like pain. Soon we start to use only the chest muscles for breathing instead of those deep down in the abdomen. This means that the large muscular diaphragm, which by its powerful action helps to knead and massage all internal structures tucked below it, is not allowed to do its work. Hence, internal and glandular upsets will tend to be aggravated because the organs are not getting their regular work out.

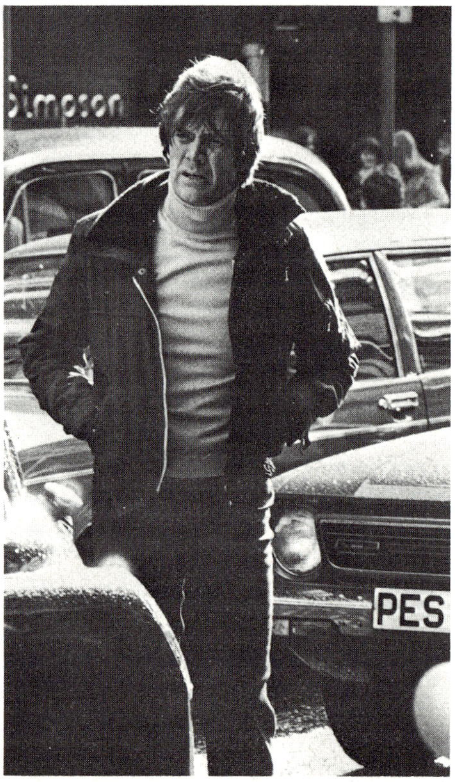

Surrounded by the fast pace, noise and crowded conditions of modern city living, we now have to look for ways of learning to relax. We have to overcome the effect of stress on our bodies, which shows itself as muscular pain, headaches, bad backs and stomach disorders

Real relaxation reverses all these trends; it allows the muscles to relax properly and breathing to function at its optimum. A concerted effort to achieve relaxation is needed. Unfortunately there is no objective measure of the state of relaxation, because individuals vary so much. On the whole anxious people sweat more – as measured by the conductivity of electricity on the palms of the hands – presumably partly because their nerves are working overtime. The tension in their muscles is on the whole greater, although the instruments for measuring this are as yet rather crude. Their blood circulation is adversely

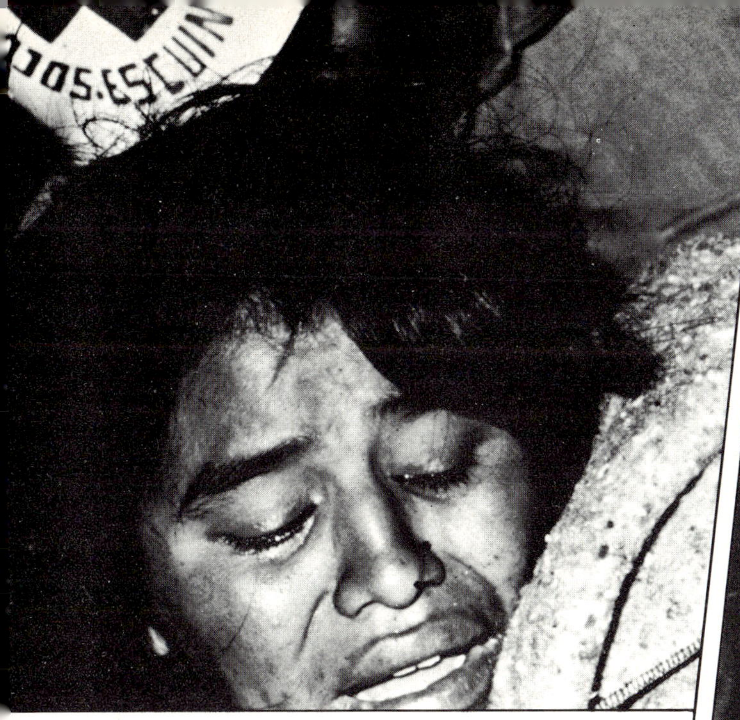

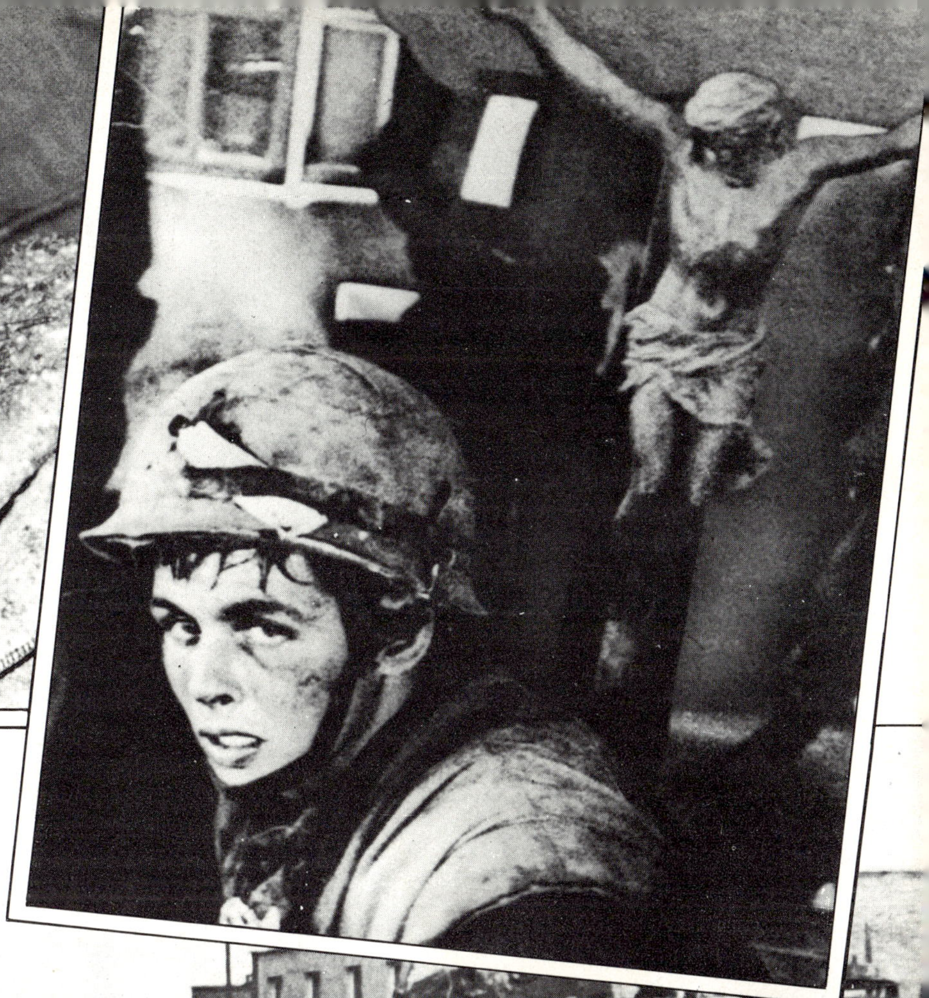

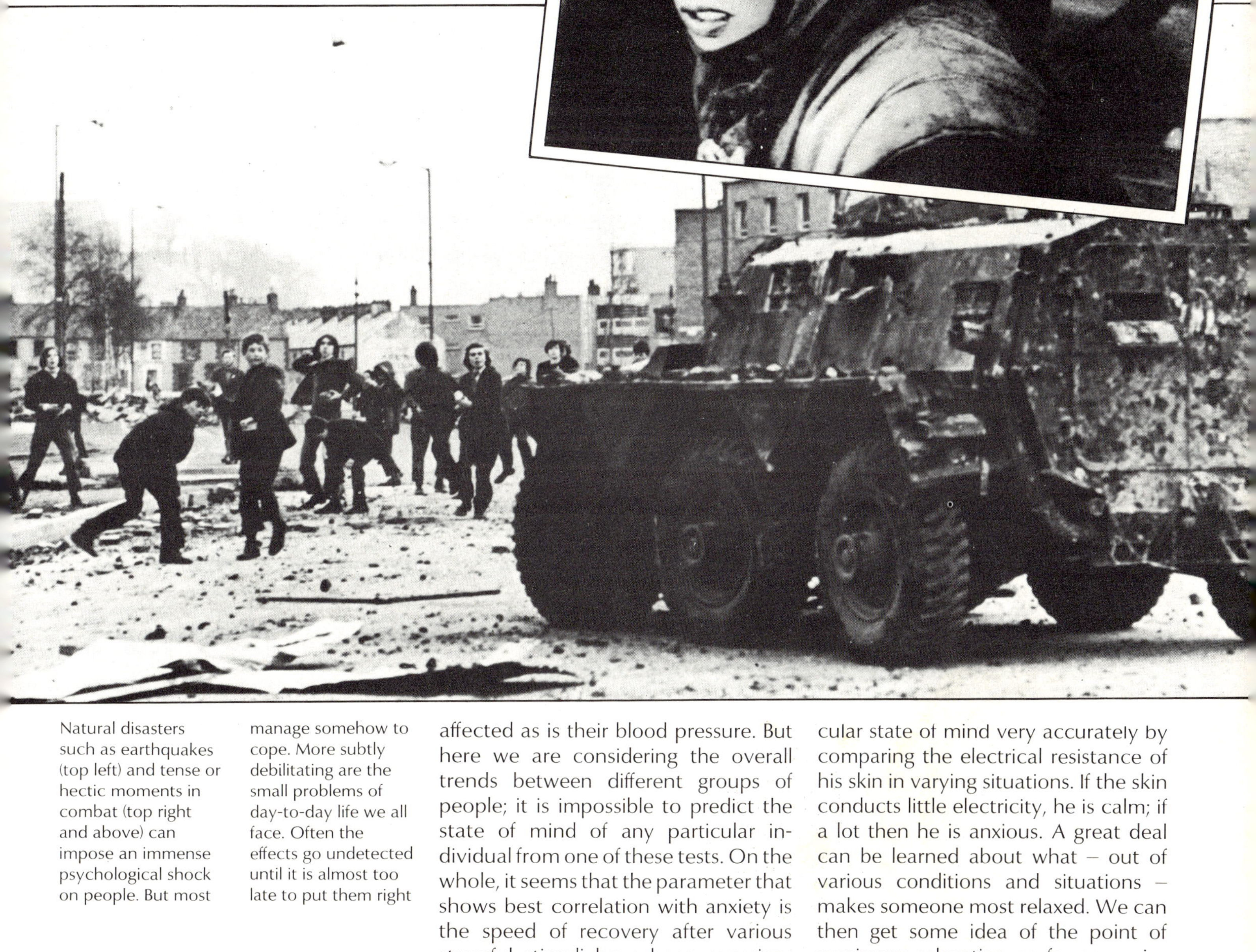

Natural disasters such as earthquakes (top left) and tense or hectic moments in combat (top right and above) can impose an immense psychological shock on people. But most manage somehow to cope. More subtly debilitating are the small problems of day-to-day life we all face. Often the effects go undetected until it is almost too late to put them right

affected as is their blood pressure. But here we are considering the overall trends between different groups of people; it is impossible to predict the state of mind of any particular individual from one of these tests. On the whole, it seems that the parameter that shows best correlation with anxiety is the speed of recovery after various stressful stimuli have been experienced. The normal, calm person recovers from the 'attack' on his system most rapidly, the anxious individual is sluggish about it and the average person falls in between. In any one individual, however, we can measure his particular state of mind very accurately by comparing the electrical resistance of his skin in varying situations. If the skin conducts little electricity, he is calm; if a lot then he is anxious. A great deal can be learned about what – out of various conditions and situations – makes someone most relaxed. We can then get some idea of the point of maximum relaxation as far as an individual is concerned; but the more we learn about meditation and other such methods and the more we delve into the inner being, the more the depth and breadth of relaxation seem to be virtually limitless.

The Pleasure Principle

The best way to relax is to be happy. This might sound very obvious, but even today a lot of people are not aware of this seemingly self-evident truth. The Puritan ethic which has permeated so much of Western thinking held that work automatically brought the greatest rewards and that pleasure was sinful. As it is clearly impossible to separate happiness and pleasure completely, it is not difficult to understand why the concept of happiness as a pre-requisite to health and physical well-being has not been understood in the western world. Now scientific evidence is emerging that happiness is the key to health, but it is interesting that Puritanism still hangs over us sufficiently to prevent us labelling the pleasure principle for what it is!

A positive attitude to life helps protect us against ulcers, against cancer, virtually any ailment you can name. The body and mind (meaning the brain) are completely interrelated, not two separate entities. They share the same blood supply, so that the same chemicals are shunted round the nervous system as pass through other parts of the system such as liver and stomach. There are a few localized mini-systems, but even they make contact with all the neighbouring parts of the total organization and transmit messages which influence the overall mechanism. Mood can be swayed by the influx of such substances which do not act directly on the nervous tissue but have a mediating effect on transmitters situated locally in the brain. Exercise, by stimulating the release of certain substances that the brain seems to need to work at top efficiency, can have a startling effect on how you feel about life. Cases of depression are being cured with great success, in the United States particularly, by a regular jogging programme; the drugs previously used had been only a mediocre boost. Of course, the need for this kind of stimulus varies from person to person but that exercise can benefit the mind seems to be universally acknowledged.

Similarly, the chemicals produced locally by the brain in response to your angry feelings about something will seep out over a period and gradually transmit their negative message down the line, until the stomach or some other part is acquainted with the idea that all is not well above. Of course, the stomach doesn't 'know', or even care, why things have gone a bit awry but merely reacts with a chronic grumble. If you are happy, then 'friendly' chemicals spread through nervous tissues and a warm glow is transmitted all over the body.

Part of this process involves a shutdown of certain nerves in the body – those that cause agitation. There are basically three kinds of nerves in the body; the first, known as the voluntary nerves, which we can consciously influence, transmit most of the messages from the brain to the outer boundaries of the body. The other two sets (together known as the autonomic nervous system) are centred in the solar plexus and control those aspects that are generally considered to be involuntary, i.e. automatic and outside our conscious control. They are known as sympathetic and parasympathetic nerves and control such processes as breathing, blood flow, digestion and so on. When one set is active, the other group is quiescent. When we are nervy, anxious, tense, fearful, angry, the sympathetic gets into gear. Adrenaline is produced and we prepare for remedial action – action which might never come leaving adrenaline and similar stimulating hormones coursing round the bloodstream looking for a target area. The parasympathetic system works in the opposite direction; it involves a clampdown on all the busy, frenetic energy–wasters and concentrates on pleasure, food and the conservation of energy.

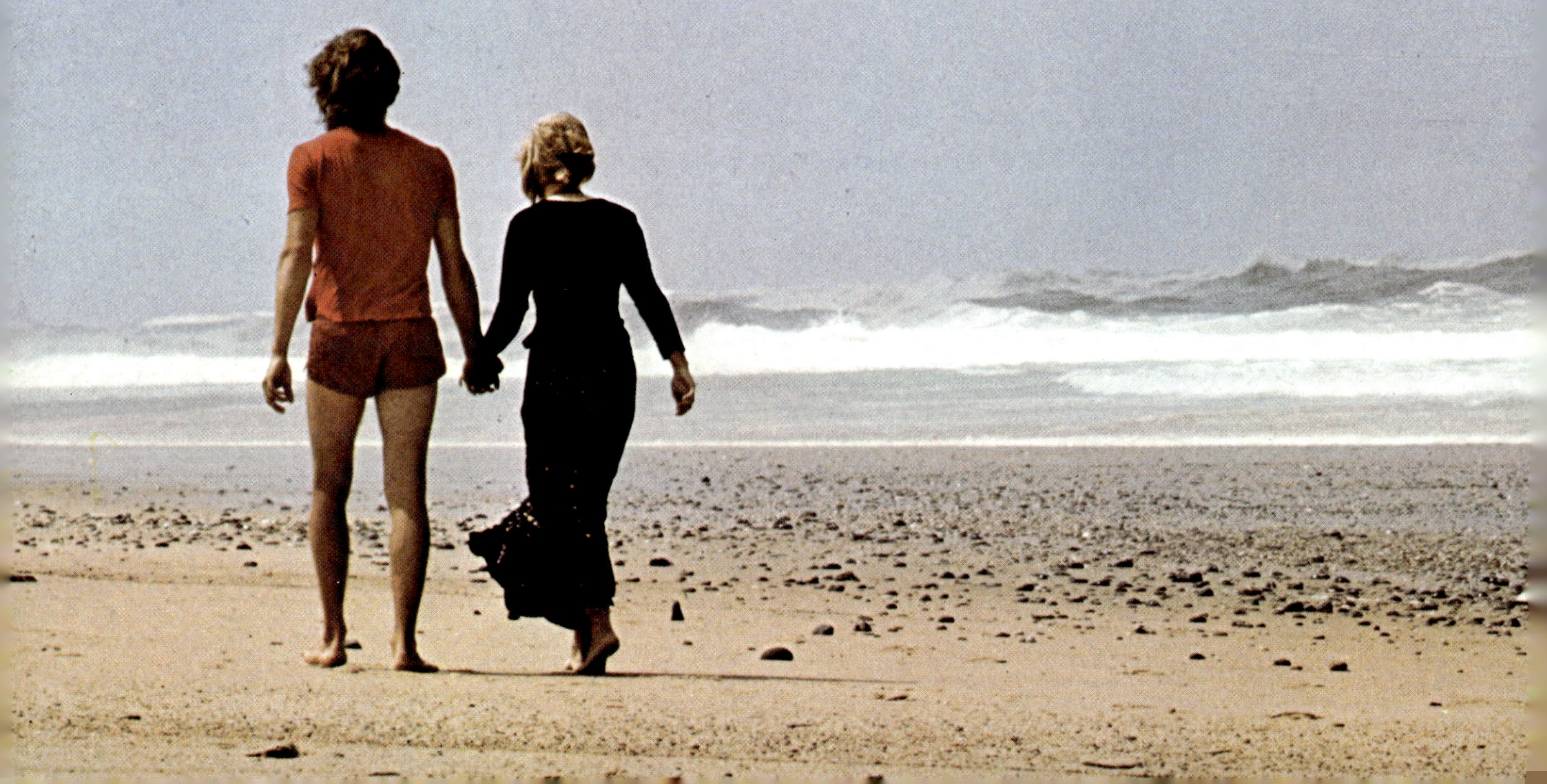

Happiness tends to harmonise with the parasympathetic nervous system, although this is a rather simplified view. It is possible for the parasympathetic to be in fine fettle yet happiness remain elusive; on the other hand, it is impossible to achieve real happiness if the sympathetic adrenaline is running amok through the system.

The chemical shutdown, represented by the ascendency of the parasympathetic, can be described as calmness or peace of mind. Peace of mind goes somewhere towards happiness but not all the way; some positive feeling that all is right with your world must be present as well. The ultimate in this respect, ecstasy, is experienced by some when they fall in love, or during a moment of exhilaration generated by flirting with life itself during some particularly dangerous sporting exploits. Many people look to food or drink or sex to find this extra experience. Meditators claim that they can remove the need to search for external stimulation by finding a way to generate internally these ecstatic peaks.

For most of us happiness is not ecstasy, nor do we need to aim so high to achieve wellbeing and relaxation. Good old contentment is probably enough, for real joy has a tendency to create its own troubles. For most of us, then, happiness is just simply feeling good, through and through. How do we reach this goal? Good health, positive health is an obvious prerequisite that needs no further elaboration here. The absence of worry over money and so forth is essential. If this seems difficult work on ways to cut your living costs: lots of our so-called necessities are really luxuries and can be discarded. You must also deal with anger, petty jealousies and fears. Then you can concentrate on the good things. Friends, family and loved ones. A good laugh. Friends play a very important role in helping us relax but we tend to take them for granted. We choose people who reflect our own attitudes to some extent and being with them reaffirms our belief in ourselves and what we stand for. Having our own internal value systems boosted by their presence provides a warm positive feeling. Similarly, helping our friends with their problems or even aiding strangers causes a warm glow, a sensation that we share fellow feelings with all human beings. That is a powerful inducement to happiness. So many of us get so bogged down in our own problems that we feel nothing but loneliness and the resultant feelings of alienation which cause anger and bitterness. You learn to have greater confidence by focusing on other people. The benefits of reciprocated love derive from the blending of the two personalities. The person who gains a lot from friends or the stranger on the street is gaining some of this benefit without the complications of the love experience. This sharing of part of your personality has a healing, synthesizing effect on the persona.

The sparkle of success for the racing driver (right) the exhilaration of sky diving (below right) or the simple contentment that can come from walking hand in hand along the beach – all are ways of relaxing. Laughing, sharing the company of friends and lovers, brings a warmth to life missing for those who concentrate on work and duty to the exclusion of everything else

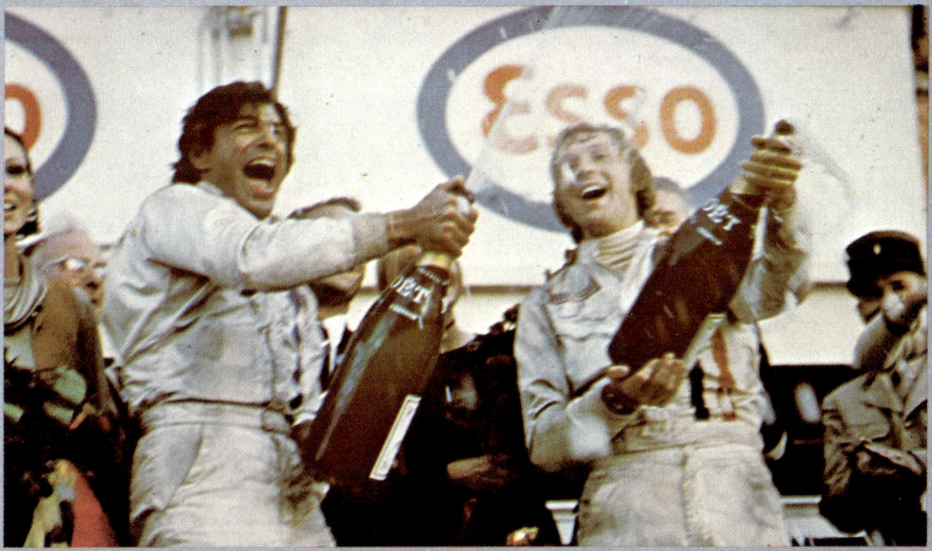

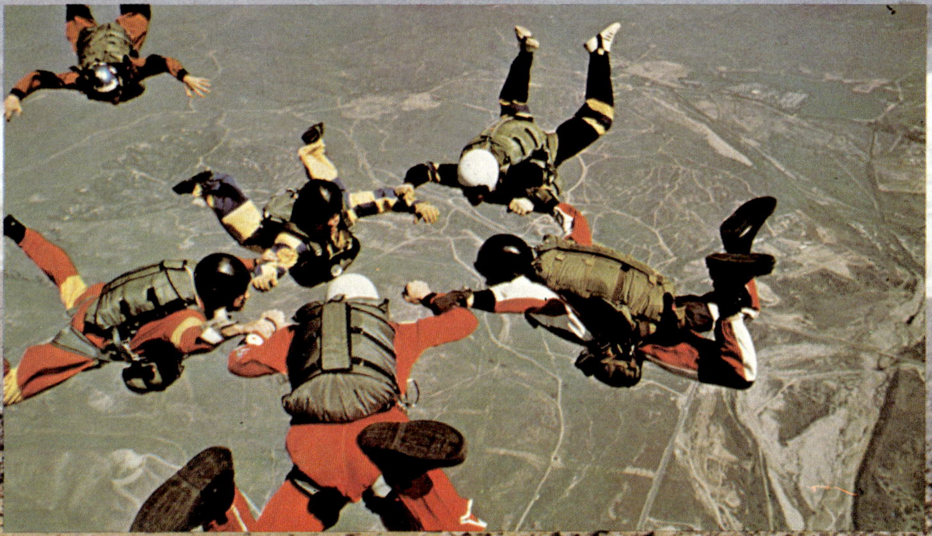

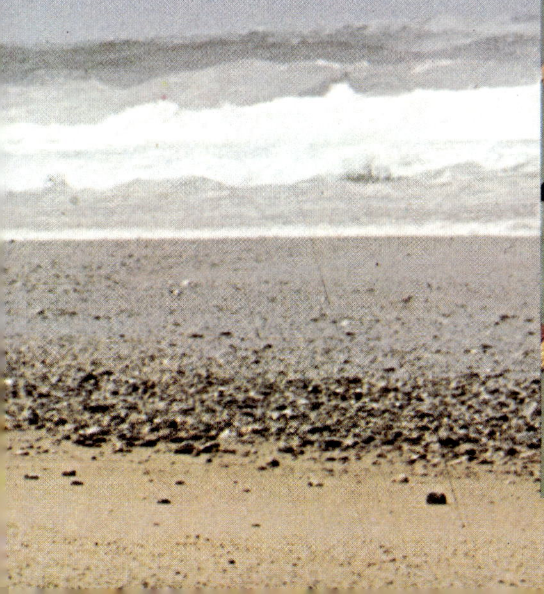

Eating and Drinking

When people sit down to eat together they are formalizing the need to be involved together; eating is one of the most basic human drives: by marrying that with the act of social intercourse we help to cement our contacts with the outside world. Eating, whether at home or at a restaurant, is generally considered one of the most pleasant ways of relaxing. The environment should be conducive to intimacy – warmth, a pleasant glowing light and conversation which reinforces, hopefully, the sharing of one individual with another. Then there is the food itself and the care with which it has been prepared. Its taste jogs the pleasure centres of the tongue and boosts the processes of digestion which stimulate the parasympathetic system or the calming nerves.

This relationship of food and that part of the nervous system which is diametrically opposed to tension explains to some extent why overweight individuals have a reputation for being calm and happy. Being gross and ugly are very negative features which can submerge the phlegmatic temperament but chemically speaking there are several reasons for the connection. Because anxious people are busy producing adrenaline-like substances they cannot digest efficiently as blood is being diverted away from the intestines. They easily feel full up as the nutrient pathway is blocked. As a result they tend to eat less. Laboratory animals refuse food when they are agitated, but eating actually helps to calm them down if they can be encouraged to take what is offered, because the adrenaline producing nerves are shut down. People who eat lots of food are keeping the relaxing set of nerves in good trim.

There are other aspects to this: calm people use energy less wastefully, their metabolism is probably more efficient and so they need less in the first place. They don't burn up the excess, so there is plenty in the bloodstream. The brain is well supplied with all its needs and the person feels replete, satisfied; even euphoric. On the other hand, the anxious person who is short on calories – for one or all of the reasons given above – might find himself with a blood-sugar level that is just below par. His hunger may go unrecognized as the tension takes away the normal urge to eat and this stress – that of hunger – pushes full relaxation even further out of reach. For an anxious individual the right circumstances for eating are very important. Not only do they relax him or her by creating an atmosphere in which he can let go his rigid self-control but this very easing back allows him to eat a square meal and to enjoy it – all factors contributing to his overall relaxation. This whole process is greatly facilitated by the use of alcohol, a drug which has been in widespread use throughout the world for centuries. It has its dangers but they

Drinking with friends can provide great pleasure and relaxation. If it is taken to excess, though, it can become an end in itself, creating more difficulties than it was intended to ease

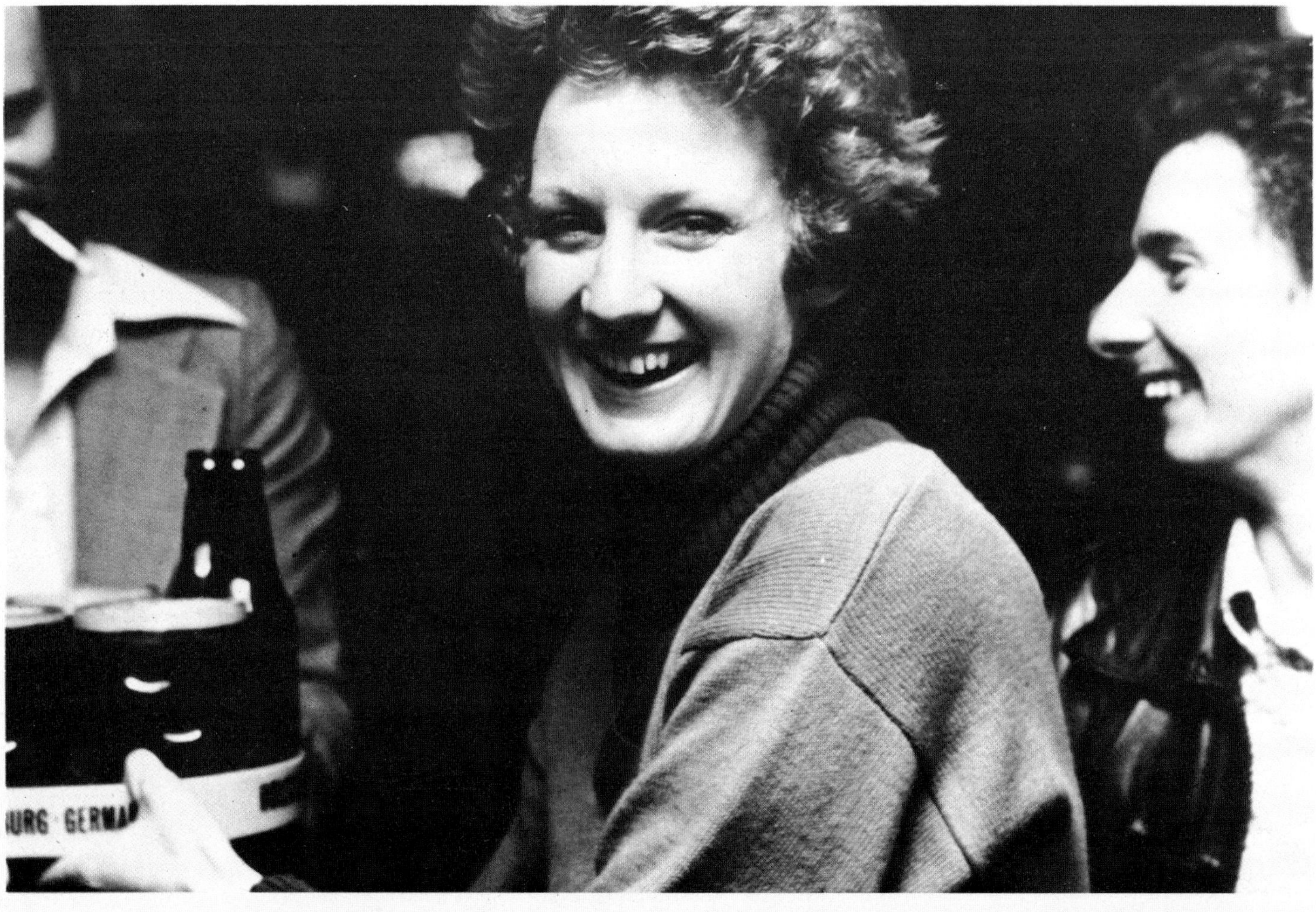

are very small and we are at least familiar with its hazards as a result of long experience. The damage is in any case likely to be no worse than what people inflict on themselves through unresolved tension and the excess circulation of chemicals that this creates. It can be taken to extremes, but there is no doubt that a small amount of alcohol, in whatever form it is taken, is very relaxing. Although the loss of control it generates makes a driver less capable than when he is sober, studies all seem to show that after one drink – and in some cases possibly two – the driver performs better. The tension, which is a perpetual life companion for most of us, is relaxed as a result of the first drink. The muscular tightness is eased, hand-muscle coordination is sharpened up, along with reaction time. After that, the disadvantages begin to outweigh the benefits.

Alcohol is, of course, a drug. Here we are taking a substance which is quite foreign to the body; we could all exist without ever taking a drop. However, it is a substance that the body seems able to cope with fairly easily, albeit slowly, because its chemical structure is relatively simple. Part of the action of a drug is to modify the body's internal chemistry – through the way it reacts with other compounds – a process we do unconsciously all the time, as we breathe or eat or get worried or even carry out relaxation exercises. Then it has a specific action all its own – alcohol depresses certain of the brain's higher centres. These are the parts concerned with stiffness, discipline and control. Many of us exert too rigid a control over ourselves, just asking for tension; after a few drinks this grip is loosened. Of course, if it is carried too far complete lack of control results, not just of behaviour but also disrupting some of the vital processes like breathing. The whole of the nervous equilibrium is rocked, with potentially harmful results.

Alcohol is not the only drug to be used for such purposes: marijuana is a very common one in some parts of the world, though it has a different action. It is not really a sedative, more a hallucinogenic substance, leaning in the same direction as LSD – though nowhere near as powerful a distorter of perception. It has a specific calming effect; it takes away anxiety and cuts out the need for the user to communicate with the outside world. In this it resembles various techniques of meditation. It turns the person inward to the relaxation of peace with oneself.

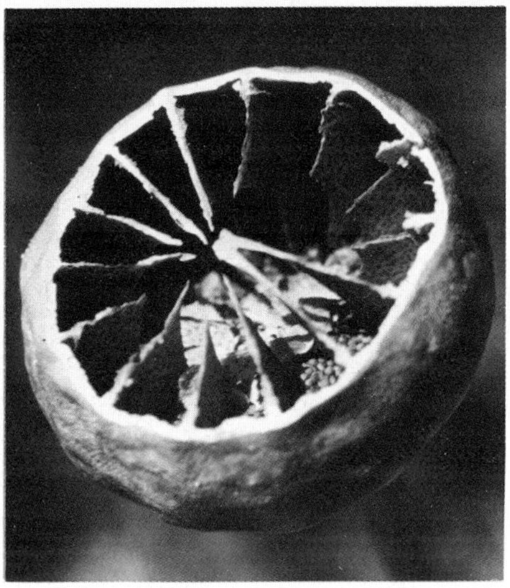

The seed from the opium poppy (above) has been used all over the world for centuries to bring pleasant dreams and a sense of well-being. But the danger of addiction is very great, particularly with its derivatives, morphine and heroin. Marijuana (below) is sold openly in the shops of Nepal, but it also causes problems

Alcohol merely removes inhibitions so that the fear of the environment is reduced, actively encouraging communication with the outside. Of course, marijuana is complicated by its legal status in most places, like opium. The latter is relatively safe when consumed in the form extracted from the poppy, that is opium itself, but becomes highly addictive in the purified form of morphine or when concentrated as heroin. As with marijuana, outside weights and stresses are transported away, so that the person feels a light and joyful floating feeling. It is interesting to find that these substances bear very close resemblance to the enkephalins, compounds found naturally in the brain, which exert a soothing effect and seem to be nature's own tranquillizers. Scientists are working on ways to synthesize these substances in large quantities, making sure that no addictive qualities exist; then we will really have sedatives to write home about. Meanwhile opium and the others give pleasure but the dangers of addiction severely limit their use and uncontrolled experimentation should not be encouraged.

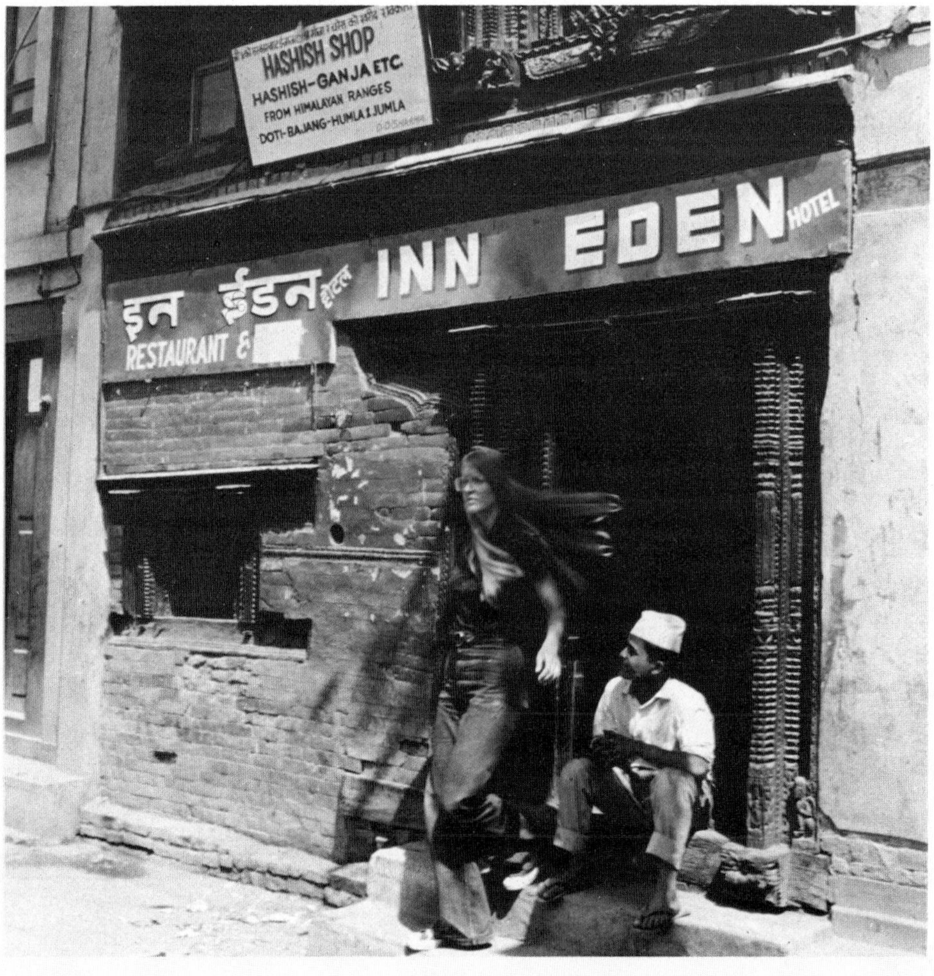

The Calm Mind

The time for rest is, or should be, while we are asleep. Unfortunately, for many people slumber is never smooth or undisturbed and they wake feeling as tired as before. They wake fitfully throughout the night. They are not properly relaxed. They fall asleep out of extreme tiredness but as soon as the fatigue disappears a little, the tension in the muscles and the attendant awkward posture impinge, the pattern of slumber can be broken. When people are emotionally upset their sleep can be disturbed. Children who wet their beds are often found to have unbalanced sleep rhythms. In their case, hypnosis – actually teaching them the art of self-hypnosis – can correct the deficiencies and help the disordered bladder control which was triggered by emotional tension.

Sleep is divided into various phases: the two most important being orthodox and dreaming sleep. The latter seems to be very necessary for us to chew over all our problems, but it is easy to disrupt the balance: if we do not dream enough our behaviour is disjointed and the brain is subsequently not able to function at its best. During this period, the eyes engage in very rapid movements, hence its name of paradoxical sleep or REM (rapid eye movement) sleep.

Most of us can forget the finer details – the point is *how* to get to sleep. The time honoured sheep-counting method does work, but for beginners the mere effort of counting tends to be distracting. For someone practised in the arts of meditation the sequence of numbers would be easy. Probably the best method for today's worriers is deep breathing. This produces real relaxation and thereby eliminates the tensions which are putting obstacles in sleep's way. Individuals as varied as opera singer coaches, yoga exponents and common or garden relaxation enthusiasts with no strings attached, all advocate this method. And it certainly can be very 'heady'. If the right technique is practised whilst standing up one can feel positively floating. Basically it involves using the muscles of the abdomen. To induce sleepiness, Yoga advocates that you 'Lie flat on the back with the fingertips placed on the solar plexus. Inhale and exhale deeply and slowly, feeling the rise and fall of the abdomen. There is an almost hypnotic effect in this movement which induces drowsiness.' Some followers of Eastern traditions suggest that both in and out movements are done slowly to the count of four and that you should concentrate hard on the counting. This is fine as a practice for meditation but may be disruptive to the untrained person seeking sleep. Yoga tradition allows you to assume other positions in bed provided that the breathing rule is always observed.

Deep breathing forms the basis of relaxation exercises. The latter are many and varied, their variety equalling the number of self-proclaimed gurus who abound today. Some are

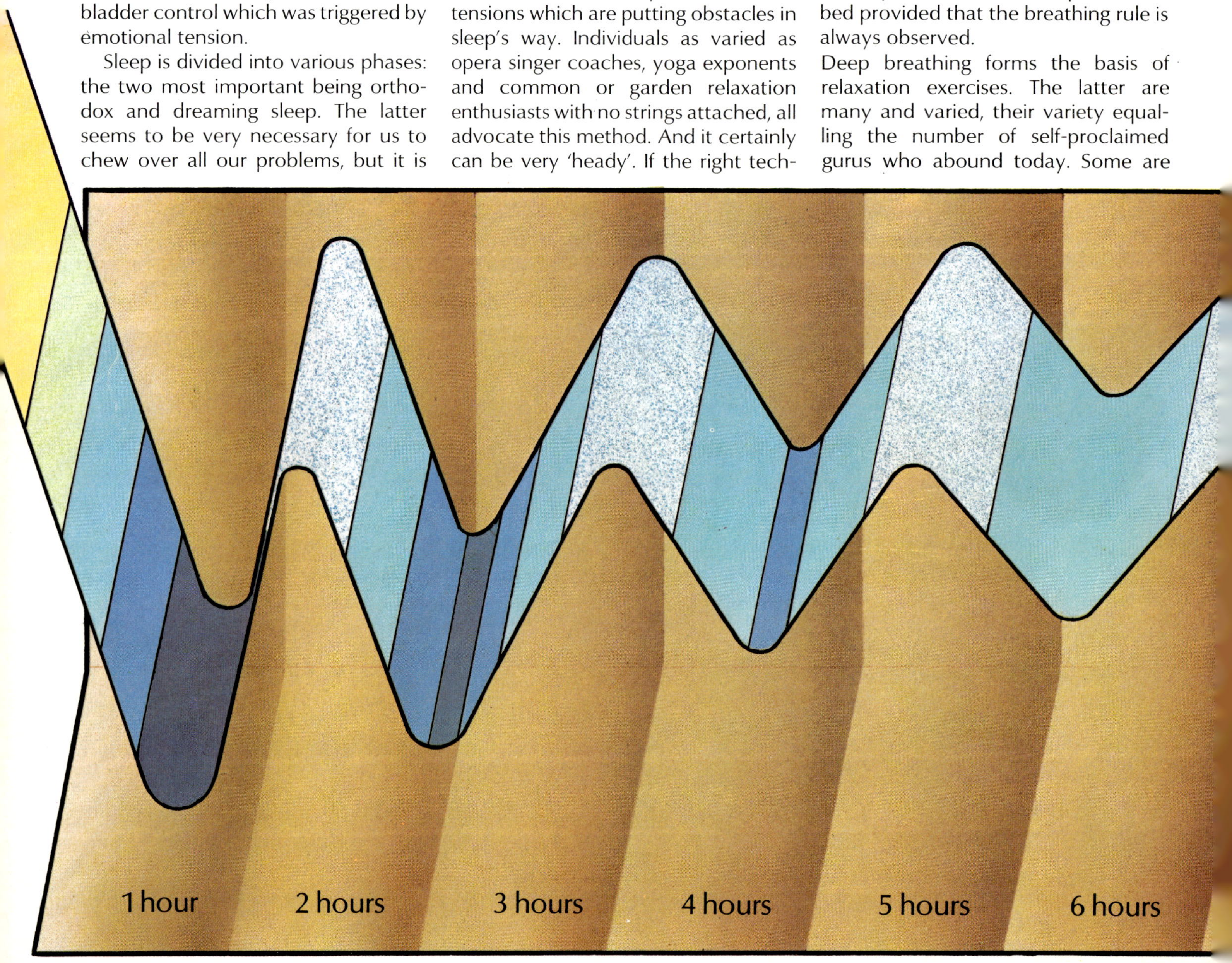

simple and involve nothing more than your head flopping loosely in front of you, or pressing on the hollow parts which separate the top of the back of the neck from the parts above. Favourite headache cures come in guises like these. The Yoga Triangular posture is supposed to soothe nervous centres at the back of the head; it can also be performed iin a rocking-type action. The Yoga mental exercises are of a different order; they are difficult for the uninitiated to master as they are so seldom written down in those tomes on the subject we find in the west.

One technique which is very effective if you are able to concentrate is 'focusing of the *chakras*'. There is an energy force called *kundalini* and all the force and power of the system stems from this; there are seven points roughly located along the axis of the spine where this energy appears to be harnessed. These centres are called *chakras* in Yoga and *lataif* in the Sufi tradition. Each has a different colour and the person trying to relax focuses first on the lowest one at the base of the spine and allows that particular colour to flood the mind. The idea is to get the colour swinging round like a centrifuge and then move on to the next highest centre and get that colour moving until the top of the head is reached. Any area that is experiencing trouble will take longer to 'ignite' than the others, but the extra effort helps to resolve the negative features current in that area producing overall harmony. It takes practice, but those westerners who are initiated swear by it.

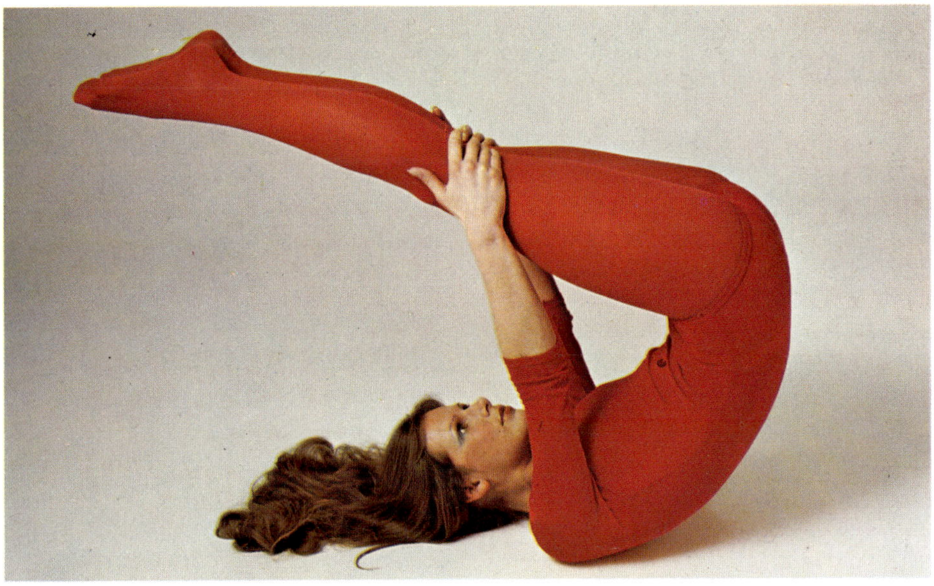

The Yoga Triangular position, lying down, looks awkward, but is not only soothing and relaxing for the mind, but exercises the neck and shoulders. A perfect way to relax and exercise

Institutions such as health farms sometimes practice their own brand of relaxation exercises. These exercises involve initial mastery of the breathing exercises. Once really relaxed abdominal breathing is assured, the muscles are given some attention.

Some hypnotists use a similar method. First tense the muscles of the right foot, hard, then relax them. Then concentrate hard on the left foot. Slowly. Tense and hold for a few seconds, then relax. This is also a little reminiscent of Yoga technique except that Yoga uses active, actual movement rather than contractions of this sort. Gradually you work up the body concentrating very hard. The very act of concentrating is enough to make this a type of meditation, to exclude all extraneous noise and allow the system to relax completely once the stimulus, tensing the muscles, is released. The breathing helps throughout. Next, you are told to let your mind wander freely. You are not supposed to concentrate on anything nor to try to free it – for the mere act of trying to make your mind a blank involves concentration and that means some effort. Just allow the mind to roam and invariably pleasant peaceful thoughts pervade the mind. Combined with diet and some positive exercise plus Yoga, maybe a regime like this can work wonders.

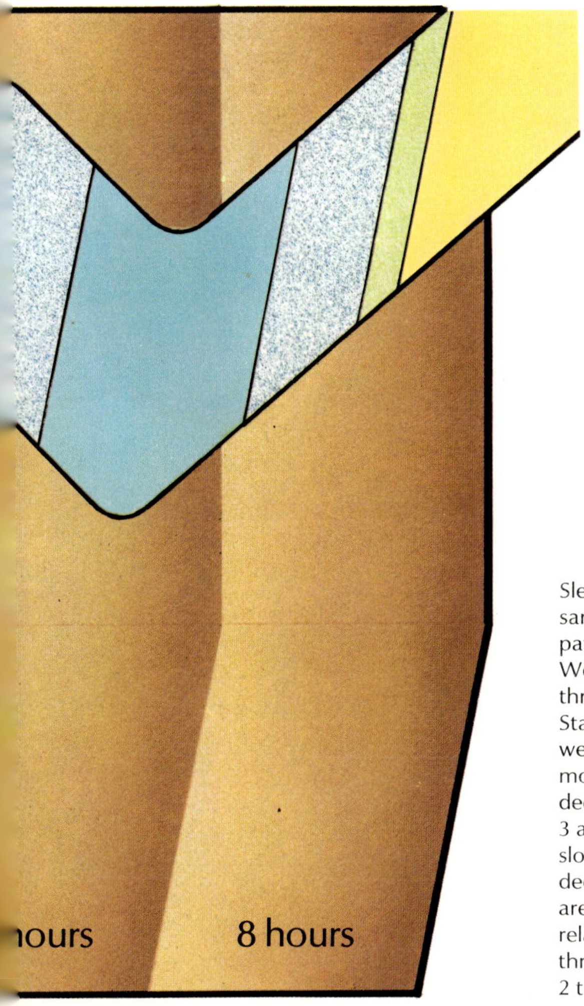

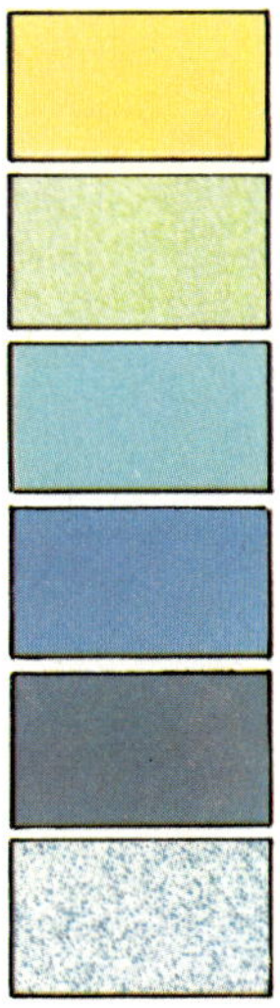

Sleep follows the same rhythmic pattern for everyone. We sink quickly through the light Stages 1 and 2, when we show many body movements, to the deep sleep of Stages 3 and 4. Brain activity slows, breathing is deep and regular, we are completely relaxed. We then go through Stages 3 and 2 to dreaming or REM (rapid eye movement) sleep, when the brain is more active, and our eyes move to and fro under the lids. Descending briefly once more to Stage 4, we spend the rest of the night in dreaming and the lighter stages of sleep, until we awake naturally. Each stage is essential to a good night's rest

Meditation

Meditation is generally regarded as an exclusively eastern practice, inextricable from ideologies grounded in a very different environment from our own. However, this is not strictly true – the tradition of contemplation does exist in the west. In conventional western religions, as well as many of our lesser known sects, meditation of a type is practiced. In early Christianity the exercise of contemplation performed a function similar to that of meditation in Zen Buddhism, Yoga and a lesser known system, Sufism. Some of the early instructions for exercises in concentration were remarkably similar to the best from the east. Prayer itself was originally designed to fulfil this purpose although that function appears to have been superceded. St John Climacus said: 'If many words are used in prayer, all sorts of distracting pictures hover in the mind but worship is lost. If little is said or only a single word pronounced, the mind remains concentrated.' The same ecstatic feeling of joy and relaxation can be achieved through Christian prayer as for an eastern mystic.

Meditation is a widespread, global phenomenon, not limited to one part of the world and one time-scale. This fact more than anything else bears testimony to the usefulness of the technique. Before drugs were available to alter consciousness and induce relaxation, human beings had to find other ways with which to remove themselves from their daily cares and find some peace, some other reality which would allow them to detect some apparent purpose in the muddle and squalor that more often than not represented their earthly life. Because of this desire for 'wider' experience of reality and of the dimensions of earth and the heavens, almost all techniques of meditation were part of an overall religion. It is interesting to note that the dogmas of these various religions, ideologies, call them what you will, were widely divergent, but the exercises through which meditation was to be achieved were remarkably similar.

This is very reassuring to the would-be meditator of today who wishes to learn this practice for its physical, mental and emotional benefits, but does not want to wade through all the confusing claims of an alien belief system. Another fairly common accompaniment is a special diet of one kind or another. This is merely part of the belief structure and has nothing to do with the process of contemplation as such, although in practice an individual may find that a bloated, or a completely empty stomach is not conducive in the initial stages.

During meditation the individual relaxes into an altered state of consciousness. It resembles the relaxation of sleep from the physical point of view but mentally the person is aware and alert, but aware of different things from those hopping through the mind in our normal conscious state. Physically, the pulse rate is lowered, the blood pressure falls and the nervous system sends out messages at a decreased rate. As a result the amount of electricity reaching the skin falls and the readings on electrical instruments on the skin surface register this slowing down and relaxing of the whole body. The blood pressure can fall so low that an unfit person in a normal aware state with this type of reading would be considered to be in a state of shock. This is a very special kind of relaxation which obviously in some people goes beyond sleep. No wonder the meditator emerges feeling relaxed – although there are always critics to be found who try to deny that revitalization occurs.

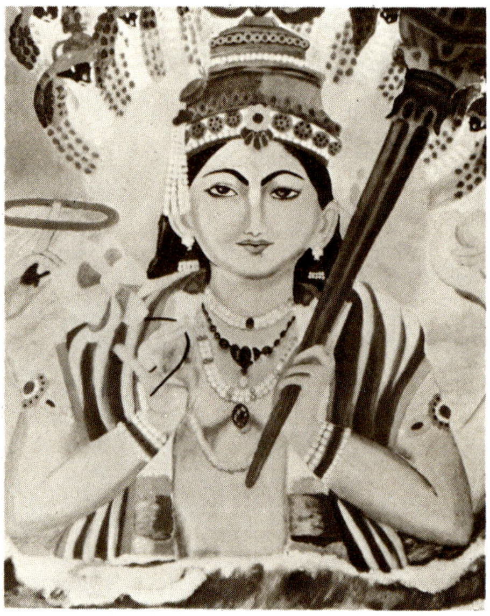

The Hindu god Radna Krishna. Meditation in the East is a regular part of religious observance; Christian prayer can be used in the same way whatever your beliefs

On the mental side, the relaxation is of a different order. The state of consciousness bears little relation to sleep and also steers the mind in a different direction than hypnosis. If hypnosis seems to move the mind downwards, then meditation pushes it more sideways. It probably depends what kind of a traffic jam exists in your cerebrum to determine which 'other' consciousness can provide the greatest benefit.

The one most important characteristic that all forms of meditation share is detachment from world activity. Other things may be superimposed, such as concentration of a particular form of energy, (known in Yoga as *kundalini*). Self-observation is a variation practiced by all three of the major proponents. However, for all practical purposes we can state that all roads to meditation involve separating the would-be practitioner from his daily activities. As our minds tend to be a bustle of conflicting ideas, it is not surprising that the concentration on one channel which is the central feature of meditation serves to quieten the mind, quite apart from the physical effects on the nervous system.

Besides endowing a welcome sense of relaxation, meditation opens up the avenues of perception that we always keep restricted within certain narrow limits. Psychological research has proved that we cannot cope with all the stimuli that hit us every minute of the day – all the mundane things we shut out, for the sake of sanity. But this necessary device limits our abilities to understand others and communicate with people materially different from ourselves. Human beings, in order to grow, need to be able to expand their perception at times.

Unfortunately of course it isn't possible to merely decide one day that you're in need of a little help from meditation. Its use requires discipline and regular practice. You have to learn to focus the power of your mind and keep your mind in training. Just what does a commitment to meditation involve? Let me quote Dr Robert E. Ornstein, an authority on the links between meditation and science. In *The Psychology of Meditation* he writes:

> Since the general state of our knowledge about the various forms of meditation within science in particular, and within the West in general, is extremely low, we should perhaps set the background and review some of the general similarities of the meditation exercises. Most involve separating the practitioner from the daily ongoing activities. He usually sits alone or with a small group in a special room set aside for meditation, or in a special place often constructed in a naturally isolated area, a quiet wood, near a waterfall, or a cave. Generally, the attempt is made to keep all external sources of stimulation to a minimum to avoid distracting the meditator from his object of meditation. This isolation is felt to be especially critical in modern cities, where random sounds or human voices can distract the person from his exercise. In most forms of Yoga or Zen there is emphasis on maintaining a specific posture, the lotus position. This is done for the purpose of keeping bodily movements to a minimum and therefore out of awareness during the meditation period. The stiff back is said, additionally, to lessen the possibility of drowsiness in the reduced stimulation setting. Incense is often burned during meditation to provide a strong consistent background odour to keep out any small distracting changes in smells.
>
> Instructions for most of the meditation exercises are to attend closely and continuously to the meditation object. This is more difficult than it would seem, and most beginners lose awareness of the meditation object quite often. Each time one notices that awareness has shifted from the object of meditation, the instructions are always to return awareness back to the meditation object. In many of the traditions, each session lasts about half an hour.

There are usually two practice sessions per day and beginners slowly work up to this level. Too much at a time can be debilitating.

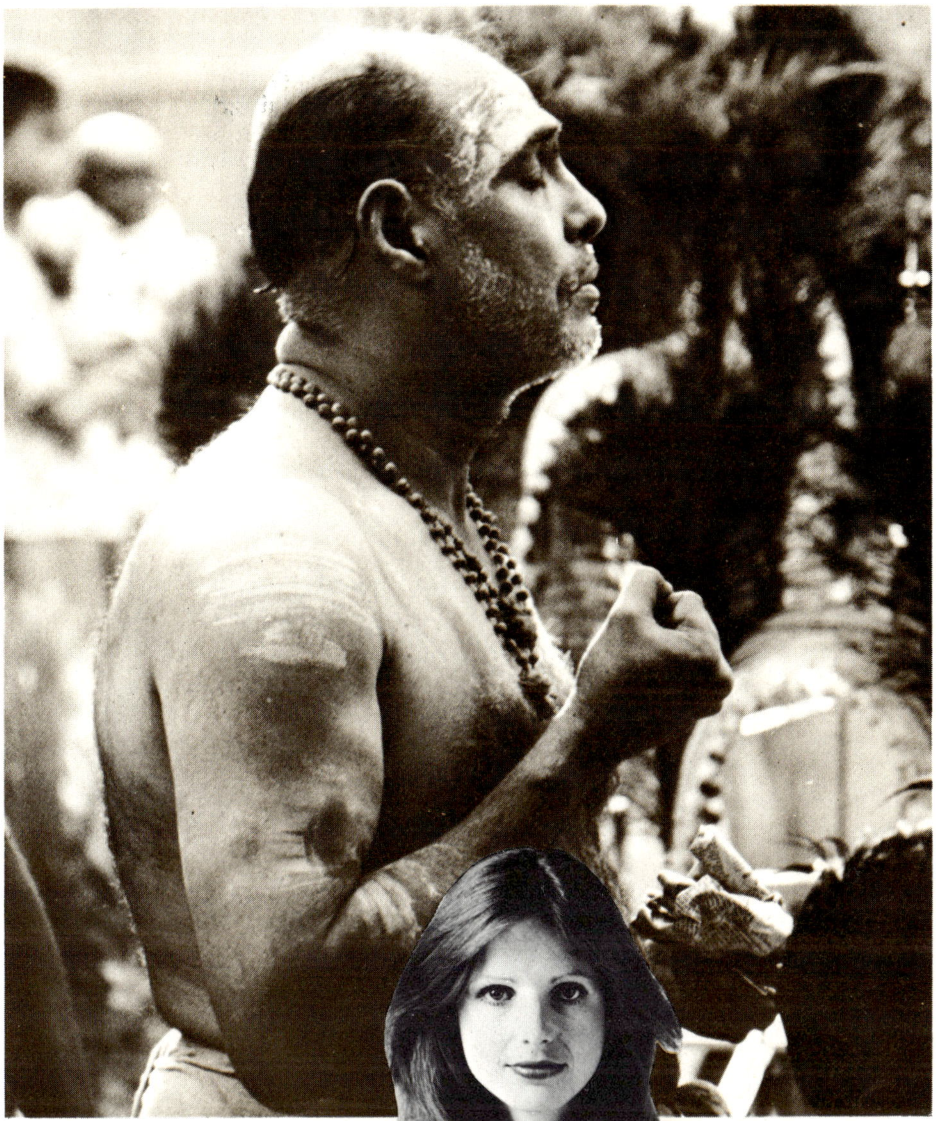

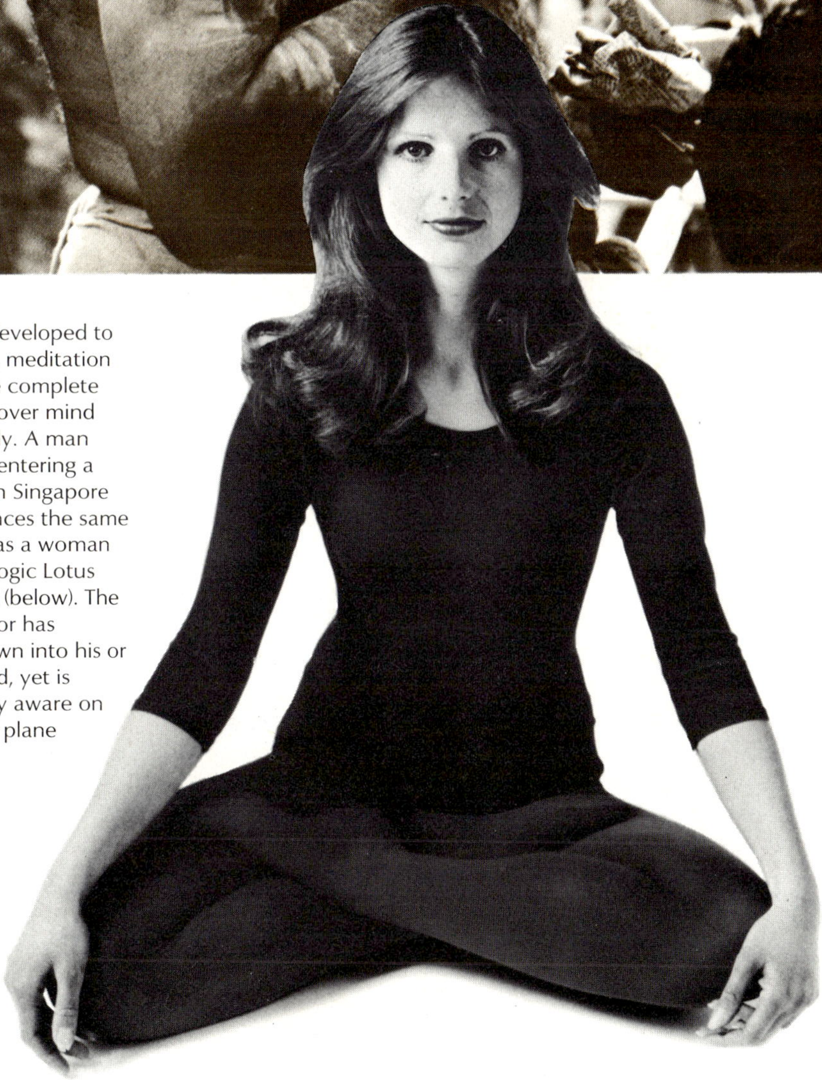

When developed to its peak, meditation can give complete control over mind and body. A man (above) entering a trance in Singapore experiences the same release as a woman in the Yogic Lotus position (below). The meditator has withdrawn into his or her mind, yet is intensely aware on another plane

Yoga

The aim of Yoga is to bring mankind to the highest state of advancement, in all his dimensions. It is an overall philosophy designed to influence every part of a person, whatever his or her calling, or way of life. As with every religion, some exponents believe in and follow every part of the creed to the letter, whereas others merely absorb those parts which seem to them personally to make most sense. Yoga aims to bring its believers to the pinnacle of mental, spiritual and physical fulfilment. As far as the two former goals are concerned, other philosophies offer roads to enlightenment which can claim equal effectiveness. Zen Buddhism, for instance, which is well known in the west has a very sophisticated philosophy and a highly developed series of meditation exercises which are, to a westerner at least, of equal value to those of Yoga. Yoga does seem to have a range that is somewhat greater and a repertoire of mental exercises which lead to a greater integration of the body's physical force. As far as the majority of westerners is concerned however, these aspects of Yoga are insignificant. The occident has fallen in love with the only aspect of Yoga which speaks out to them, which has a relevance to today's hectic pace.

It is the physical side, known as Hatha Yoga to the initiates, which is of overwhelming interest to us today. And it is also something which seems to be unique. The other eastern roads to enlightenment, bountiful as they are, seem to have nothing like this. There seems to be no doubt of the popularity of this form of activity. Yoga is on the crest of a wave. To some extent this trend must at least partly be a reflection of current fashion, thus ensuring that its popularity will wane when the next fad comes along in accordance with the generally accepted maxim of the fickleness of popular opinion. But even when the fanfare is over and its value as a news story has been eclipsed, Yoga will still remain as a valuable adjunct to western culture.

On the whole doctors are concerned with the physical benefits of this 'new' discipline. Similarly, most of the Yoga clubs or classes up and down the country put the physical side of the question first, but none of them ever forget the other, more mental, aspect of the story. All of them report the increased feeling of wellbeing, the feeling of relaxation that the Yoga exercises create. Yoga involves the mind: there is absolute silence during a Yoga class; it's not a contrived silence but a genuine feeling of unity with what one is doing with the body. It is a *physical* activity but it is sensual too. It is not hard work like the hard jerky muscle straining of other physical activities, instead the movements ripple and glide throughout the system, tickling the muscles as you go.

From a scientific point of view Yoga involves stretching exercises rather than actual physical work. There are those who say that both stretching movements and sheer work, destined to get the blood bounding round the system, are needed for perfect health and fitness. This may be so, if ordinary stretching movements are used. But in Yoga's case the movements seem to be done in such a way that all the glands and internal organs get a gentle pummeling, to ease the blood through the bodily backwaters which don't normally get the benefit of a clear-out, except possibly during times of great physical excitement. It is interesting in this connection that physical parameters of the body can be profoundly affected by the Yoga gyrations. For instance, blood pressure can fall considerably, to the point where doctors are frankly amazed as the reading goes below what is generally considered

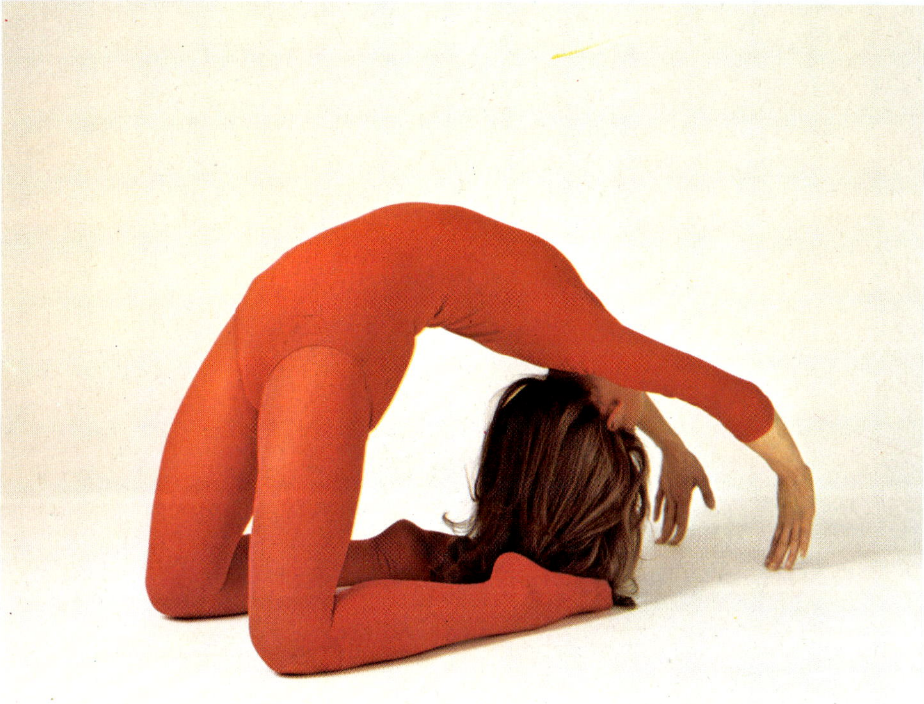

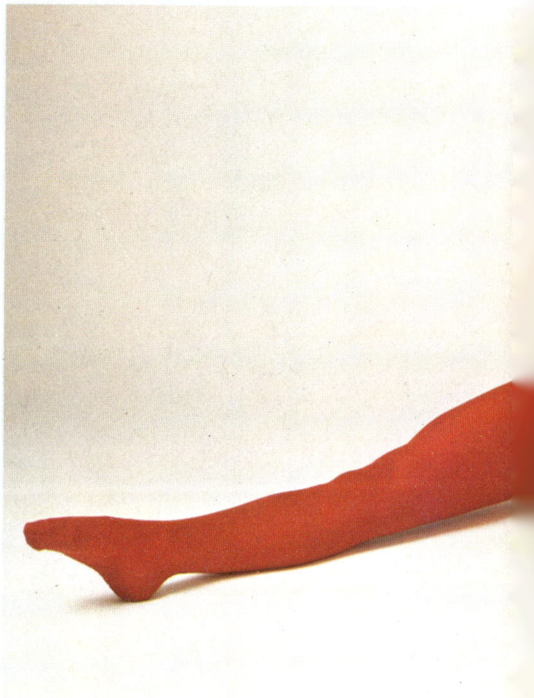

normal in a person who is very clearly quite the opposite of ill. The diet and appetite regulating mechanism seems to be miraculously retuned in certain individuals so that the once permanent battle of the bulge is won. Of course, if the practice of Yoga is stopped then the benefits are gradually lost, but even this regression can take place over a surprisingly long time.

However, Yoga fans claim that this discipline exerts a greater than usual effect, that goes beyond that experienced from mere physical fitness; the most obvious difference lies in the mental arena. The muscles are not as capable of great feats as they would be if you had spent your time at a gymnastics club but then powerful muscles are not top priority for most of us today. However, fine control is greatly helped by Yoga, as is balance. The ability to sustain a position with say the legs just an inch or two above the floor – normally a most difficult position – is transformed from what it probably was before. But, as stated before, the attitude of the performers to the exercises they undertake is quite different from other exercise buffs. They feel relaxed and peaceful throughout the experience; they feel marvellous afterwards and experience no stiffness of the muscles. Instead of tiredness as a sequel, they tend to feel just marvellous. How is this all achieved?

First of all, the subject must relax – in what is known as the pose of the dead man, an exercise that is common to practically all exponents of relaxation techniques. Then the exercises themselves are started – known to real Yoga addicts more properly as *asanas*. They have been carefully worked out so that every movement has a point, caressing in turn every part of the body. The movements are done slowly, with some teachers very slowly indeed. This has the effect of stretching the muscle fibres very gently, a small part of each band of muscle fibres at a time. Most advocates also encourage slow controlled breathing. To do these movements slowly requires real concentration, not just cursory attention to what is going on. If the breathing has to be watched the need for concentration is even greater.

If a movement is performed slowly, it involves concentration. Here we are approaching the techniques of meditation Secondly, the Yoga position is held quite still for a few seconds – frequently to the slow count of five. Then slowly again one returns to the starting point. The gentle rippling movements resemble the sensual touching of massage or of sexual activity, except that this time the sensation comes from within and not from outside of the skin. A heady feeling bears some resemblance to certain stages of sexual desire. The slow rhythm plus the warmth and comfort act in a way akin to self-hypnosis. Here we seem to have a little of several ingredients all of which contribute towards relaxation, namely massage, hypnosis and meditation. No wonder Yoga can be such a powerful relaxant. And at the end of the session, again a couple of minutes of complete rest, the pose of a dead man, enables the body's natural equilibrium to come back at its own pace.

The more the person is stretched and the more she or he is forced to immerse herself in it, the more profound the effect. As a result the discipline of a class is very valuable and even one hour a week can be enough to transform the system over a period of time. The group obviously has a potentiating effect, which is possibly even hypnotizing, and is difficult to mimic on one's own.

The brief spurts of punishment we call exercise seem to the Yoga practitioner to be a way of fighting the body rather than caring for it. Yoga teaches you to get to know your body, its limits, and to recognize its internal rhythms. Success is to be found in trying, in reaching towards the positions. Each part of the body is gently brought toward its peak working condition in a natural way. The camel position (left) promotes flexibility of the trunk. Centre and right, these positions stretch thigh and leg muscles

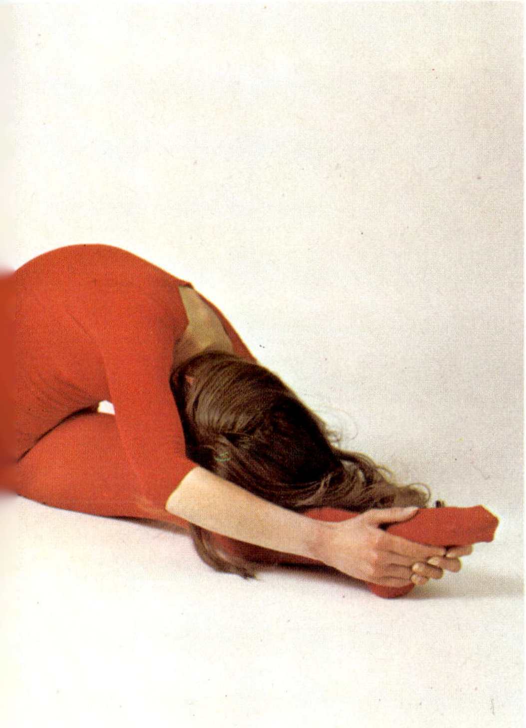

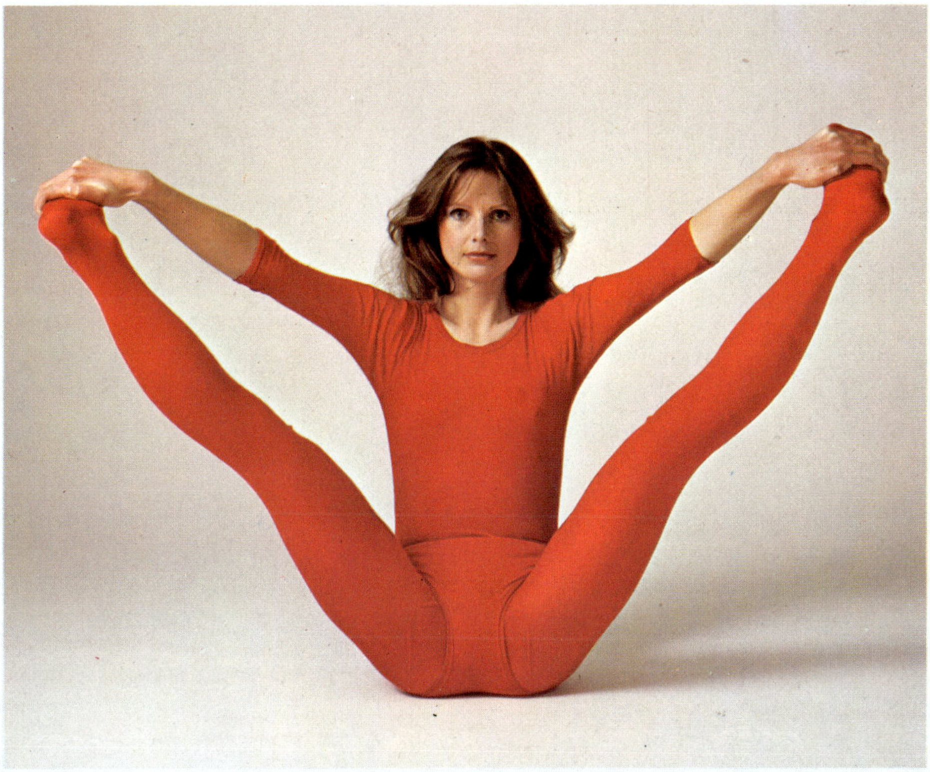

Yoga for Relaxation

One of the best and most complete methods of relaxation is to regularly practice a studied schedule of yoga movement. There are countless positions, techniques and exercises all aimed at revitalizing one or several areas of the body. Here we have presented a few basic movements which will form the basis of a relaxation programme.

Under no circumstances should you take a competitive attitude when performing these movements. Yoga must be relaxing, devoid of any painful or strenuous elements and always carried out at your own pace. Ease yourself into a rhythm that lets you produce fluid, precise actions. Study the exercises carefully and then attempt to perform them slowly and effortlessly. Hold each position as long as comfortably possible then proceed to the next one. Do not let yourself become tired. Twenty minutes a session is perfectly adequate but adjust time and frequency to suit your own needs.

2. This is a good exercise for stretching the back and and especially good exercise for those who sit all day. There are three basic positions. Start in the prone, or corpse, position and relax. Then, using your elbows, forearms and head push the chest upwards, drawing your arm back at the same time. Thus raising yourself off the floor.

2

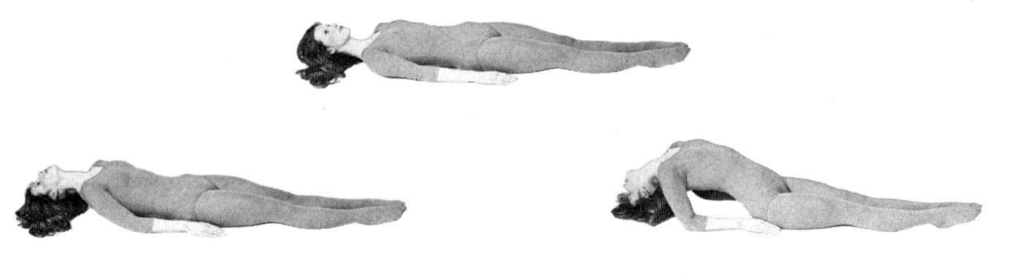

4. This movement is good for the legs and hips. Start lying on your back in the prone position with your arms alongside. Lift your legs slowly upwards then, using your hand arms and back, raise your body until your legs are fully extended. Come down by drawing your knees into your chest and then roll the body until your feet touch the ground.

4

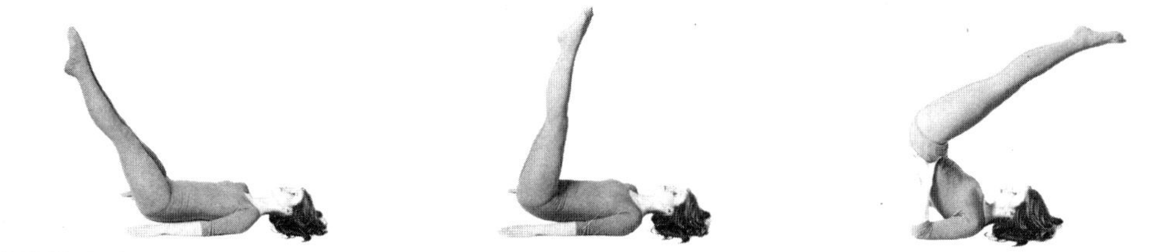

5. This movement is known as the Cat and is very useful for relaxing the spine. Start on your hands and knees, raise your head and push downwards arching the back as shown. Then reverse the procedure lowering your head and raising the back to arch in the opposite direction.

5

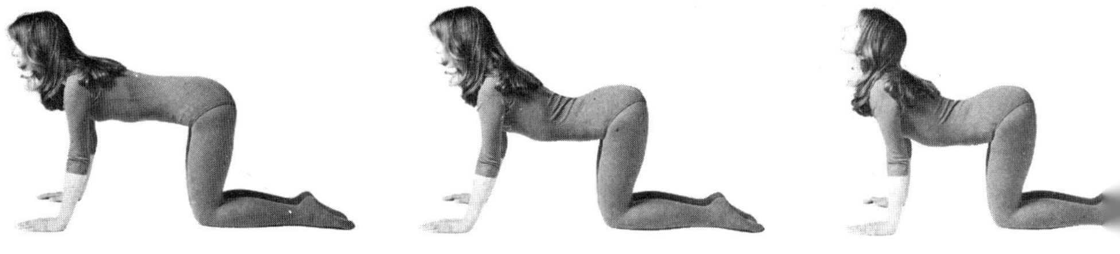

6. The backward push-up is an extremely good overall exercise. It requires good concentration and also helps to firm the abdomen and hips. As always, start in the prone position. Pushing, first with the legs, raise your body off the floor; then pushing downwards with the hands try to lift your head and shoulders off the ground.

6

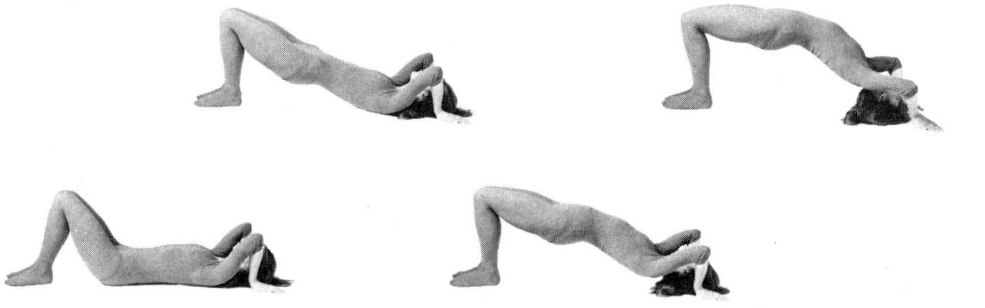

7

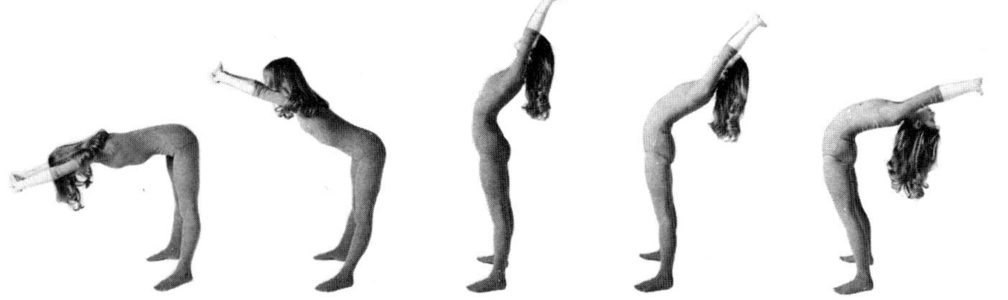

Finally, move with feet apart, from side to side stretching and firming the body.

1. Rolling your neck when in a comfortable sitting position helps ease aches and pains and relieves tension in the neck. Start in a good upright posture, cross your legs and put your hands on your knees. Hold the movement in each position and let the head do the work.

1

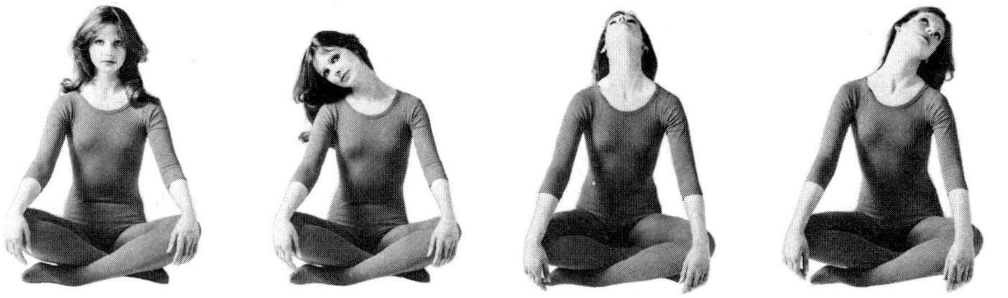

3. The Backward Bend is another good back movement. Start by sitting back on your heels in an upright pose. Then place your hands behind you and gently lower your head and trunk backwards. Finally, if possible, shift your hands right back and hold the position before slowly and calmly recovering to the initial pose.

3

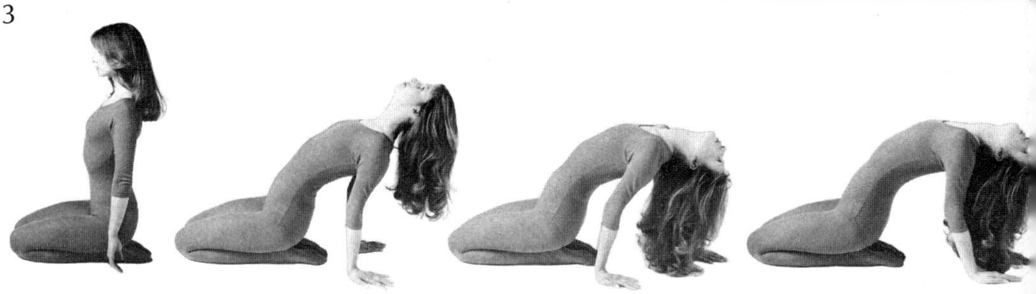

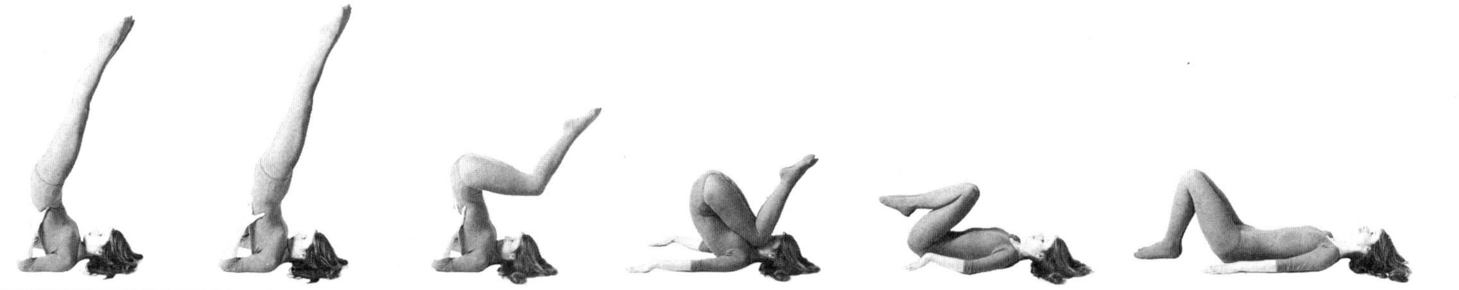

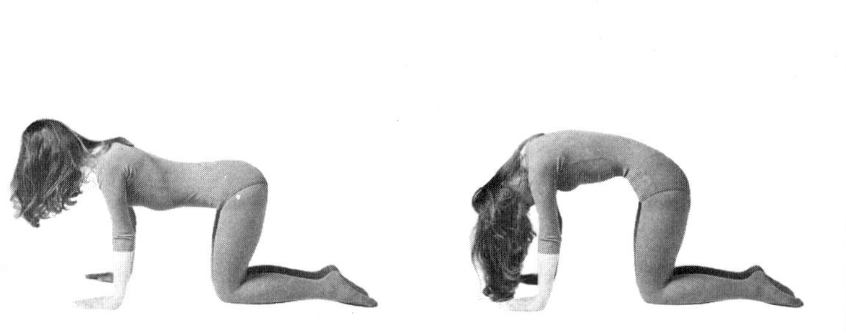

7. These movements flex and ease the body into a relaxed state. Start by clasping your hands in front of you and then swing them up to hold over your head, arms straight. Then lean forward and backward in a slow steady way.

7

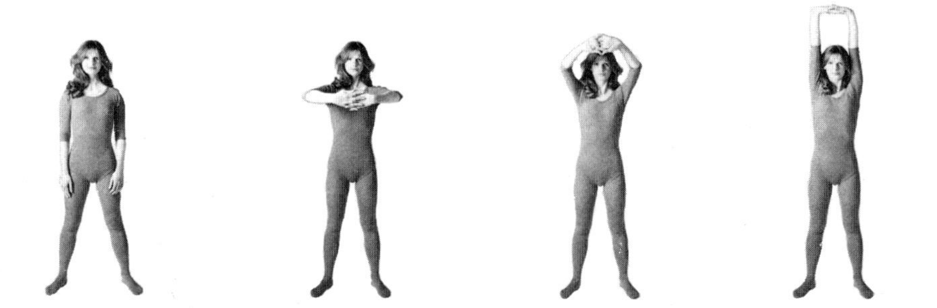

7

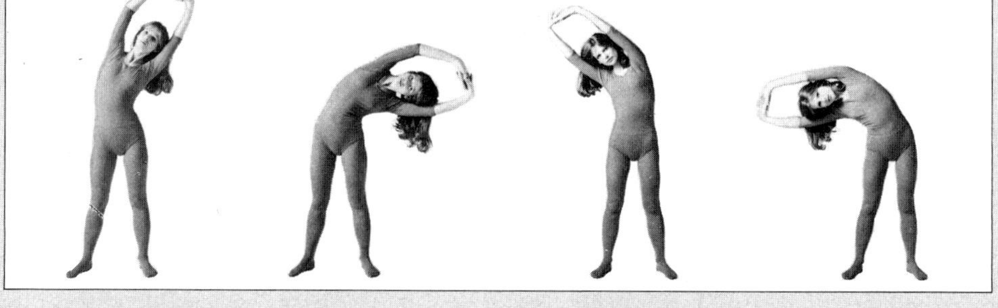

Massage and Sauna

Whereas some routes to relaxation look at first sight to be too much like hard work, because of the investment of time and effort, massage is very clearly a technique which leads immediately to a feeling of wellbeing and relaxation. The masseur has to work hard, but provided he or she performs his task in the right way, a feeling of relaxation should always accompany his labours. If he concentrates on his task to the exclusion of everything else and becomes positively integrated with what he is doing then he can gain some benefits by mimicking the meditation techniques. However, this type of role is considered elsewhere; here we are concentrating exclusively on the joy that can be experienced by the person who is receiving the massage. He or she should be very passive and merely lie back and enjoy what is happening to him, concentrating on the body's sensations. Sometimes the recipient is tempted to try and help the masseur by voluntarily moving a limb, by changing positions in some way. This tends to defeat the object of the exercise, which is to lose oneself completely in the sensuality that is generated; to lose oneself to the exclusion of everything else. For massage to be beneficial, it is important that you feel good, that all the aches and pains which you did not know existed are whisked away temporarily. This feeling good allows the whole nervous system to relax, allows the muscles and all the other components to completely let go at the same time.

Common sense as well as several thousand years of pseudo-medical records suggest that massage is most effective when it is a sensual experience. The Victorians ignored this aspect of the art, endeavouring to make it a purely scientific phenomenon. Gordon Inkeles and Murray Todris in *The Art of Sensual Massage*, berate the Victorians whose

> massage specialists spent years in dusty libraries poring over gigantic treatises on anatomy and physiology to learn the 'correct' way of touching other people. Massage ... was transformed from a common folk-healing technique to a science whose secrets were supposedly only available to the initiated ... Their conclusions regarding technique are usually nothing more than the translation of ancient massage methods into a modern idiom, the language of science.

To some extent this pseudo-scientific attitude seems to have persisted in the west: there is now an emphasis on qualifications – and the girls in massage parlours are encouraged to go through extensive training sessions. Fortunately this aspect of the craft is not worrying as yet because the courses are very short and do enable the teachers to point out a few basics which might easily be otherwise overlooked. However, there is a danger that some practitioners might start to take themselves too seriously and try and make too much of a science out of what they do. It does not matter very much how the massage is performed, provided

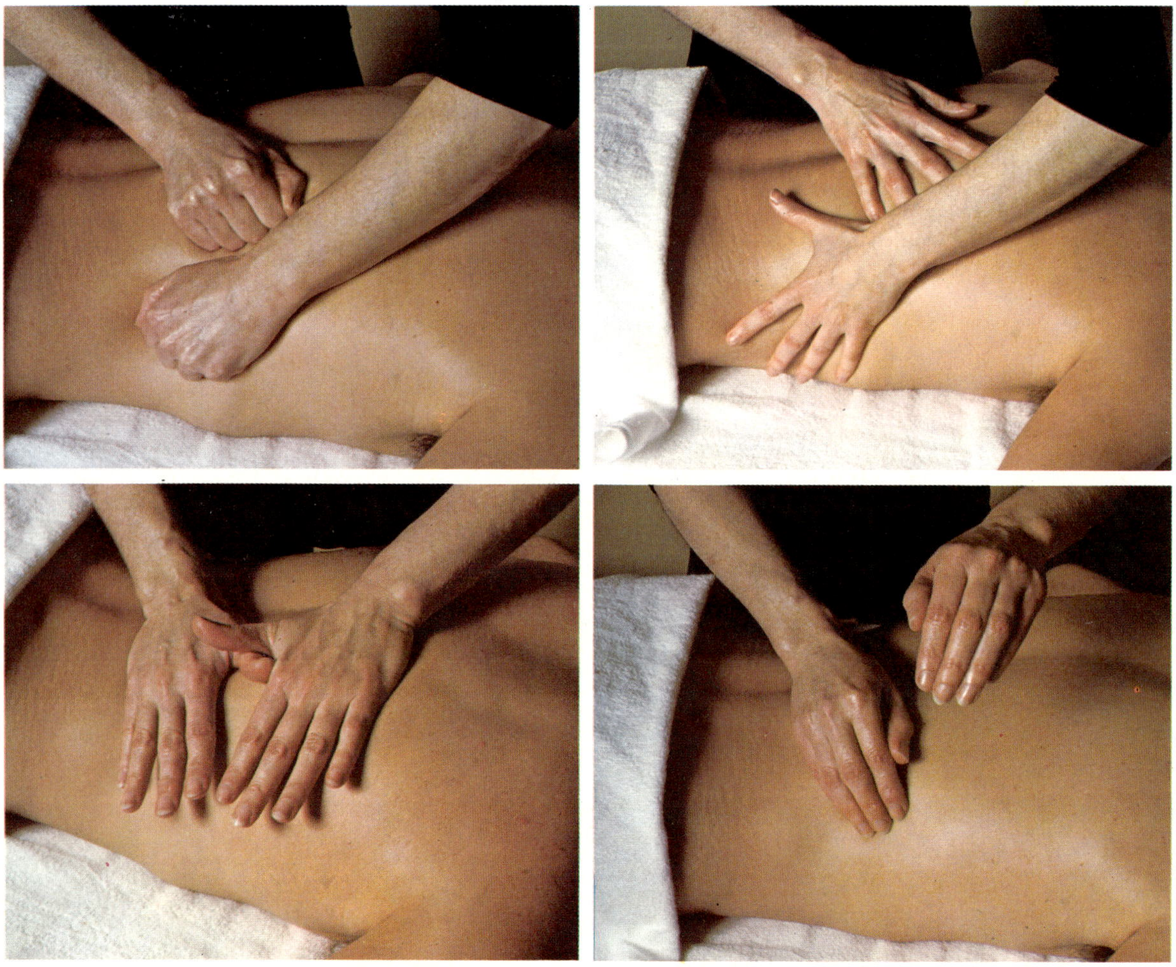

In massage, the contact between bodies through the hands is as important as the smoothing of tense muscles. It should never be a painful experience. Massage (top left) with the knuckles provides good skin friction. Leaning across the body (top right) pull your hands up from the side across the back in a rotating movement. Firm pressure (below left) is applied as you stroke both hands together across the back. Cupping (below right) is a percussion stroke. Cup the hands, fingers together, and slap them smartly on the body. This is particularly good for either side of the spine and for the circulation

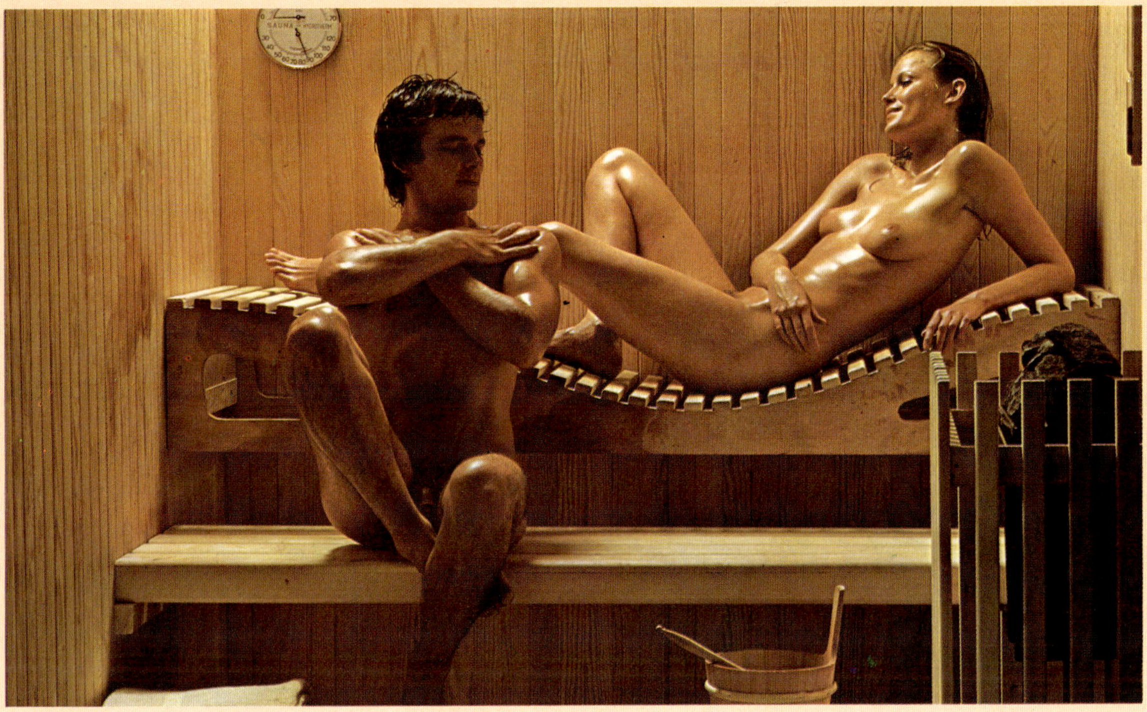

Relaxing in the gently steaming heat of a sauna, with a friend, not only opens the pores, deeply cleansing your skin, but helps you forget the cares of daily life. Caring for your body makes *you* feel loved too. The tingling sensation of the cold shower afterwards, washing away the sweat and dirt, brings the whole body alive, so that you want to repeat the process. A swim after a sauna can also be very exhilarating, as long as you make sure not to overtax the heart

real attention is paid to the feelings and wants of the person receiving the treatment. If what is happening feels good, then that is the way to continue a little longer. Of course, certain methods can be learned but that should by no means be allowed to exclude all the other possibilities which arise out of each interaction between the two individuals involved in the massage process. It is the subtle giving, the imaginative touches that allow one personality to respond to the other that mark the truly great, the truly sensuous massage.

We are only just relearning what an overall feeling of wellbeing massage can provide, a relaxation that will lead to sleep in some people – if they are tired; or will lead to sexual excitement if the body is ready and anxious for that kind of stimulation. The important thing is that the normal constraints holding us tense and active are released, allowing the system as a whole to move in whatever direction it wishes. This ability of the nervous system to express itself in its own way only happens if the experience is very pleasant, allowing full release.

The second important thing about massage is to just let it happen – so often we try to achieve a certain bodily result – we try to chase away that tension; the sheer effort can make things worse. These pleasant feelings are there and sooner or later you will be able to acknowledge them. Whatever the initial resistence in your head the pleasant feelings in your skin will win through and the body will start to respond. The more insistent these sensations become the more the ugly nags will tend to disappear. The only two essentials of massage are gentle touch – to make sure that no harshness is allowed to break the mood – and time. As the nervous system becomes overwhelmed by the pleasant sensations, its messages to the muscles become as repetitious as they were during the most strenuous moments of life. Now, instead of screaming hysterically for action, they murmur 'relax' and the muscles follow suit.

Massage can have other effects too. The blood supply to the part being manipulated is increased and improved by the action. This will come primarily to the skin, which actually needs it less than the muscular parts of the body, especially if the latter are all knotted up through years of unabating tension. The circulation to the muscles is increased through deep massage, pressure and kneading of the muscle fibres. However, this is of unlimited value; the most chunky, least healthy bits are most resistant to the entry of blood; they can only be reached by repeated but very gentle attempts. Too vigorous pummelling can cause pain and even inflammation which can be counter-productive to the desired overall effect. This is where technique comes in – for a clever practitioner can have maximum effect on the muscle fibres with minimum trauma. However, detailed descriptions are beyond the scope of this book. As far as the average practitioner is concerned, it is enough to remember that touch, when it is gently and smoothly executed, is the most important factor.

You must make the recipient of your caresses feel that they really are caresses, that you genuinely want to give pleasure and that time is no object. If you are caught looking at your watch then the effect will be ruined (although any person receiving a massage who is able to notice such a thing is probably not as completely involved in his own physical feelings as he should be). But here we touch on another aspect of massage that adds to its overall effectiveness. It is a way of showing caring. The touch from one human being to another is a way of showing fellow feeling, of showing that we care. Animals nuzzle and stroke each other all the time. We tend to do it only in a sexual context, which means we miss a lot. The touching of massage, even if performed entirely as a ritual between complete strangers, is a way of saying each to the other, 'We are both in it together, we feel for each other as people.' This transmission of a common bond has very healing properties which are impossible to measure.

Back massage
Oil the part of the back you are working on first – safflower and coconut, scented with lemon or cloves, are especially suitable. This reduces friction, giving greater sensuality. The lower back suffers most from muscle tension, so spend more time on it than any other part of the body. Smooth the small of the back (top left) with both hands then knuckle massage down the side of the body (top right). Apply pressure as you press across the lower back hands pointing inward (middle left). Push firmly up the back towards the head (middle right) massaging the muscles around the spine. Finish with circular strokes around and across the shoulders

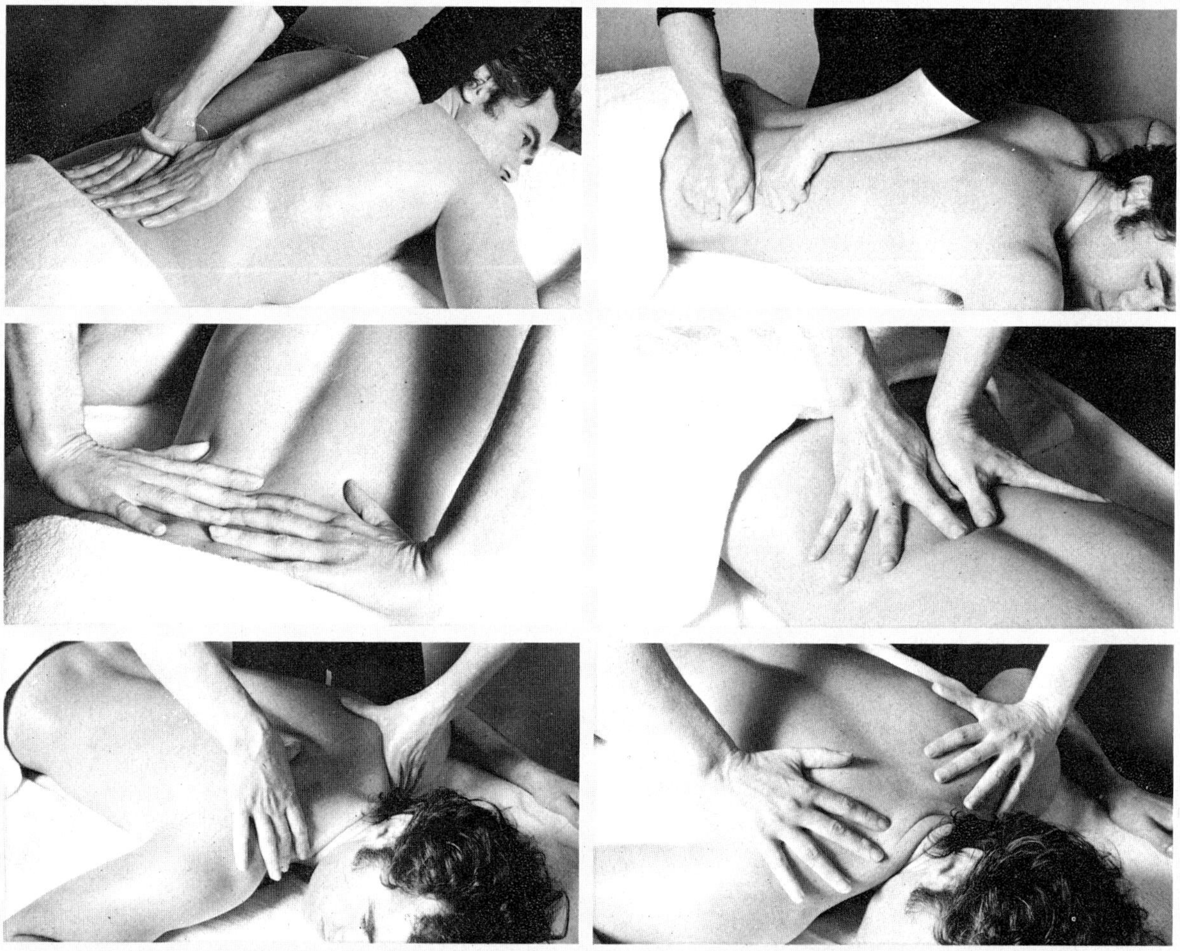

Front massage
A warm, quiet and dimly lit room with the phone off the hook is the perfect setting for massage. A firm surface, table or floor, gives support. Massage the stomach (top left) clockwise to help digestion. Continue down the sides with the knuckles (top right). Gently knead, pushing up the flesh and smoothing it down between thumb and fingers (middle left). Stroke the hands alternately up from the back across the stomach (middle right, bottom left) which produces very pleasant sensations. Hacking (bottom right) is a light pummeling with the edge of the hands, the little finger slightly extended, reducing the weight of the hand

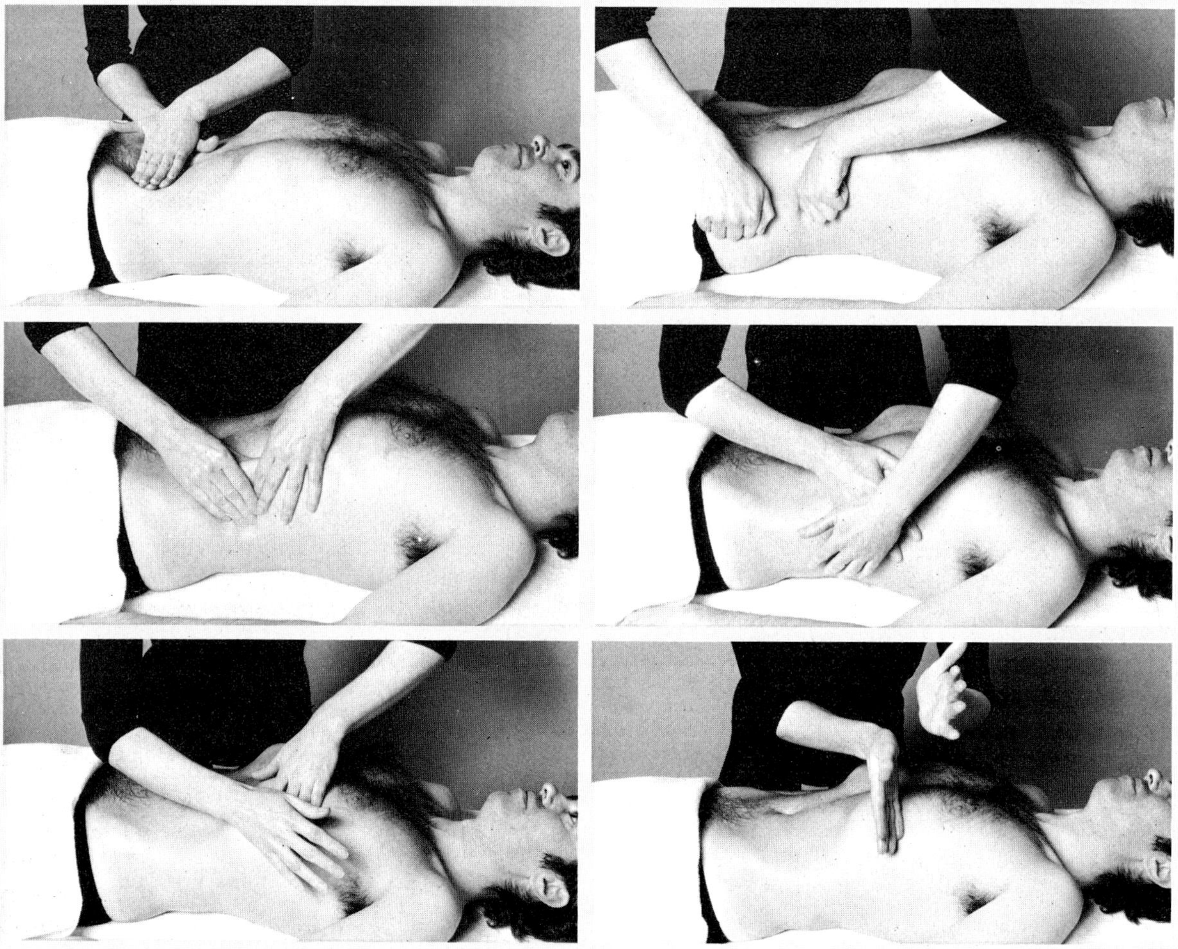

Legs and feet
You should be completely relaxed during a massage, the masseur doing all the lifting and moving. Massage is a two-way experience, and both should think of the comfort of their bodies, breathing deeply and regularly. The feet are especially important, so spend some time on them, easing away the tension from toes, soles and tops (top left). Then gently hack the calves (top right) before holding the whole lower leg and smoothing up towards the thigh (middle left). Repeat these strokes for the front of the leg (middle right, bottom left). The thick muscles of the thigh should be kneaded, and also smoothed towards the head, (bottom right)

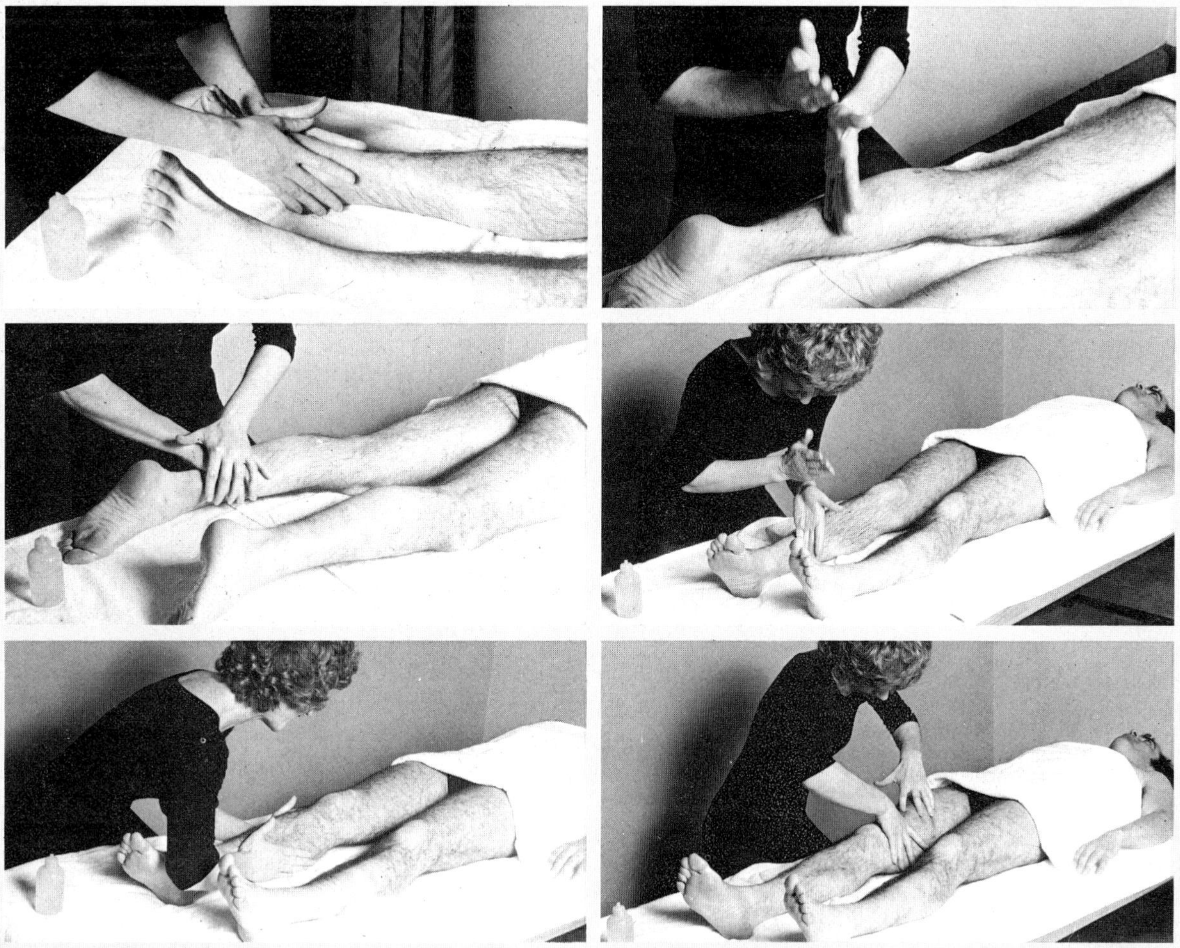

Arms and hands
The masseur applies firm but gentle pressure, using the weight of his own body, moulding his hands to the contours of the other's body. The upper arm needs firm pushing up towards the head, to drain the blood (top left) and firm kneading of the biceps (top right). The hands are also very important (bottom left), each finger as well as the palm and back needing attention (bottom right)

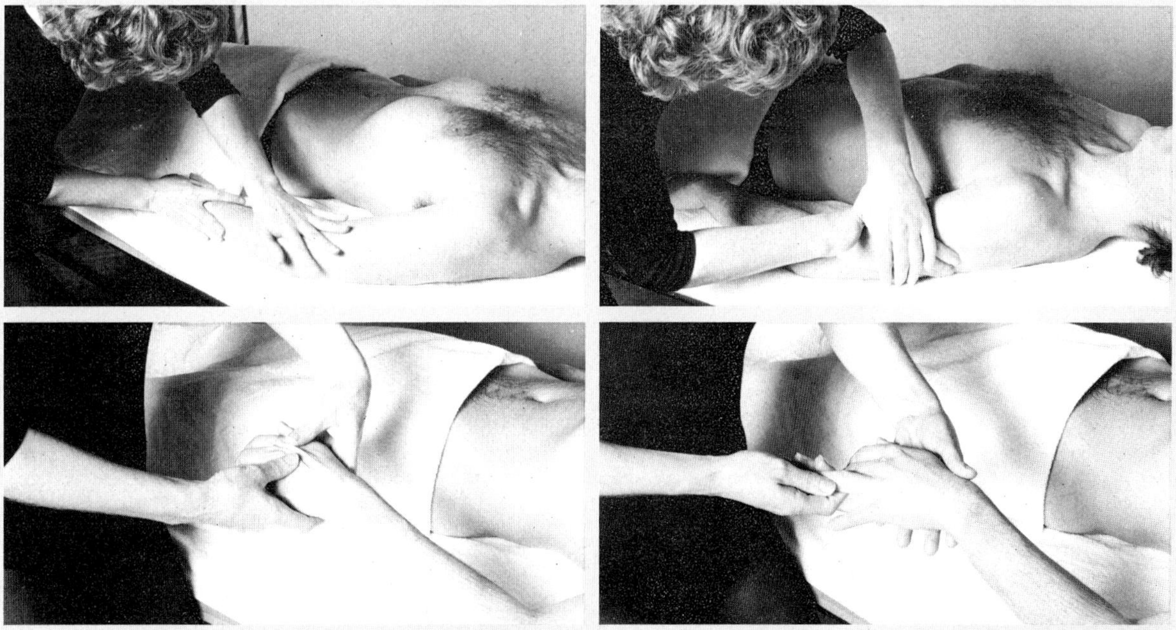

Head and neck
Deep finger-tip massage for the scalp, continued down to the base of the neck and then to the shoulders can soothe away headaches. The face can also be gently massaged

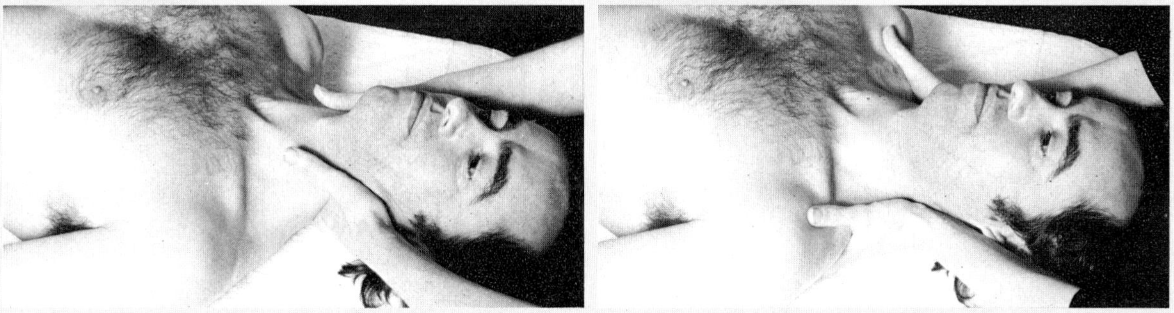

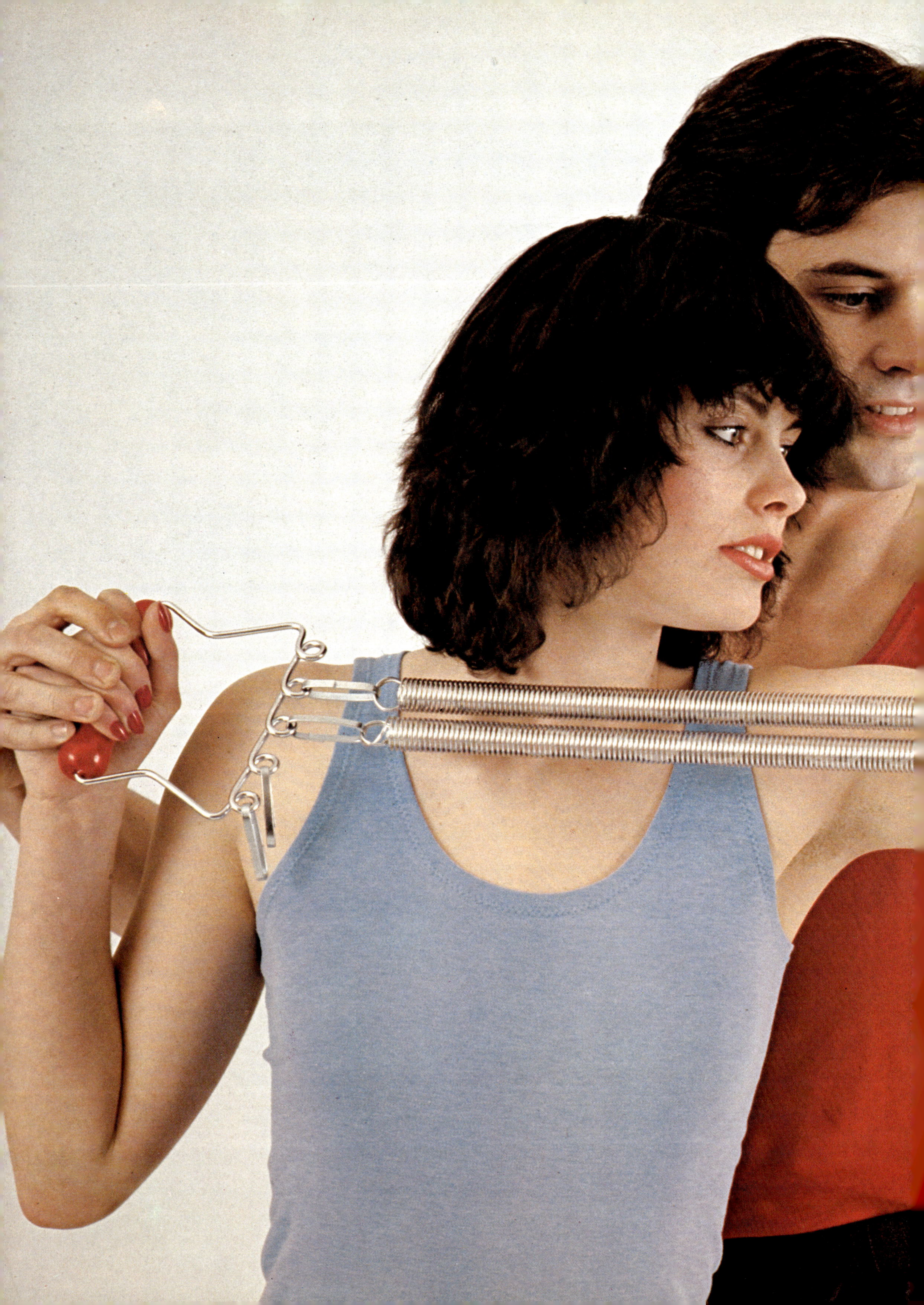

EXERCISE AND HEALTH

Sensible exercise can save your life. With our tendency today to overindulge, muscles become soft and eventually useless. The heart is a muscle–a very special muscle–so we must learn to respect and look after it. Exercise is the ideal solution. It is not meant to be strenuous or exhausting, in fact exactly the opposite–easy, relaxed and enjoyable. The many myths of needing pain and sweat before any good is achieved are now dispelled. Over the last decade we have developed schedules and techniques to meet every requirement. Speed, stamina, strength and suppleness are the areas that need attention. This section gives instruction and advice.

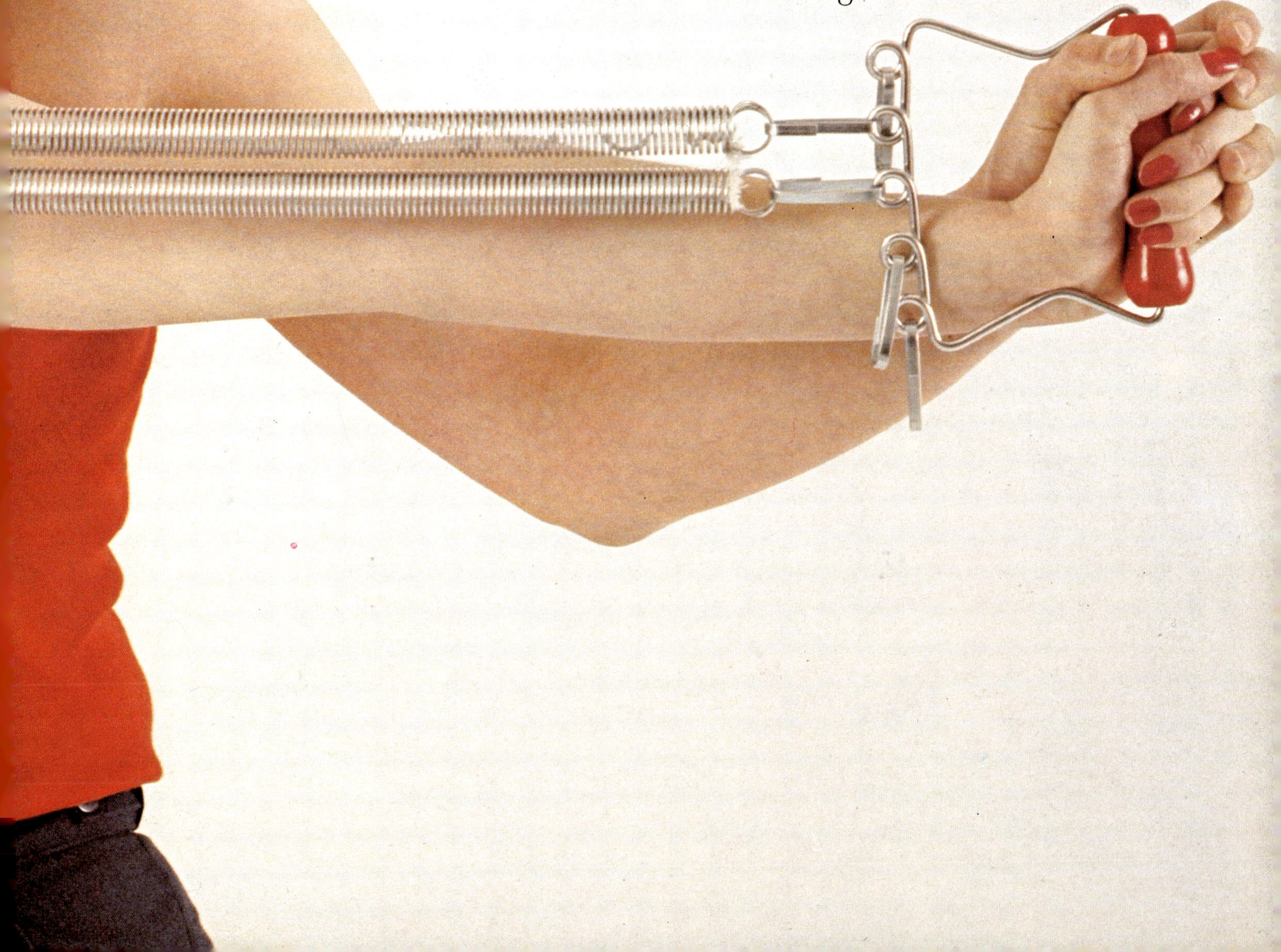

Why Exercise?

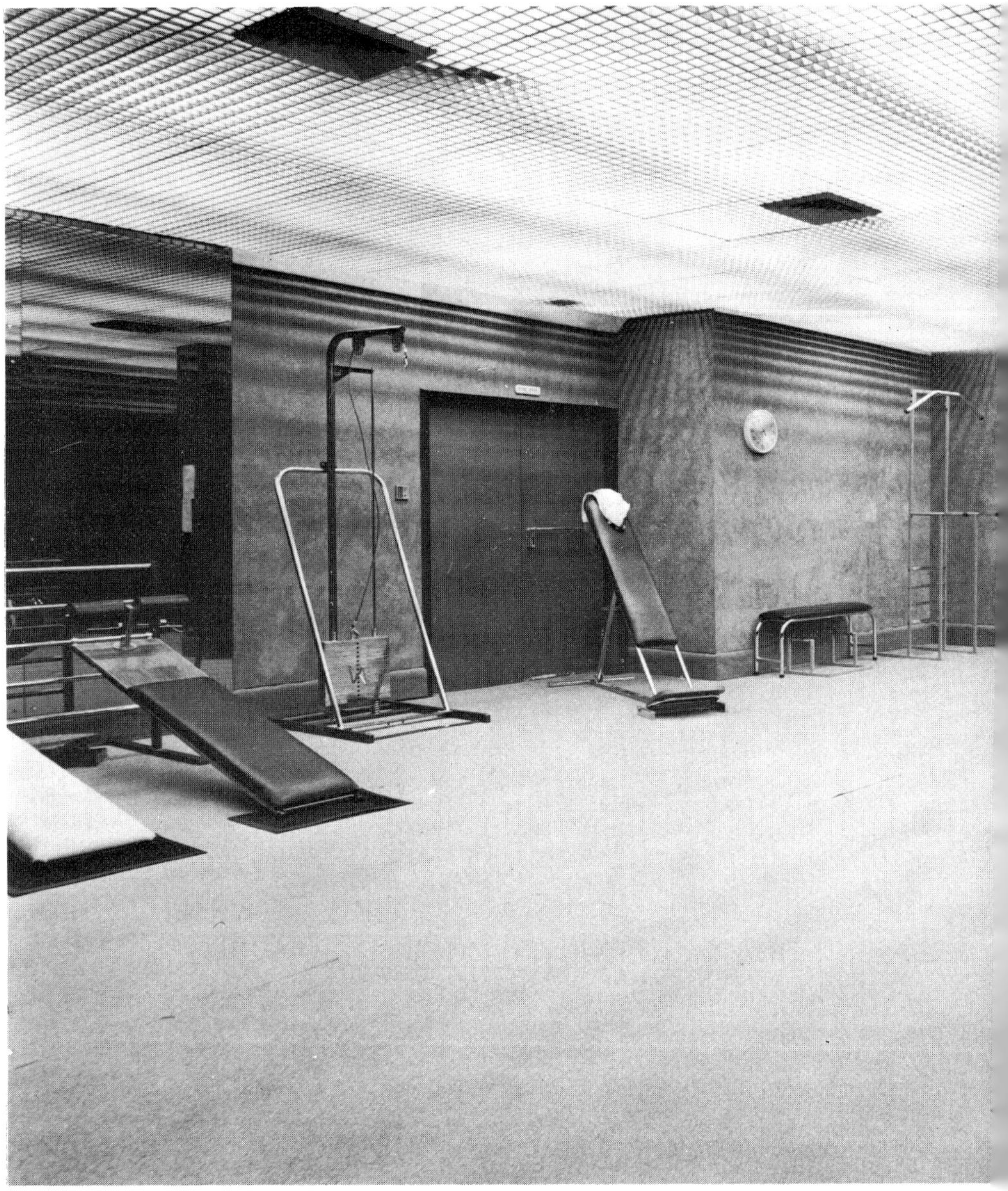

Most people take exercise because they enjoy it. However, there is plenty of medical evidence to support the view that exercise helps to combat a number of serious illnesses, particularly high blood pressure, strokes and coronary thrombosis, the cardiovascular diseases. Statistics from the Registrar General demonstrate that in Britain these attacks are the largest single cause of death between the ages of 45 and 65. Moreover, this incidence is increasing. In the United States, this trend is even more pronounced: deaths from cardiovascular weakness account for more than all the other reasons for death added together. There is also a distinct association between obesity and early death. Obesity is a strain on the heart. The heart is muscular, and so weakens if it is not exercised. Superfluous weight makes the heart work harder even though it may not be strong enough to cope. Fat deposits increase in the blood vessels, making it difficult for the blood to reach the body tissues and the heart has to beat more quickly to force the blood round the body. Consequently, the blood pressure rises. High blood pressure is often associated with a cardiovascular weakness and obesity.

Exercise can protect the body in a number of different ways. Combined with a sensible diet it can help you to lose weight, eliminating unnecessary strain on the heart. Certain types of exercise can strengthen the heart so that it is less liable to coronary attack. Regular, steady training provides what is termed the cardiac reserve: the blood vessels grow larger, ensuring a liberal supply of oxygenated blood to the heart considerably reducing the probability of heart failure. As a conditioned heart grows larger, it beats more slowly since it is pumping more blood with each stroke. After a few months of regular exercise or training, the resting pulse rate is often less than the customary 75 per minute. Top athletes, particularly cyclists, swimmers and runners, sometimes have a pulse rate in the low 40s.

There are other beneficial effects. An excessive and constant intake of cholesterol leads to hardening of the arteries (arteriosclerosis). Although the human body can withstand a reasonable amount of fat, it nevertheless circulates in the blood stream for some time after consumption. The better physical condition the body is in, the quicker the fat will be eliminated from the blood stream. If you are inclined to consume large quantities of animal produce, the prime source of cholesterol, you can partially offset this through regular exercise.

This, of course, does not mean that, if you exercise, you are immune from heart attacks or from other associated conditions, but it does mean that you stand a better chance both of avoiding them and of combating them should they occur.

On a less serious level, exercise also makes life easier. For instance, after a steady series of running sessions, you can chase after a bus without excessive breathlessness. Weight-training helps you to cope easily with heavy tasks in the garden, shifting furniture and suitcases. Indeed, ordinary back pains are often caused by weaknesses in the muscles surrounding the spine. A slipped disc is invariably related to abuse of the back. A regular course of weight-training can prevent undue suffering.

Some people get exercise during their jobs. Farmers, through their daily walking and work on the land, may well get sufficient exertion to give them a healthy body. On the other hand a clerk, working in an office, will not get similar opportunities. An interesting piece of research, conducted by Professor J. N. Morris on London Transport employees, compares bus drivers with conductors. It indicates that drivers –

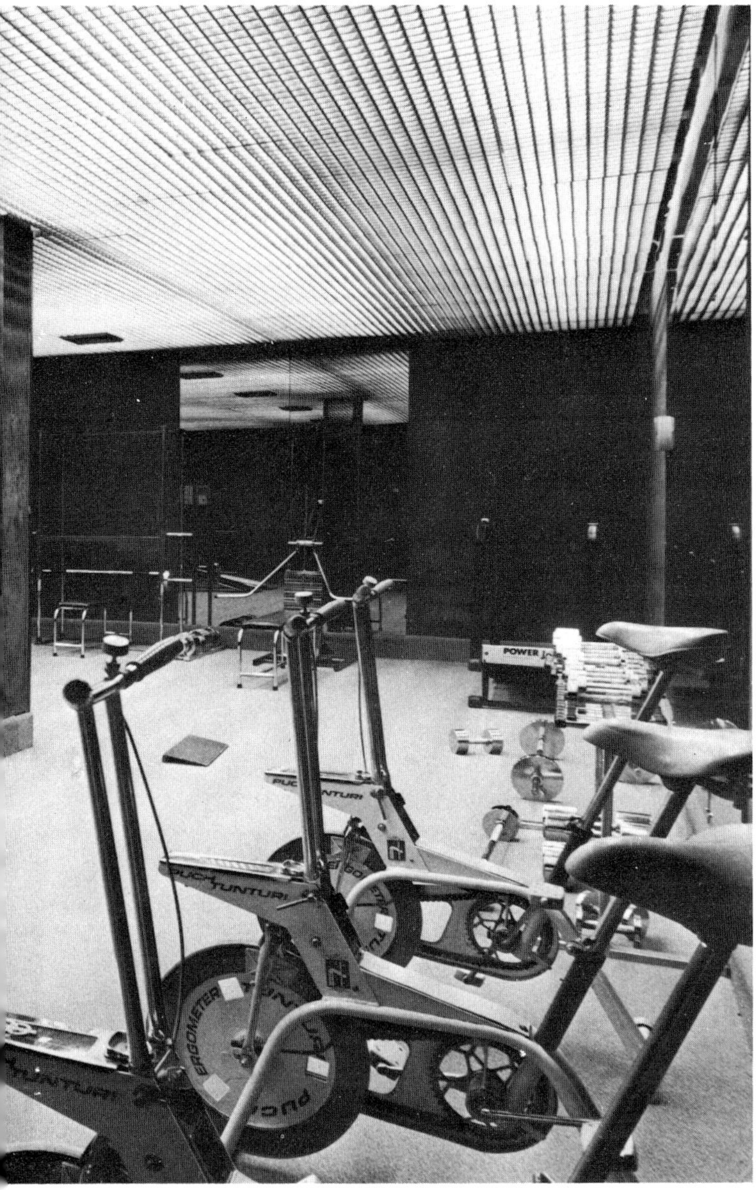

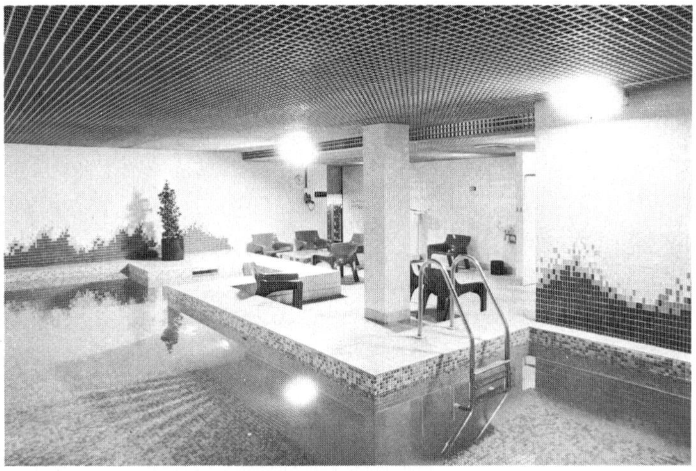

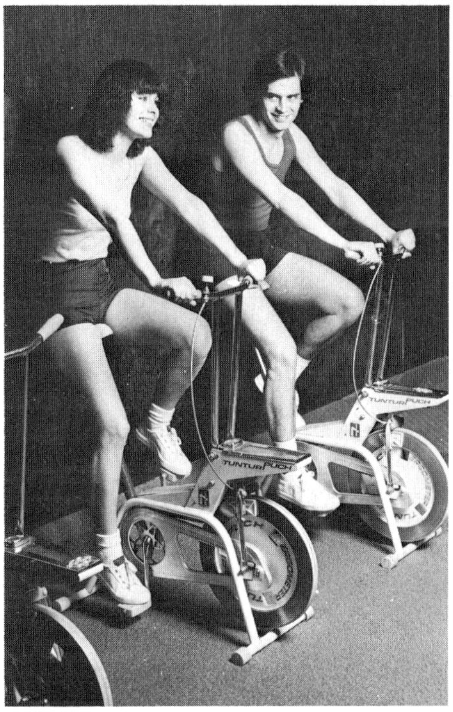

The old-fashioned concept on exercise, namely that it was something akin to punishment, to be carried out in unpleasant and primitive surroundings no longer hold true. Modern gymnasia, swimming pools and exercise machines provide valuable activity in attractive and sociable surroundings

who sit throughout their duty – suffer more heart attacks than their more active colleagues, who have to climb stairs many times a day. In the United States, examination of workers on the railway was equally significant. Clerks suffered twice as many coronary thromboses as did plate-layers and signalmen between them. The evidence is substantial – if you have no physical exertion in your jobs (and very few jobs provide it) you should exercise carefully and regularly if you want to diminish your chances of suffering a heart attack.

In the affluent west, most people lead a sedentary life. One of the most pleasurable ways they can exercise their underused bodies is through sport. The seduction of sport is that it is primarily a recreation, a relaxation from work and study. If there were no more Olympic Games, no more World Cups for soccer, no more World Series for baseball, those sports would still survive because people enjoy playing them. Different sports suit different temperaments, climates and times of life. Some people like mountain-climbing, or scuba-diving, others weight-lifting or tennis, but there can hardly be anyone in the world who has not participated in at least one sport at some time in his or her life.

Sport can keep people comparatively healthy throughout their lives. Sometimes the two motivating forces contend; the sport you enjoy is not always the one that keeps you healthiest. It is up to you to compromise between the two because it may be valuable for your health to give up one round of golf to have two running or swimming sessions a week. Best of all try to keep that extra round of golf but add more testing exercise.

However, sport is not the elixir of youth. There is little evidence that it helps to prolong life. Indeed, in three American surveys – by Louis I. Dublin (1932), Henry Mantoye (1956) and Antony Polednak and Albert Damon (1970) – it was found that Harvard students who participated seriously in major sports at university tended to die earlier than non-athletes. The first two examinations reported that the difference was about two years. However, the most recent survey did not find the difference so statistically significant. In addition, it stated that athletes competing in minor sports like fencing and swimming generally lived longer than non-athletes and athletes taking part in big sports such as football, rowing and baseball. It concluded that the man with the mesomorphic build (muscular) dies noticeably earlier than the ectomorphic (skinny) man; an endomorph (person inclined to fat) rated in between. However, much of the evidence is based on conditions 40-50 years ago and there has been no detailed research published which deals with longevity related to those people who exercise (or don't exercise) in middle age. The fact that people took part in serious sports 40 or 50 years before their death may not be relevant to the time of their death.

Sport does not always promote health. People die from accidents at events: between 1931 and 1965 a total of 642 fatalities occurred in American Football alone. Injuries are a perpetual problem for many sportsmen from the jogger suffering from a tendon strain to the professionals who sometimes have injections so that they won't feel the pain when they are playing with a damaged limb. Nor is exercise necessarily a preventative against some diseases: the death of Britain's Lillian Board from cancer in 1970, two years after taking the 400 metres silver medal at the 1968 Olympics is tragic and convincing proof of this.

Regular exercise into adulthood should be a carry over from the games of one's youth; but in America specifically, the lavish standard of living has deprived many children of the physical qualities of their European counterparts. In 1954, Professor Hans Kraus of New York University published a study comparing the muscular fitness of 4,264 American children with that of 1,036 Italian, 1,156 Swiss and 678 Austrians of the same age. Only 8 per cent of the Italians failed the test with the other Europeans achieving almost similar scores, but 57.9 per cent of the Americans failed. Professor Kraus commented:

> The major difference between these groups is the fact that European children do not have the 'benefit' of a highly mechanised society; they do not use cars, school buses, elevators or other labour saving devices. They must walk everywhere – even to school, frequently a long distance. Their recreation is largely based on the active use of their bodies In this country the children are generally conveyed in private cars or by bus, and they engage in recreation as spectators rather than as participants.

American P. E. departments reacted determinedly to this research by instituting their own series of tests and programme of training. Although the gap between the Americans and Europeans may have now narrowed, this may be because increasing numbers of European children have unfortunately adopted many of the American habits condemned by Professor Kraus. The insidious comfort of modern life brings its dangers to children as well as to adults, because they are not taught sensible and healthy habits when they are young.

Principles of Exercise

You can exercise through specific training or through games. Certain sports put a premium on some physical attributes and ignore others. For instance, competitive weight-lifting emphasizes strength, whereas long-distance running stresses stamina, or cardiovascular endurance. For American Football you need size and speed, but not the suppleness and dexterity which are essential to gymnastics. Therefore you must consider a number of factors before you decide what sports and exercises you need to do. Firstly, do what you enjoy. You are more likely to continue practising a pleasurable activity than one you dislike. However, there is a tendency to believe that your favourite sport demands and trains all the physical qualities necessary to maintain a healthy body. This is rarely so. Consequently, try to be as objective as possible when looking at the chief physical recreations, and be prepared to supplement them either with other games or with specific training to exercise those faculties not sufficiently tested.

Ideally you should work at speed, stamina, strength and suppleness each week. All sports are made up, to a greater or lesser extent, of these attributes, in addition, of course, to the specific skills. However, through disinclination or lack of time, few people will be able to train all their physical qualities. Therefore, it is important to get the priorities in the correct order to see what should be emphasized in your physical life. Then you can look at these four fundamental talents and examine how best to develop them to reach a good level of fitness.

The need to exercise the heart is vital. Although the acquisition or retention of strength and suppleness is useful, it is not as important as stamina – the ability to carry out prolonged work without undue fatigue. Later, ways that strength, suppleness and speed can be maintained or even improved will be suggested, but the primary requirement is to improve cardiovascular endurance. This is promoted by continuous activity of various kinds. Although a game like tennis will strengthen the heart, it will not do it so efficiently as one of the aerobic (literally 'with air') activities of running, swimming or cycling. Dr Kenneth Cooper, in *Aerobics* states that:

> The training effect benefits begin about five minutes after the exercise starts and continue as long as the exercise is performed. If the exercise is not vigorous enough to produce or sustain a heart rate of 150 beats per minute, but is still demanding oxygen, the exercise must be continued considerably longer than five minues, the total period of time depending on the oxygen consumed.

Often in a game like tennis the heart beat will exceed 150 but also it will invariably drop down to below 120 because there are slack periods when changing ends or collecting balls. To get the same benefit therefore, tennis would have to be continued for far longer than a period of running.

Walking is an extensive form of exercise. The pulse rate will rarely reach even 120 beats per minute and therefore will not have the conditioning effect of running unless it is carried out for several hours. However, it is invaluable as an adjunct of exercising because it can be practised anywhere and become part of ordinary life. In addition, it can form an ideal preparation for running, and for elderly people is often more suitable. Done regularly, and for long periods, it is an invaluable feature of many people's fitness. Although people should not be dissuaded from activities like playing tennis or walking, they must recognise their limitations. Young people, in particular, could be doing something more vigorous than, say a 30 minute walk, although this could be a convenient extra to the regular exercise programme.

Although the best results in cardiovascular conditioning come from continuous intensive activity, fixed-duration games should not be forgotten. Just how valuable certain games are to physical fitness can be seen from the charts at the beginning of the next chapter. Some will clearly need supplementing with some continuous aerobic work; others provide sufficient effect by themselves if they are carried out persistently.

Because of different lifestyles, interests, requirements and environments of people it is impossible to set down exact schedules for all readers. However basic guidelines can be established. It is important to achieve a balance between those activities that are enjoyable, but give only a limited physical benefit, and those that will drastically improve fitness and health. Both must be contained within the time available. For instance, a person wishing to maintain a reasonably high level of fitness, is prepared to spend 10 hours a week (far more than most people are willing to devote); but he can only play two rounds of golf in this time because 18 holes take three and a half hours and his nearest course is 30 minutes drive away. He also spends half-an-hour changing and having a quick drink, making a total of five hours. Do this twice a week and there is 10 hours spent in activity which has only restricted physical benefit. In this case, unless the person is prepared to extend the amount of time exercising, he should play just one round of golf and supplement this game on other days with three sessions a week of aerobics. Each of these aerobic sessions will take a maximum of an hour, even allowing for changing at home. Therefore, he is now spending only eight hours a week on his physical activity (five hours for a round of golf plus three one hour sessions of aerobics). He has saved two hours and is fitter as a result.

The frequency of exercise is entirely a personal matter. Daily intensive training is ideal but rarely possible. A target of three sessions a week, with some regular gentle exercise (such as walking) on the other days is reasonable. These three sessions should be, if possible, separated by a day's rest although this is not compulsory. They must be serious workouts, for instance a three set game of tennis, a 30 minute jog, a 25 minute swim or 20 minutes circuit training. Since people often enjoy variety it is quite permissible to

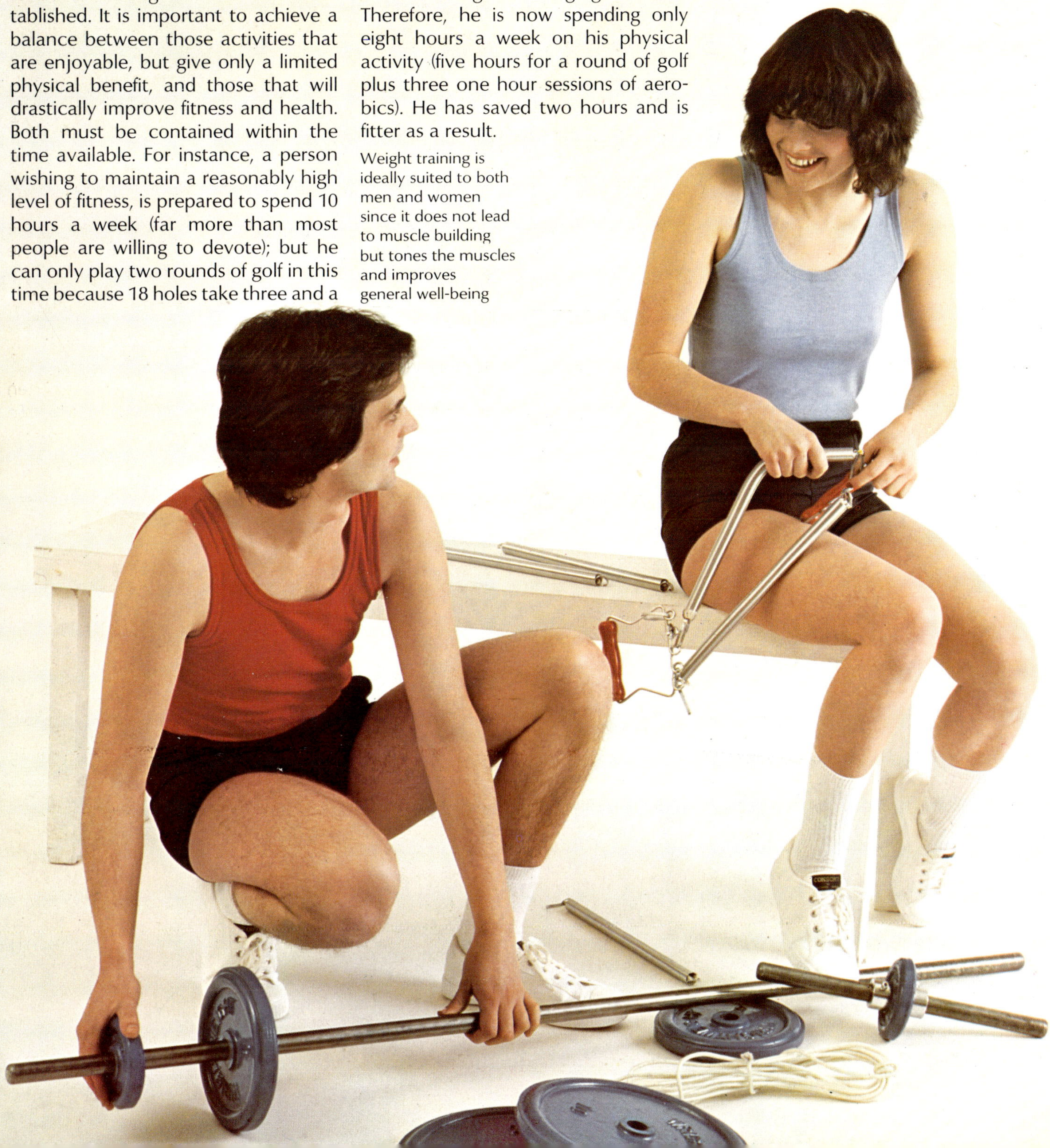

Weight training is ideally suited to both men and women since it does not lead to muscle building but tones the muscles and improves general well-being

do different activies each week. A change of sport confers both physical and mental benefits. Let us look at some of the wide variety of permutations which three hypothetical people could do.

Mr Adams, aged 45, likes to play golf every Sunday and is rightly concerned that one round a week is not giving him enough exercise. He decides to follow a plan of training a minimum of three times a week. He has not exercised seriously for 25 years and so, after a physical check-up by his doctor, who encourages him in his determination, he begins swimming two days a week in his lunch hour and one walk/jog (graduating to jogging after some months) once a week in the evening. Perhaps during the summer he will prefer to swim three times a week rather than do any jogging; that's fine provided he trains three times a week.

Mr Bright, aged 30, plays squash twice a week after work. They are intensive 45 minute workouts and certainly count as serious session, but he should have a further workout – and obviously running would be suitable. He is used to the activity while playing squash and therefore a steady jog at week-ends will give him all the exercise he needs. Perhaps, to his pleasure, he will find that like Jonah Barrington, the former British Open squash champion, the running will increase his stamina for the game.

Finally, Mrs Cutliffe, 38 years old, who has not played sport since her schooldays. She has the opportunity to play badminton and plans to do it twice a week. Understandably and rightly, she is concerned that the sudden activity might cause her some physical distress, particularly since she finds that she easily becomes breathless if she has to carry shopping any distance. So, after consulting her doctor, she starts a course of gentle walking but finds it rather boring if maintained for long periods. Since she lives in the country she can use a bicycle, initially for short trips but eventually building up so that she rides it for up to five miles. Then she feels she is ready to start badminton, but continues to use her bicycle, going out once a week for a 30 minute spin. In this way she gets in three serious sessions a week.

There are many ways of fitting in these three sessions a week, depending

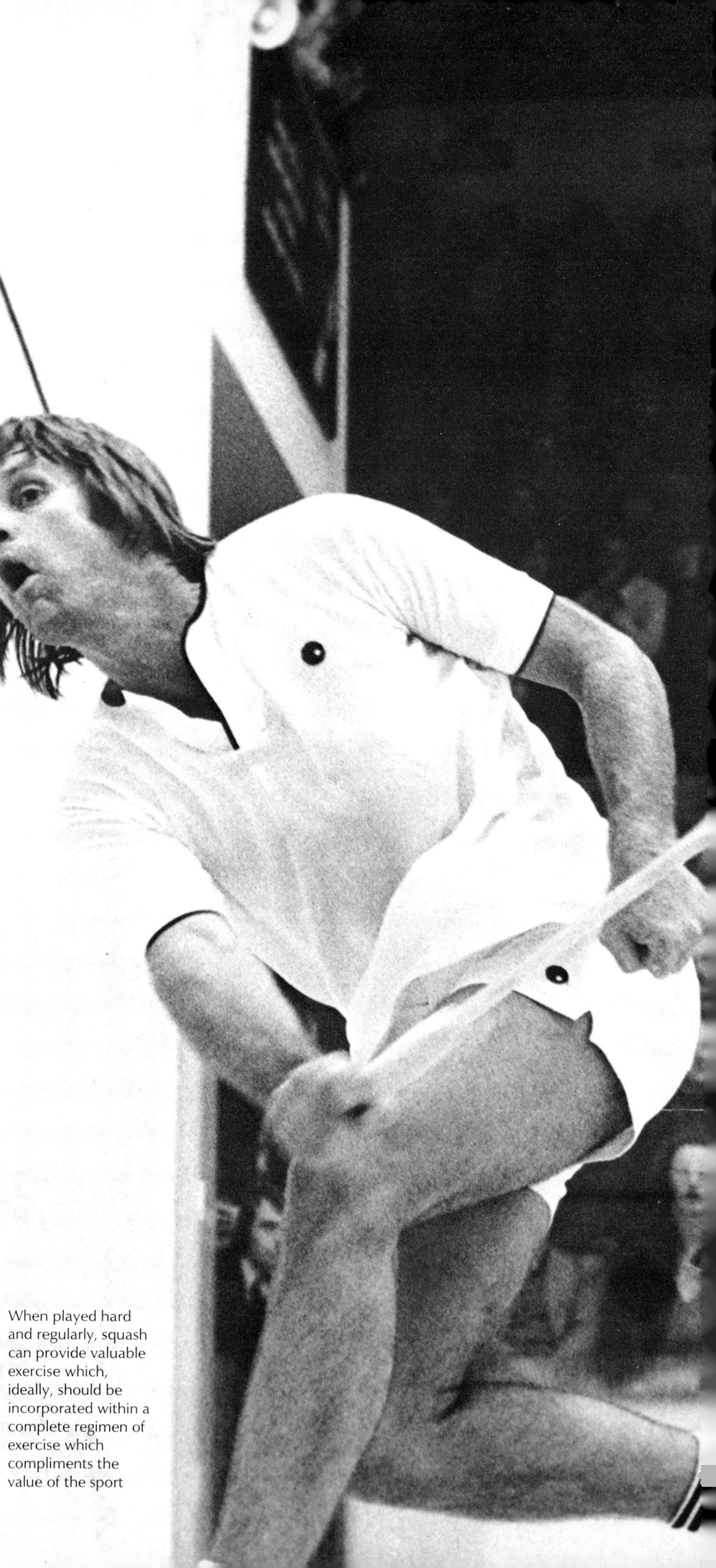

When played hard and regularly, squash can provide valuable exercise which, ideally, should be incorporated within a complete regimen of exercise which compliments the value of the sport

on available facilities. Do what is handy and pleasant. However, the sessions should be supplemented with walking, wherever possible, instead of using transport (for short distances in city centres it is invariably quicker anyway). Walk upstairs instead of taking the lifts for a few flights. You will feel better and be healthier as a result.

Supervision and Care

Before embarking on an exercise programme, particularly if you have not done any serious sport for some years, it is essential that you should have a complete medical check-up. Explain to your doctor what you plan to do. If, for any reason he is concerned about your health, you should follow his advice and perhaps do a modified course under strict medical supervision. In any case, you must be extremely careful how you exercise. It is far better that you do too little rather than too much in the early stages. There should be a gradual increase of activity. Those accidents that do occur invariably happen because the intensity of the programme has been made too severe too early. This is particularly true with people who used to practise a sport seriously. They believe that they are still capable of the same level of performance and their pride often pushes them to attempt efforts which are now beyond their powers.

Perhaps the greatest bugbear of sport, even at the non-professional level, is the incidence of injuries. You must rest the damaged limb until it has recovered and then return gradually, to full activity. In some cases medical advice or physiotherapy may be required. However, where a serious runner will have his training set back through a leg injury, an amateur can switch sports and practise swimming. He is not training for the Olympics and therefore will receive equal benefit from another aerobic activity which does not aggravate the injury while it recovers. One of the principal advantages of swimming is that, because it is a non-weight bearing exercise and there is no body contact, the incidence of injuries is only slight.

Many injuries can be avoided by keeping warmly dressed and by slowly increasing the severity of the exercise. Everyone should warm-up the body before training to diminish the chances of torn muscles or tendons. It is also important to allow food to be digested properly before exercising. Often as much as three hours should elapse between the last large intake of food and the exercise to avoid stitch or a stomach upset. This is a personal matter. Some people can train seriously within a shorter time of their last meal. Others require longer especially if the effort is to be prolonged and the meal has been heavy.

One result of exercising is that people often require slightly more sleep than previously. This is because the body needs more rest to help repair the tissues which have been broken down in training. However, as a bonus, people also find that they can get to sleep more readily then hitherto.

Smoking, alcohol and diet

The evidence against smoking cigarettes has been extensively and increasingly documented in recent years. It certainly cannot aid anyone's health and there is massive evidence that it is harmful, sometimes fatally so. The best thing is never to start smoking. If you have, give it up if you possibly can. It is expensive and probably lethal.

Alcohol, in moderation, is less debilitating. A few glasses socially brings the benefit of relaxation. On the other hand, in excess, it can be dangerous. Alcohol is also high in calories and can grievously increase your weight.

Many people believe, wrongly, that provided you exercise regularly you will lose weight. This is not necessarily true, unless you eat the same amount of food that you did before training. Vigorous exercise does burn up the calories more quickly than ordinary living, but not to the extent that is generally believed. For instance, a 16 kilometre (10 mile) run in 60 minutes (a respectable time even for a serious competitive athelete) will only burn up 1200 calories. If the individual then consumes 2 litres ($3\frac{1}{2}$ pints) of beer he will have replaced the weight loss he earned from the run. Exercise should be part of a calorie controlled diet. But it usually can't maintain a permanent weight loss unless sensible eating habbits are also observed.

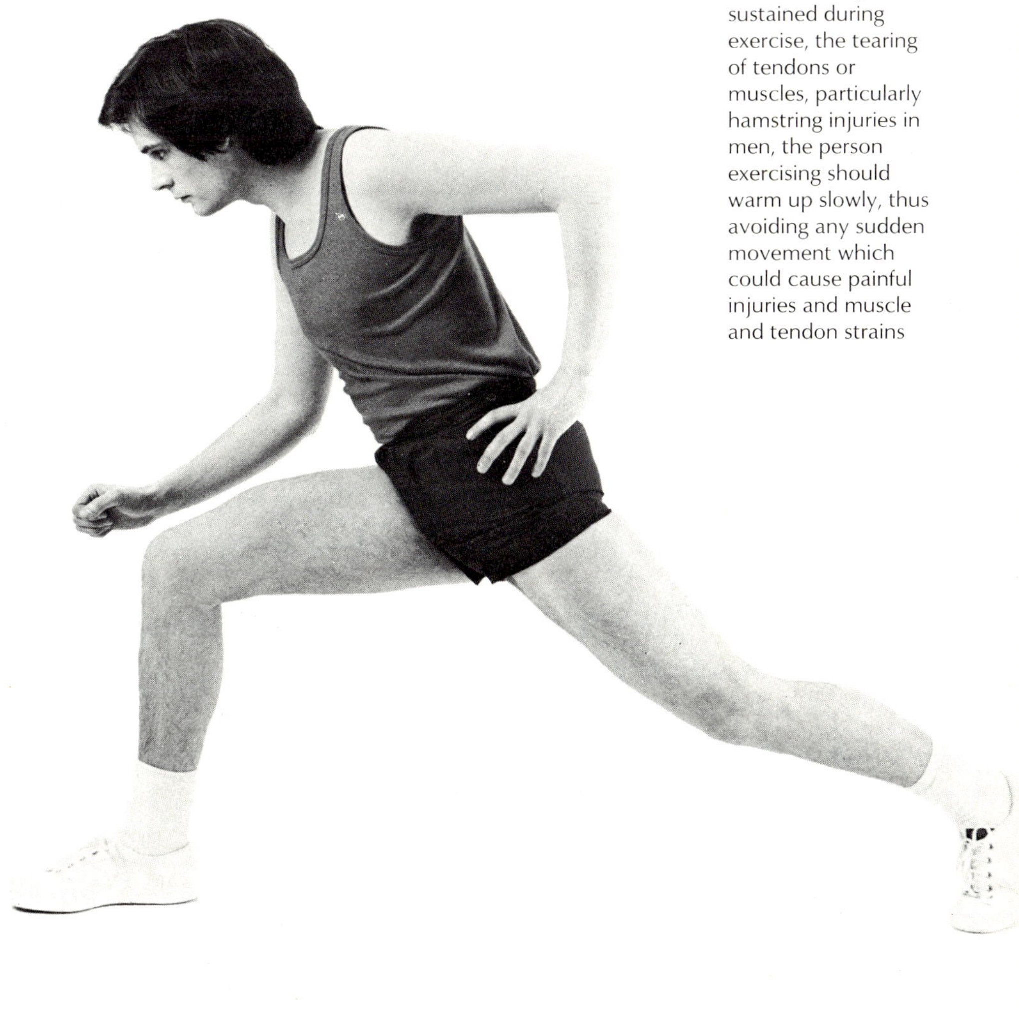

In order to avoid the commoner injuries sustained during exercise, the tearing of tendons or muscles, particularly hamstring injuries in men, the person exercising should warm up slowly, thus avoiding any sudden movement which could cause painful injuries and muscle and tendon strains

Suppleness

Suppleness permits increased mobility and allows a full range of movement. The ability to turn quickly and stretch the limbs easily are essential criteria for many recreations. A sport like gymnastics demands an extraordinary degree of suppleness. Unless you have trained persistently and have always possessed a naturally flexible body, many of the movements are virtually impossible. Modern competitive gymnastics largely require special apparatus and an ordinary person would have had to have started the sport young enough to learn many of the difficult movements. Mobility, unfortunately, decreases drastically with age. Unless they already possess it, or are prepared to devote many training sessions to acquiring it, the technical skill demanded by gymnastics is beyond the ability of most adults. Sufficient suppleness can be more readily obtained by performing a complete and easy series

1. Stand with feet about 25cm (10in) apart and clasp your hands overhead, reaching up as high as you can. Keeping your head between your arms, turn to the left as far as you can; bend down to the left side. Change over the to right side, letting the hands sweep past the feet. Raise the body so that you are facing to the right. Keep your heels on the ground. Bend your knees slightly if you want to. This movement stretches the whole body.

1

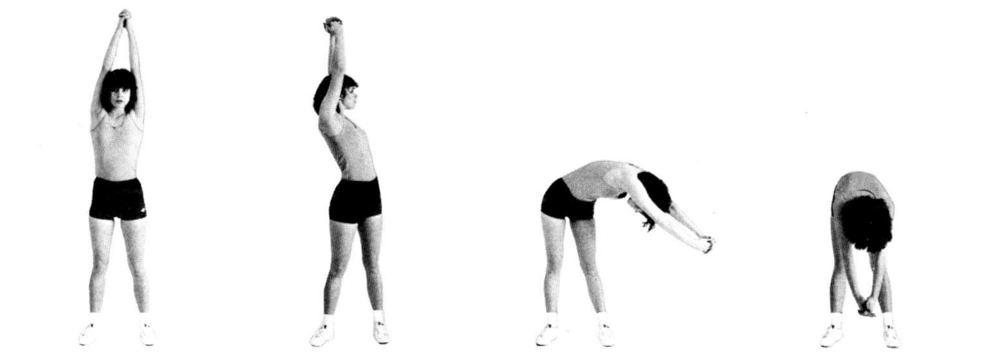

2. Stand upright, keeping your head still. Roll or shrug your shoulders forwards, backwards, upwards and downwards. Then in the reverse direction. Then do it with one shoulder at a time. use your elbows to lead the movement. This loosens your shoulders.

2

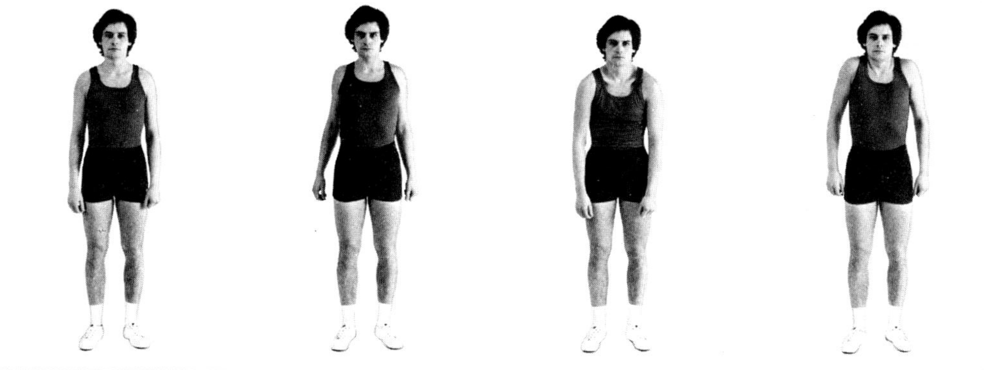

3. Stand upright, keeping your shoulders still. Roll your head forwards, backwards, sideways and downwards. Then move your head in the reverse direction. This loosens your neck.

3

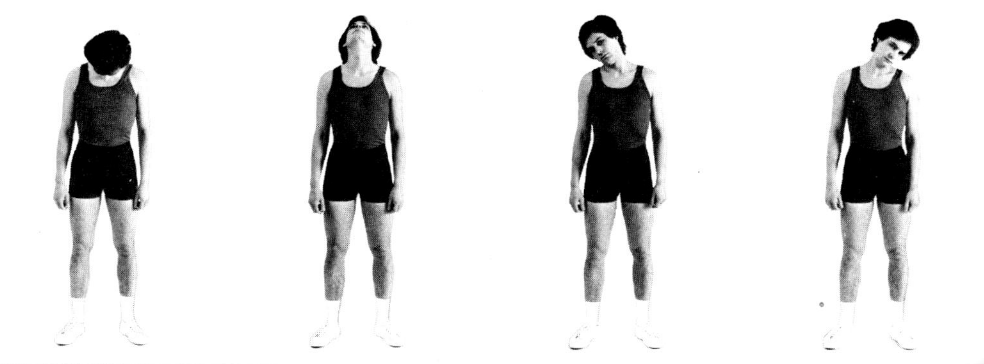

5. Grasp your right wrist with your left hand and move it through its complete range of movement, rotating the joint and then moving it up and down. Repeat with the other hand. Then do the same on both ankles while sitting down.

5

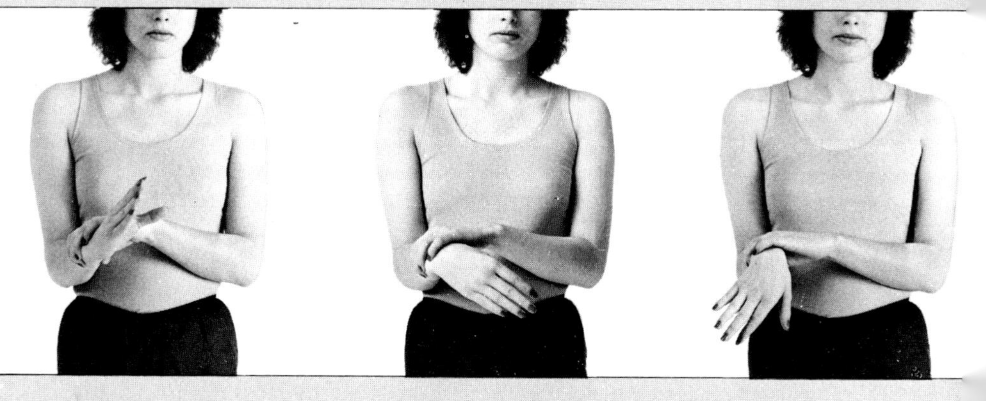

of free-standing exercises.

The schedule below has a number of advantages: no apparatus is required; the session would be useful as preparation for more severe exercise, thus forming the basis for a warm-up; in addition, it has a flexibility value of its own. Carried out once a week, the schedule would only take about eight minutes. It is important, especially if you are not accustomed to these movements, not to strain yourself to begin with. Do the exercises carefully, gradually increasing the severity over a period of months. For instance, in the simple movement of touching your toes you should feel a slight tingling at the back of your hamstrings but not a severe pain. You are training your body not straining it. Do each exercise for 30 seconds before moving onto the next. Relax as you do the early ones.

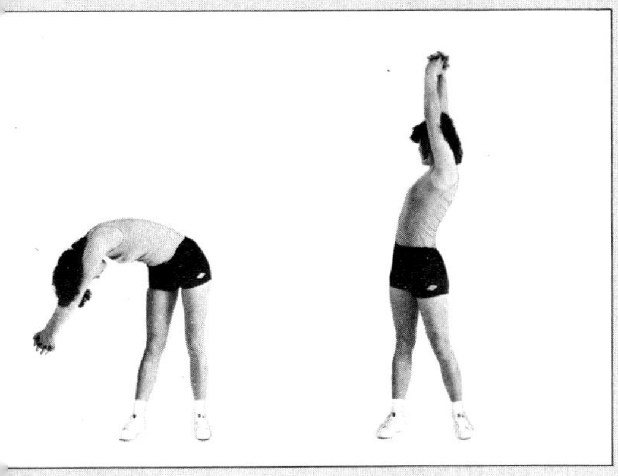

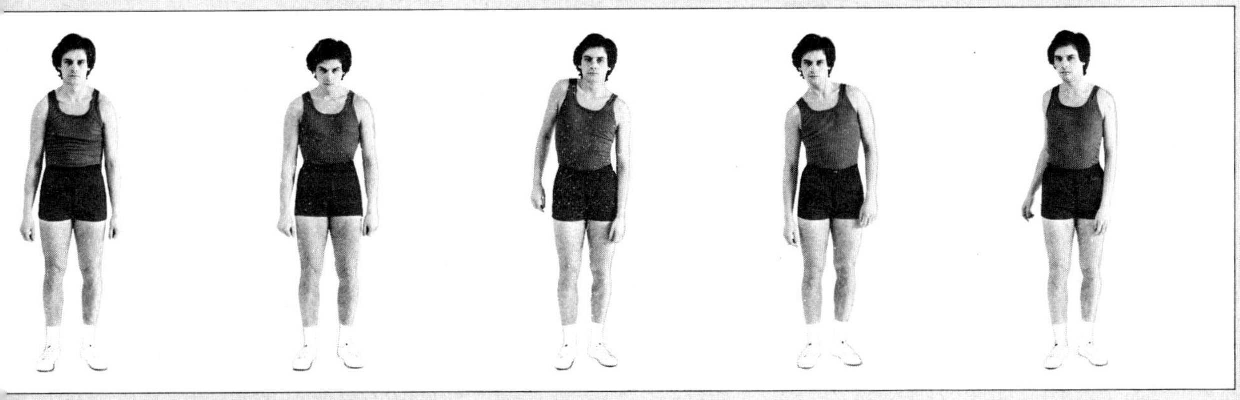

4. Bend your left arm behind your back as if someone were trying to put a half-nelson on you. Your knuckles should now be against your back. Swing your right hand by your right ear and over your back. Attempt to clasp hands. If you can do this try to grasp your wrists with your other hands. This is excellent for keeping shoulders supple.

4

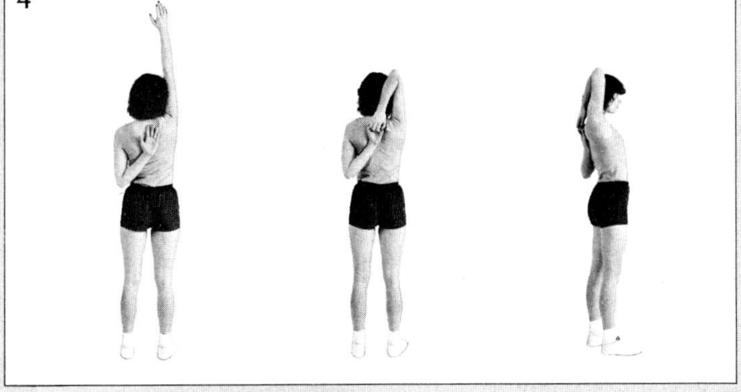

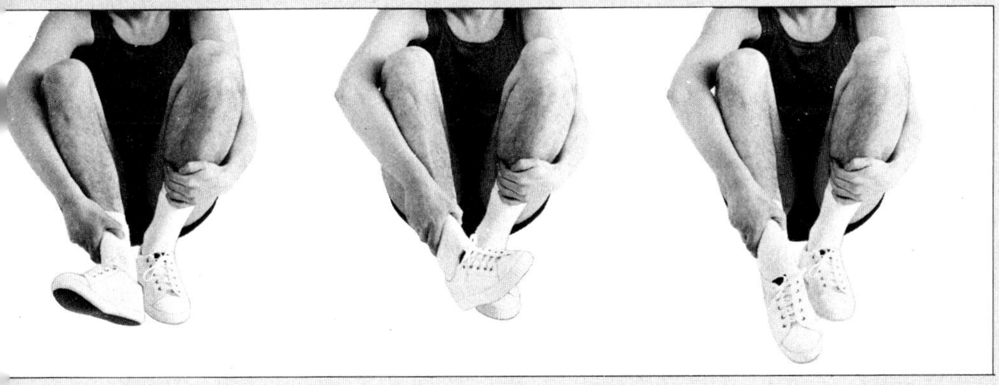

6

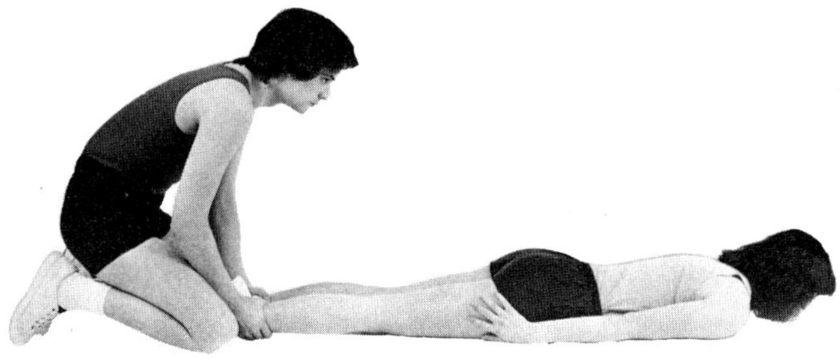

6. Lie on your front with your feet firmly anchored underneath an object (a barbell, wall-bar or partner clasping your ankles is ideal). From this prone position raise your body upwards, bending at the waist. This exercises the lower back.

6

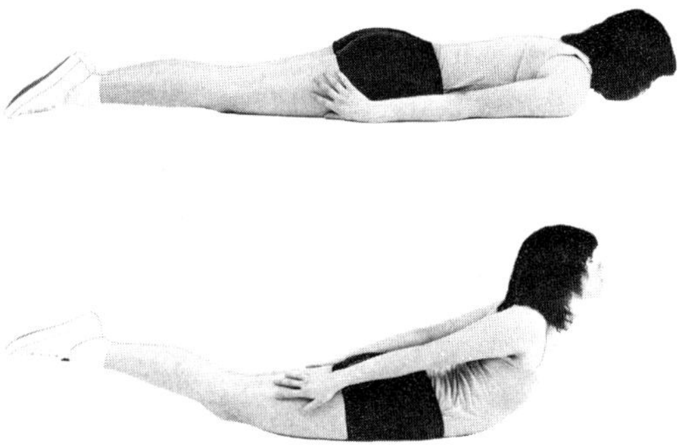

9. Stand upright and then bend at the waist to touch the toes. If you can do this without bending your knees try to put your hands flat on the floor. This stretches the hamstrings.

9

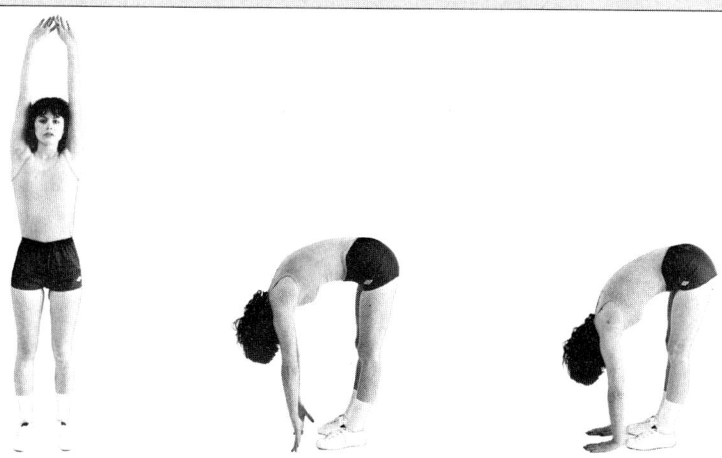

11. Sit down with your legs outstretched. Bend your knees so that your ankles are close to your crotch and your knees are splayed out. Place your right hand on your right leg and left hand on left leg. Press your knees down. This again loosens the muscles and tendons inside the top of the thigh.

11

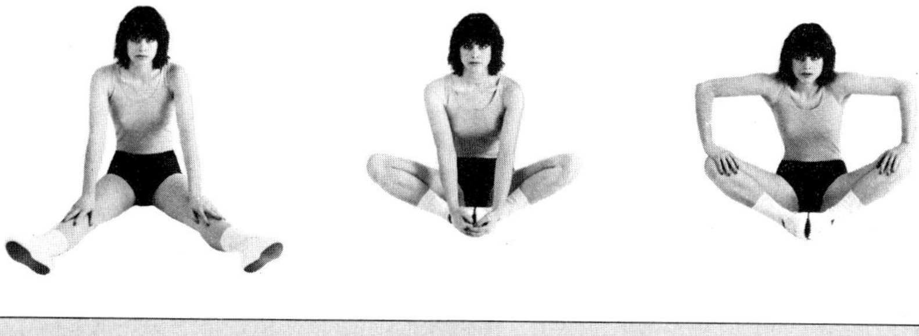

7. Stand with feet about 25cm (10in) apart, toes pointing forwards. Allow your knees to bend forwards as you bend backwards and twist your body round to the left to try to touch your right heel with your left hand. This relaxes the trunk and sides of the waist.

7

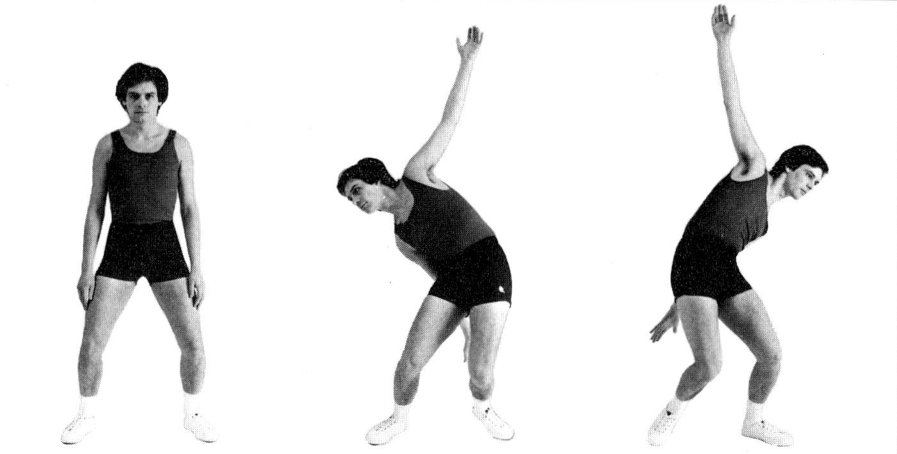

8. Kneel on the ground with your legs bent, splayed wide behind you with the feet facing outwards. From this position try to sit your bottom on the floor. If you can reach this position then lie down, and sit up again. You probably can't – so keep working on just sitting down. This loosens the hips.

8

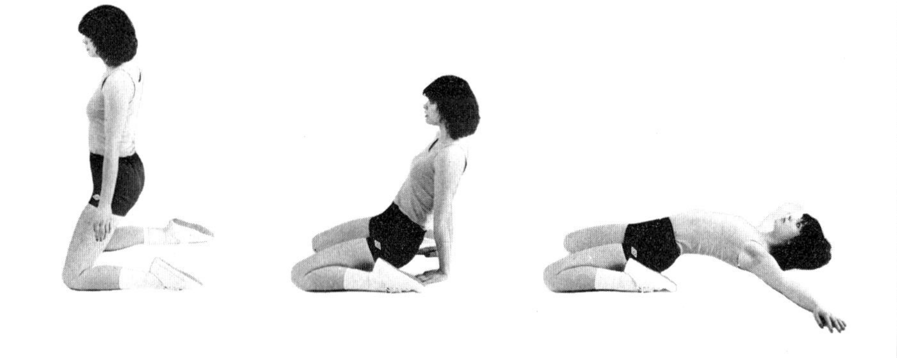

10. Stand upright and with your right foot always facing to the front swing your leg sideways. Raise your leg as high as it will go. Keep the leg straight and face the front. This loosens the muscles and tendons inside the top of the thigh.

10

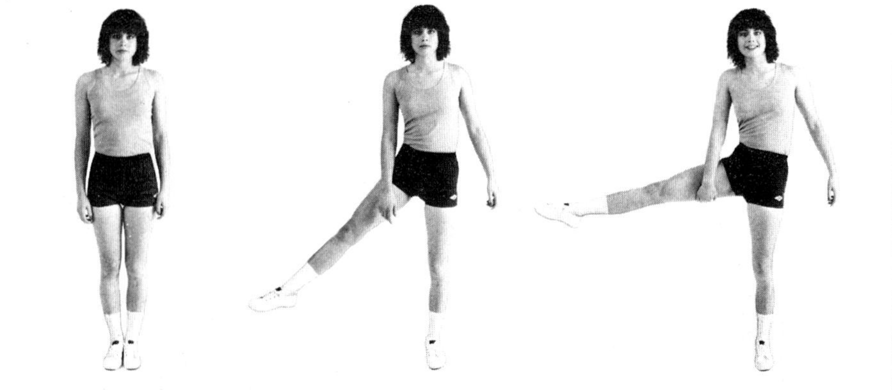

12. Stand upright with your knees slightly bent. Bend over and using your hands rotate your knees so as to loosen them completely.

12

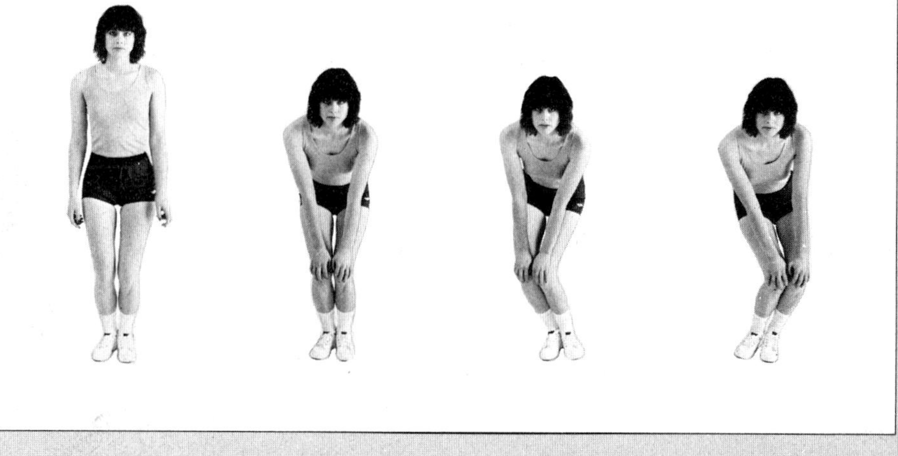

Many people like to do these exercises on getting up in the morning, and then follow them with some more strenuous exercises like press-ups and sit-ups (see section on strength). This routine is an addition to, not a replacement for, a session aimed at cardiovascular exercise.

Speed

Although speed is a crucial feature in many sports and games, it is something that is largely inbred in a competitor. The adage 'A sprinter is born not made' has considerable validity. Great increases in strength and stamina can be established through assiduous training but the ability to move quickly cannot be developed to the same extent. For this reason, sprinters in track and field athletics have to spend far less time on training than long-distance runners or throwers. For an ordinary person, therefore, there is little point in spending long periods trying to improve speed so as to be, say, better tennis or squash players. Much of the speed in these games derives from the reactions which are developed during the game.

Neither is the ability to move fast associated with a noticeably healthy body. Don't spend long periods of time developing this faculty. What increase of speed is possible often comes from exercises emphasising mobility and strength-gaining movements from weight-training. Speed has some relation to power. The fastest sprinters are powerful men

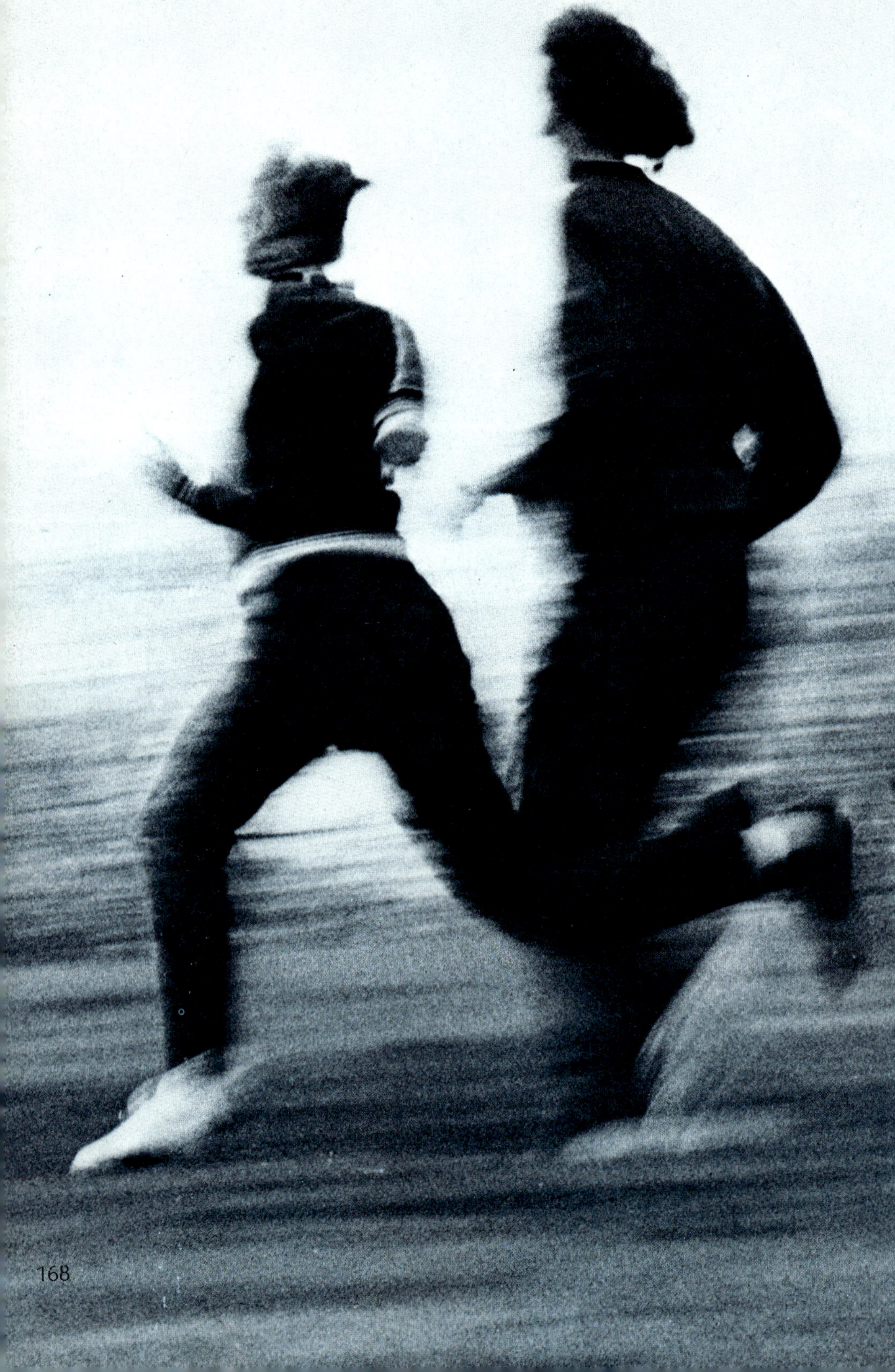

Strength

From Hercules and Samson to the present day world weight-lifting champions, strong men have always been glamorous personalities for the public. Many people who are interested in keeping fit are attracted to the different ways of becoming strong. Leading weight-lifters, who take part competitively on the Olympic lifts look tremendously healthy. This is even more true of the top bodybuilders, who attempt to train their physiques so that every muscle is in proportion to the rest of the body.

However, appearances are particularly deceptive in weight-lifing and body-building. Although competitors are often phenomenally strong, they are invariably less fit than many other leading sportsmen. Since they don't require a high level of cardiovascular fitness, many lifters and body-builders would feature only moderately in aerobic activities. This is especially true of heavyweights and super-heavyweights, some of whom are as unfit, in cardiovascular terms, as an untrained person.

For the purposes of any person who does not wish to compete seriously in weight-lifing and body-building but is only interested in maintaining a healthy body, strength training should not be allowed to dominate a programme. Certainly not more than half the number of weekly sesssions, preferably less, should be devoted to strength exercises. One disadvantage of weight-training is that it takes a long time to complete a session (often over an hour) which is why conventional weight-training should be used as a preparation for circuit-training. By doing this, moderate benefits to physical strength combine with sufficiently long duration of exercising the heart to provide all-round benefit. The circuit can be completed quickly, often 20 minutes.

There are those people who are attracted to or enjoy ordinary weight-training, an extraordinarily satisfying sport in itself. Nevertheless, they must be urged to complement their work in a gymnasium or at home with serious cardiovascular exercise. It may even, as leading weight-lifters have now found, benefit their weight-training because they can raise weights more intensively.

Weight-training is based on the work of a man called De Lorme, who found that his patients improved the strength of the muscles in an injured limb only if the weight they were moving was progressively increased. The fundamental rule of strength-gaining is that the body becomes stronger to cope with the increased resistance, either through more repetitions or with heavier weights. Although an exercise like press-ups is a form of weight-training, with the body as the weight to be raised, the expression is more commonly used to describe the raising of barbells, a long bar evenly weighted at either end, or dumbells, shorter bars which are often lifted in pairs. The advantages of weights are obvious: the resistance can be accurately assessed and increased as the muscles grow stronger. Furthermore, although an increase in the number of times the exercise is repeated does add to your strength neverthless when a very high number (over 15) of repetitions are used, the premium is on muscular and eventually on cardiovascular endurance.

Most weight-trainers practise the 'set' system, since research has shown that muscles grow more quickly when each group of muscles is subjected to intensive exercising before one moves onto the next group of muscles. Let us take a simple movement like press-ups. Someone who might be capable of a maximum of 16, may conveniently perform 10 repetitions of the exercise then rest for a few minutes, perform another 10 rest again and then perform another 10. This is three sets of 10 repetitions, often written as 3×10. It has been found that low repetitions with heavy weights are best for increasing strength, that repetitions from four to eight promote muscular bulk, and that above 10 put an emphasis on muscular endurance. Higher repetitions, particularly when part of a circuit, chiefly promote stamina. For beginners 10 repetitions are recommended.

The exercises that have been selected are the basic ones which can later be incorporated into a circuit. For the first month, the complete beginner should perform just one set of each exercise; in the second, two sets; and in the third month he can do three sets. During the third month of training he will expect to spend about an hour and a half at every session. He should train three times a week, exercising on alternate days. Although anyone can train alone, it is better to join a gym where you can get advice and assistance. Both are invaluable in the early stages. The equipment will be better than that available for use at home and there is much benefit from training with other people. Many gyms have special pulleys and multi-gyms (one piece of apparatus on which a large variety of exercises can be performed). These are expensive and difficult to store in the home. It is important that the techniques should be carried out satisfactorily and that the competitor does not strain himself by trying to raise too heavy poundages. Train sensibly. It is better at this stage for the weights to be too light than too heavy. The approximate starting poundages are at the end of the descriptions of the exercises; this includes the weight of the bar 7 or 9 kg usually (15 or 20 lbs). These may be increased by a little over a kilo ($2\frac{1}{2}$lb) each week if you find it comparatively easy to complete the exercise without struggling. It is important to be warm while training; a track suit and tee shirt are recommended clothes. Warm up with some light exercises, such as the suppling routine given in the previous section, before beginning training. Add some free-standing squats, press-ups and jogging, either on the spot or, preferably, outside. Then you are ready to start.

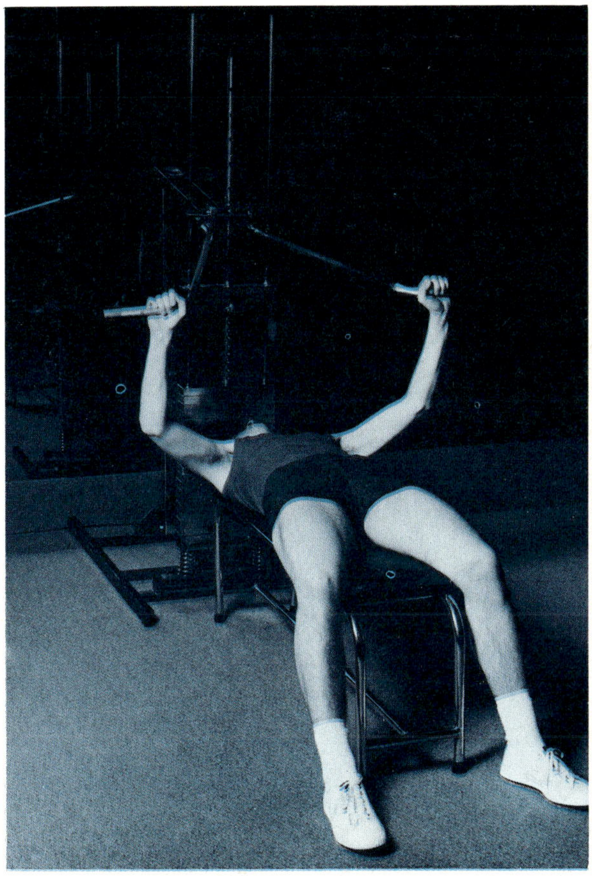

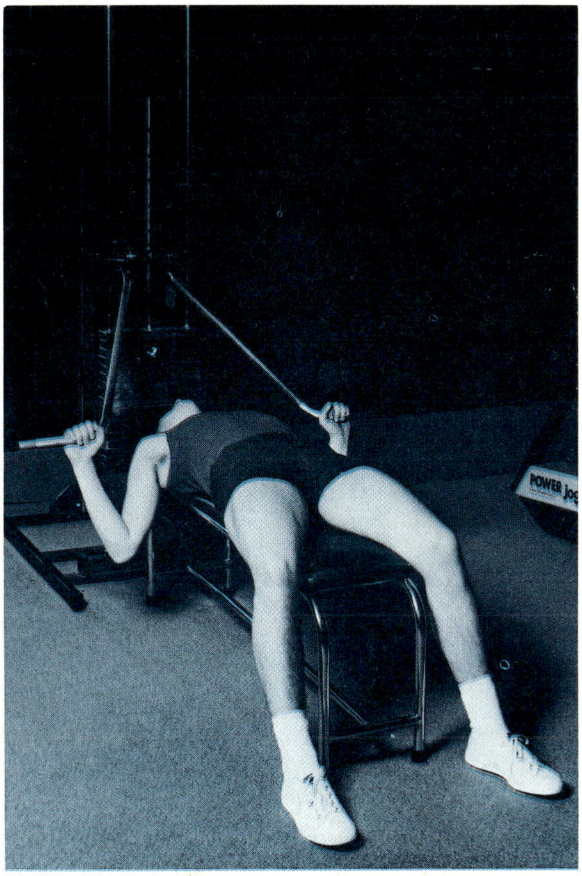

A modern gym will have various kinds of weights available. In this case the weight training machine works on a pulley system where the athlete can adjust the amount he wants to train with. This is an extremely safe method of using weights as well as being very easy to use.

Lifting position from the floor.
The legs should be about 30cm (1ft) apart, close up to the barbell, back straight, head up, arms locked and the shoulders a little forward of the barbell. It is important that the weight lifter should use his legs, as otherwise too great a strain would be placed on the lower back.

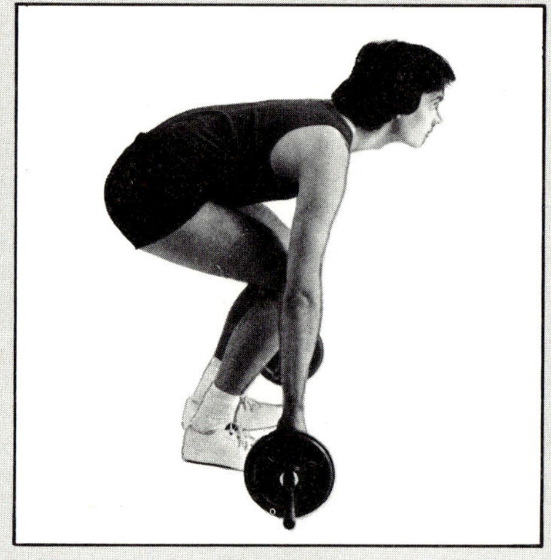

1. Power Snatch. Use light barbell since this exercise serves as an excellent warm-up for the later exercises. Use a wide grip to facilitate raising the bar overhead. Pull the weight from the floor, close to the body to locked arms in one smooth, swift action (11kg/25lbs).

2. Abdominal Sit-up. A free-exercise movement. From the lying position with hands behind neck, raise the trunk upwards. After a few weeks' training the number of repetitions can be comfortably increased from the starting number of 10. Later make it more difficult by performing the routine on an inclined board (head at the bottom of the slope) which increases the resistance. Similarly, if you find it impossible to sit up on a flat surface at the beginning, make it easier by putting your head at the top of the board to decrease the resistance.

2

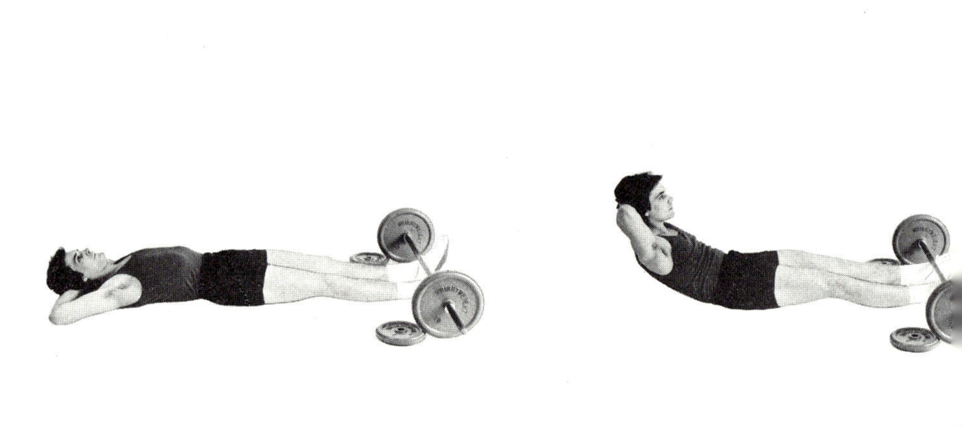

2

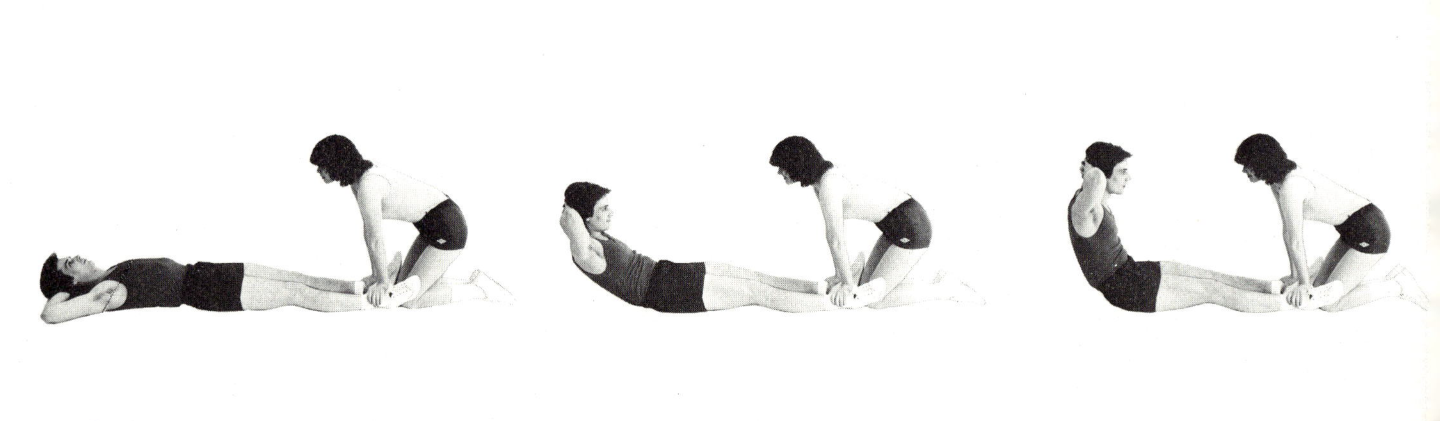

3. Bench Press. The major exercise for the upper body and one which heavy poundages can be safely used. One advantage of training with other people is that 'catchers' (other trainers or partners who convey the bar from the ground or racks into the lifter's grasp and then take it off him after he has finished his set) can be employed. You can do without catchers by using racks and pulling the bar into the starting position yourself and returning it afterwards. Press the barbell from the chest directly upwards to locked arms and then lower (13.5kg/30lbs).

3

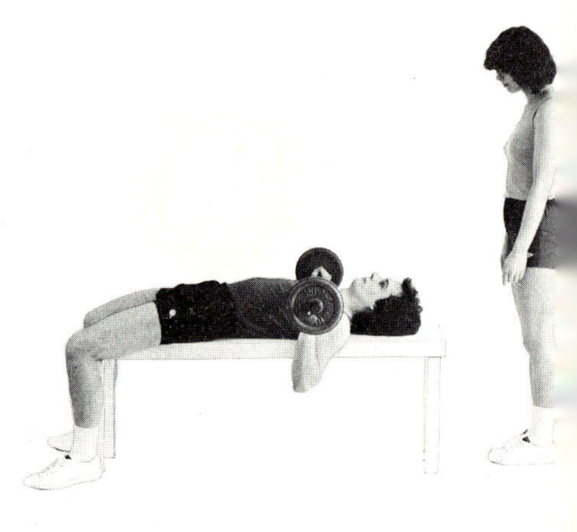

1

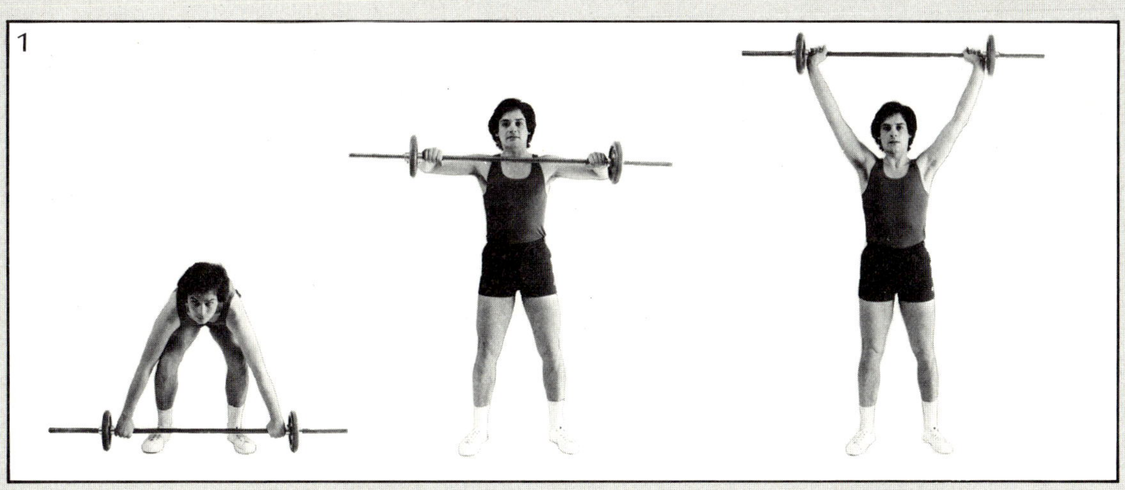

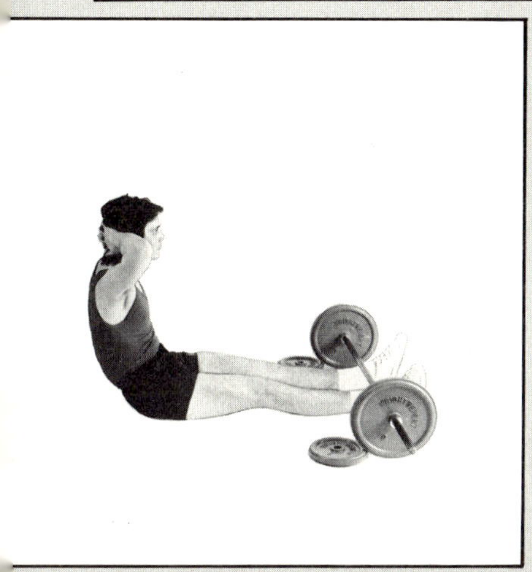

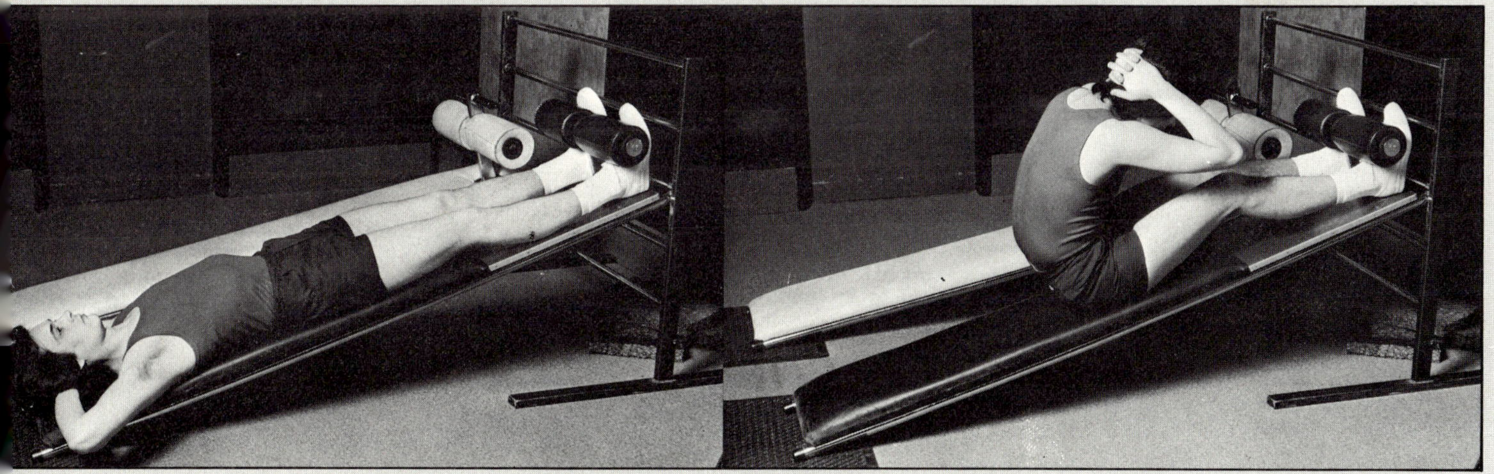

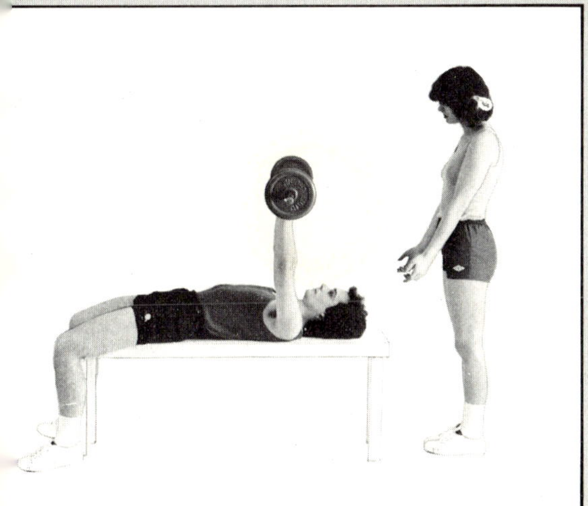

4. Alternate Dumbell Press. Hoist the loaded dumbells onto the shoulders and then press alternately overhead, one lowered as the other is raised. This is a fine exercise for the triceps and shoulders. (7kg/15lbs) each dumbell.

4

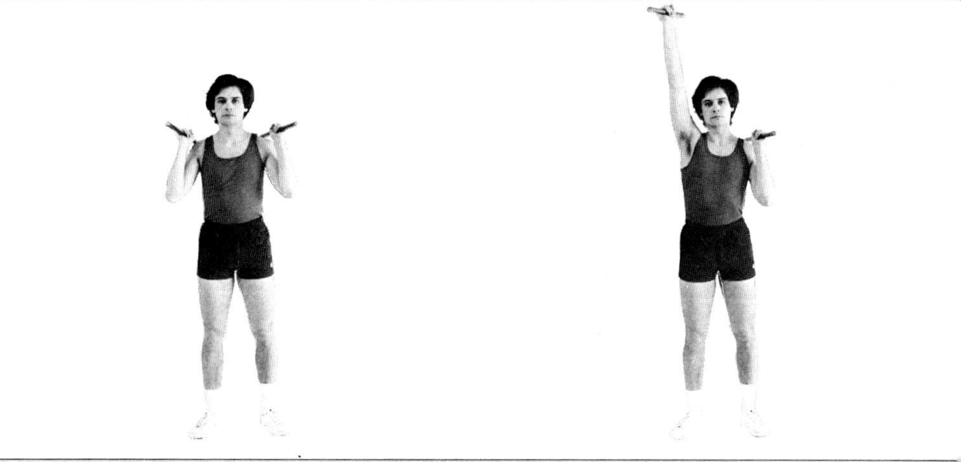

6. Power Cleans. Pull the barbell from the floor to shoulders in one clean, swift movement, the legs bending a little as the weight is received. This exercise is good for strengthening the back, and also the legs and shoulders.

6

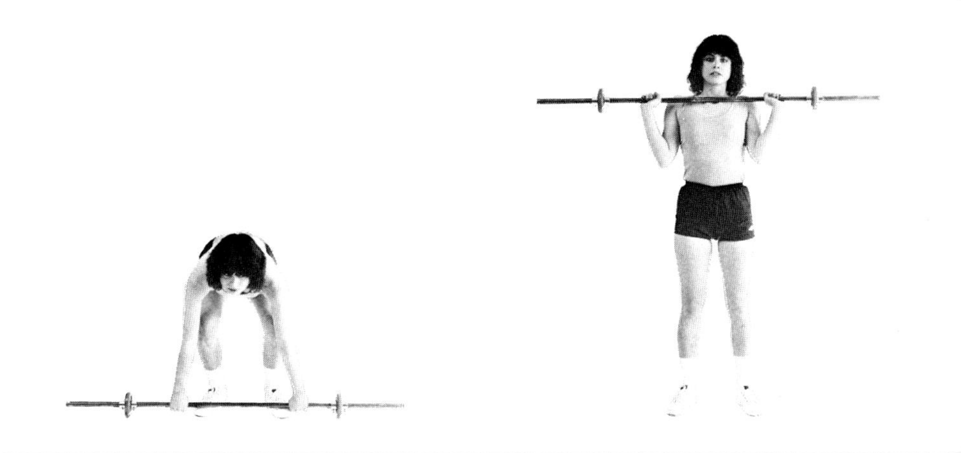

8. Half Squat. From a standing position the lifter squats to touch the bench with his backside. The movement can be continued so that the lifter rests on his haunches but this can affect many people's knees. Heavy weights can easily be used in this movement, in which case the bar can be loaded onto stands and removed from them before beginning to exercise. When this occurs 'catchers' should usually be employed. Squats primarily strengthen the legs and back. Begin without a weight before using an empty, and then loaded bar.

8

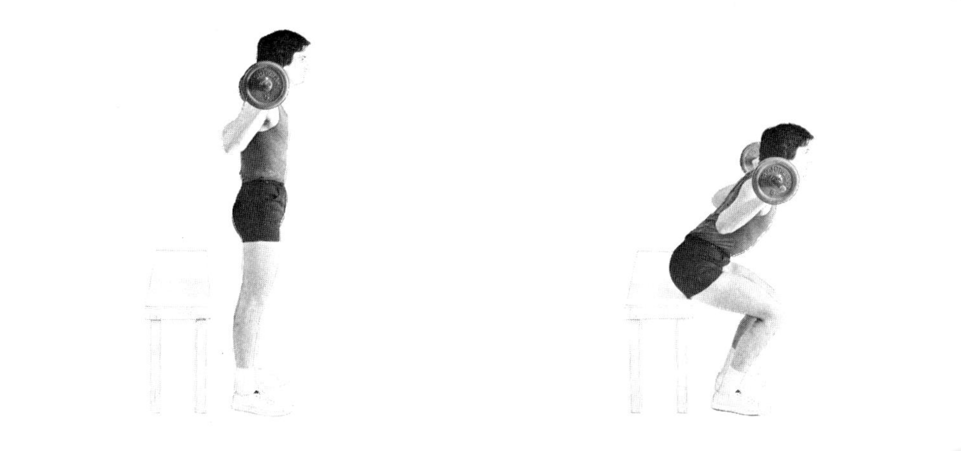

Those who wish to practise weight-training at a more advanced level should get expert advice, but, for the person who just wants to keep fit circuit-training should be added to the routine.

Circuit-training

Here the exercises are done continuously with no pause between the sets. Do one set of each exercise to complete the circuit before going round again and then a third and, perhaps eventually, a fourth time. The important thing is to train without any pause. However, unless you are already experienced and comparatively fit, you should begin gradually with one circuit and then the next month add a second and so on. The poundages will

5. Bent-over Rowing. The body should be bent at 90° at the waist and the knees unlocked. With the body and legs maintained in this position pull the barbell from outstretched arms to touch the chest. This exercise develops the *latissimus dorsi* muscles of the back and also the shoulders. (11kg/25lbs).

5

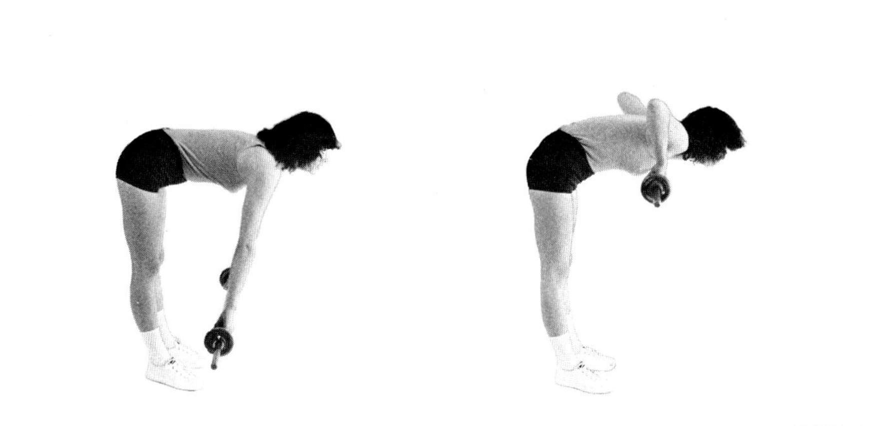

7. Two Hands Curl. With the palms uppermost, the bar rests on the thighs of the lifter. From there it is 'curled', using only the upper arms, onto the top of the chest. This movement principally activates the biceps (11kg/25lbs).

7

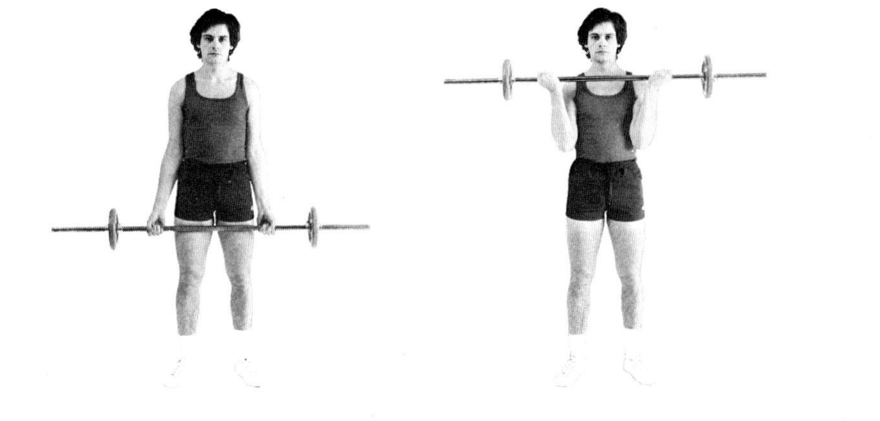

9. Straight Arm Pull-over. This exercise should be performed between each set of half squats. After the 10 repetitions of half squats the lifter performs 10 repetitions of straight arm pullover. This is called a 'super set' and is carried out three times. Squats tend to compress the body while straight arm pullovers stretch the body, thus acting as a relief. Hold the barbell with straight arms above the chest, then lower it backwards, keeping the arms straight, until parallel with the floor. From there steadily pull it back to the starting position. Begin using an empty bar.

9

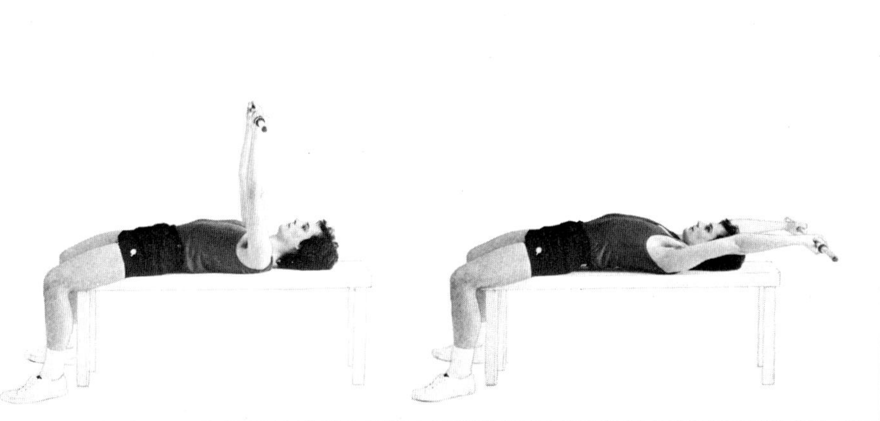

be much lighter than in ordinary weight-training, so that muscular weakness won't occur before the cardiovascular system has been tested. Don't rush at the weights but it is occasionally valuable to time yourself over the whole session. Use between 10 and 20 repetitions for each exercise.

It is best to do circuit-training in a group, but this can often be difficult – unless it is carefully organised – because there are problems in proceeding quickly from one exercise to another when someone else is still using that apparatus. This produces bottle-necks and much of the value is lost because pauses in the session are necessary. Gymnasiums often do not cater for circuit-training as such, being principally concerned with weight-training. It is best either to find a time and place where you can go immediately from one exercise to another without the interruption of other trainees or to train at home. It is worthwhile exploring every avenue because circuit-training is extremely valuable for promoting all-round general fitness. A session can maintain strength and yet make a substantial demand on one's cardiovascular system. It is not necessary to use weights for circuit-training – the Canadian Air Force during the 1950s invented a system called the 5BX (basic exercises) plan which only involved the body-weight as resistance. However, the use of weights does give better all-round exercise.

Strands and Isometrics

Strand-pulling, using a chest expander, is often popular with people who are forced to travel regularly, as they are easily transported and sessions can fit in with a busy routine. It can be incorporated with free-standing exercises into a valuable session. An expander consists of two handles with either metal or rubber strands between them. The degree of resistance of these strands is measured in the pulling strength instead of the weight, but all the strength-gaining principles of weight-training apply. However, strands can only satisfactorily exercise the upper body and, since they come in a minimum strength of 10 lbs, slight increases are difficult. Therefore, to increase the severity of the exercise, increase the number of repetitions before adding resistance and the revert to a fewer number of repetitions. Here is a routine, incorporating free-standing exercises, which gives an all-round workout. In the early sessions use one set of 10 repetitions, progressing to two and finally three.

1. Front Chest Pull. Hold the expander taut in front of the chest with the knuckles facing outwards. Pull the strands evenly apart until they rest against the chest. Return to the starting position. Keep the arms locked as the movement is made with the inhalation preceding the effort (7kg/15lbs). This affects the shoulders and back in particular.

1

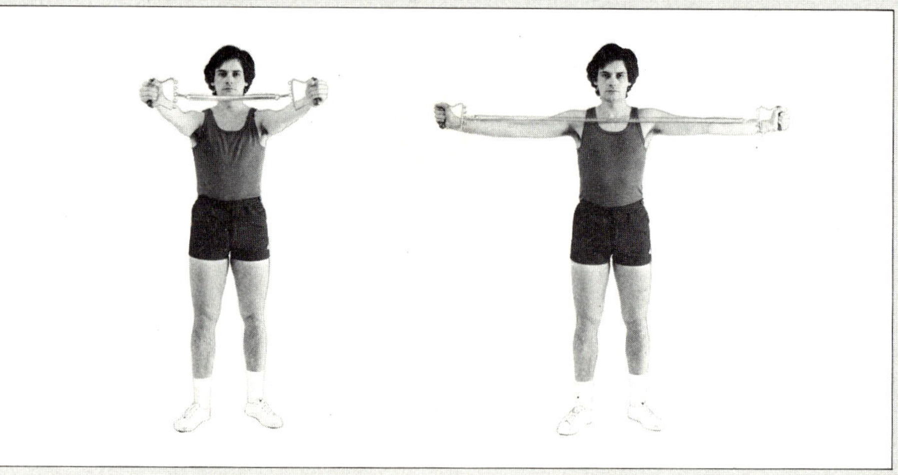

2. Downward Pull. Hold the strands overhead with the palms facing outwards. Then pull the expander slowly apart and let it rest on the back of the neck before returning it to the starting position. Breathe in as the effort is made. This exercise works the shoulders and back. (7kg/15lbs.)

2

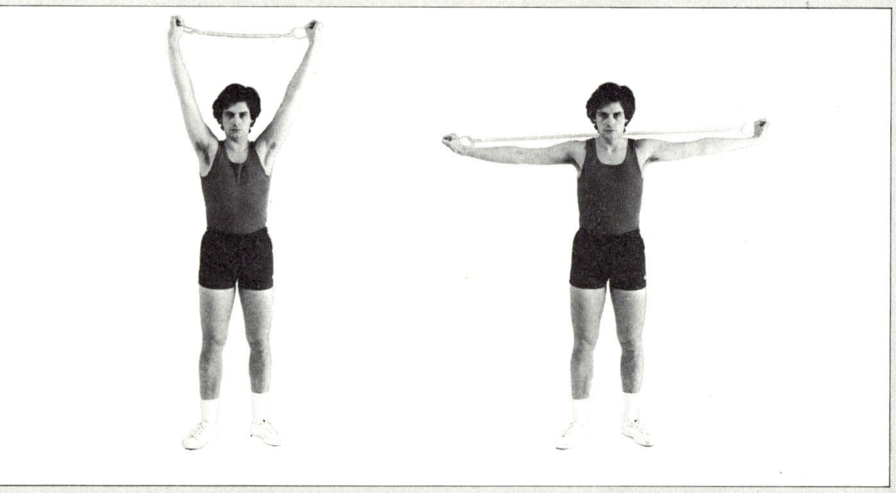

3. Triceps Extension. Place the expander behind the neck and with the palms facing outwards stretch it to the limit of the arms. Breathe in as the effort is made. This exercise affects the shoulders and triceps (7kg/15lbs).

3

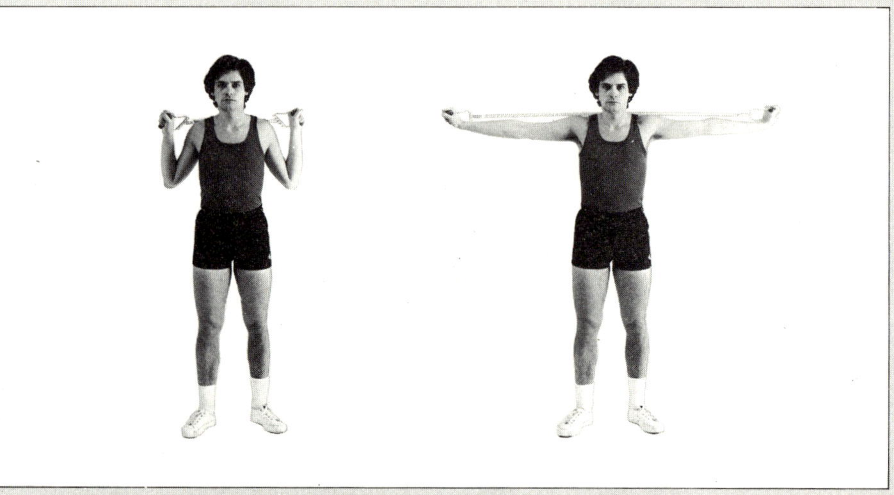

4. Single Arm Curls. Lock one of the handles of the expander underneath the foot. Then, grasping the other end with the palms uppermost, curl the weight to the shoulder, trying to keep the elbow close to the body. After the required number of repetitions switch to the other side. Breathe in gradually, as the aim is a smooth exercise. This works the biceps and forearms (4.5kg/10lbs).

4

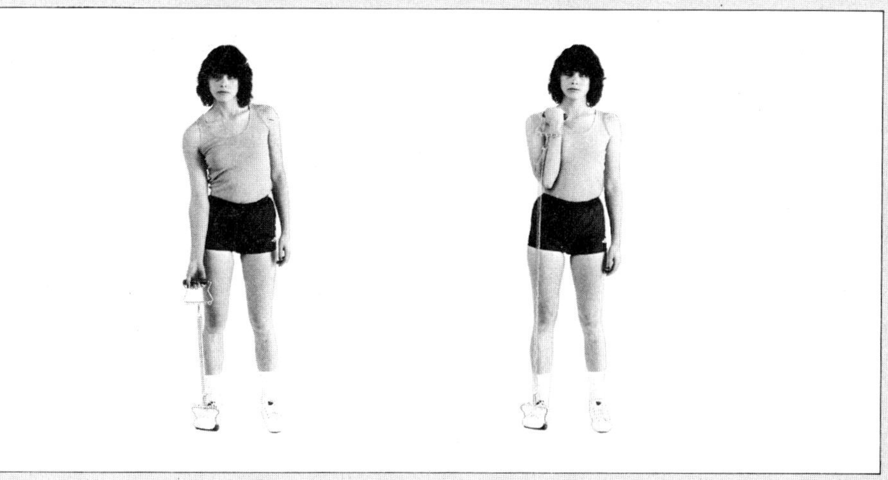

5. Press-ups. Adopt the front support position with the shoulders over the hands, body straight and only the hands and toes in contact with the ground. Unlock the arms until the chin touches the ground and then push evenly upwards. This exercises the chest, shoulders and triceps. It has a similar effect to bench press.

5

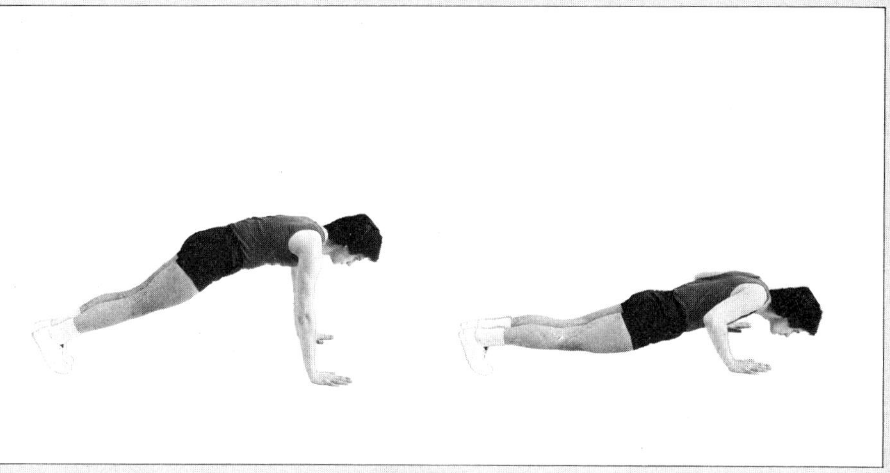

6. Step-ups. Place the left foot on a chair or bench and step up until the body is erect and both legs are together. Step down. Repeat with the right leg leading. Repeat 30 times, building up to 100 repetitions.

By doing these exercises without a pause you can improvise a circuit quickly and effectively whenever you feel like it. As with circuit training involving weights, the resistance must necessarily be kept light so that the individual can put stress on his heart and lungs.

6

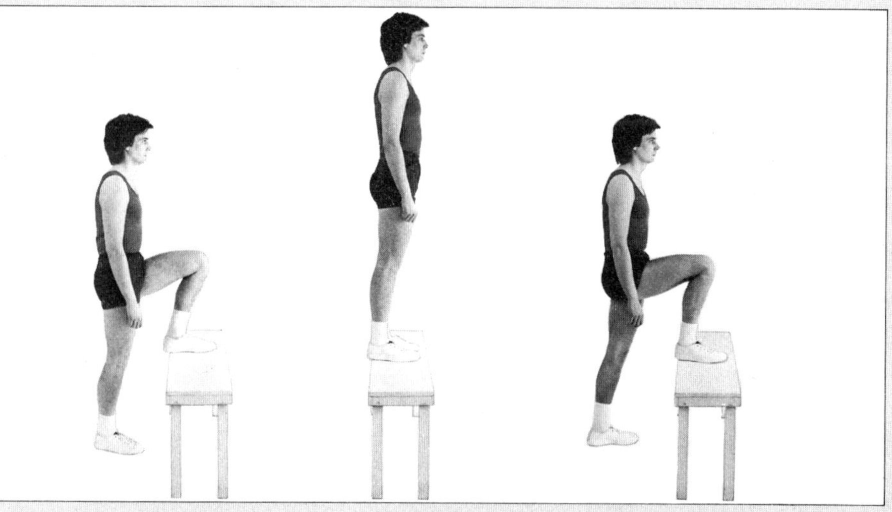

Isometrics

Isometric (literally 'equal measure') exercises contract muscles, –either against each other or an unyielding object. The credit for the introduction of this training method is attributed to two German physiologists, Professor E. A. Muller and Dr T. Hettinger, who claimed that an increase in strength of 5 per cent per week could be obtained. Since 1953 when the method was first introduced this figure has been widely challenged, and it would appear that weekly increases of 1-2 per cent more accurate. Hettinger has since modified his early claims. Considerable concentration is necessary during the contraction which should be held for six seconds. It is believed that two thirds of your maximum strength must be employed. Since the exercises take up very little time – although there is little motivating purpose as in weight-training when there is the stimulus of raising the weight – many weight-trainers have adopted them in addition to their regular training. However, they cannot be adapted to circuit-training and have even less effect on the heart than pure weight-training. If you enjoy isometrics, continue using them but do some aerobic exercises, such as running or swimming as well.

Aerobics and Stamina

Stamina, or cardiovascular endurance, should be the centre of any physical fitness programme aimed at maintaining health at a high level. Although other sports will promote stamina, three activities are particularly valuable – running, swimming and cycling. In none of these is the heart-rate allowed to decrease from a steady state of exertion. In other sports the particular techniques and rules of the game and the presence of an opponent mean that cardiovascular endurance is rarely full stretched. This is why so many sportsmen use running as part of their preparation for their particular game. It gives them greater endurance for their special interest: boxers and wrestlers run in the early morning; soccer players lap the field or go on cross-country jogs.

The reason they run, rather than swim or cycle, is because running is closer to their own sports and as well as training the heart, activates the skeletal muscles they will need. This points to a fundamental fact about endurance training, and indeed about all exercise – that it is partly specific to the activity you are doing. Thus, no long distance swimmer can immediately transfer his endurance capacity to running. However, as numerous biathlon (running-swimming) events have shown, outstanding swimmers are invariably at least good runners. It is less common the other way round because swimming is an acquired skill which many leading runners find as difficult to do efficiently as untrained people. This is why leading runners, swimmers and cyclists will do almost all their endurance work in their chosen sport, only venturing into the other activities for recreation or in recuperation from injury.

As a preparation for these more intensive exertions, walking is valuable. For anyone who has not exercised regularly, at least three months of regular walking is suggested. A great advantage of walking is that it can be easily fitted into a person's day without ever looking like training. Walking to and from stations and to the shops, instead of taking the car or bus, can be a useful preparation to longer walks building up, for a normally healthy 40 year-old male, to two hours steady exertion at week-ends. Older men and women should aim at less ambitious targets. Walk slowly in the early weeks concentrating on breathing deeply and maintaining a good posture. Preferably do your walking in the country, where the natural environment is pleasant and diverting. Even if you advance to more strenuous activity you may care to spend days in the country, walking for long periods as a relaxation from the more taut atmosphere of your life in cities. A day's hike has much to recommend it.

The three activities of running, swimming and cycling are all governed by the same fundamental principles. The training required is that which enables the heart to deliver oxygen-rich blood to the working muscles as fast as possible. Thus a feature of the endurance type of athlete is his exceptionally low pulse at rest. Gordon Pirie, the 1956 Olympic silver medallist at 5,000 metres, often had a resting pulse as low as 40 beats per minute. This means that a heart with a resting pulse of 40 is able to distribute the same amount of blood round the body as someone with a resting pulse of 80: but with half the effort. To discover your

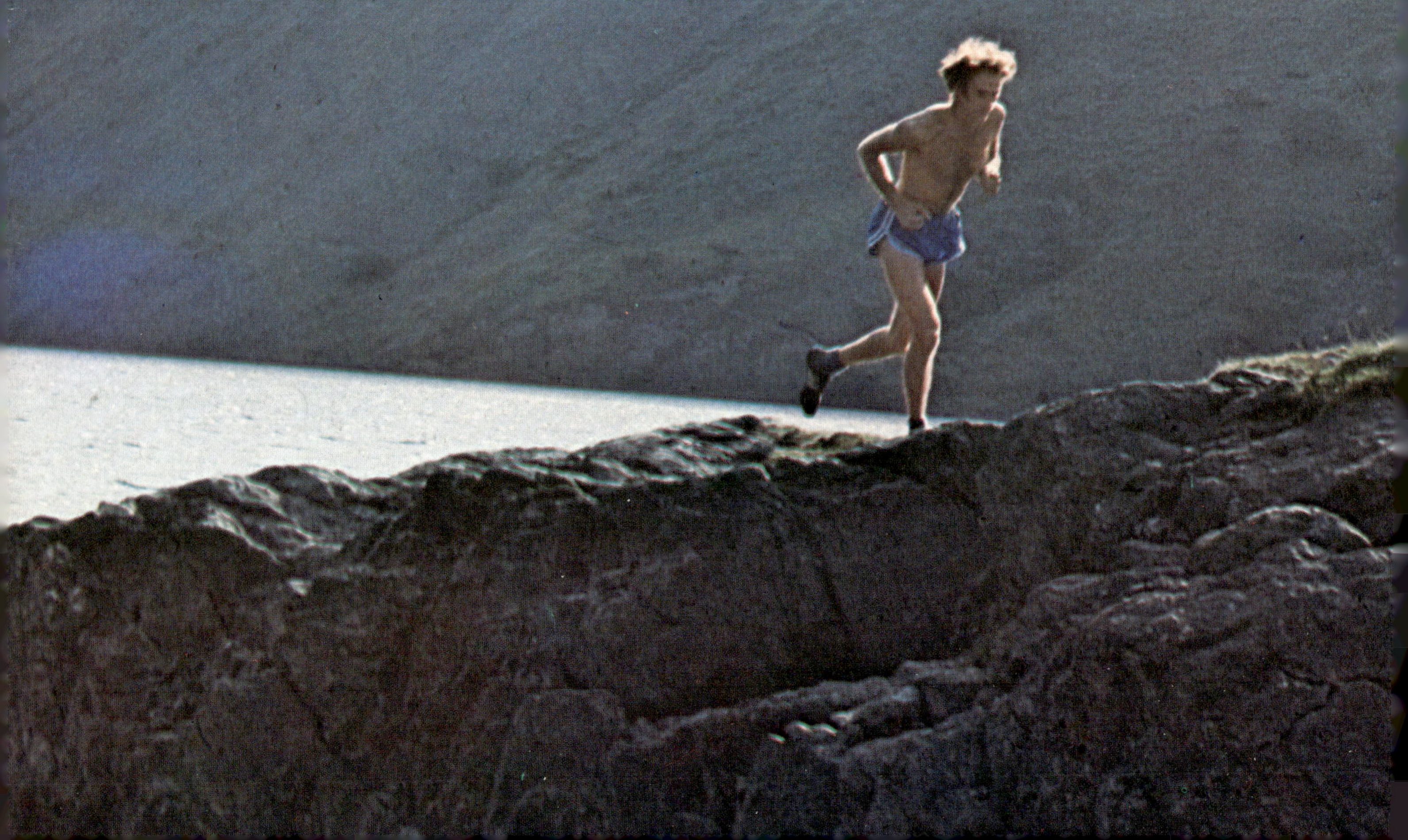

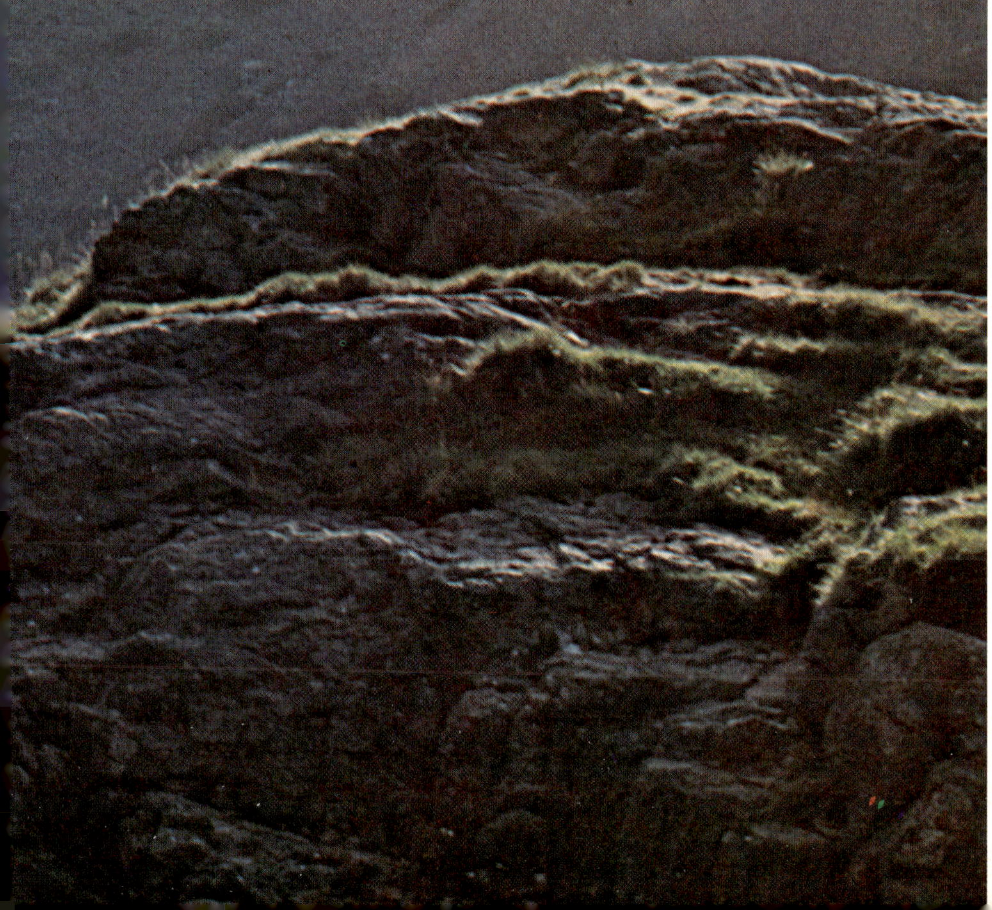

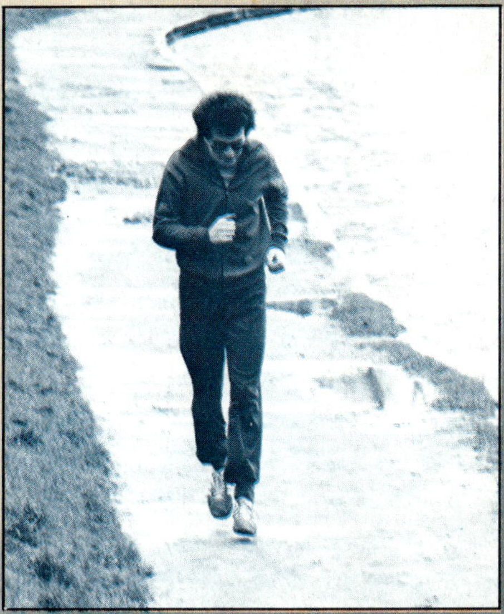

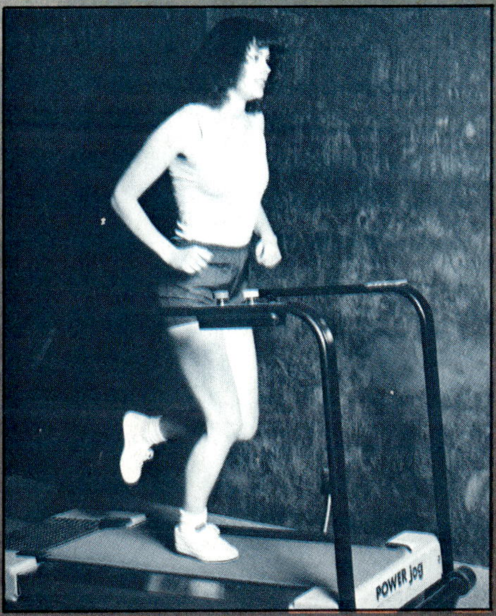

Jogging is a particularly effective form of exercise since it requires no equipment and can be done anywhere. Its value lies in the fact that it tones up the cardiovascular system, exercises the heart. As the illustrations show, you can jog outdoors on a hard surface, or on a machine in the gymnasium or you can push yourself to the limit by fell jogging over basically hostile but rewarding terrain

resting pulse, measure it on waking in the morning. Place the middle three fingers of the left hand on the inside of the right wrist, just below the base of the right thumb and you will be able to feel your pulse. Count it for a minute. Most people have a rate of 70-75 but, if it is higher, your heart is having to pump harder than its normal rate. It is weaker than it should be. If you are starting training, it is worthwhile taking your pulse regularly in the mornings. You will see how it gradually becomes slower as the months pass – an indication of how your heart is becoming stronger . The speed of your ability to return to a pulse rate reasonably close (i.e. up to a third more) to your resting beat is an excellent indication of your fitness. When you are training your pulse should be between 120 and 160 beats per minute. This can be checked at the end of a session, often more conveniently at the side of throat than at the wrist. Count for 10 seconds and then multiply by six, a quick and efficient way to get your rate for a minute.

The training effect should be continuous, building up the length of the effort over a period of time. Specimen schedules will be shown later in the chapter. You will, in fact, be doing a modified version of what outstanding competitors in these sports practise in their preparation for international events. Many of them will also be doing a different kind of training from aerobic work – termed anaerobic (literally 'without air'). Here they do a series of very hard efforts interspersed with a rest or lesser activity like gentle jogging, cycling or swimming. The pulse rates are frequently higher than 160 at the completion of the intense activity thus forcing them to decrease the effort because they go into what is termed 'oxygen debt'. However, this is geared to competitive sport and, since it can cause unnecessary distress, there is no need for an ordinary person interested only in keeping healthy to practise it. What is needed is a steady exertion so that after a year's gradual preparation it should not be beyond anyone below 45 years of age to continue their chosen activity for 30 minutes without undue fatigue. Many people over 45 should also be able to continue exercising for this period of time. It is nothing at all unusual.

Jogging

The principal advantage of running over cycling and swimming is that it can be pursued anywhere without special equipment. Since skipping is a suitable substitute, it can even be carried out indoors. Unlike swimming you don't have to travel to a pool, and you don't risk the greater traffic hazards of cycling. The main disadvantage is that you are more prone to injury than in the other two sports and may have to miss the occasional session through leg strains. These can be largely avoided, if correct shoes are worn and the start of the run is slow enough to allow the body to accustom itself to the movement. Another thing that puts people off running is public ridicule. Trainers feel that they look ridiculous jogging round their neighbourhood, a feeling that is not present while swimming in a pool or cycling. However, if you can withstand this, it is the most convenient way of training your cardiovascular endurance.

Most people prefer to jog on grass, in parks or preferably through the countryside. It is less wearing on the legs than running on roads. However, some people do not live near suitable terrain and so jog to and from their homes (thus saving travelling time). One should always dress warmly and even more important keep warm after the session. Try to wear something lightly coloured if you run at night so drivers can see you, and always jog towards the oncoming traffic. In the summer, shorts and a vest are all that are necessary; gloves and a 'bobble' hat are useful during the winter. A watch with a second hand is essential for timing the length of your runs. Shoes should be selected with care and the advice of sports shops considered. The best shoes have reinforced soles to prevent jarring and you should buy those you can afford. Generally avoid cheap plastic shoes and go for the ones with nylon or suede uppers. Blisters are a bugbear of running. Many experienced runners wear two pairs of socks, a thin inner pair and a thicker pair on the outside to accommodate any rough edges of the shoes. Vaseline spread on the toes is also useful.

Provided you have a hot bath immediately after jogging, and then keep warm, it is perfectly possible to train in wind and rain. Ice is more dangerous and it may be better to restrict your sessions to the grass or skip for an equivalent period of time. The secret of jogging is to go slowly. Far too many start their run quickly and then get depressed when they can't maintain the pace. Try to build up the length of the activity rather than taking a set distance and attempting to go faster each time. Minutes spent on one's feet are what is required.

Here are two schedules for people of different ages and sexes who have already spent more months walking daily and now, after clearance from their doctor, wish to move on to jogging.

Mr Adams, 45, has been walking daily for three months. He will now be supplementing this with jogging. He has increased the hardness of his walking gradually so that at week-ends he is now able to cover an hour, without stopping as he does when playing golf. He hasn't run for many years and, therefore, must take things slowly. He mixes jogging with walking to begin with and his jogging should be very slow, hardly faster than his walking:

Week One (three sessions): Walk 10 minutes. Jog one minute. Walk five minutes. Jog two minutes. Walk five minutes.

Week Two (three sessions): Walk 10 minutes. Jog two minutes. Walk five minutes. Jog three minutes. Walk five minutes.

Week Three (three sessions): Walk 10 minutes. Jog three minutes. Walk five minutes. Jog four minutes. Walk five minutes.

Week Four (three sessions): Walk 10 minutes. Jog four minutes. Walk five minutes. Jog five minutes. Walk five minutes.

Week Five (three sessions): Walk nine minutes. Jog five minutes. Walk five minutes. Jog six minutes. Walk five minutes.

Week Six (three sessions): Walk seven minutes. Jog six minutes. Walk five minutes. Jog seven minutes. Walk five minutes.

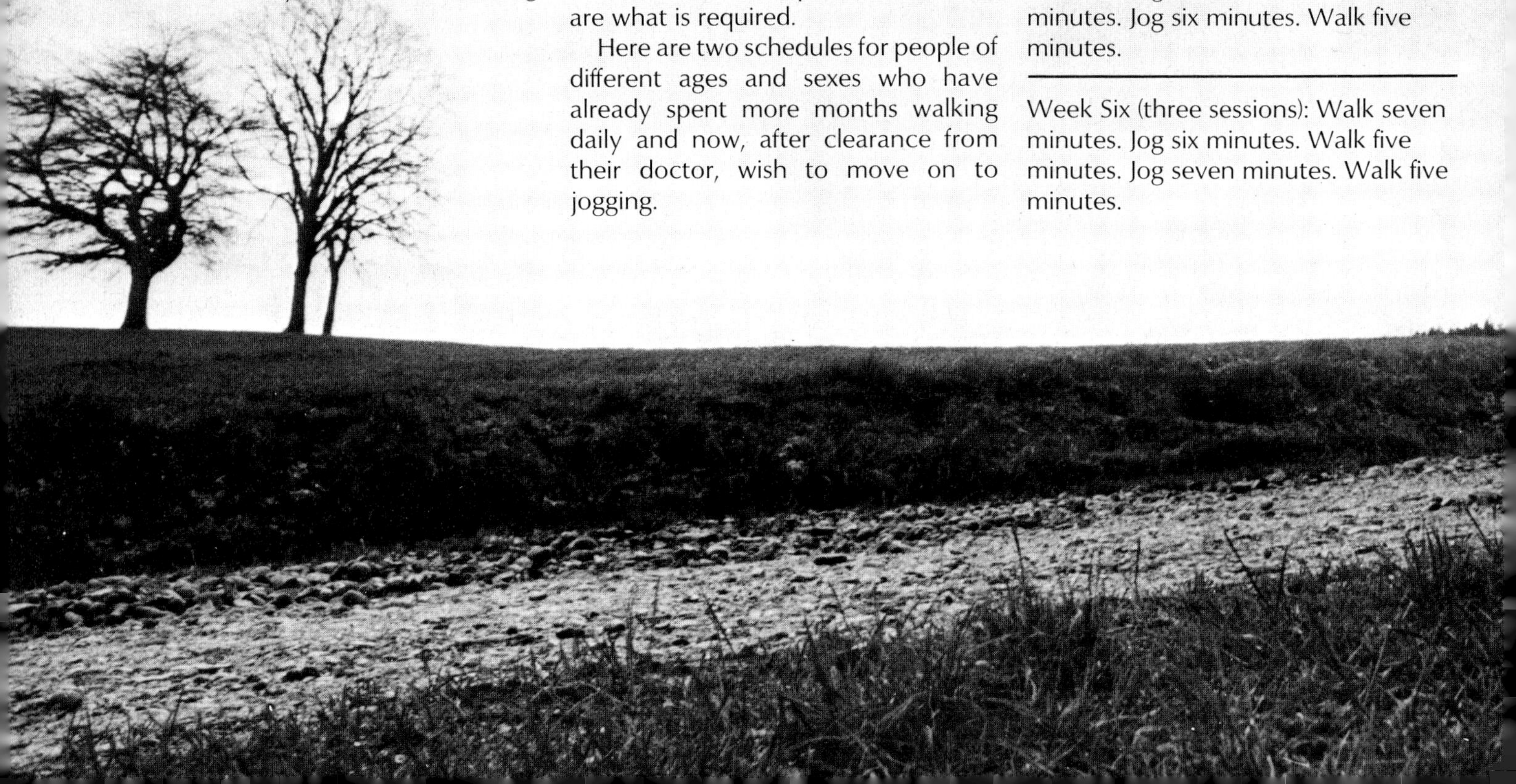

Week Seven (three sessions): Walk six minutes. Jog seven minutes. Walk five minutes. Jog eight minutes. Walk five minutes.

Week Eight (three sessions): Walk five minutes. Jog eight minutes. Walk five minutes. Jog nine minutes. Walk five minutes.

The idea is easily grasped: you gradually decrease the amount of walking and increase the amount of running as the months pass, but you always exercise for 30 minutes. Younger, fitter men can progress more quickly. Older men may have to go more gradually. The important thing is never to strain yourself. You should complete three sessions of each set before moving onto the next workout. If Mr Adams prefers to have a swimming session instead of a running workout that is perfectly satisfactory but he must complete three sessions of each running group before moving onto the more strenuous routine.

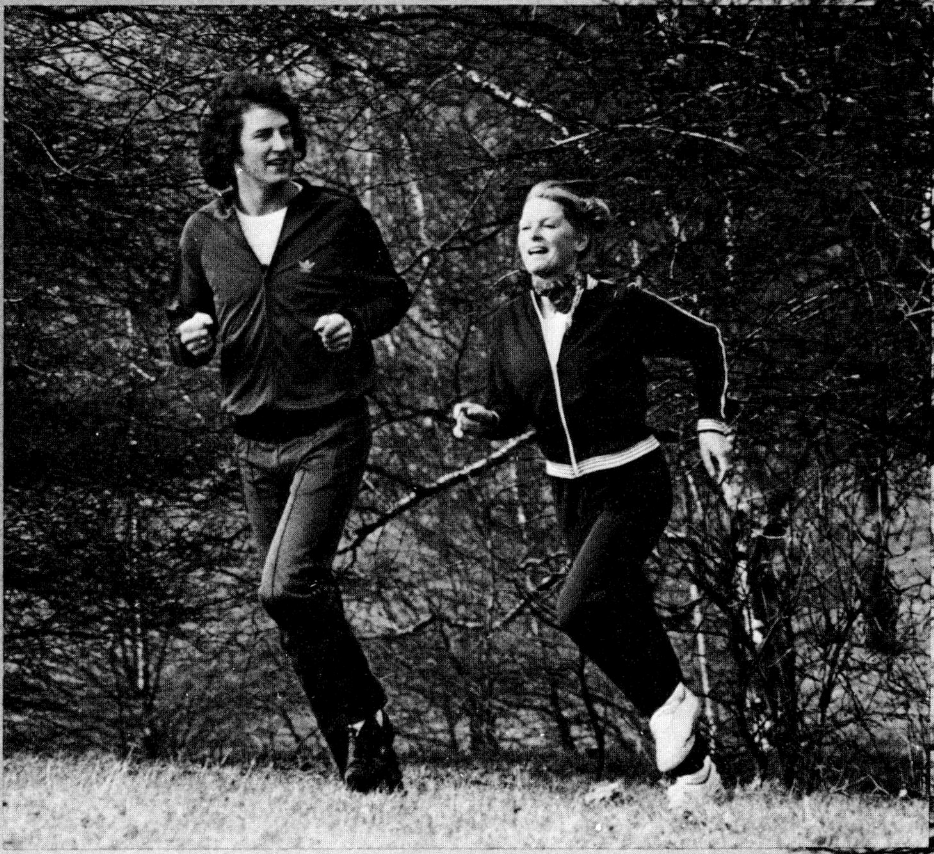

Jogging is *fun* and should not be seen as some form of punishment. It is an ideally simple and satisfying way to exercise that lends itself to social enjoyment as well as the improvement of your body and its health. Exercise should *always* be taken as an enjoyable activity

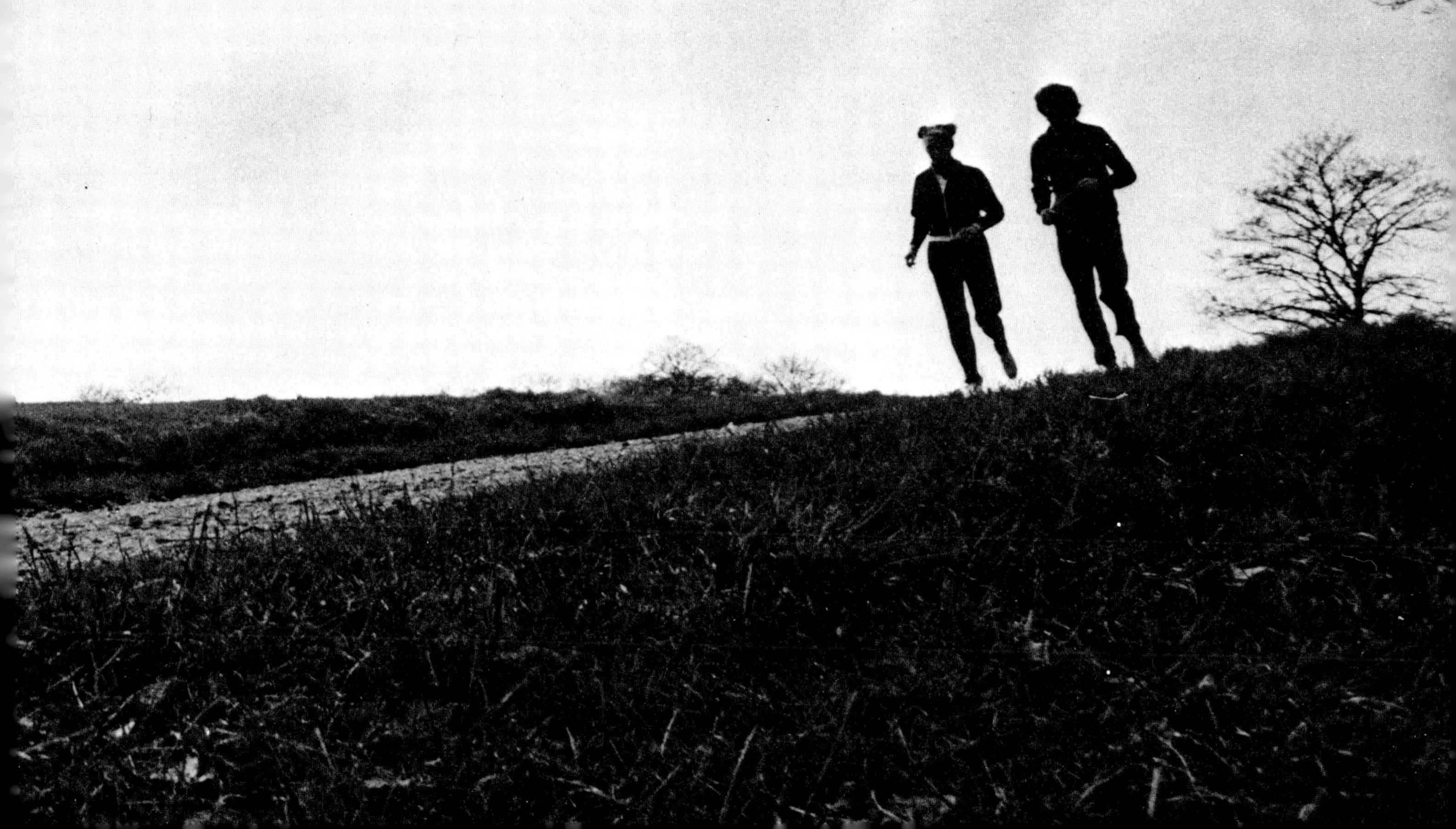

Swimming

There is much to be said for the superiority of swimming over jogging as a method of keeping healthy. It exercises a wide range of muscles and yet does not strain the tendons because it is a non-weight bearing movement. It can be practised in any weather provided that a pool is convenient. Furthermore, many people who are embarrassed at the thought of jogging through their neighbourhood will willingly travel to a local pool and swim because it does not appear to be training. Unfortunately, the majority of people who use pools do not wish to swim, but use pools as a playground. Therefore, a swimmer has to put up with hordes of children jumping on each other or diving across his path. Try to choose times and places when you can swim in reasonably clear water. The only special equipment you may need are goggles, which prevent the eyes from being irritated from the contact with chlorine.

It doesn't really matter which stroke you use but many people run courses to improve your technique. The fastest is front crawl or freestyle, and, if you are young, it is worth becoming proficient. However, you can use breaststroke of even backstroke. Unlike running and cycling where it is possible to time the length of your exertion, in swimming you should count the number of laps, having discovered the length of the pool. Here is a typical schedule for Mr Adams, who sometimes prefers to swim in his lunch hour to running in the evening. The rest periods need not be exact and can be counted.

Week One (three sessions). Swim 25 yards. Rest one minute. Repeat four times.

Week Two (three sessions), Swim 25 yards. Rest one minute. Six times.

Week Three (three sessions). Swim 25 yards. Rest one minute. Repeat eight times.

Week Four (three sessions). Swim 50 yards. Rest one minute. Repeat three times. Swim 25 yards. Rest one minute. Repeat twice.

Week Five (three sessions). Swim 75 yards. Rest one minute. Swim 50 yards. Rest one minute. Repeat three times.

Week Six (three sessions). Swim 100 yards. Rest one minute. Swim 50 yards. Rest one minute. Repeat three times.

Week Seven (three sessions). Swim 150 yards. Rest one minute. Swim 50 yards. Rest one minute. Repeat three times.

Week Eight (three sessions). Swim 150 yards. Rest one minute. Swim 50 yards. Rest one minute. Repeat once.

Week Nine (three sessions). Swim 250 yards. Rest one minute. Swim 100 yards. Rest one minute. Repeat once.

Week Ten (three sessions). Swim 300 yards. Rest one minute. Swim 100 yards. Rest one minute. Repeat once.

The build-up is similar to the running programme, a slow increase in the severity. Many people are amazed at the improvement that is possible if the training is done steadily and frequently.

Swimming is an ideal form of exercise since it is suitable for men and women of all ages, and can be carried out at a pace to suit the individual. Swimming also has the great advantage of exercising *all* muscles, and is simple and fun

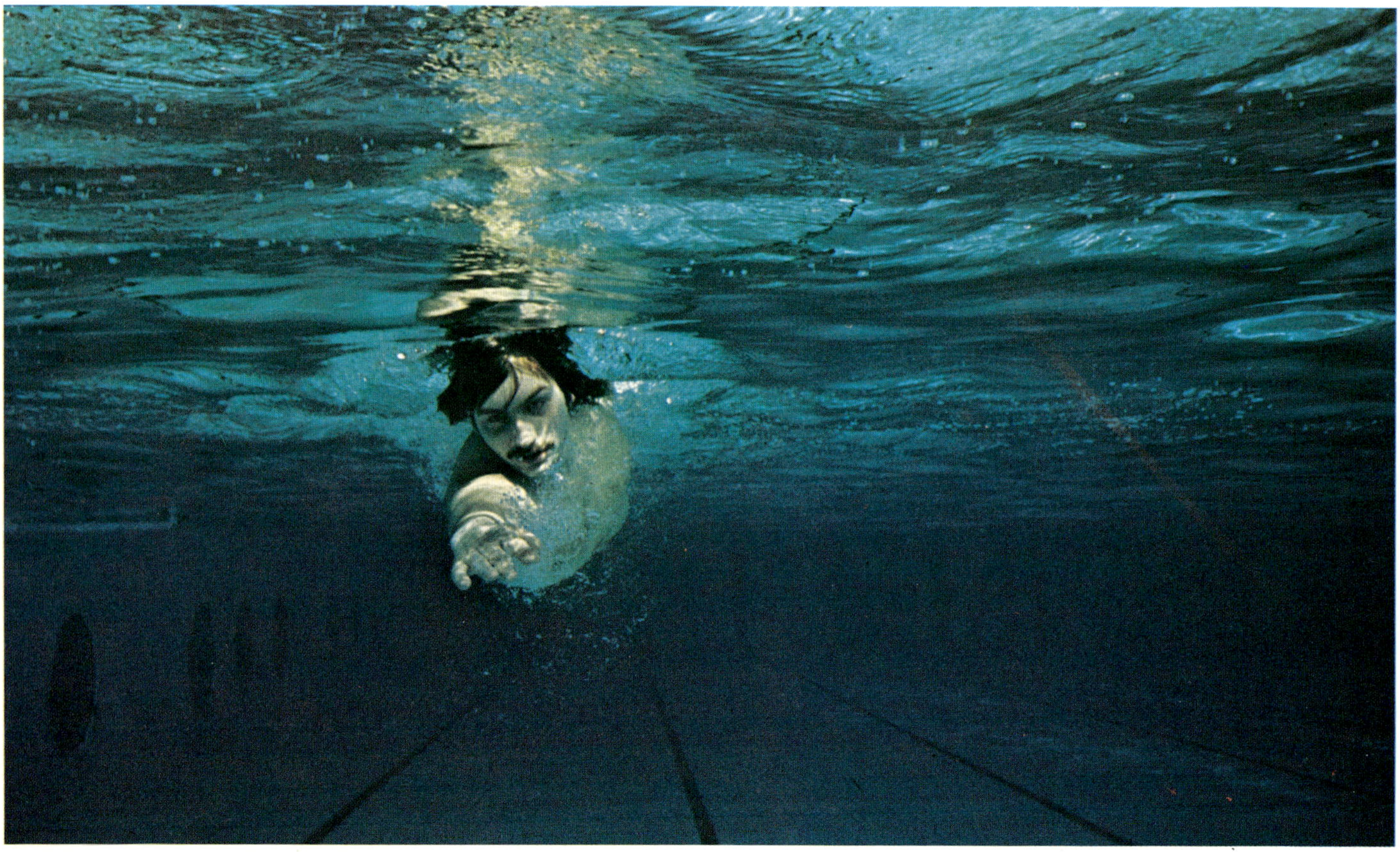

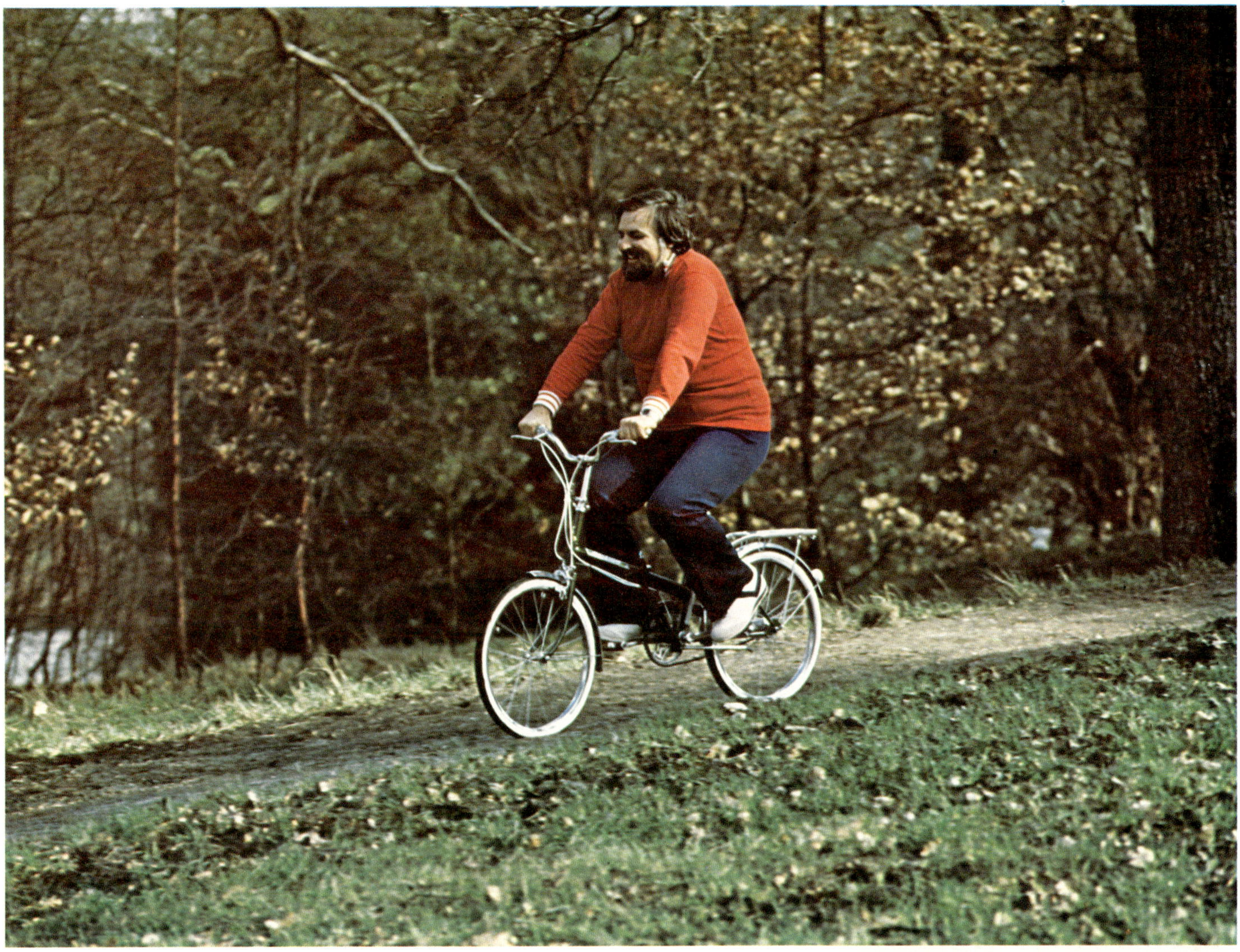

Cycling

Cycling shares with swimming the advantage of not appearing to be training. You can use a bicycle as a means of transport in daily life as well as riding it specifically for exercise. Busy streets are unsatisfactory and it is obviously best to ride in quiet areas and at times when there is little traffic. Although some bikes are expensive sufficient exercise can be gained from cheap models. Lightweight machines are used by serious cyclists but they don't have mudguards to prevent you from getting splashed in wet weather. Indoor static bicycles can also be obtained. However, regular use tends to be as boring as long spells of skipping since it provides neither the pleasure of movement, not the changing scenery which outdoor riding furnishes.

A track suit and windcheater are suitable clothes for bicycling, with a waterproof cape and trousers for wet weather. The rider should be as conspicuous as possible, so these garments ought to be a bright colour like orange or red. Baskets are easily fitted on the bike for carrying things but tend to make the machine awkward to manoeuvre. Many people prefer waterproof packs.

Someone concentrating on cycling as his or her only method of keeping fit, should build up to 30 minutes sustained riding three times a week. In the initial stages, bicycling should be used for short journeys, for shopping or transport in your immediate environment. After this preparation for a few months people can start building up the distances. For people over 45, 30 minutes would be sufficient, but younger people can try eventually to ride continuously for an hour or more.

Cycling provides both first rate exercise and great pleasure, whether outdoors or indoors on a static machine, and can be included as part of a planned regimen. Cycling is suitable for all ages

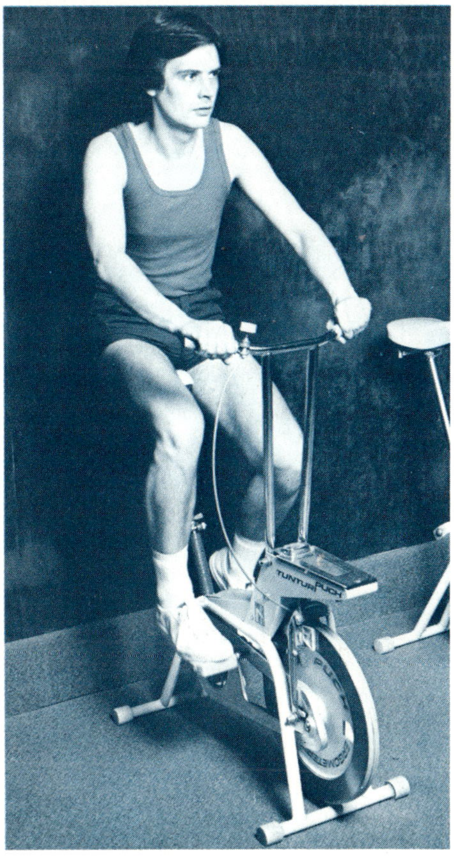

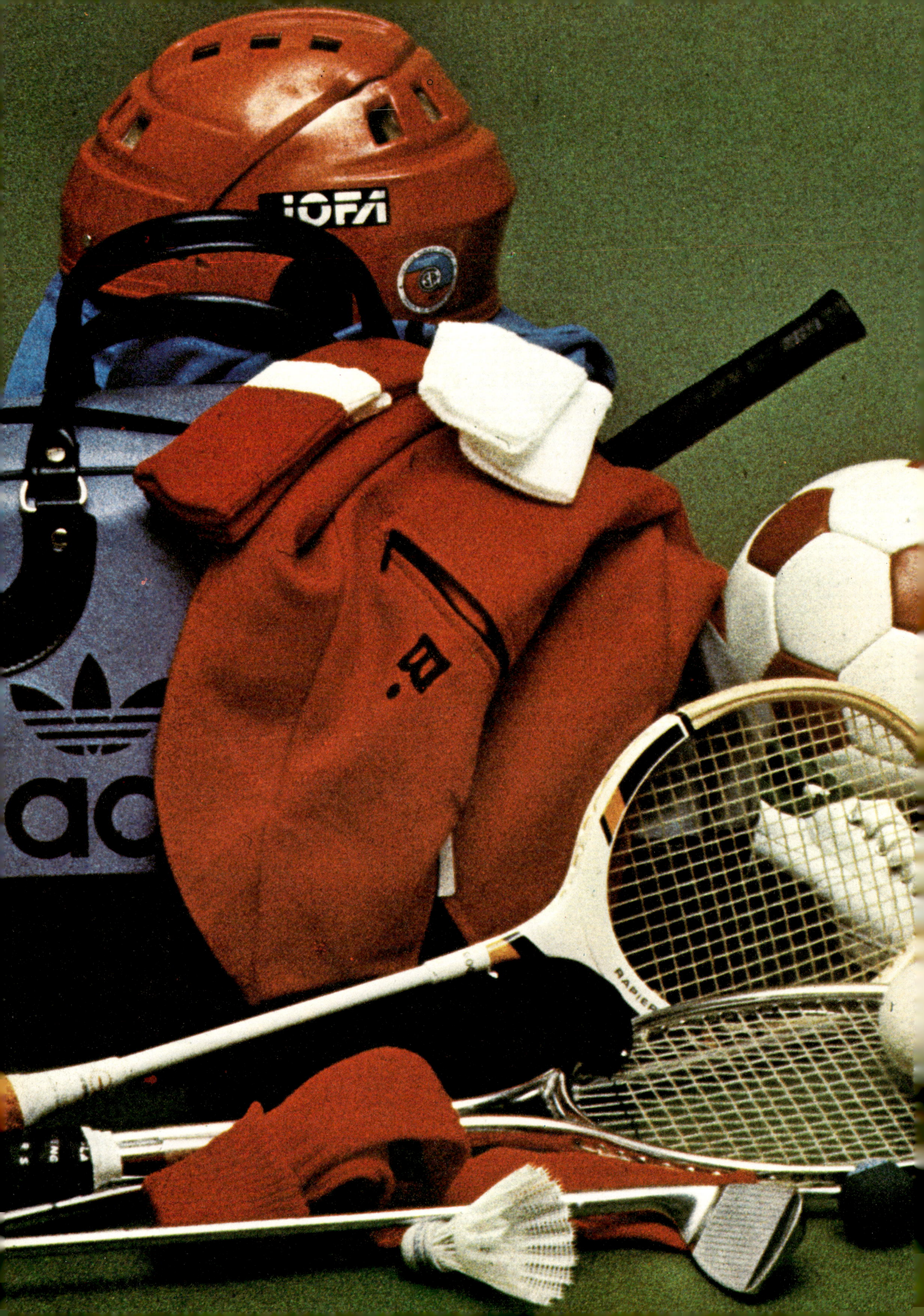

SPORTS AND GAMES

Hundreds of games are played all over the world. Some need specialized buildings or equipment, others can be played in the back yard. As well as being pleasurable recreation for all the family, sports provide essential exercise. Full physical fitness can be attained from one, or a balance of games, played regularly throughout the year. This section analyzes a carefully selected group of games, both team and individual, competitive and recreational, some of which provide all-round fitness, and others which need supplementing.

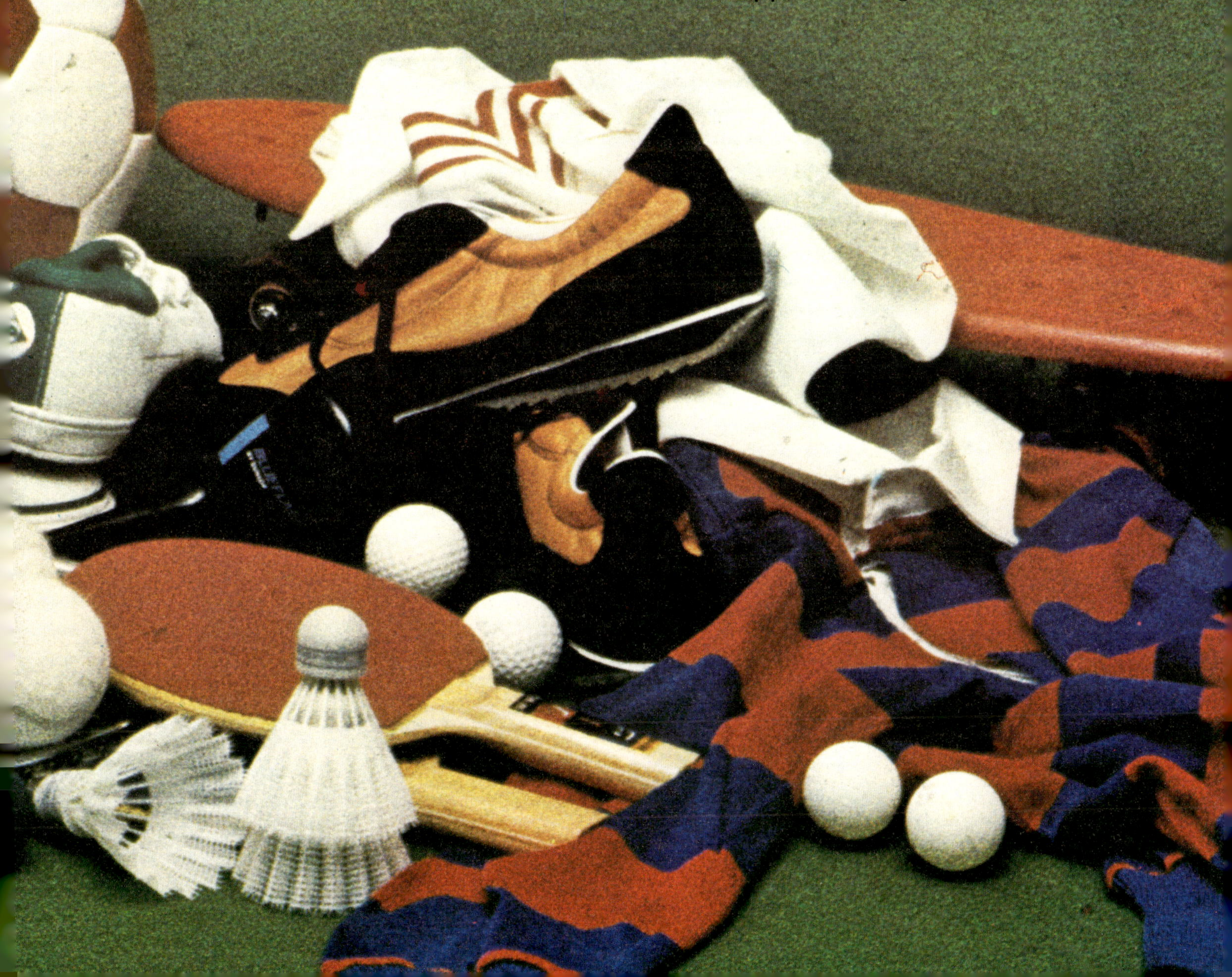

Selected Sports for Fitness

Any activity that provides recreation or relaxation must be of some benefit. If these activities are sociable and take place out of doors then the value increases. Organized games, of course, are an inevitable and natural carry-over from those of our childhood. But the playing of games often produces dangers. For many people the winning becomes more important than the taking part, the feeling of triumph in defeating an opponent overshadows the pleasure in the competitive struggle. Games played in this way create tension rather than release it. This is particularly true of professional and serious amateur sport, but in recent years it has increasingly filtered down to recreational level. Too many people take part in a sport to win, rather than just to participate, and what is worse, too many winners despise losers, not accepting the fact that however good they themselves are, they too will lose one day.

There is a difference between losers and people who just don't try. Losers are often the hardest triers. They are just less talented. So for the preservation of games at all levels it is vital that there should be comradeship in the competition rather than just antagonism. Perhaps the attitude which should be adopted was that voiced by a famous American boxer Jersey Joe Walcott. The former world heavyweight champion said after one especially gruelling, and much appreciated fight: '*Together* we made a great contest.' Without an opponent so courageous and determined that bout would not have been possible and Walcott was as grateful as the spectators that the experience had been realized.

In the last chapter, we examined which physical qualities were most valuable to exercise in order to maintain a really healthy body, but clearly anything that takes a human being out of doors and places him, or her, in contact with nature must be beneficial. Activities like gardening or rambling should not be ridiculed because they lack the intensive competition of many games. The selection of what games to play is entirely an individual matter. Clearly the body-contact sports like American Football, rugby and boxing can only be pursued in youth. Therefore, if you enjoy these activities it is useful to recognize that you should develop at least an interest in other games or else you could be without a physical recreation by your early 40s. Moreover, many games cannot be enjoyed by all ages and sexes, and it is often an advantage in maintaining the family as a unit that one activity can be enjoyed by the whole family. Children respond especially well to example and, if both parents enjoy, say, skiing, they will naturally and rightly encourage their children to join them.

However, the parents should also encourage their children in healthy habits and they can exert a worthwhile influence over their children by getting them to accept, as part of their everyday lives, those games which are most likely to benefit them in the future. These, of course, are primarily the aerobic ones and there is much to be said in favour of parents taking their children on long walks, cycling expeditions, hill climbing, swimming session and even regular jogging sorties with other families.

The following charts are a guide to some physical qualities needed for different sports, but they should not be taken to indicate the relative level of all-round fitness of leading competitors in these sports. For instance, competitive cycling puts perhaps a greater stress on the cardiovascular system than any other sport but it requires very little physical strength or supple-

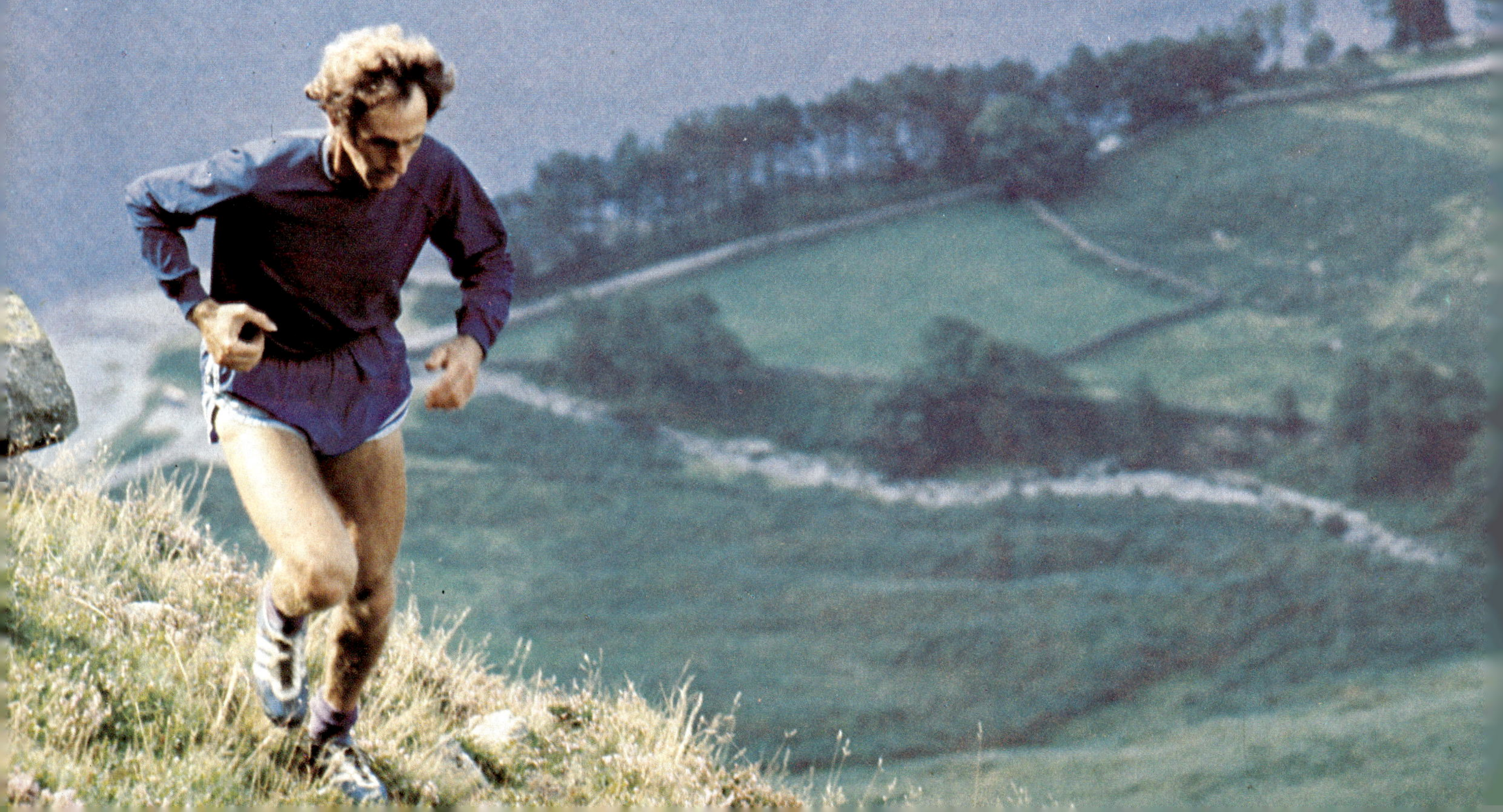

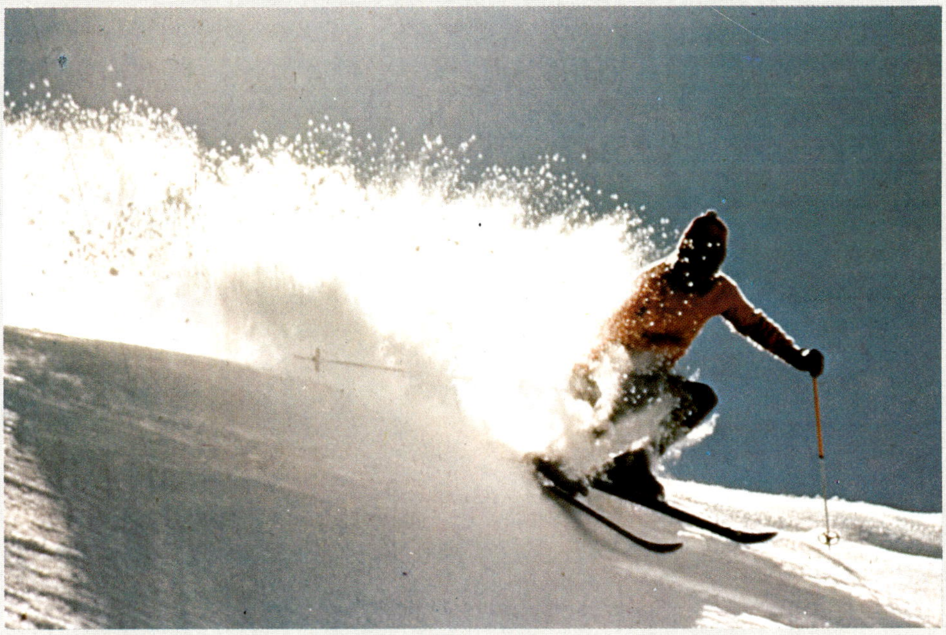

ness, certainly nowhere near the level of the performers in weight-lifting and gymnastics respectively. Judo fighters and wrestlers, however, have a superior balance of physical properties but neither strength, stamina or suppleness to any remarkable degree. It is impossible, therefore, to say that any sportsman or women is fitter than a person from another sport which is often equally strenuous – but in a different way. People are fit for the game they play. Although one is fit for swimming or running, it doesn't necessarily follow that one is ready for even supposedly far less arduous sports like cricket or baseball. An afternoon's intensive bowling or pitching would inflict on people unsuited to these activities severe muscular and tendon strains. There is also the question of concentration, since many sports demand intensive mental application to the event. This is especially notable in the case of top-class sport. Golf, for instance, is a sport which may make limited demands, but does require acute concentration. Even success in weight-lifting, which supposedly is such a pure physical activity, depends ultimately on the competitor's mentality – his belief in his capacity to raise heavy weights.

However, there are certain physical properties, particularly cardiovascular endurance, which it is vital to engender. There are also those people who are interested in losing weight. They may be interested in selecting a sport which is valuable for this reason because certain games burn up more calories than others. If we limit ourselves, therefore, to exercises demanding a high degree of cardiovascular endurance we find a number of different tests that have been carried out by different authorities in recent years. One early one was the Harvard Step Test, which measures the capacity of the athlete to recover from exertion by a simple method. The person being tested steps up and down off a 52cm (21in) step at the rate of 30 times a minute for five minutes. Then the subject's pulse is taken on three occasions during the first three and a half minutes following the exercise. From these measurements a formula is worked out to assess the ability of the athlete's pulse to return to normal. The higher the number the more quickly

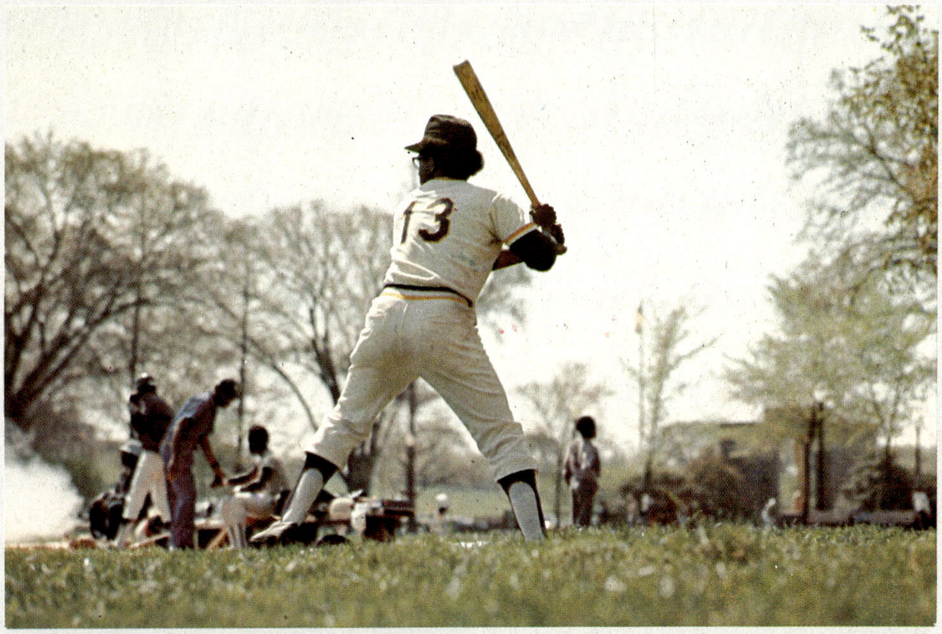

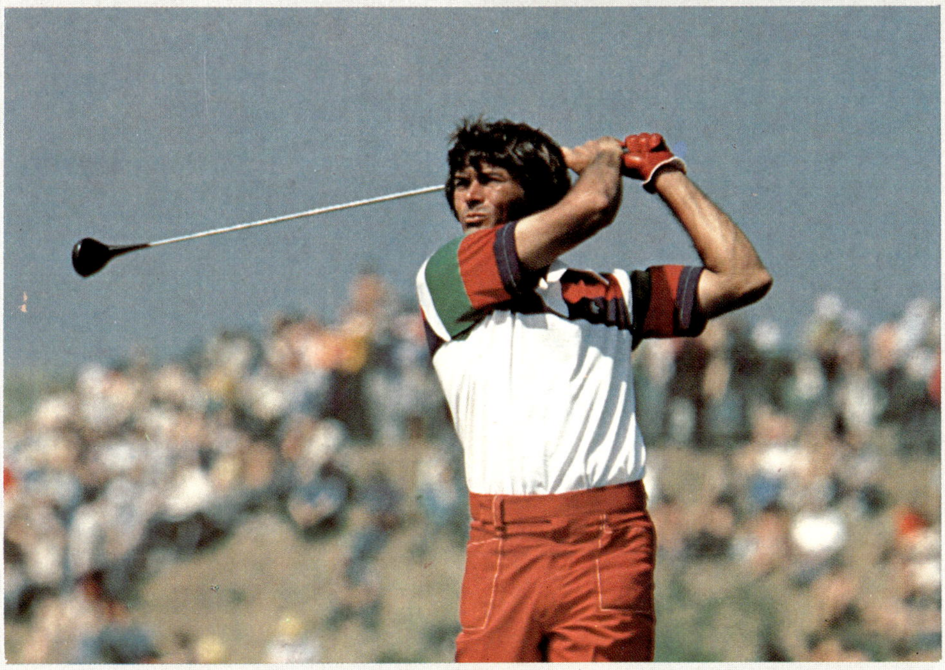

the subject's heart-rate has adjusted. Dr Vaughan Thomas, writing in *Science and Sport,* listed the capacity of leading performers in various different sports to recover from this simple test. From this we deduce how these sports condition the cardiovascular system.

Pentathlon	154	Volleyball	112
Basketball	128	Judo	111
Rowing	123	Hockey	106
Swimming	122	Track & Field	105
Cycling	121	Fencing	96
Football	117	Weight-lifting	95
Canoeing	115	Gymnastics	93
Boxing	115	Yachting	92
Wrestling	114	Equestrianism	86
Water-polo	112	Shooting	83

However, it is important that these charts be considered in the light of certain factors. Firstly, the capacity to score highly in a test is specific to that test. Even such a simple requirement as stepping on and off a bench or step is a more physiologically familiar movement for certain sportsmen than for others. Runners and basketball players have to possess highly conditioned legs, but not arms.Therefore they are bound to have an advantage over wrestlers and judo fighters, whose exercise principally requires strength and local endurance in the arms, together with cardiovascular endurance. It is a mistake automatically to assume that a better score in the Harvard Step Test proves superiority.

Two other well-known scientific tests related to recovery from exertion involve a bicycle and treadmill. Clearly the former will favour the cyclist and the latter a runner. Similarly, it doesn't necessarily mean that superiority in any gymnasium test will be followed by superiority in that aerobic sport. A gymnasium test only has strong associations with a particular aerobic activity, it is not the same thing. If you took an Olympic marathon field and assessed them for cardiovascular endurance a week before the race it wouldn't follow that they would finish in that order in the actual event. A large number of other factors such as the ability to translate one's cardiovascular superiority into running technique, tactics in the race, response to competition and so forth, have to be taken into consideration. So all these tests should be regarded with caution. They can only be a guide, not a rule. Where they possess greater (but again not complete) validity is in assessing one individual's improvement over a period of time.

One test that has greater value was that carried out by Dr Kenneth Cooper, (the author of *Aerobics*). He scrutinized the relative demands on the oxygen system of the human body during 30

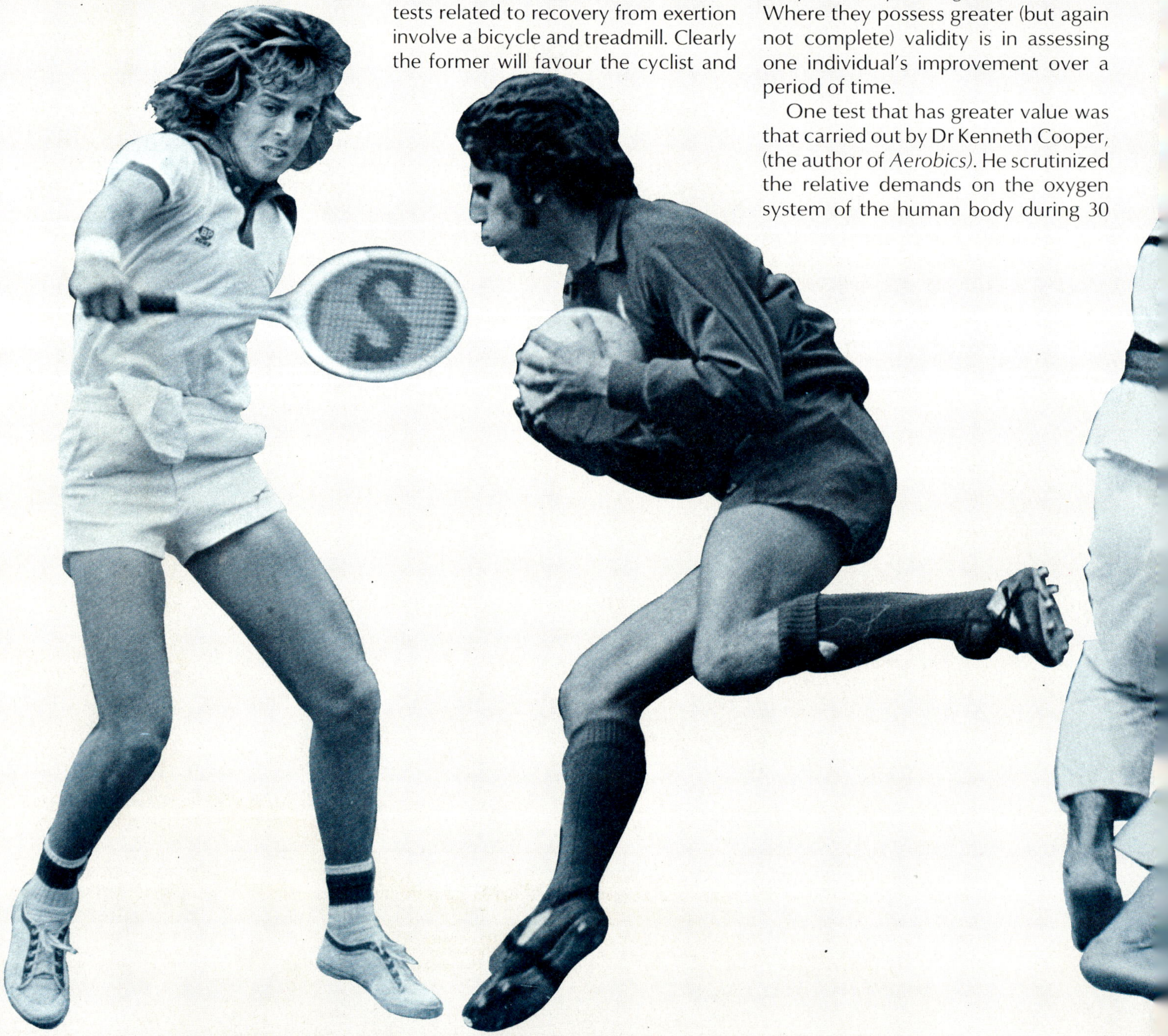

minutes of active participation in various chosen sports. Since competitors were taking part in their own sports, and not in a test which would suit some people to a greater extent than others, it is a more useful guide. The relative demands were:

Wrestling	12	Lacrosse	3
Rope-skipping	9	Tennis	3
Rowing	5	Fencing	3
Hockey	4.5	Soccer	3
Handball	4.5	Volleyball	2
Squash	4.5	Skating	2
Basketball	4.5	Baseball	1
Skiing	3	Golf	0.5
Soccer	3		

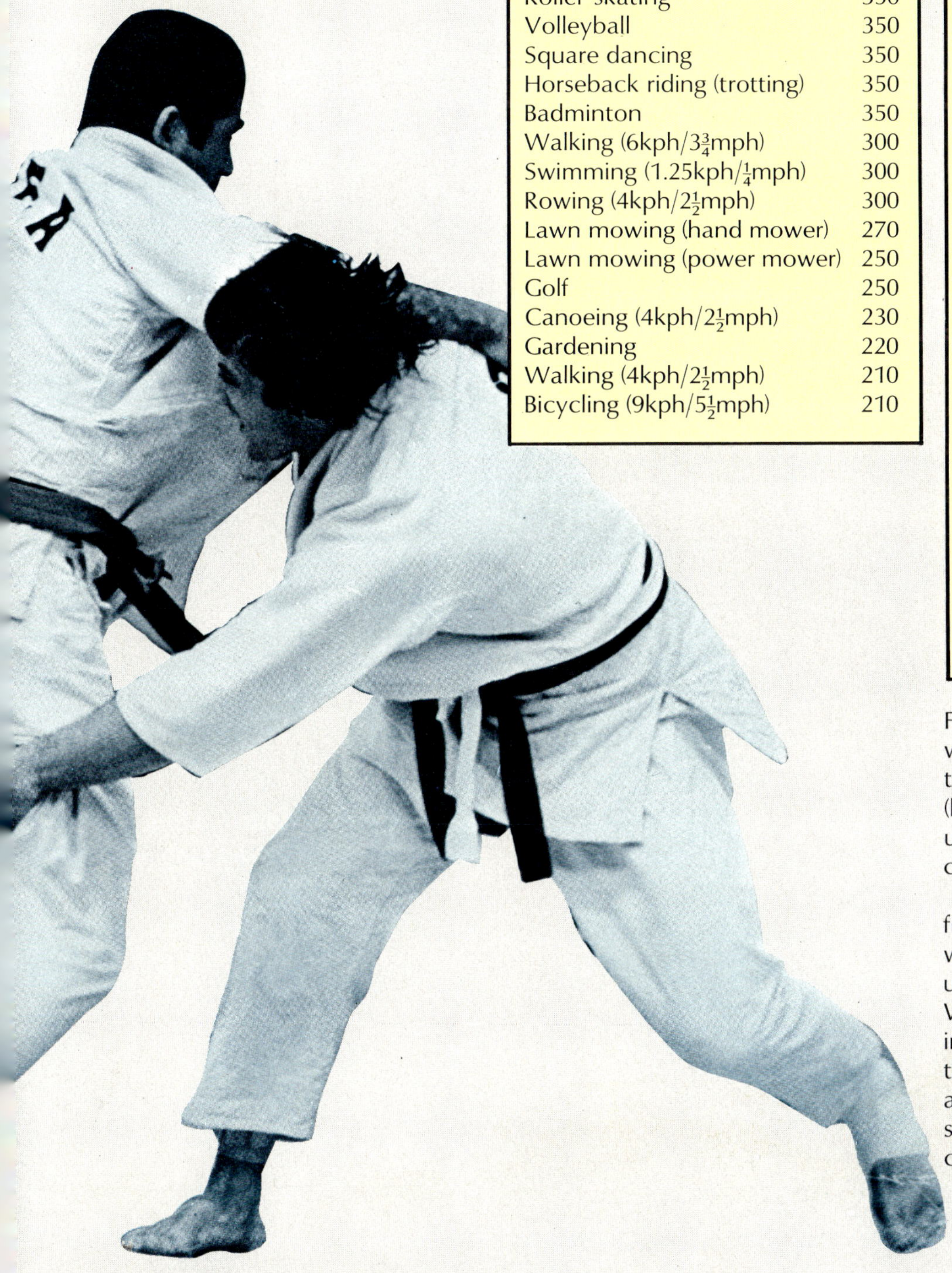

There remain two further tests, which will be of value to people interested in the capacity of sports to burn up calories. The first was by Dr Robert Johnson, a lecturer at the University of Illinois, who listed the activities in the following order:

Running (16kph/10mph)	900
Scull-rowing (race)	840
Bicycling (21kph/13mph)	660
Squash and handball	600
Skiing (16kph/10mph)	600
Hill climbing (30m/100ft per hr)	490
Water-skiing	480
Tennis	420
Woodchopping or sawing	400
Table tennis	360
Roller-skating	350
Volleyball	350
Square dancing	350
Horseback riding (trotting)	350
Badminton	350
Walking (6kph/3¾mph)	300
Swimming (1.25kph/¼mph)	300
Rowing (4kph/2½mph)	300
Lawn mowing (hand mower)	270
Lawn mowing (power mower)	250
Golf	250
Canoeing (4kph/2½mph)	230
Gardening	220
Walking (4kph/2½mph)	210
Bicycling (9kph/5½mph)	210

The other was by two Scotsmen, John Durnin and Reginald Passmore, whose data originally appeared in the publication *Energy, Work and Leisure*. They worked out the expenditure of energy during recreations and sports and recorded it in kcals per minute.

Archery	3.2 to 5.7
Badminton	6.5
Basketball	9.0
Billiards	2.7
Bowls	4.1
Boxing	9.0-14.4
Canoeing	2.5-7.0
Climbing	7.0-10.0
Cricket	5.0-8.0
Cross-country	10.6
Cycling, easy	4.0
Cycling, Tour de France	20.0
Dancing	4.0-8.0
Fishing	4.0
Gardening	2.7-8.6
Golf	4.0-7.0
Gymnastics	2.5-12.0
Hockey, field	8.7
Horse (walking)	3.0
Horse (galloping	10.0
Judo	14.6
Mowing lawn	9.1
Music playing	2.0-4.2
Rowing	4.1-11.2
Skiing cross country	18.6
Skiing, mixture	5.4-10.0
Soccer	5.0-15.0
Squash	10.1 to 18.2
Swimming	5.0 to 15.0
Table tennis	3.6–5.2
Tennis	5.7-8.5
Volleyball	3.5
Weight-lifting	8.2

From this chart you can see that if you wish to lose weight you will have to do two hours intensive lawn mowing (hand not machine I'm afraid) to burn up the equivalent of an hour's cross-country skiing.

You now have a reasonable basis from which to plan the sports you would like to practise and the frequency with which you should do them. We now move onto a closer examination of these sports and examine their benefits and defects. Obviously to assess them comprehensively you should always bear in mind these four charts.

Badminton

Badminton, which has many devotees in Europe and South-East Asia, is an exciting game which can be played by both men and women, until almost any age. The often lengthy rallies give it an absorption which demands intense concentration. Leading players need both the power to smash the shuttlecock at over 160kph (100mph) and the delicacy of touch to flick it across the 1.50m (5ft) net so that it seems to hover and drop almost vertically on the other side. Although it attracts some interest as a spectator sport, it is primarily a participation activity. It can be played indoors or out with inexpensive equipment; the racket is the only major item of expenditure. Unlike tennis, badminton courts can be used regularly for other pursuits. The singles' game demands stamina so that the player can quickly cover the 6 × 3.90m (20 × 13ft) area on his side of the net for the whole of the game. Sustained rallies place a premium on manoeuvrability as players attempt to lure their opponents out of position. In doubles the players play side by side, either covering equal ground or one up at the net and one behind. In mixed doubles the women is usually close to the net to take anything short while her male partner maintains a barrage of low shots from the back of the court. Badminton plainly requires the ability to change direction swiftly and also jumping power so that high shots can be comfortably reached. However, the activity would have to be sustained for some hours to make a genuine demand on the cardiovascular system. Since the court is smaller than tennis, the requirement to run for long periods is not so pronounced. Clearly badminton, by itself, is not usually enough exercise for a person wishing to maintain a high level of fitness. Additional activities must be practised.

A fast and exhilarating game which demands great agility. Whatever your age, badminton is great fun for men and women.
Below: court, racquet and shuttlecock

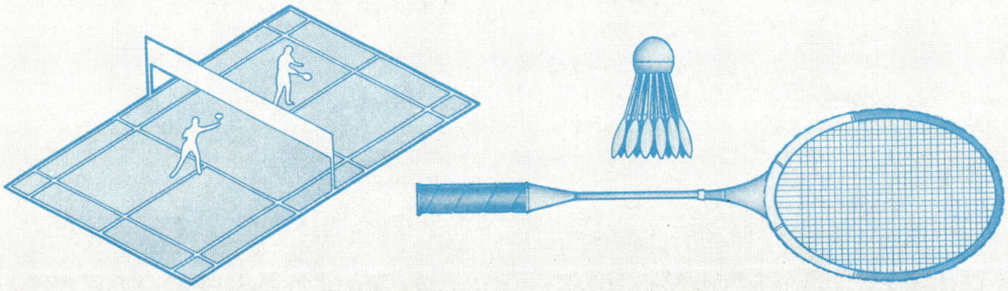

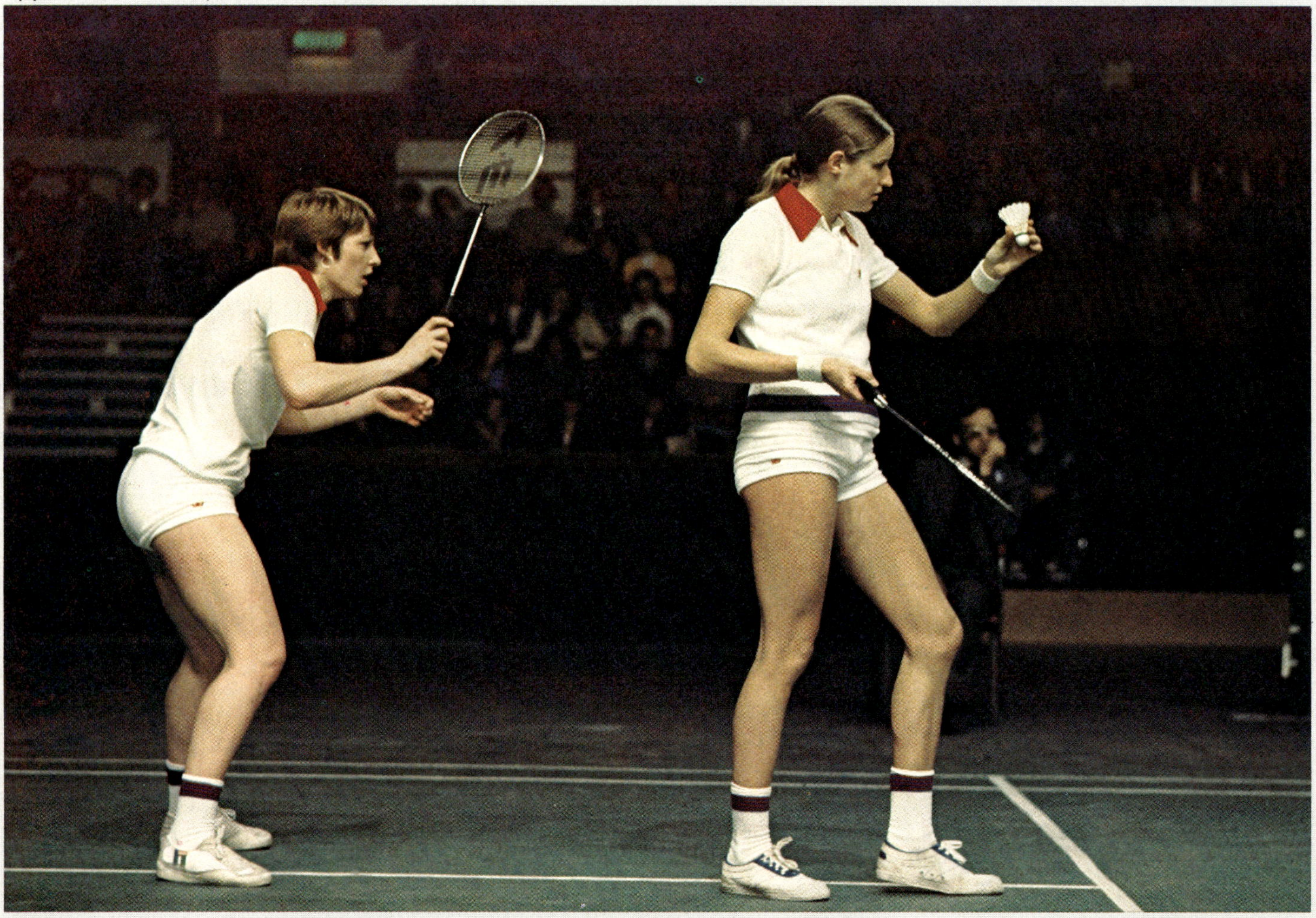

Baseball

The tremendous attention given to professional baseball in the United States sometimes overshadows the interest in the sport for participants, not only in this country but also in Mexico, Japan and Australia. It is the major recreation during the summers for millions of boys, and, although serious baseball is restricted to males, girls can enjoy it as an entertainment. The prime qualities required for hitting the ball is a good 'eye' and excellent technique. The pitching and throwing have been highly developed. Injuries to key pitchers can grievously affect leading teams; the frequency of games means that the player has got to be durable as well as talented. Baseball players have to be strong, but not particularly heavily built, in order to generate the power required for hitting and pitching. Mobility is an essential feature of fielding the very fast ball.

Equipment is not exorbitantly expensive and the game can be conveniently played in many open spaces. Although many league fixtures take place indoors, this is less common for local games because of the vast area that has to be enclosed. Because of the weather it is largely a summer game.

Baseball by itself does not develop cardiovascular endurance. The short periods of action involving comparatively few players with pauses in between mean that the sport should be complemented by something more arduous. Regard baseball purely as recreation – unless, of course, you are talented and fortunate enough to take part in it professionally. Play it, by all means, but play it just for fun, without pretending that it has any stamina-producing qualities, or special abilities to increase general fitness.

This summer sport has spread in popularity from America. A big spectator game, women are now showing interest in playing. It requires strength, endurance and accuracy but although good recreation is not enough to produce peak fitness

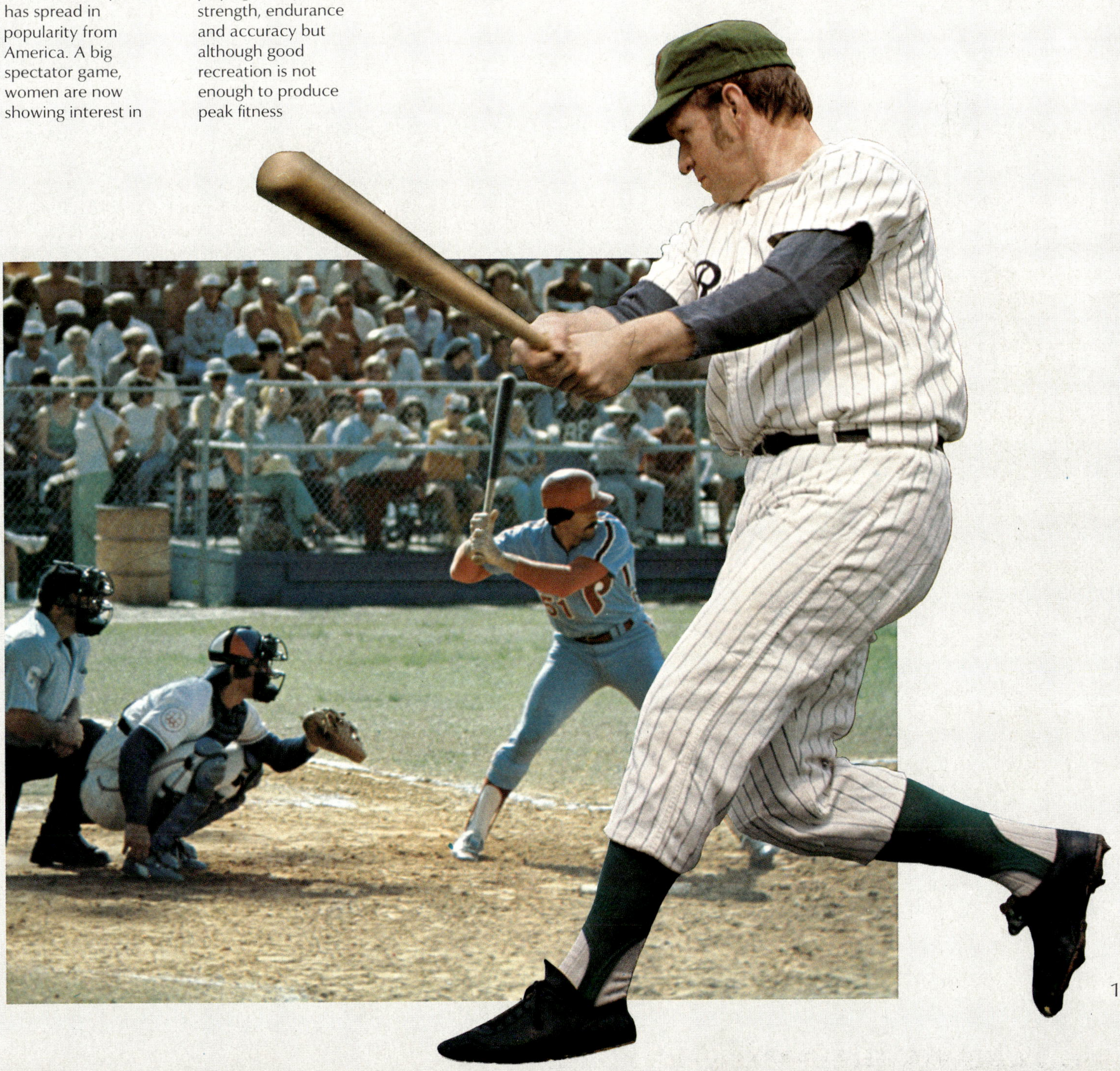

Basketball

Basketball is a serious competitive game in over 130 countries, making it a rival of soccer in popularity. Games are usually played indoors, although this restricts the number of possible spectators, because it is invariably highly appealing in countries where winters are severe. In the United States, for instance it is the principal sport for the first few months of the year. Many team games, like soccer and rugby football, require large area and therefore are unsuitable for indoor stadia. The flexibility of basketball means that it can also be staged outdoors and the cost of the equipment is minimal: rubber-soled shoes, shorts and a singlet, a ball, two baskets and a flat playing area. Most schools, colleges and sports centres have regulation courts. Women can play, but also have a less boisterous relation, netball, common in English schools.

Basketball requires great dexterity with the hands and keen appreciation of positional play. It provides considerable training for speed, stamina and agility and develops the leg muscles and body spring. Although there is sometimes harsh body contact in the competitive game, the real disadvantage of the sport is that to be really successful you simply have to be extremely tall. Almost all the leading professionals and amateurs are at least 1.90m (6ft 4in) tall thus precluding more moderately-built men from aspirations of success. The exceptions are so rare as to be noteworthy. However, as a recreation, lack of inches should not hamper an ordinary person wishing to take exercise. Provided he takes part with spirit and determination, hard play for over an hour will give him a severe session. It is also a handy training session for other team games since it teaches positional play and accuracy of throwing. American football and rugby are sports that can benefit in this way.

A team game played all the year round, indoor and out, the fast running it requires makes basketball first-class exercise

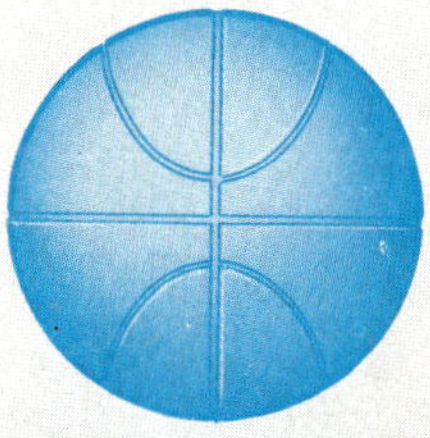

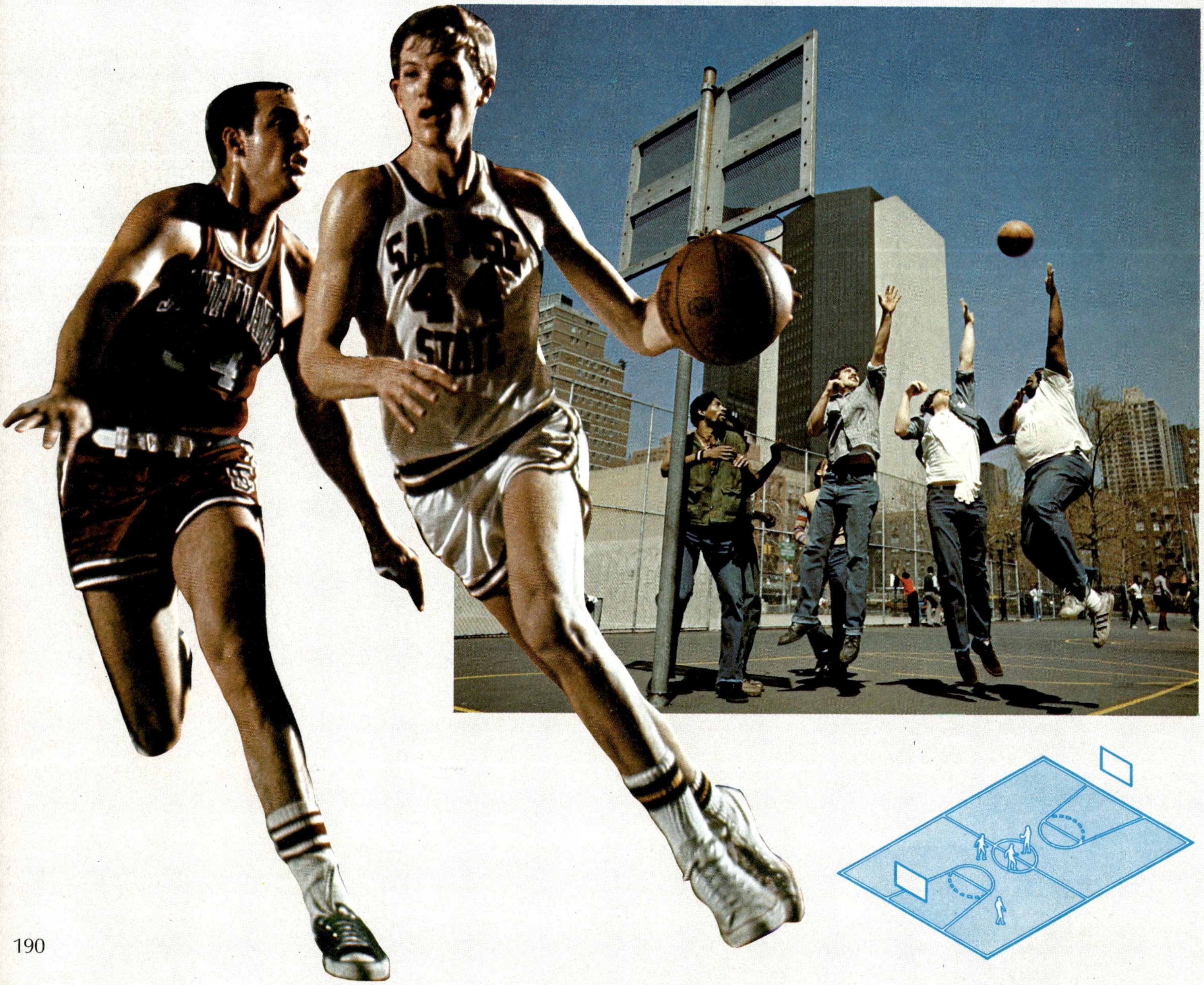

Canoeing

Although canoeing is an Olympic sport, it has many non-competitive features. From hunting seal by kayak and shooting the rapids of mountain rivers, to leisurely paddles up slow-moving stretches of water, canoeing enjoys many facets. Obviously proximity of water is essential, but some swimming pools cater for enthusiasts who are unable to reach a river, lake or sea easily. Men and women both take part competitively in the sport, which at its highest level requires much physical strength in the shoulders, as well as cardiovascular endurance. In addition, considerable judgement is required for the deft handling of the body in slalom and wild water events. The major expense is the cost of a canoe, the design of which differs according to the requirements of the event. Slalom canoes, for instance are made of fibreglass and are designed for manoeuvrability as well as for speed. Kayaks, however, for sprint racing or long distance events, often have rudders. Many clubs hire boats to members.

It is important to differentiate between canoeing gently as part of an outing and a serious session in which the individual feels physically stretched. Both have a place in an enthusiast's life. Although legs have to be used to assist in the steering of the boat they do not get the strenuous exercise that is experienced in rowing. There also is little need for suppleness, but carried out seriously for long periods, canoeing can make a contribution to overall fitness. Certainly it makes a pleasing alternative to progression by land if you are exploring unfamiliar country. It is preferable in these circumstances, partly because a canoe can pass where a rowing boat could not, and also because you can always see the way you are going and direct yourself accordingly. Some canoes can carry sufficient equipment to camp on the way. Whatever aspect of canoeing you wish to pursue, you must be a competent swimmer.

No longer a specialist competitive sport, canoeing can be combined with enjoyment of and exploration of the countryside. It entails fresh air and exercise for arms and shoulders, but the legs tend to be underused

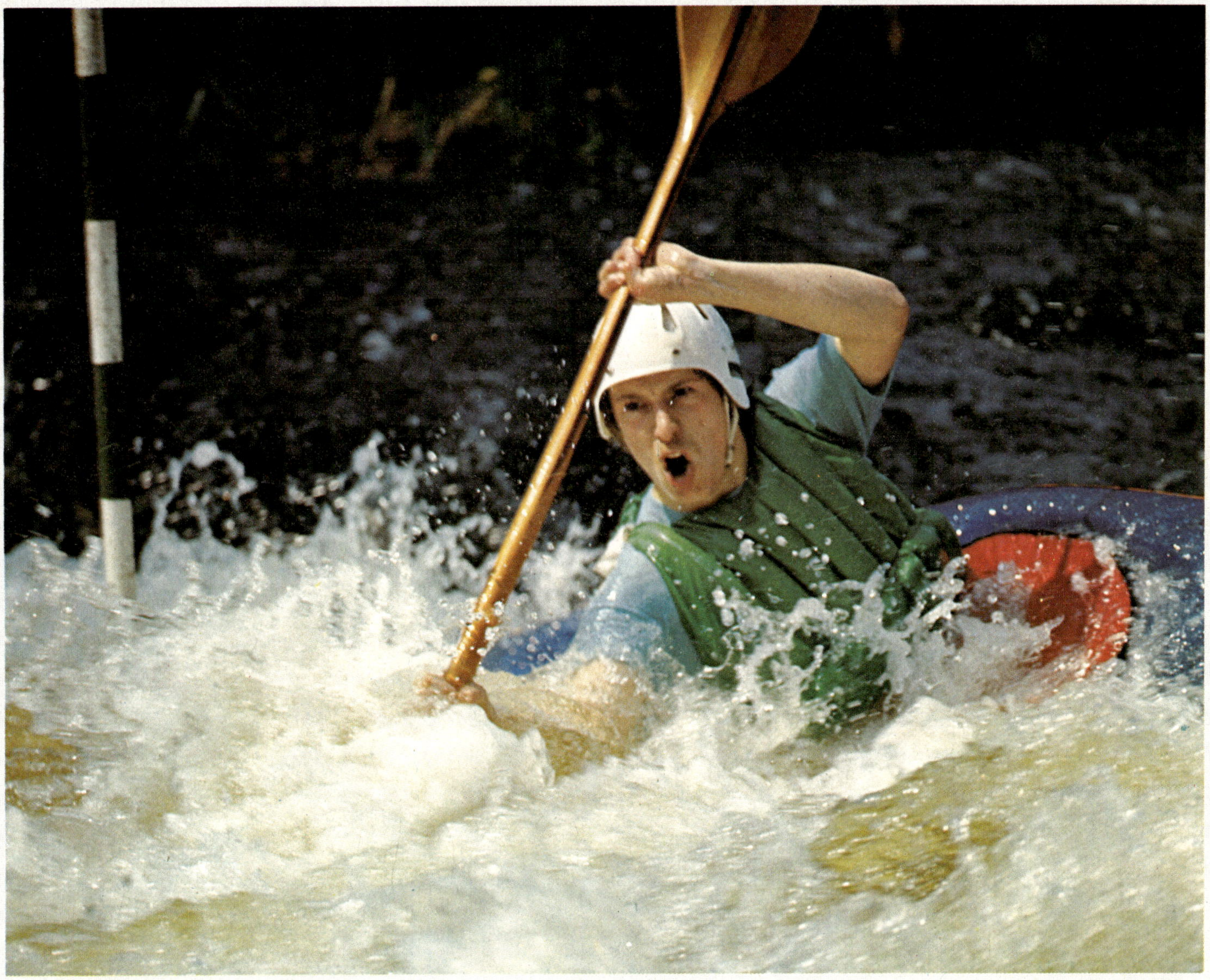

Cricket

Cricket is a major game in the British Commonwealth. The subtlety of the tactics and technique attract many people, both as spectators and as participants. Part of the interest in the game is aroused by the length of time taken to complete it, which generates intense and detailed analysis of every move by the players and captains. Yet despite this , cricket does not place an excessive demand on the physical stamina of players. The breaks for meals, the fact that only 13 of the 22 players are on the field at any one time and the generally leisurely tempo of the matches give it a restrained, civilized quality. The chief demand is on the mental concentration of the players to cope with the unexpected demands on them – to intercept a ball after a long period of inertia. Although cricket is predominatly a male game women play at a national level and locally. Sometimes there are mixed matches, but they are not serious.

Although cricket is ideally played on perfect grass wickets, with good equipment, it is nevertheless possible to get considerable pleasure out of a spontaneous game in the street, on the beach or in the garden. The emphasis in cricket is on skill and no physical quality is stressed except fast reactions and a good 'eye'. It is possible to play serious cricket into middle age; Jack Hobbs, one of the most successful batsman in history, had his best season at the age of 42. Assiduous practice and coaching stimulates people's natural talent rather than constant attention to physical fitness.

For the maintenance of physical fitness, therefore, cricket has little value. This is especially true if the individual does not spend much time in bowling, which is comparatively arduous. Cricket must be supplemented by the three serious sessions which have been recommended. The game puts a strain on individuals' joints and tendons and therefore participants should consider doing plenty of stretching movements, especially in the off-season. The suppling routine could be followed with advantage. In these ways, the genuine and unique pleasure which cricket brings can be balanced by something more directly advantageous to health.

Cricket can be played by all the family and, because it demands little physical energy can be played into middle age. It requires concentration and mental alertness and players should supplement with other exercises for full physical fitness

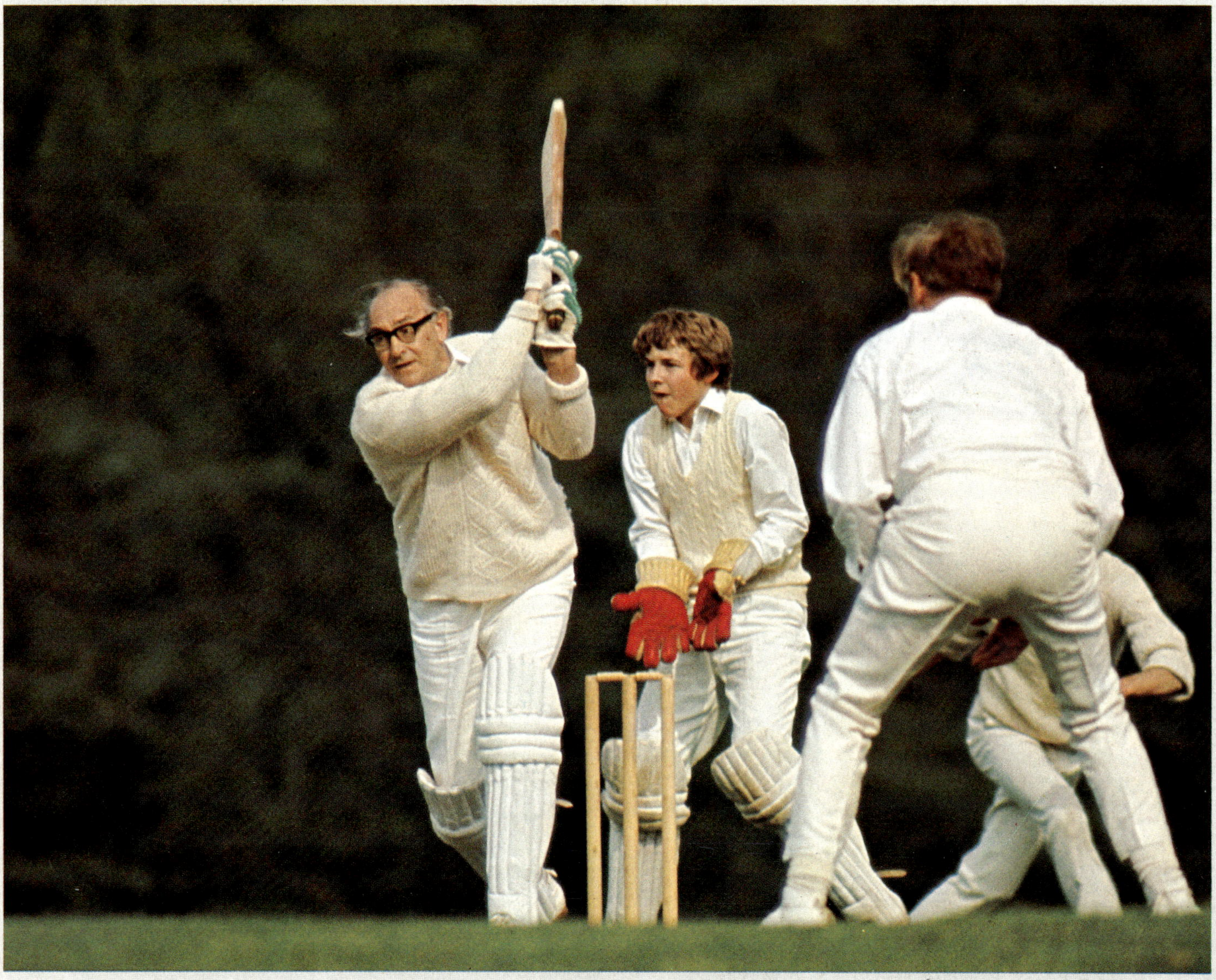

Equestrian Sports

Although equestrian sports are enjoyed by thousands of enthusiasts all over the world, the attention of the public has usually centred on the specialized events. These include flat racing, harness racing (trotting) and steeplechasing, polo, hunting, show-jumping and dressage. Yet, the sport can also be non-competitive, with such features as the pony clubs, that teach children to care for and appreciate their animals, and to practise the techniques of correct riding. For the adult whose time is limited and who rides more for pleasure than profit there are a number of equestrian clubs. There is little enjoyment in riding in towns, so much of the activity takes place in the country. Some large cities, however, do have stables and 'rides' in large parks. Often the enthusiast may have to travel a long way to enjoy the activity in pleasant surroundings.

Besides developing a love of nature, the equestrian sports also demand a good sense of balance, together with the technical skills of riding. The rider's legs have to grip the flanks of the horse to guide the animal, thus encouraging strong thighs. Courage is also needed in many of the more difficult events. however, equestrian sports do not exercise the body as much as is desirable. People interested in one or other of the sports and not intent on competition should regard it as the delightful relaxation that it is. If you enjoy riding at week-ends in the country, spend three sessions during the week in serious aerobic activity. Horse riding does not noticeably improve overall strength or suppleness: it is the horse who is gaining much of the physical benefit from the exercise. The rider should try to get his or her exercise from another source.

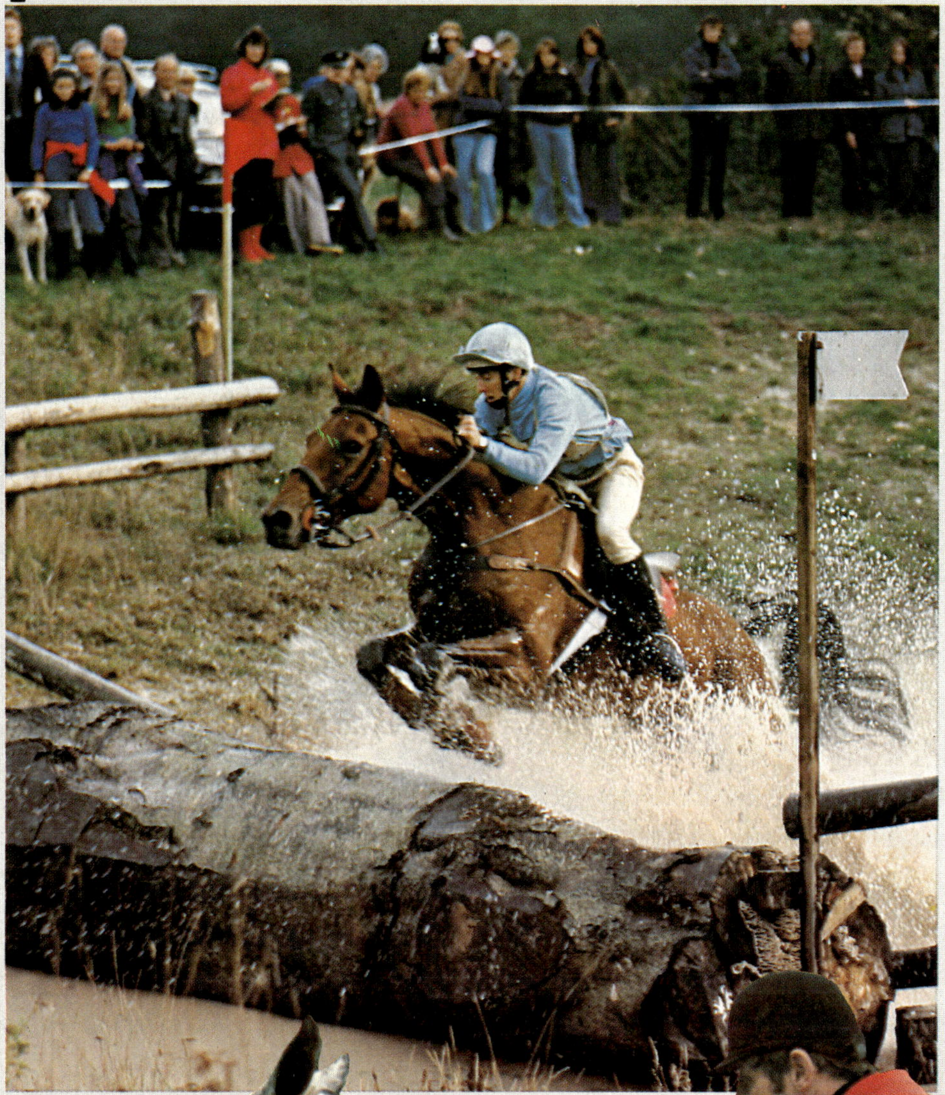

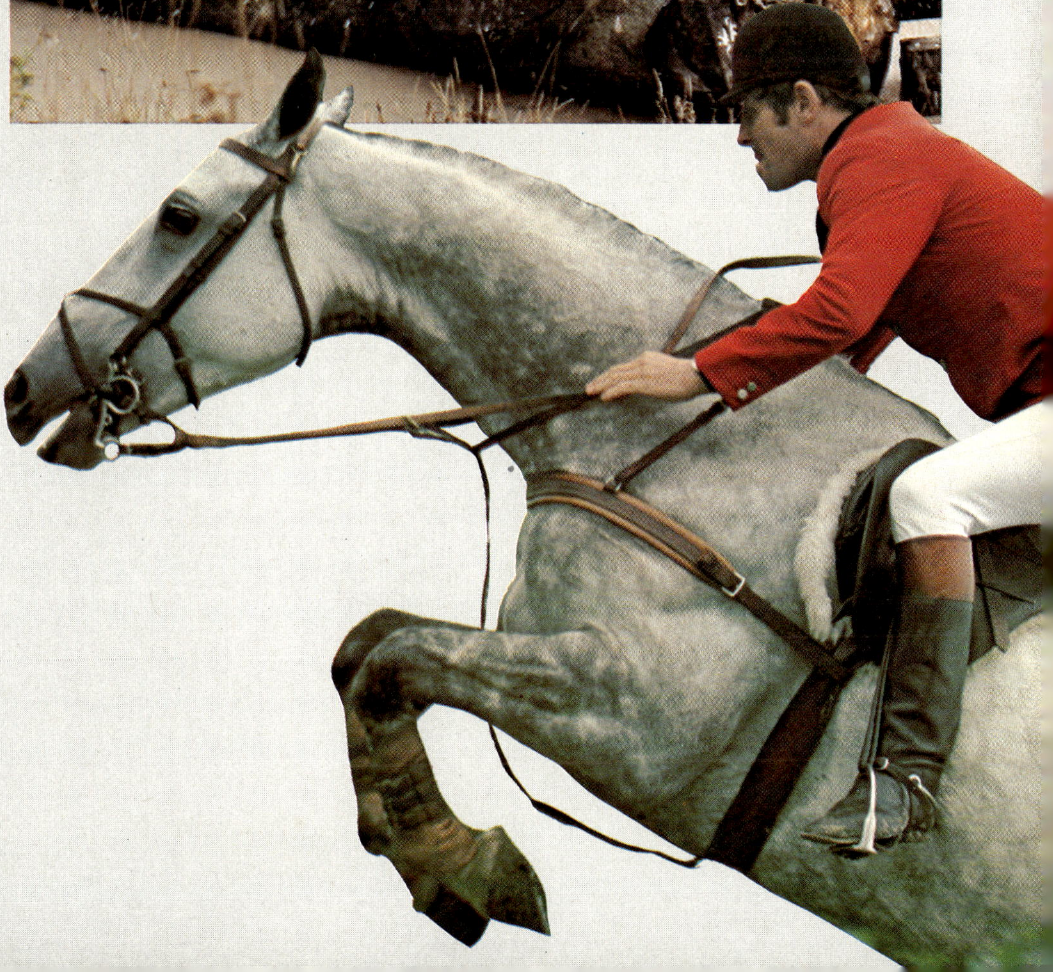

Any pastime which involves the outdoors and gives pleasure is worthwhile. However in terms of exercise it is the horse rather than rider who gains in equestrian pursuits whether it is show-jumping, cross-country racing or hunting

Fencing

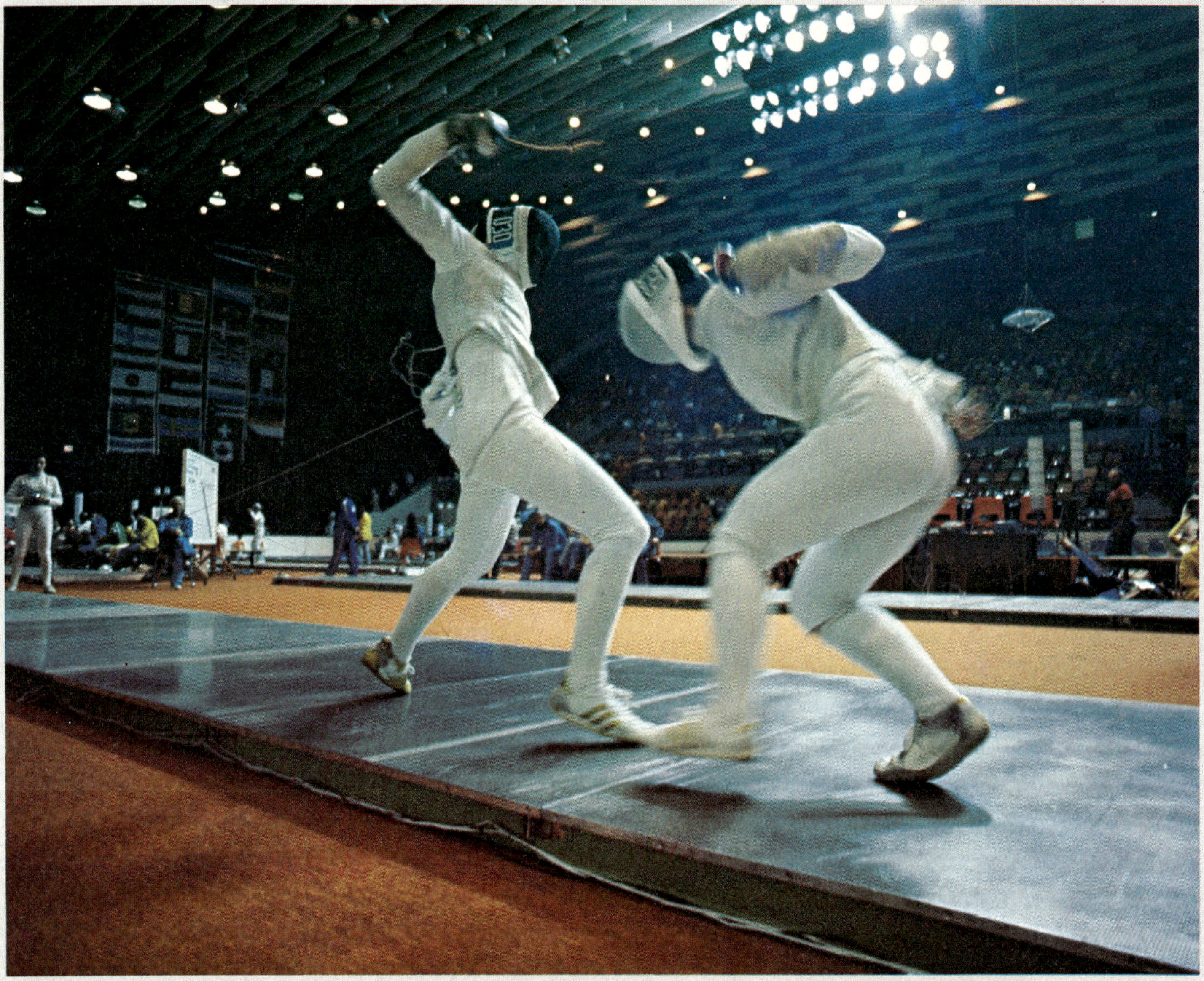

Fencing requires great concentration and flexibility rather than brute strength, and men and women are well-matched. The bouts are too short, however, to really build up stamina and develop muscles, so fencers should also follow some other form of exercise

Fencing, which derived from the need to practise swordsmanship for duels and warfare, is now an international sport in its own right. Its origin confers a distinct glamour because of its associations with chivalry. If this provides the initial impetus for taking up the sport, fencing itself gives the participant concentrated exercise in a short space of time, no matter what the weather is outside. It is a suitable sport for those who live in towns. Nor does it require a large location – any reasonably large room can be employed – or expensive equipment. The system of lights which flash when a fencer strikes his opponent may have to be confined to use in clubs since this does cost a lot of money, but practise can be carried out without these luxuries, and any multiple of two can practise together.

Fencing develops balance, poise and muscular control together with a high degree of reaction speed. A bout brings a sense of freshness to both mind and body, because it is so concentrated that it is impossible to fence and think of anything else. It furnishes a medium for swift thinking, speed and finesse, and since there is no advantage to be gained from mere strength, differences of physical attributes such as height and strength are largely levelled off. Consequently, men and women can fence together at foil on far more level terms than is possible in most other major sports. The other weapons used internationally are the sabre and epee, in which men have a more marked advantage over women.

Because of the emphasis on technique and speed, there is little contribution to physical strength. The constant lunging develops and stretches the legs but the short (although intense) barrages of fencing do not make a substantial contribution to your stamina. Many fencers run or exercise in addition to their chosen sport. Anyone fencing, however seriously, twice a week could carry out an aerobic activity on another evening.

Golf

Golf is probably the most popular participation sport for men over 25 in the western world. How much this has to do with the amenities provided by the 19th hole is debatable. Although, on a professional level, it is the most commercialized of all outdoor activities, its appeal partly derives from its attraction to people of all ages and both sexes. People can play into old age with only slight deterioration in their ability when compared to participants in American Football and rugby. There is an emphasis on skill rather than physical powers. The handicap system, whereby everyone taking part at golf is rated in relation to 'par' (the number of strokes an excellent performer should require to complete the 18 holes), means that participants of different ages and ability can gain satisfaction from playing together. A further feature is that it is not necessarily dependent on the performance or interplay of an opponent for its enjoyment. On a smaller, but no less genuine scale, the humble golfer can experience all the emotions of the game – the pleasure of a well-hit stroke, the frustration of missing a short putt – that a professional does.

The emphasis on skill must not be allowed to obscure the physical qualities that assist to make some professionals so outstanding. Gary Player, one of the most successful players of the 1960s, trained assiduously off the course to match the leading Americans, who were bigger and more powerful than he was. However, too many men and women who play for recreation, believe that the six kilometre (four mile) walk involved in playing most rounds of golf and the swinging of the clubs is sufficient exercise for them. It isn't. Golf makes only a mild demand on the heart and lungs and little on the capacity for strength or suppleness. Although championship golf does need a high standard of physical fitness, this fitness is not acquired by the playing of the game. Therefore, if you wish to maintain a high level of fitness you should supplement your round of golf with some more vigorous activity. A couple of steady runs, in addition to a week-end game, seems a reasonable balance.

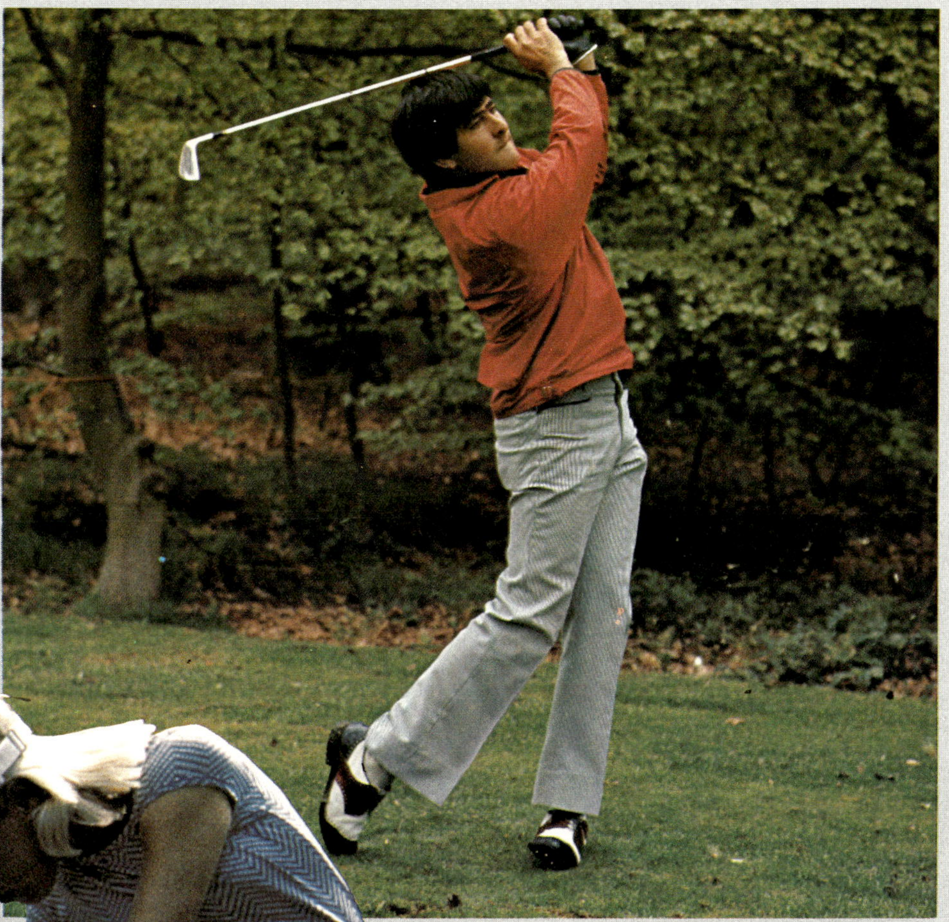

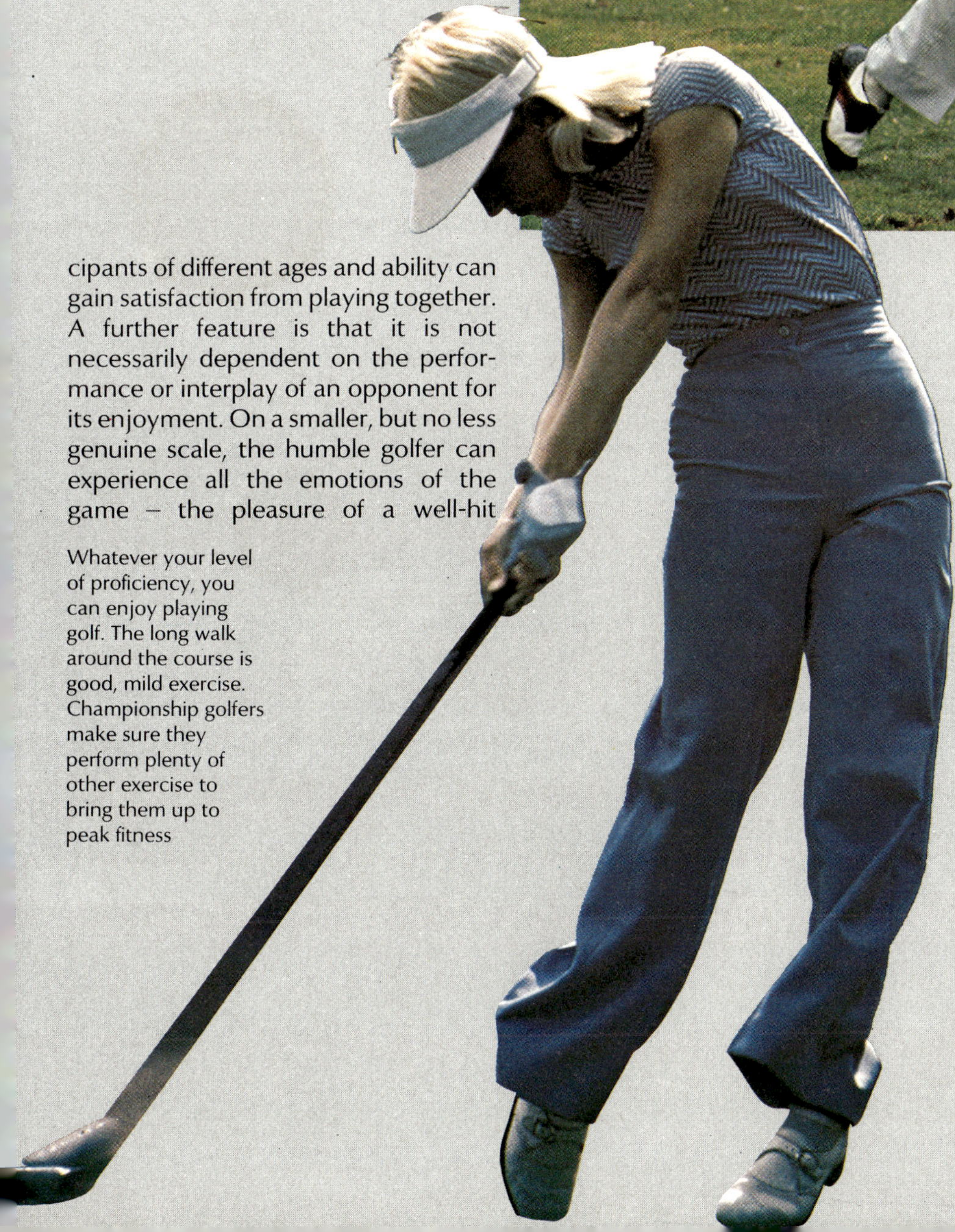

Whatever your level of proficiency, you can enjoy playing golf. The long walk around the course is good, mild exercise. Championship golfers make sure they perform plenty of other exercise to bring them up to peak fitness

Gymnastics

There are few more entrancing sports than gymnastics, in which the combination of strength, dexterity and artistry makes it both an enthralling event and a suitable training for other games. Successive Olympic Games have generated enormous interest in womens' gymnastics because it is so visually appealing. Consequently the growth in popularity of the sport has been astonishing, especially amongst teenage girls. Mens' gymnastics has lagged behind, both in spectator appeal and in participation. Both need intense technical application from a young age when facility of movement is more readily acquired than during adulthood. Careful coaching is needed to graduate through the routine. Men operate on the pommel horse, vault, floor exercises, high bar, rings and parallel bars. Women perform on the floor exercises, beam, asymmetric bars and vault.

Although equipment can be bought it is simpler to practise at gymnasiums where you can obtain advice and encouragement. Most gymnasiums are inside, but in places like California there are open-air versions. Men wear singlets and trousers; women wear leotards, the feet usually bare.

Gymnastics clearly develop mobility, strength and local muscular endurance to a high degree and, if an adult is already skilled at the sport, he should maintain his interest. However, a newcomer may find it awkward to learn some of even the most straightforwards routines, especially if he or she is heavily built. Some modified movements of the floor exercises would be valuable since they need no apparatus and can be readily learnt with reasonable proficiency. The one thing that gymnastics does not exercise extensively is cardiovascular recovery, so keen gymnasts should add some aerobic work to their training.

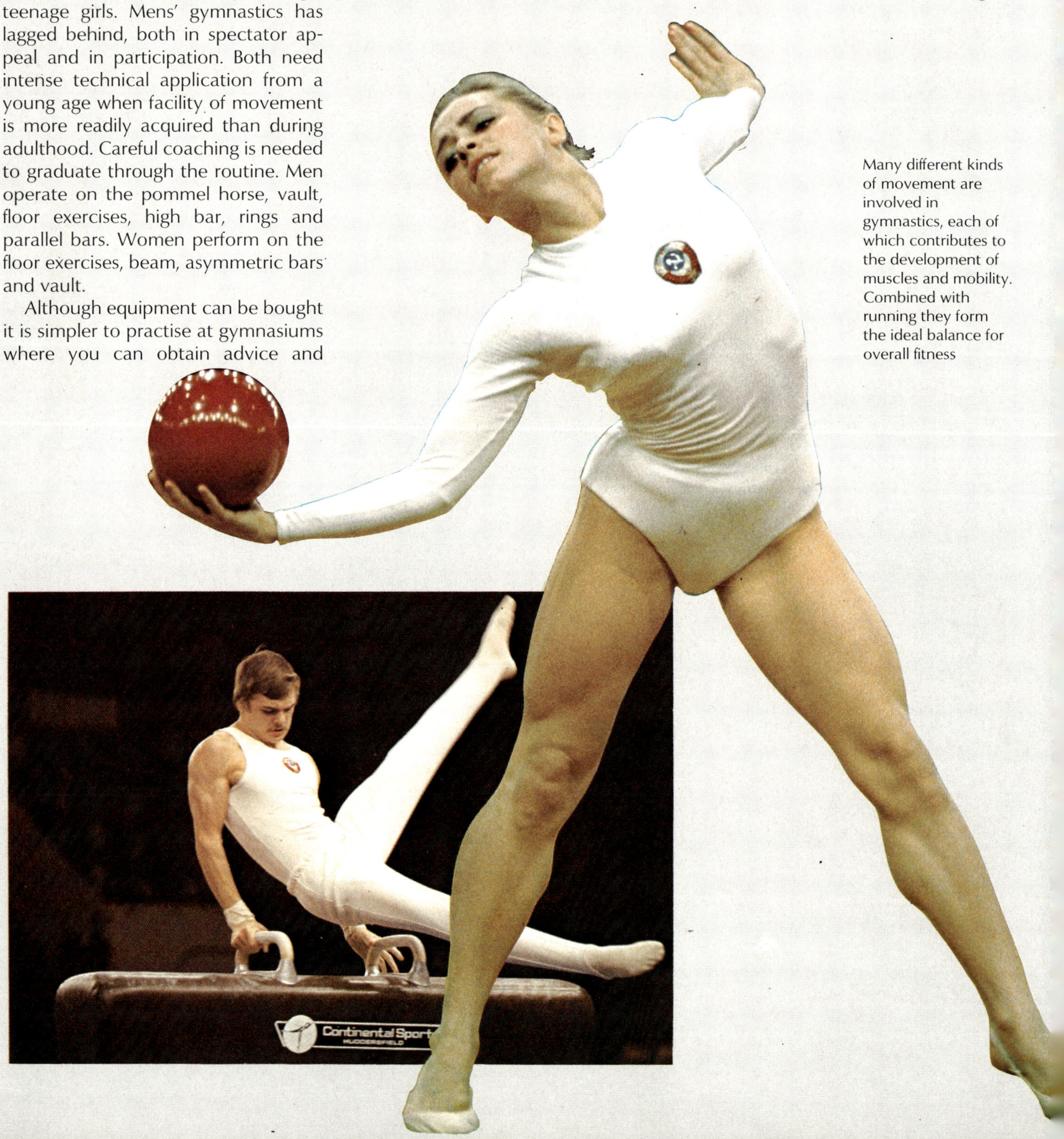

Many different kinds of movement are involved in gymnastics, each of which contributes to the development of muscles and mobility. Combined with running they form the ideal balance for overall fitness

Handball

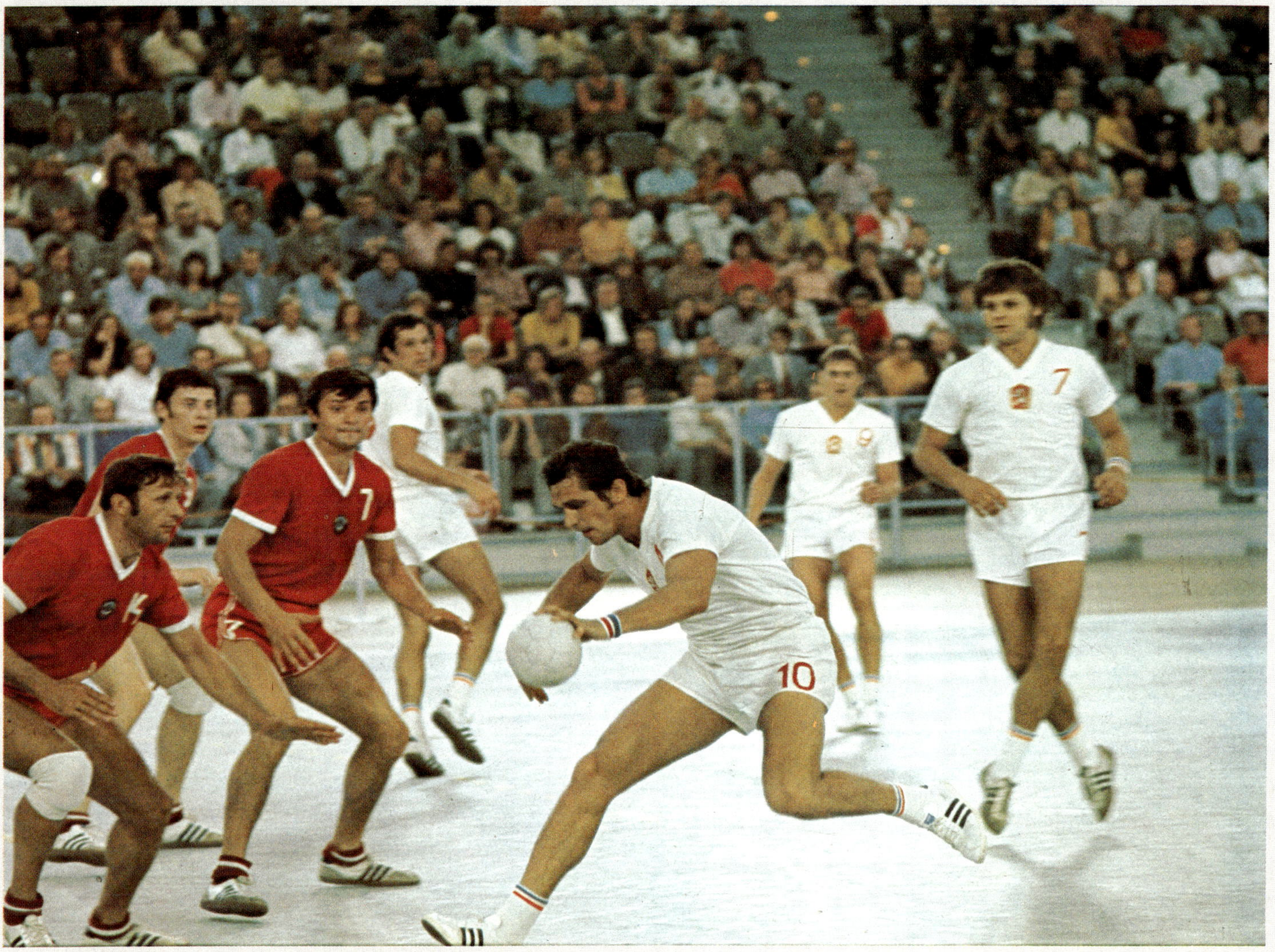

There are two completely different games which are called handball. In many English-speaking countries, the term is usually employed to describe the Irish version, which is closely related to Spanish *pelota* and English fives. Irish immigrants introduced it first to England, and subsequently to America (there are now more than a thousand one-wall courts in New York alone). There are different variations throughout the world (as there are in fives) but they all involve hitting the ball against a wall. Both singles and doubles can be played. Like fives and squash these versions of handball need dexterity of turning and the ability to move swiftly to position yourself properly to complete shots. As the charts show, it makes a considerable demand on the oxygen system. Since many gymnasiums possess courts a game of handball can often by fitted in with another activity as part of a multi-sport workout. For instance, an hour's weight-training followed by three quarters of an hour handball seems a pleasantly balanced session.

The other major branch of handball is a no-contact game played either out of doors (field handball) or indoors by teams of seven-a-side or five-a-side (adapted to a smaller court). One or two hands are used to catch, inter-pass or throw the ball. It is a fast-moving pastime, which devotees claim is the second fastest international game after ice hockey. Acute positional sense and accuracy in throwing are prime requisites. A round inflated leather ball, weighing 425-480g (15 to 17oz), a flat area and two goals are all that is needed. Like soccer, it can be a testing activity on the cardiovascular system if the competition is sustained for over an hour. It also requires considerable suppleness to spring for high balls and intercept passes.

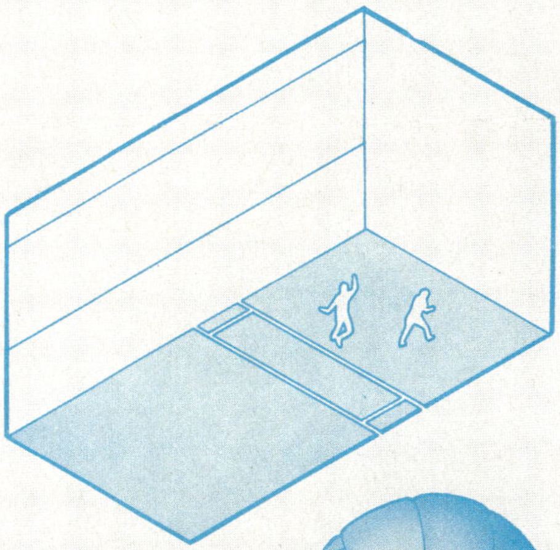

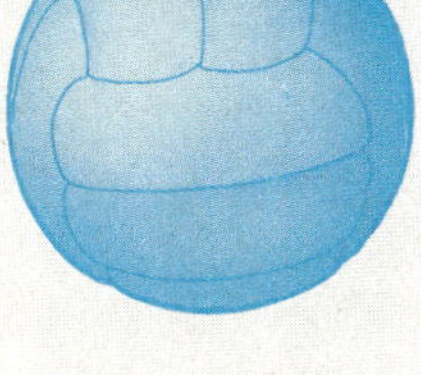

A fast and exciting game demanding an eye for the ball, speed and suppleness. Played indoors or out, handball is excellent exercise for heart, lungs and legs.
Above: court handball
Top: team handball

Hockey

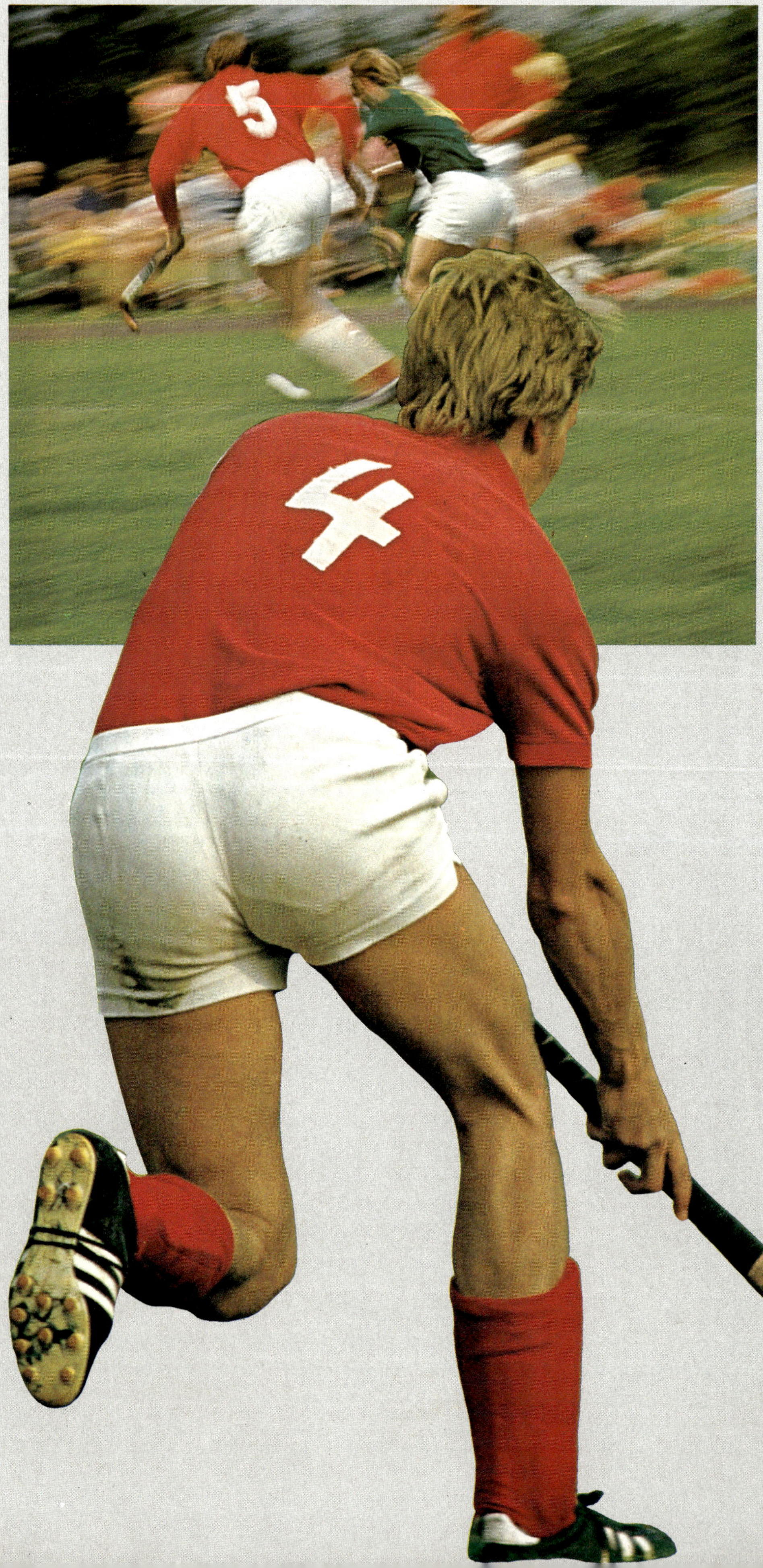
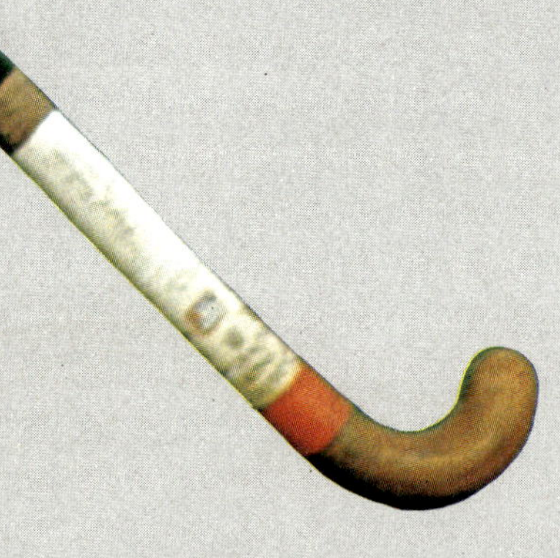

Field hockey can be a superb game both to watch and play. The great European and British Commonwealth sides often display a consummate technical mastery of the ball as well as athletic prowess. Although hockey is one of the few team games in which the two sexes can play together, they rarely do so except in recreational fixtures. Women's hockey lacks the boisterous qualities of the men's game. Hockey is best suited to warm weather when the ground conditions provide a 'true' surface. Sticks and balls are not excessivly expensive and the only disadvantage of the game is that one must have a large, smooth surface to play on. Indoor hockey has also been developed and become popular.

Probably fewer injuries are suffered in hockey than in soccer where there is stress on the legs from tackling. Played seriously, it exacts a high degree of speed and stamina as well as mobility. Unlike soccer or handball, there is little need for body spring and agility because the ball is largely restricted to the ground. It also needs little physical strength. The slightly round-shouldered stance over the ball can increase the tendency of anyone who stoops. Some exercises to develop the chest muscles which would promote a more upright posture might be advisable in these cases.

A good game to watch or play, hockey is for men and women and does not require much expenditure on equipment. It develops stamina and strength and provides good exercise as long as round shoulders are not developed from stooping over the ball

Lacrosse

Lacrosse was probably invented in North America where it was played as a tribal activity by the Indians and was a method of preparing warriors for battle. Matches went on for three days and the goals were two trees, sometimes 450m (500yd) apart. Modern lacrosse is ball and goal sport, played with the crosse, a curved, netted stick, one to two metres (three to six feet) long by teams of ten-a-side. It flourishes chiefly in America, Australia, Canada and Britain. Men and women take part separately and their respective rules vary. The robust nature of lacrosse – body contact and checking are permitted in the mens' regulations – dictates the wearing of protective equipment – arm pads, gauntlets and a helmet with a visor. The goalkeeper also wears a body pad. Positional play is important and speed and stamina tested. Because of the long, sweeping movements an indoor version is not practical. The outdoor field measures 110 yards long, the pitch specially marked out on grass.

Great skill is needed for catching and hurling the ball from the crosse. The player also needs to know how to keep the ball in the crosse while he is running. He can also be checked or intercepted by an opponent striking his crosse. Lacrosse is a vigorous sport, which probably provides equal exercise value to soccer. Because the crosse is employed instead of the body for contact with the ball, there is less need for mobility, but there is compensation in the exercise of the upper body and arms, which have to carry the crosse.

A body contact sport, hence the protective visors and gloves, lacrosse makes you run, twist and leap. A vigorous and robust game

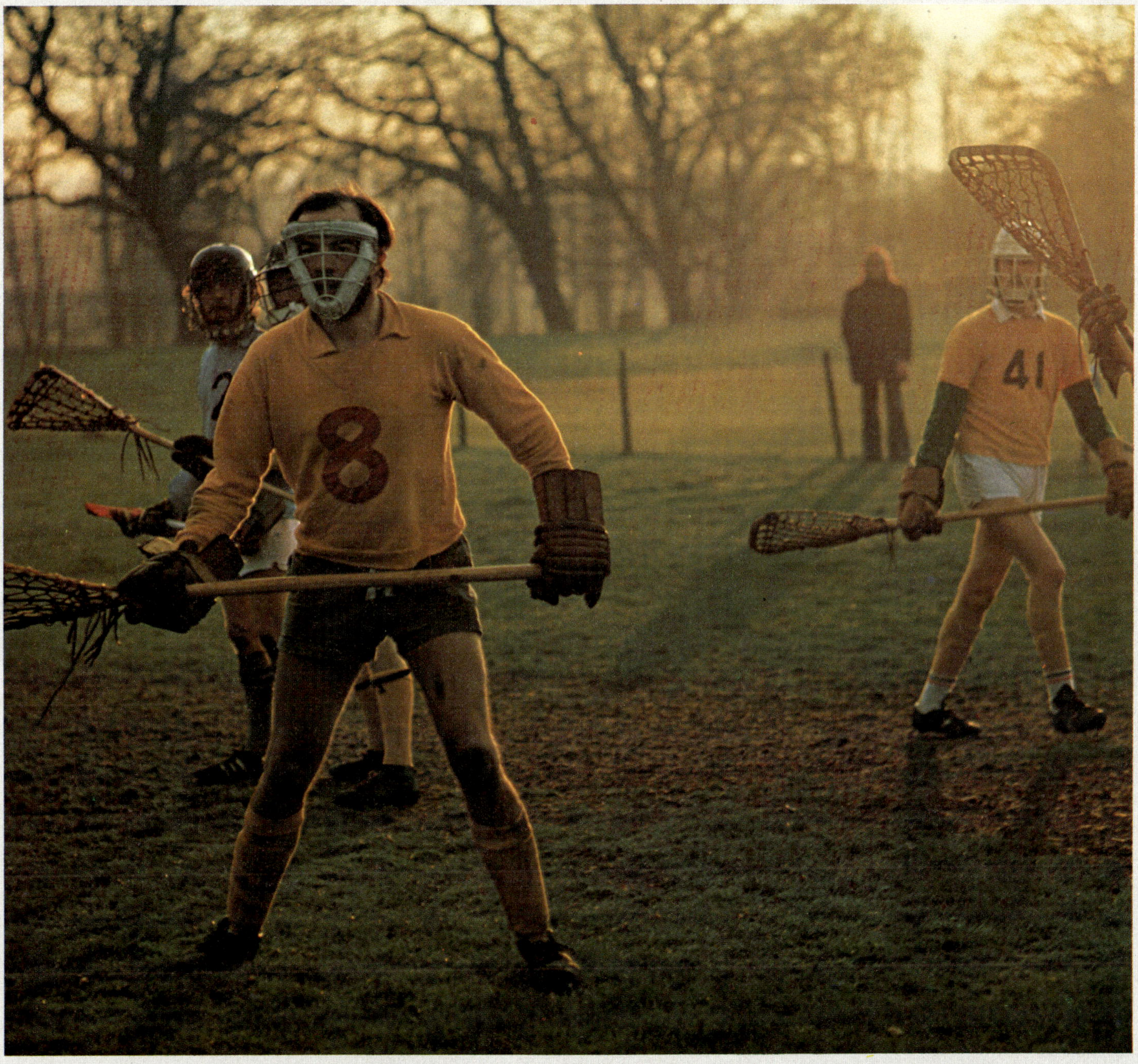

Lawn Tennis

Although tennis is technically so termed, to distinguish it from Real Tennis, part of its success has been its adaptability to a number of different surfaces – clay, cement, cinders, asphalt, gravel, wood and, of course, grass. If it became popular in the last century because it was a diversion for the English middle class, it has subsequently grown to be a truly international game, being particularly popular in Europe, the United States and Australia. Although it is possible to play indoors, there is a shortage of courts because of the area needed for the game. Therefore, tennis is chiefly played outside, restricting it to the summer in many countries. Men and women can play separately or together and this has given tennis an engagingly social atmosphere. Some houses possess their own tennis courts and they are commonplace at country clubs, schools, colleges and sports centres. However, sometimes in city centres there is a shortage of courts. The equipment is fairly inexpensive – a racket and balls are the only things essential to the game's enjoyment.

Tennis requires speed and mobility particularly. Many leading players tend to be fairly tall with long arms so that they can generate enormous power. Even five set matches demand a considerable amount of stamina despite the periods of inactivity. The chief problem for tennis players is how to continue taking exercise during the winter when they may not have access to courts. During this period of inactivity they could go jogging.

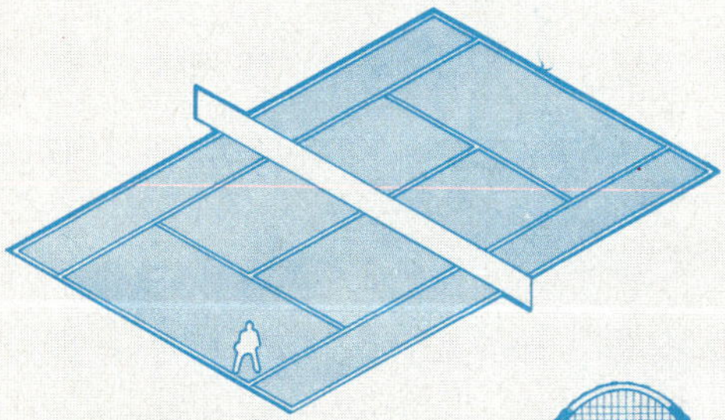

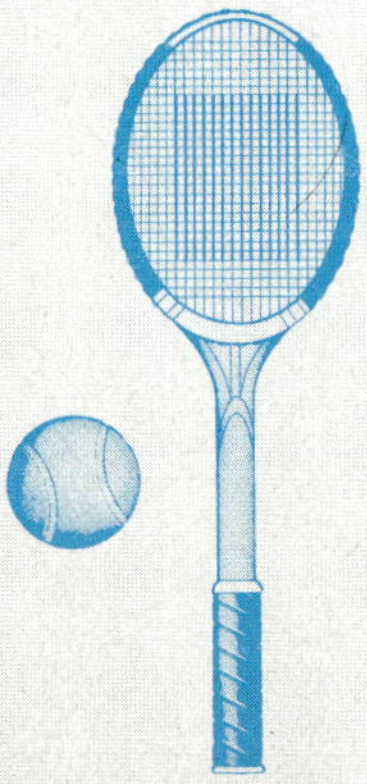

A popular game for all ages and nations, tennis has been adapted to many playing surfaces, and most people should have access to a court. As well as concentration, speed and stamina tennis involves many different movements, and is good exercise

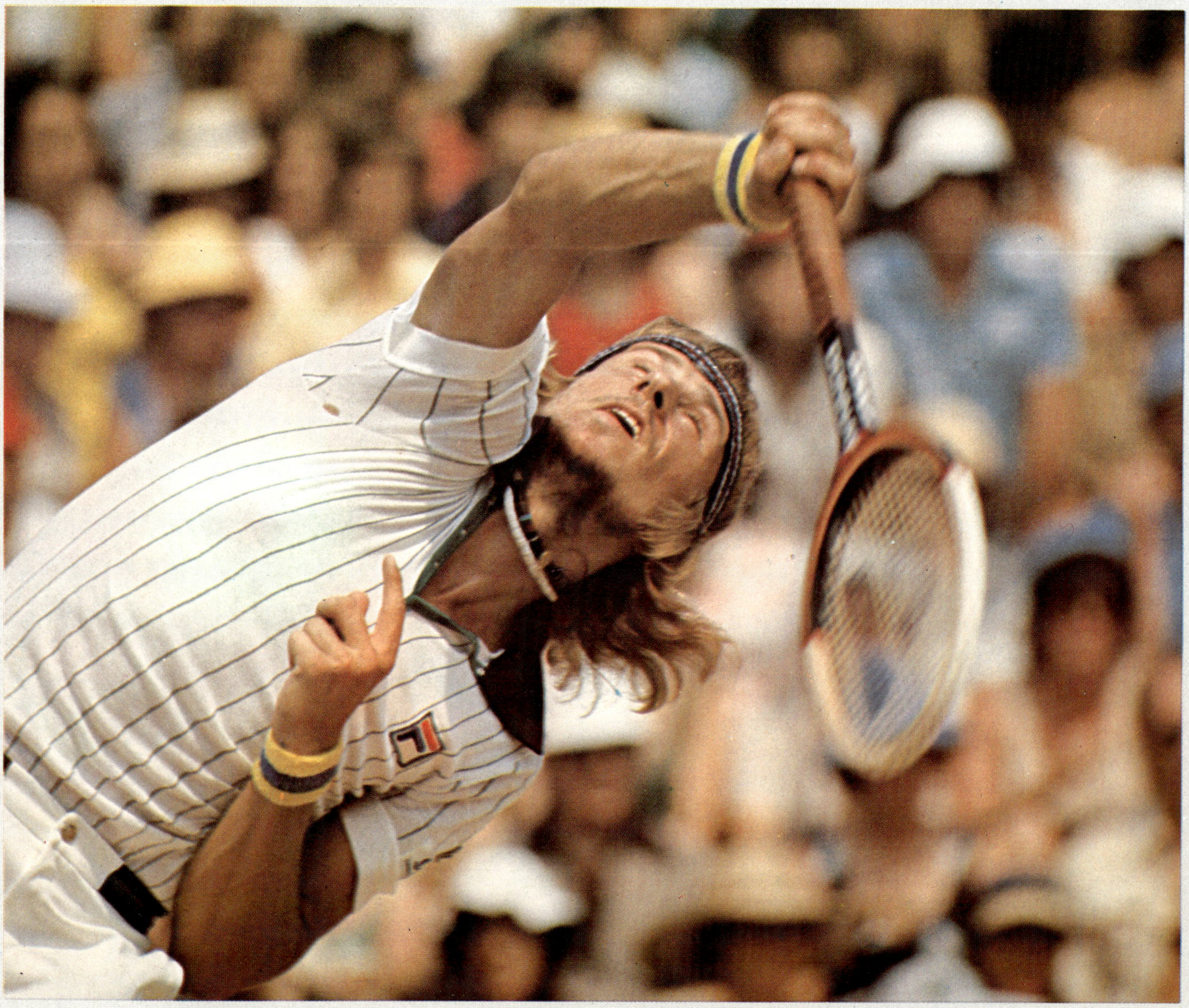

Martial Arts

The term, the Martial Arts, is usually taken to refer to such Oriental fighting skills as judo, *karate* and *aikido* from Japan, *Kung-fu* from China and *tae-kwon-do* from Korea. All have become increasingly popular in the west. Men and women of all ages can practise them, but the serious competitive aspects are usually restricted to the ages of 18 to 35. One feature that they share is a need for responsible instruction. Too many people are badly taught by coaches whose qualifications are dubious. Make sure you find a responsible club. Furthermore, in judo in particular, ability can only be developed if different partners are used. Skill in defence and attack largely derives from adapting your repertoire of moves to different styles. All the Martial Arts require special suits, but other equipment is supplied by clubs.

Judo, which is a grappling sport, usually needs a heavier build than the striking skills of *karate, tae-kwon-do* and *kung-fu*. There is incidentally a 'soft' form of *kung-fu,* called *tai-chi,* which is eminently suitable for middle-aged and old men. In Hong Kong and China, it is practised by enthusiasts on their way to work. But all of the Martial Arts, when practised assiduously, demand stamina and *karate, kung-fu* and *tae-kwon-do* require tremendous suppleness. For instance, most serious competitors can do the 'splits' sideways. In all the sports a good level of strength-weight ratio is developed. Furthermore, unlike many sports, no part of the body is especially favoured. The Martial Arts, therefore, can be thoroughly commended as an all-round exercise. What makes them also valuable in life is that part of their philosophy stresses the importance of acquiring mental attributes to balance the physical features of training.

Once you have found a responsible club which gives good tuition, the martial arts – including judo, karate aikido and Kung-fu – provide excellent exercise. The emphasis is on balanced training for both mind and body

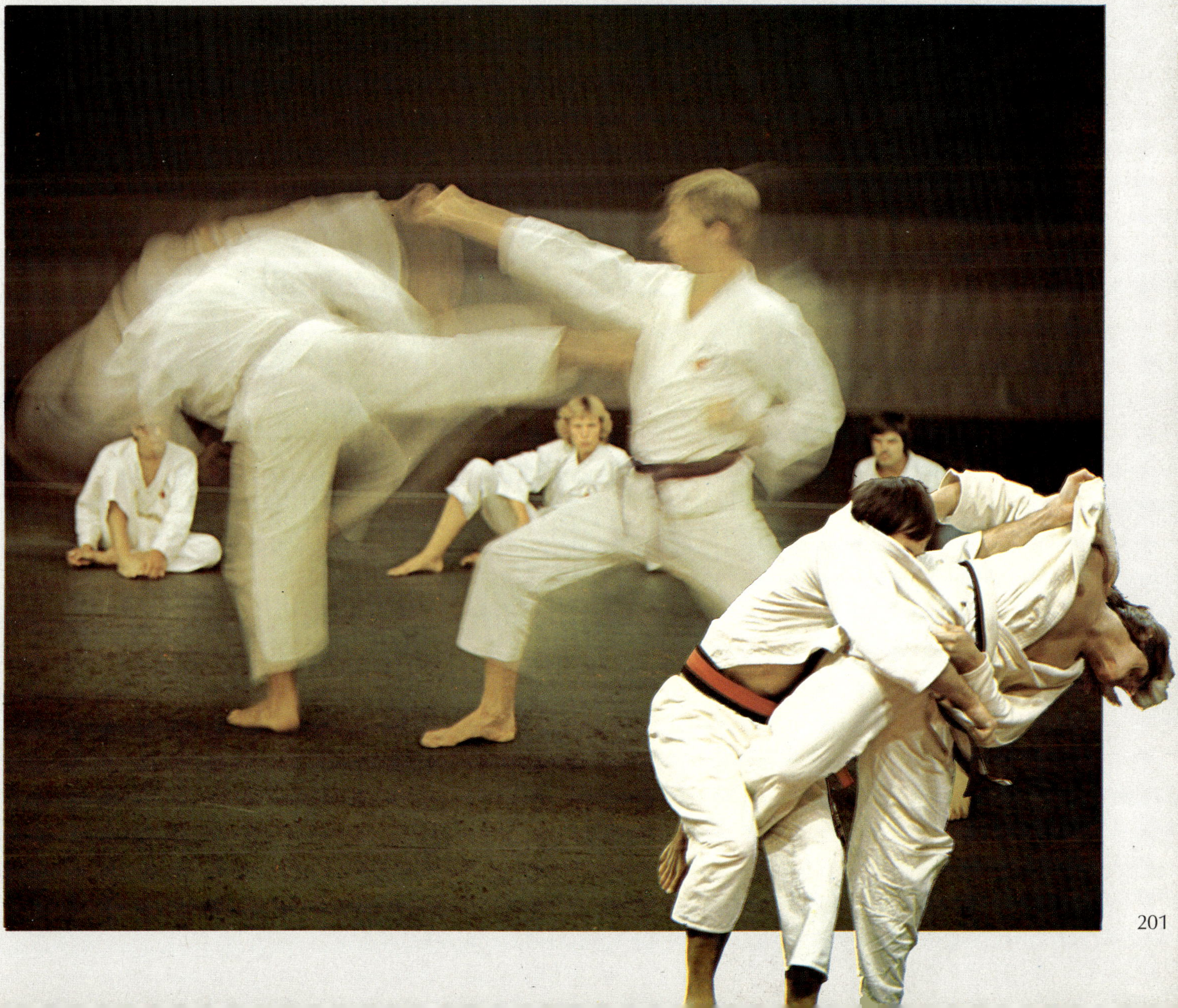

Orienteering

Orienteering has been described as motor-rallying on foot. It is a sport akin to cross-country running, but staged in less open terrain, in which runners compete in negotiating routes between isolated control points set up at defined positions within the area of competition. In most types of event, controls must be approached and visited in the correct sequence and the winner is the competitor completing a full circuit in the fastest time. A successful orienteer needs the legs and lungs of a runner and the skill of an expert map reader. He must also be able to make quick judgements as to which is the best route to take round the circuit – the most direct route is not necessarily the fastest. Orienteering combines athletic and mental skills in a way that is rare in a competitive sport and it is the joint stimulus of physical and mental exercise, in the attractive natural surroundings of woods, hills and moors that has been responsible for its growth, particularly on the European continent.

Men, women and children can take part in events which, by their nature, have to be at week-ends. This is one of the few disadvantages of orienteering. It cannot be a spontaneous affair. Everything has to be planned beforehand and the event has to be staged well away from cities, thus involving many people in a lot of travelling time. On the other hand it provides everyone with a great deal of exercise. Of course, before attempting this exacting sport, it will be necessary to do a considerable amount of running. Men have to learn to run up to 14km (9 miles), women and children have much shorter courses. It is perhaps ideal for a family outing, a serious runner who wants a change from the rigours of training or a moderately fit man eager to try a new sport.

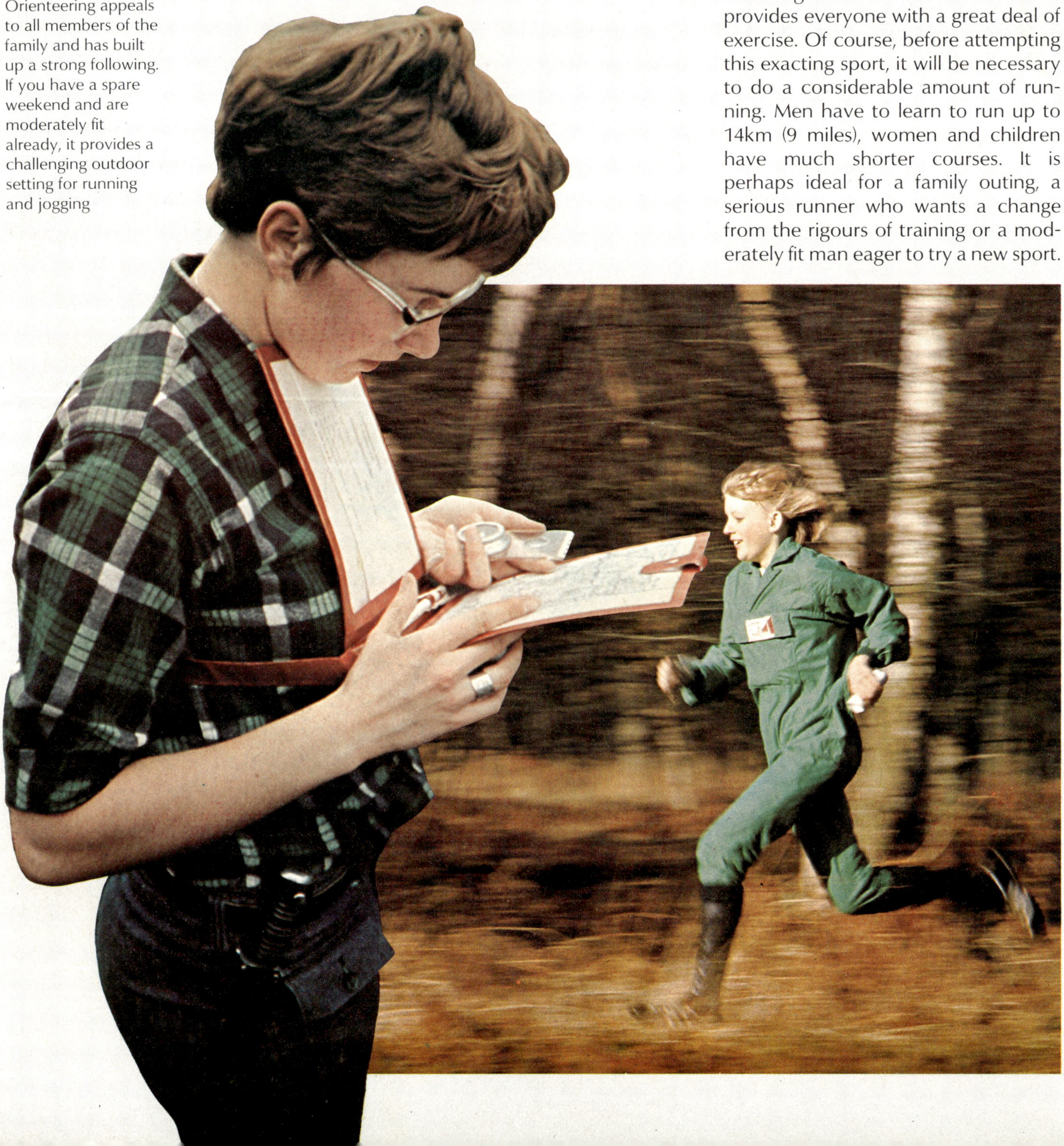

Orienteering appeals to all members of the family and has built up a strong following. If you have a spare weekend and are moderately fit already, it provides a challenging outdoor setting for running and jogging

Rowing

Although Lord Mancroft once said 'Rowing is a sport the French rightly reserved for their convicts and the Romans for their slaves', the sport has nevertheless much to commend it as exercise. Besides requiring many differing physical talents it also promotes a love of the water and boatmanship. Since boats are of various sizes one can combine with different numbers of people into small or large crews. The usual allocations are single sculls, pairs, fours – with or without coxes – and eights. Both sexes row competitively and in both Britain and the United States it is practised in schools. Because it flourishes on inland lakes, canals, rivers and sometimes on the sea, facilities are restricted for many people. Most clubs and universities who practise the sport seriously, do so because of their proximity to water – a decided advantage.

Although anyone can enjoy the sport, top-class rowing is almost entirely restricted to tall, broad-shouldered people. There are comparatively few international oarsmen under 2m (6ft tall), simply because they need the height and length of arm to provide sufficient range to propel the boat quickly. Although many international oarsmen in eights are over 95 kilos (15 stone), single scullers are often lighter. Rowing is an excellent all-round exercise. Strength and local endurance are needed, especially in the legs and back to provide sufficient force to pull the oar quickly through the water. A carefully-honed technique helps to prevent your movement from deterioration in a long outing, and stamina is essential so that the power can be maintained. Rowing has much to recommend it.

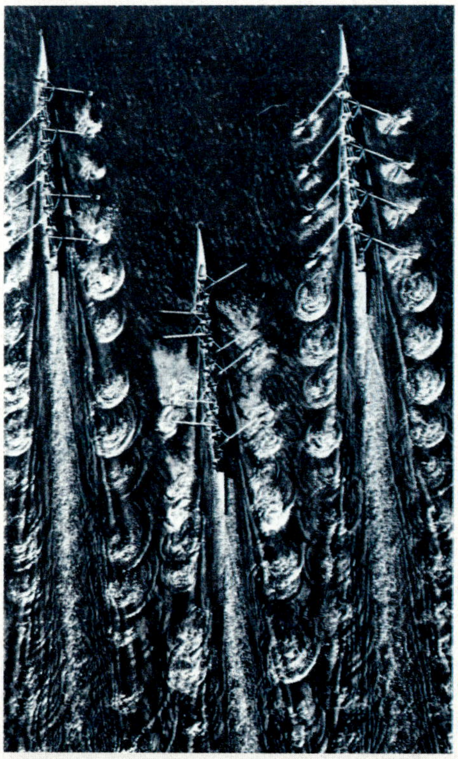

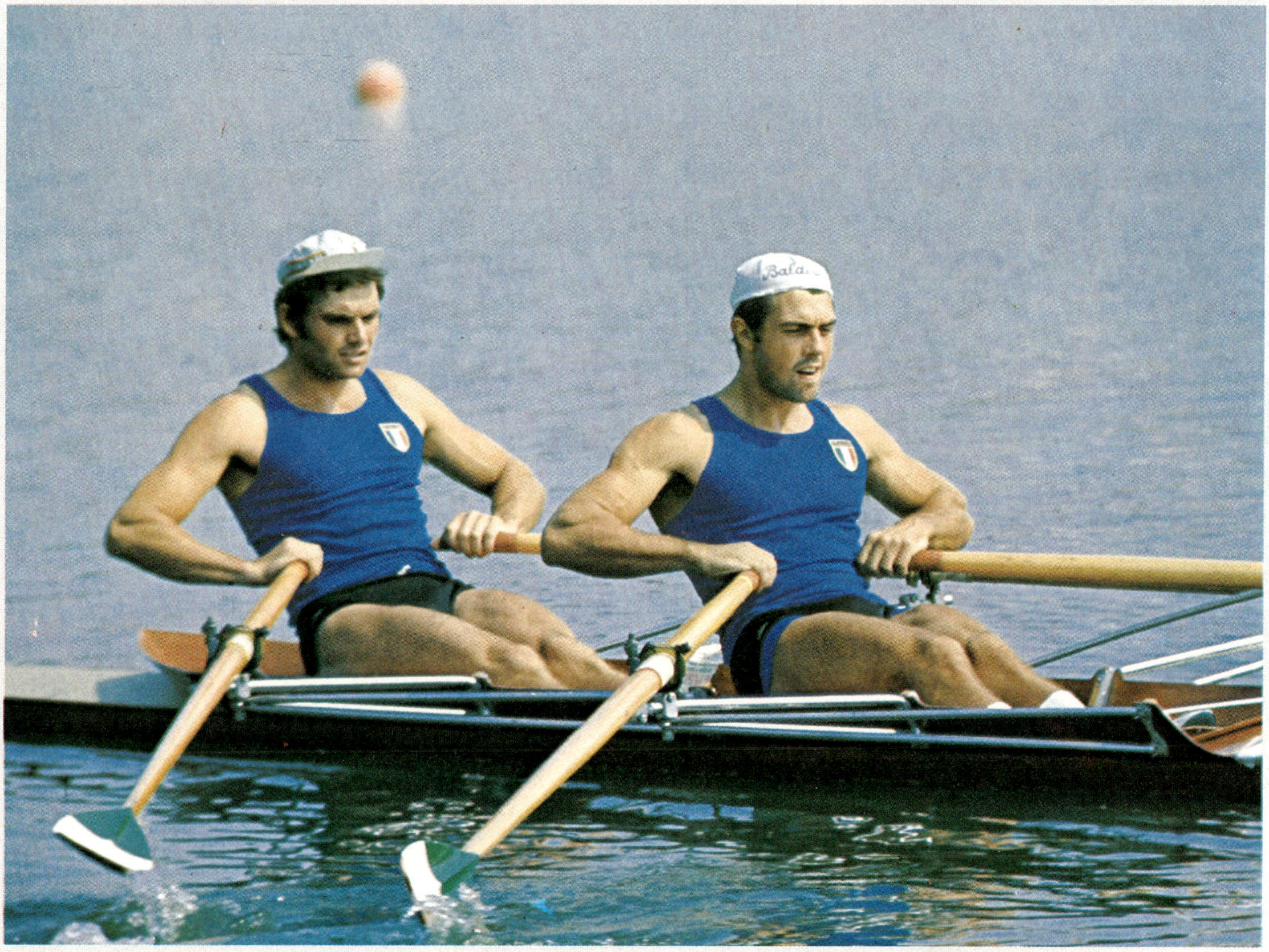

Arms, shoulders and legs are all developed by rowing, and serious rowers tend to be tall and strong, and often heavy

Recreation Sports

These are pastimes in which the emphasis is on diversion rather than on serious competition. Most of these games require partners. Many serve as additional training for sports or at least are a pleasant break from the more serious business of competition or maintaining a healthy body.

Some, like deck quoits, in which a rope or rubber quoit is thrown over a 1.5m (5ft) net, can be played in places like a ship where ball games would be awkward. Horseshoe quoits is another game which can be played by all the family. Some, like 'pig-in-the-middle', have a valid training aspect for games like soccer, rugby and basketball. The 'pig' tries to intercept a ball or quoit being passed between two other players. A variation of the game can be performed with the players kicking the ball; a development is to have two 'pigs' against three passers. The game is useful for teaching those players without the ball to move into anticipatory positions to receive passes.

Other pure amusements include kite-flying, which many people enjoy, and frisbee-throwing, where people throw a light, plastic discus to each other. Skilled participants can make the frisbee twist and spin in the air. Some recreations like darts take place indoors. But this for some people is highly competitive.

On a more exhilarating theme there are several recreational sports which require a great deal of nerve and skill although the expenditure on equipment is fairly high. In the forefront of these activities are skydiving and hang-gliding. Both are extremely exciting although perhaps not to everyone's liking. In each, the price of a mistake is the highest. However, with the proper training and instruction the sport becomes as simple and as relaxing as any other pastime. Concentration, good reactions and athletic ability are the qualities required for good performance. Both sports are suitable for men and women and have a worldwide following, Equipment must be carefully looked after and kept in perfect order at all times.

For children and young adults a wonderful new activity, skateboarding, has been developed. Here again, the equipment must be kept in good condition. Knee and elbow pads plus protective gloves and a lightweight helmet are all necessary and must always be worn. For the skateboard itself an enormous range is available catering for all tastes. The activity is usually performed outside in a special purpose-built park, although many children find ingenious ways of improvising. The activity helps promote fitness but is really only for recreation. All these recreations, therefore should be regarded as fun and not something which contributes towards maintaining a healthy body.

Hang-gliding, below, skateboarding, right, are two recent popular pastimes. Quoits, ball games like pig-in-the-middle, kite flying, frisbee throwing have long been family favourites. All take you outside, are fun and develop skills useful in serious sports

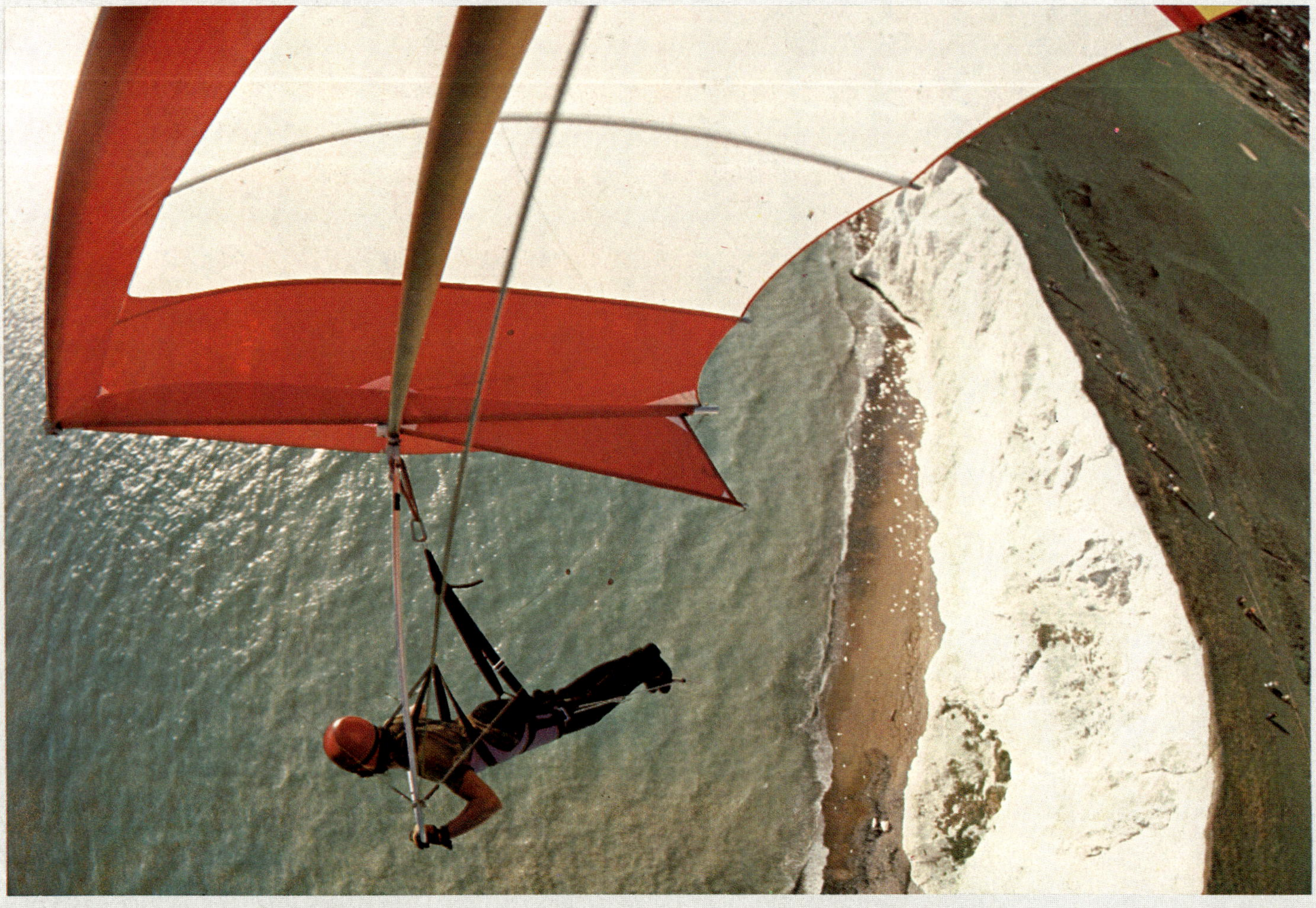

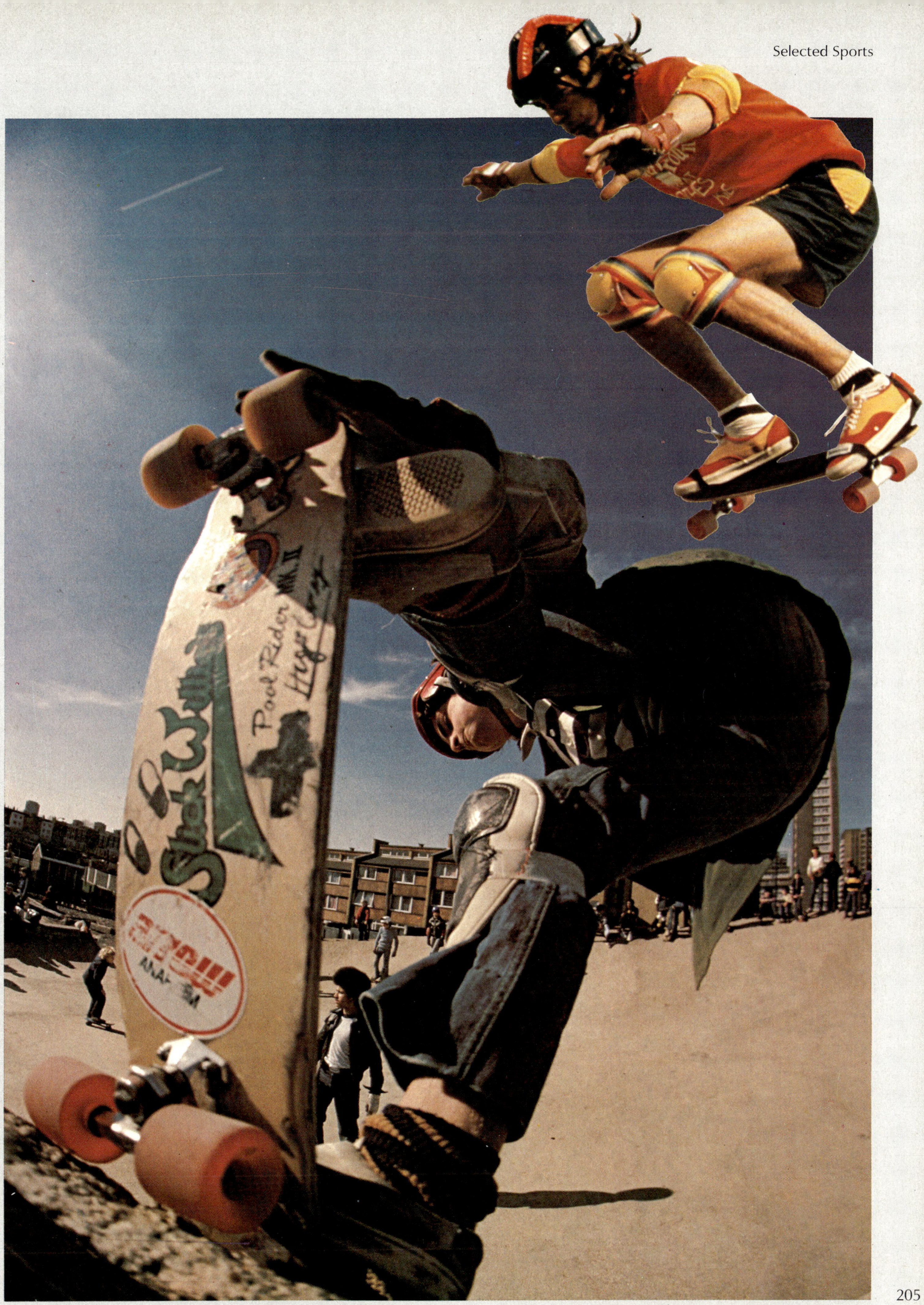
Pool Rider

Skiing

Skiing, like swimming, is often pursued as a sport by people, who have no intention of competing. For many it forms a holiday or week-end relaxation rather than a pursuit which is enjoyed all the year round. This is its major disadvantage. Although it is not confined to countries in higher latitudes – some unlikely regions like the Lebanon, Greece and Turkey have resorts in the mountains – nevertheless many enthusiasts do have to travel a long way to enjoy the sport. It is true that when the weather lets the skier down the snow can be 'manufactured', but this is usually only possible in mountain areas. In lowland regions artificial ski slopes are used, but are only good enough for elementary skiers.

There are many ways at using skis; ski-jumping; ski-racing; the biathlon, an exhausting cross-country race on skis with rifle shooting; ski-bobbing, in which a person sits astride what looks like a bicycle, with skis where wheels would ordinarily be; and water-skiing, which has many features of the dry-land version, but is carried out on the sea or lakes. All have distinctly social attractions and are practised by men and women.

Any kind of skiing is quite expensive because the participants may have to stay in the vicinity of their interest. The hire of the boat in water-skiing can also make a day's exercise costly but charges for mountain skiing tend to be cheaper. All the sports demand technical proficiency allied to an excellent sense of balance. Physically, skiing can be arduous on the legs, requiring both suppleness and strength. The rate of serious injuries to the lower limbs is unfortunately very high. If the exercise is sustained for long periods, it is very taxing on the cardiovascular system but this must include some cross-country work. The real problem for enthusiasts is to find other sports to enjoy when they cannot ski. Otherwise their physical activity may be confined to a few days a year.

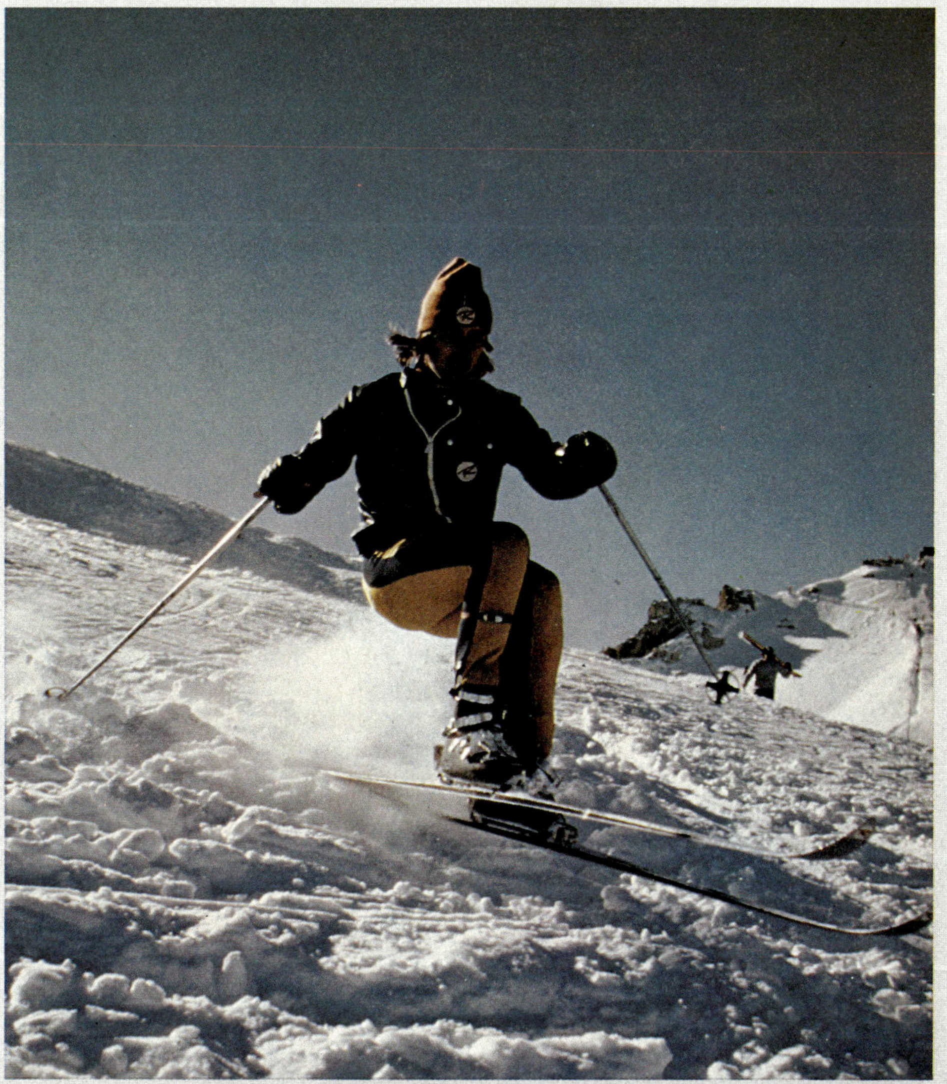

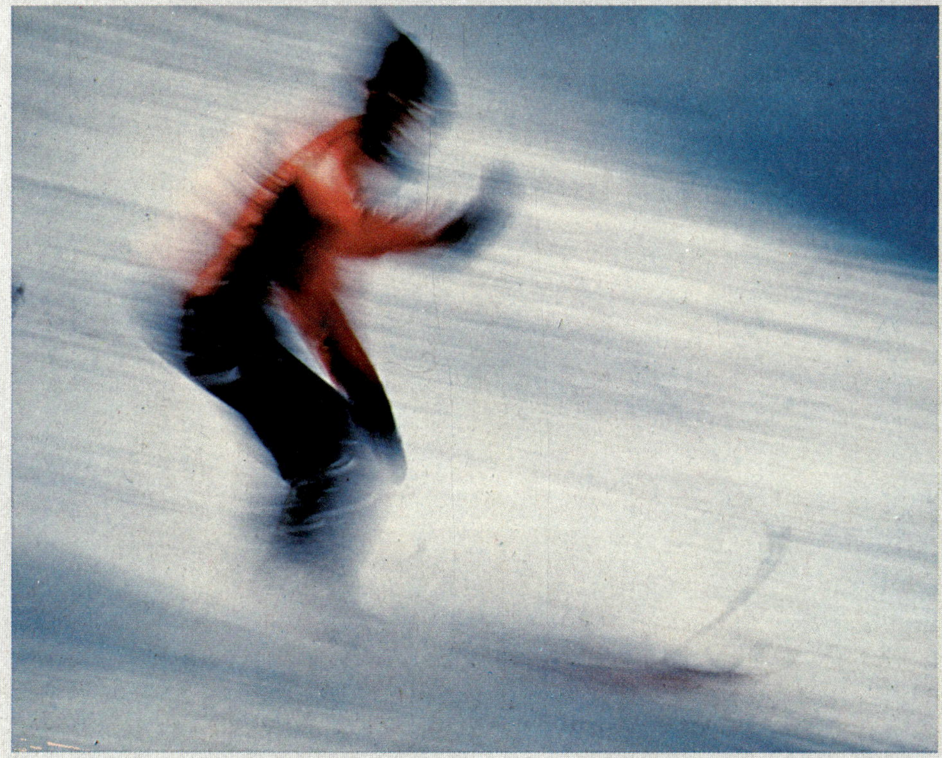

Skiing, once learned, is fast and very exhilarating – when weather permits. It can provide good, if intermittent, exercise

Soccer

Soccer or association football, is the most popular team game in the world. Professional matches are watched consistently by huge crowds and as a recreation it can be played on any surface and with only a ball as equipment. It is the most natural of team games, played everywhere from the beaches of Brazil to the backstreets of Glasgow. Although it is a highly professional sport, football remains a relaxation for millions of Europeans and South Americans, something to play in lunchbreaks and after school. 'Football was what we did when they set us free' wrote Maurice Edelston and Terence Delaney in *Masters of Soccer,* talking about how schoolboys turn inevitably to the game as a joyous release.

Although football is primarily for young men, it can be enjoyed by men into middle age, and by women. Full scale matches are eleven-a-side but organized five-a-side fixtures flourish on smaller pitches. Since the game is so simple there does not have to be extensive equipment and therefore it has the enormous advantage of being able to be played almost anywhere – parks, yards, gardens and even streets. Unlike basketball, one does not have to be tall or necessarily robust.

Speed over very short distance is essential, and mobility useful, but the most important requirement is a high level of skill, both in controlling the ball and in passing it to your team mates. The ease and accuracy with which this is done, combined with speed of perception in assessing situations, mark the outstanding footballers. Football demands a high, but not excessive, amount of stamina, since there are periods in the game when players are able to relax from all-out running. However, a full 90 minute game will give most players 8km ($4\frac{1}{2}$ miles) running as well as a variety of stretching, jumping and turning movements. A game a week provides one intensive session – and could be supplemented advantageously by two runs, both as training for the game and as possessing value in itself.

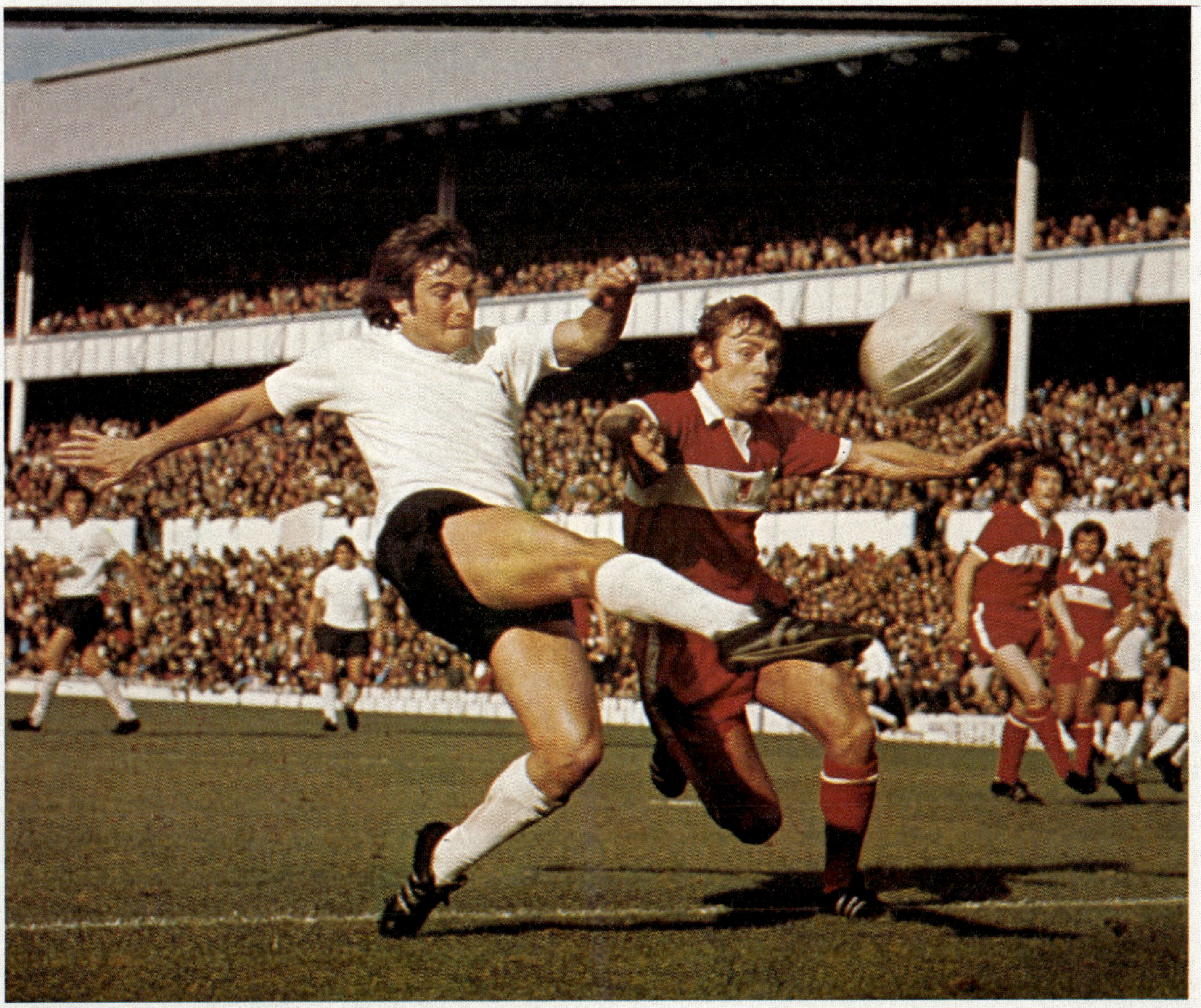

Deservedly the world's most popular team game soccer provides excitement and all-round exercise for the body

Squash

Few games in recent years have been more appealing for people wishing to maintain a high level of fitness than squash. It is the newest of the racket and ball games to have become universally popular. This is curious because it is basically so simple – give any small boy a ball and a piece of wood and he will soon discover what fun there is to be had by hitting the ball against the nearest available wall. As the size of the court and the height of the boundary lines afford a tremendous margin of safety against hitting out, an average club session of 45 minutes furnishes a great deal of concentrated exercise. Even novices do not find the aim of the game – to hit the ball above a 50cm (19in) strip on the front wall so that either the opponent cannot reach it until it has bounced twice or is forced into striking it beyond the boundary lines – difficult to learn. Within very few sessions men and women can enjoy sustained rallies. Singles and doubles are played. For many people squash is a perfect game.

Unless you belong to a very exclusive club, costs are not exorbitant. Rackets are the only substantial outlay and, although they sometimes break after a particularly sharp contact with the wall, they can last for years. Most major cities in the United States and Britain have courts so that many people work within a short distance of playing areas. Perhaps the greatest disadvantage of squash is its very popularity. In some areas it is extremely difficult to play the game, simple because courts get so booked up. Some people get disheartened and turn to another, less valuable recreation or, worse still, don't practise any game. This is a pity because squash is thoroughly to be recommended. Although it makes little contribution to physical strength, it needs dexterity of movement and considerable skill. More important, it makes demands on one's heart and lungs in pleasantly competitive circumstances.

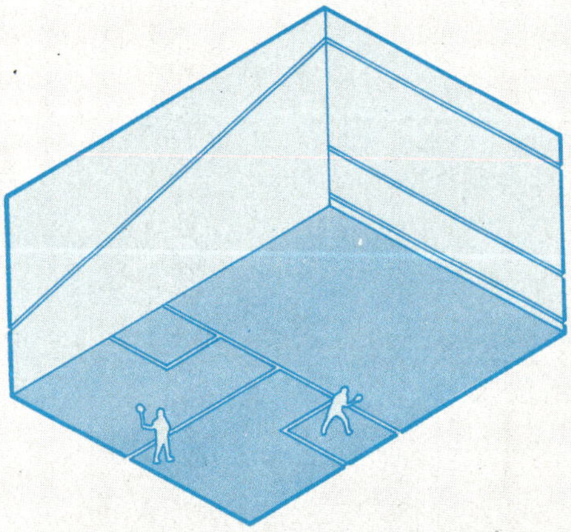

Very fast, physically exhausting, squash is one of the fastest-growth sports. More courts are now available and men and women can both play. Keeness of eye and dexterity of wrist, as well as fast running, are demanded, a set giving good physical workout

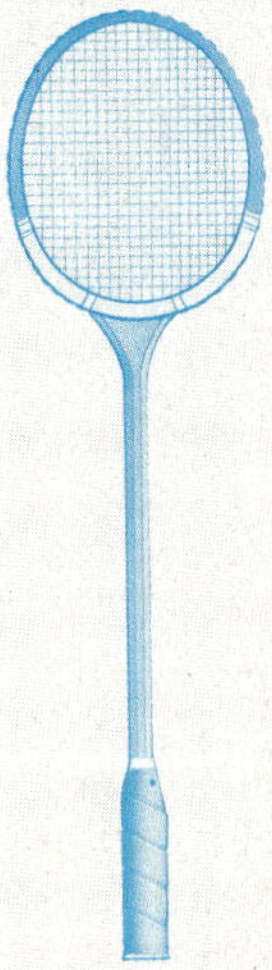

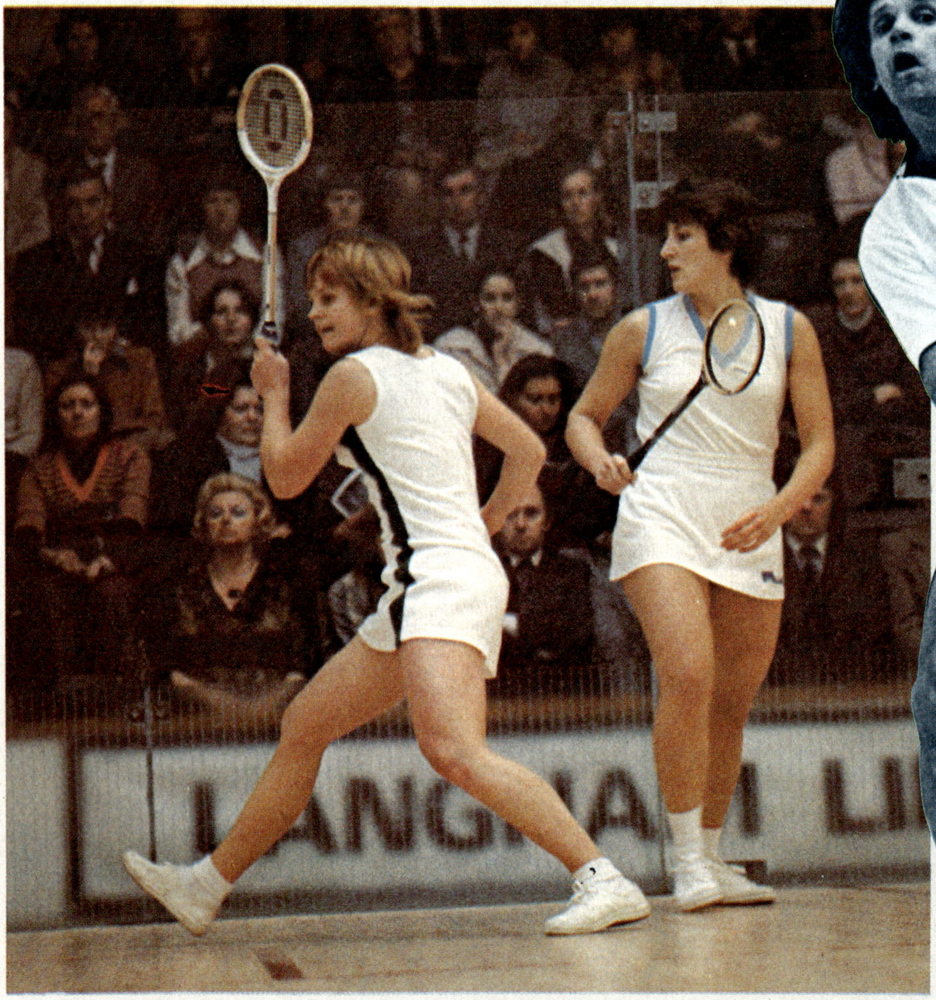

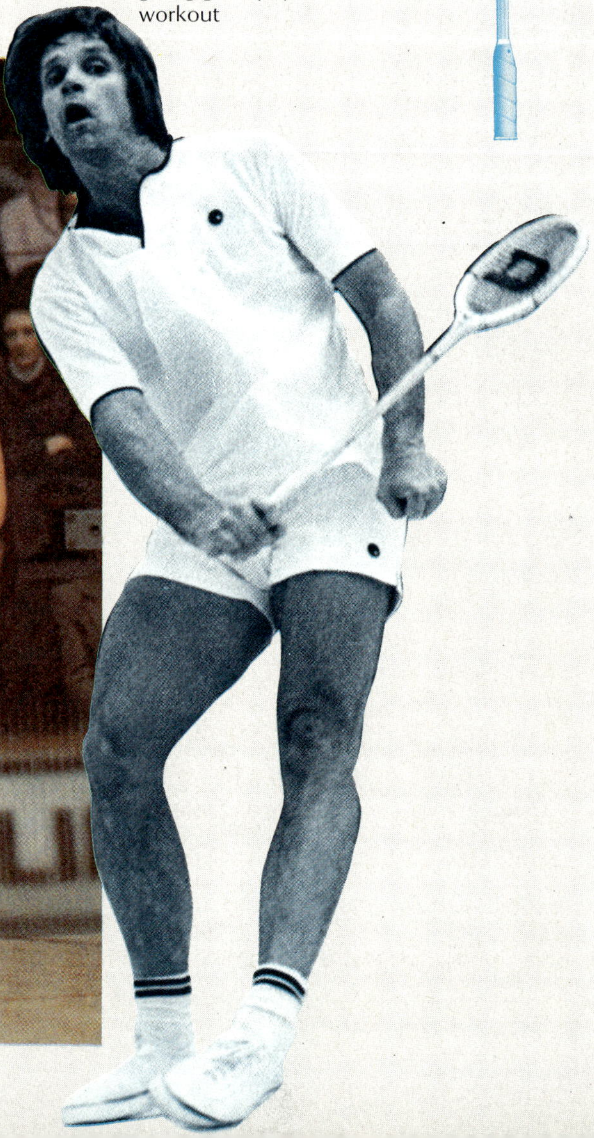

Table Tennis

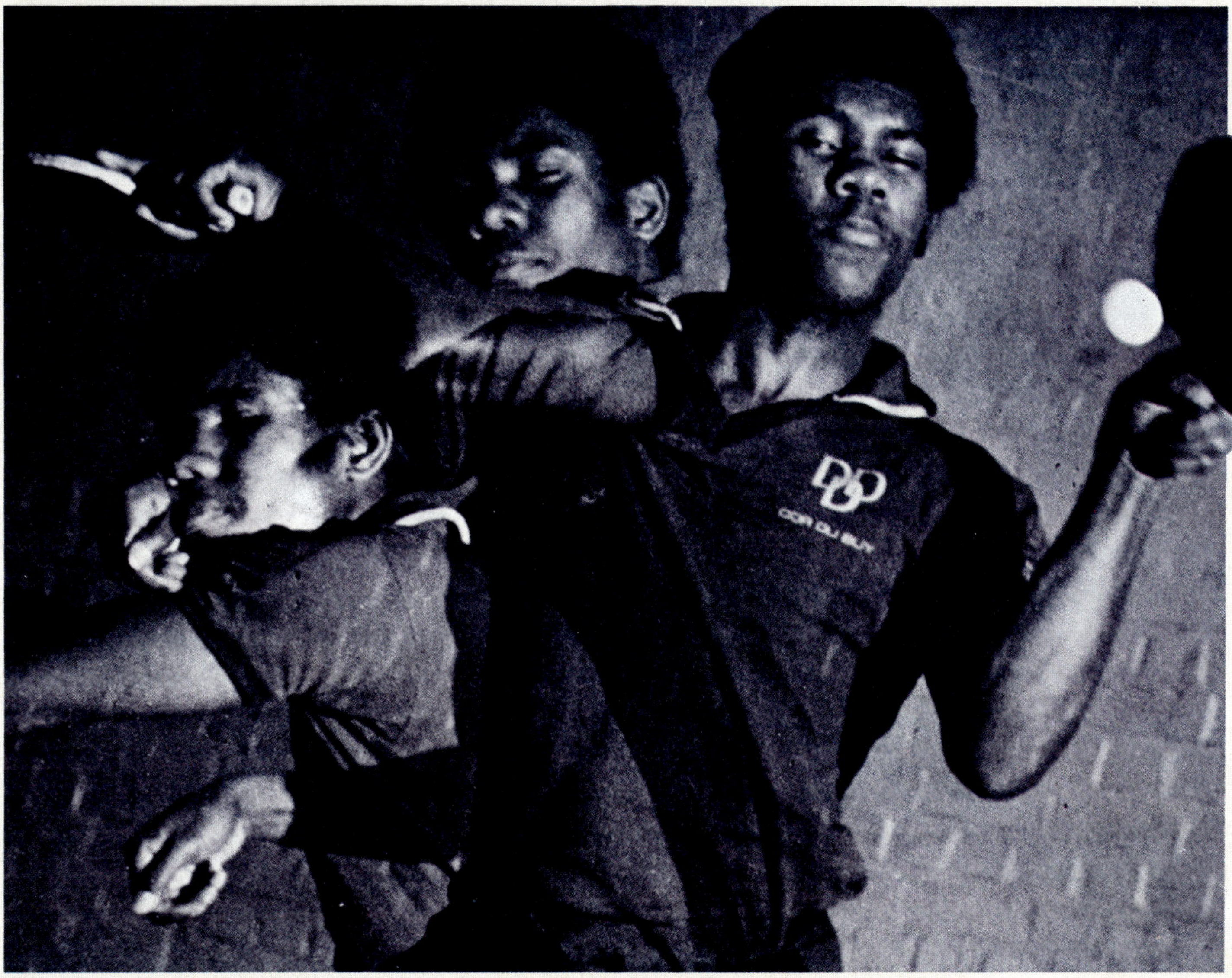

Competitive table tennis is an athletic sport; recreation table tennis is not. To take part seriously one needs a high degree of agility and speed from static positions because the players are forced to leave the rectangular table and use the 7m × 7m (22ft × 22ft) area on either side of the net to retrieve their opponents' shots. One of the main factors accounting for the participation popularity of table tennis has been the simplicity of its principles, the relative cheapness of its equipment and the moderate demands upon space when played at a minimum standard. Unfortunately, this also restricts its value as exercise since players stand close to the table and make almost all their shots from there. Men and women both play the game in which singles, doubles and mixed doubles are possible. Table tennis can be played outdoors, although the wind will affect the flight of the celluloid ball. Usually, however, it is performed indoors, in clubs, schools and country clubs. Because the equipment is so simple many people either own or have made their own table.

The Chinese, Japanese and Koreans have usually proved supreme at table tennis largely because of their small frames and deftness of movement. Strength and power is neither required nor trained in table tennis. What is principally needed is neatness of techniques, the ability to place shots carefully, quick reactions and speed of eye. Therefore, although table tennis is to be commended as a relaxation, it does not produce (below top-class competitive play) sufficient demand on the cardiovascular system. It should be played as an extra.

Agility, care and neatness are important due to limited space and lightness of ball in table tennis. A skilful and exacting game, but not one that develops muscle power. It is good training for quick reactions

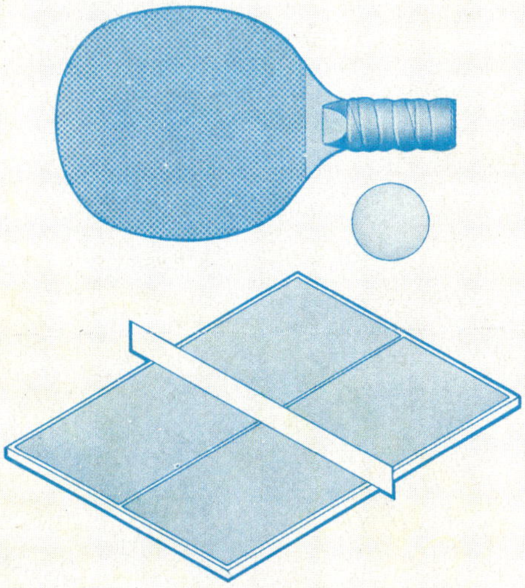

Tenpin Bowling

This indoor recreation is principally concentrated in popularity in the USA, although there are also bowling centres in many other parts of the world including Britain. It often has to compete with the longer established sports like Lawn Bowls in the British Commonwealth or Boules in France. However, being able to play tenpin bowling all the year round has given it an enormous advantage over its rivals. The sport was revolutionized in the 1950s. Automatic pinspotters eliminated pin boys (people employed to stand the pins up), speeded up play and ushered in the epoch of air-conditioned arenas which often stay open all night. The attraction of tenpin bowling is its evident simplicity – even a novice can score a strike (all the pins knocked down by the first ball). Women can compete with men and handicaps can make matches more interesting. Team events are also customary.

The equipment is always laid on by the bowling centre and many hire the soft shoes which should be worn to prevent slipping in the alley, the lane of maple and pine boards. Bowling centres are situated in most big towns, ranging from the one in Tokyo, which has 258 lanes situated in a nine-storey building, to small local clubs. Constant practice is needed to acquire the skill to bowl a hook ball and curve ball, in which the bowler twists his wrist as the ball leaves his hand, and also in the removal of single pins if the bowler has not scored a strike. Outstanding physical qualities are obviously less needed and consequently tenpin bowlers must see their sport as something that is not going to help them maintain healthy bodies. One advantage of the sport is that one can continue until very old age. A tenpin bowler never retires; he just steps down in class.

Whatever your age, this game gives great enjoyment without demanding too much physical exertion

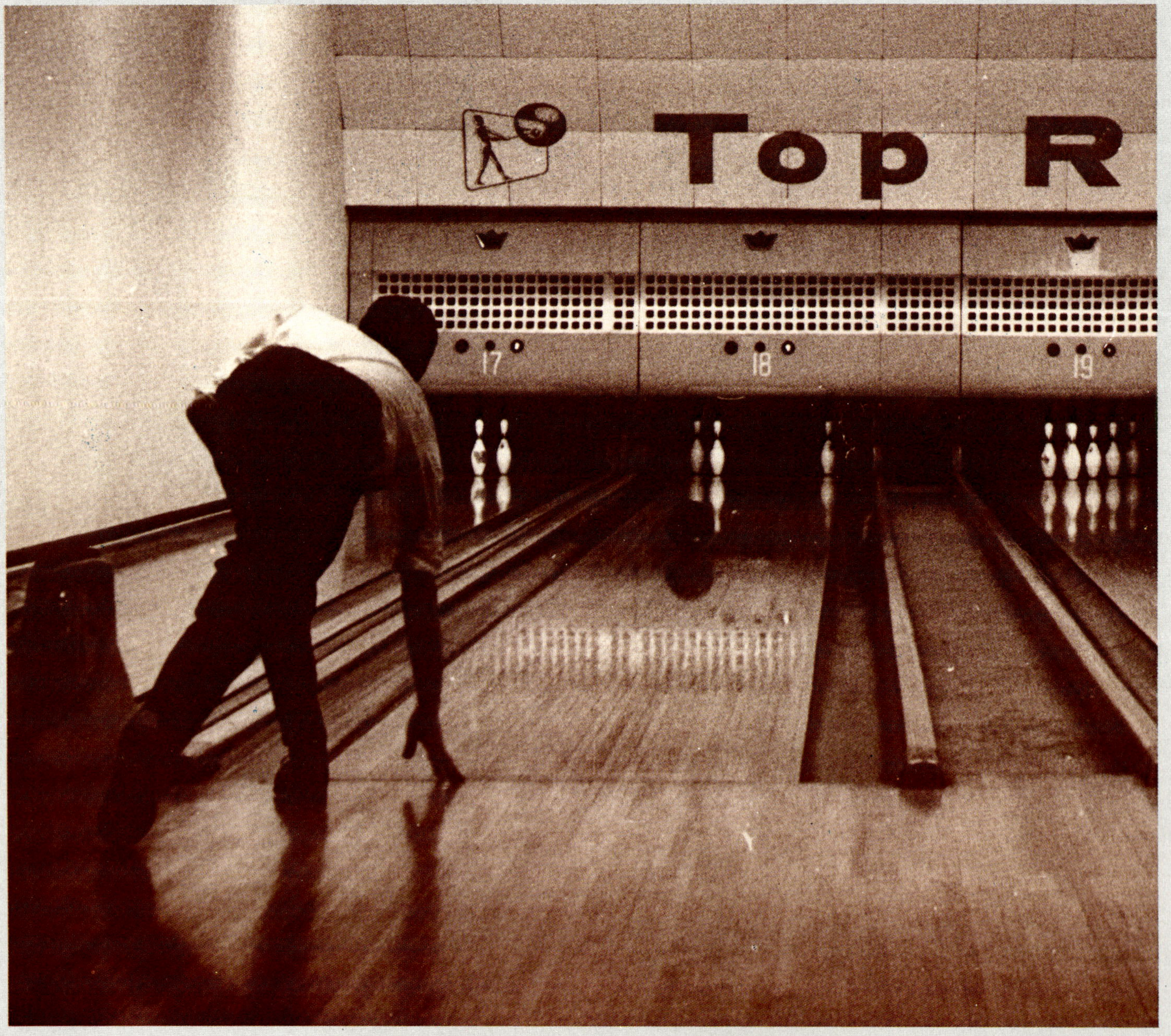

Trampolining

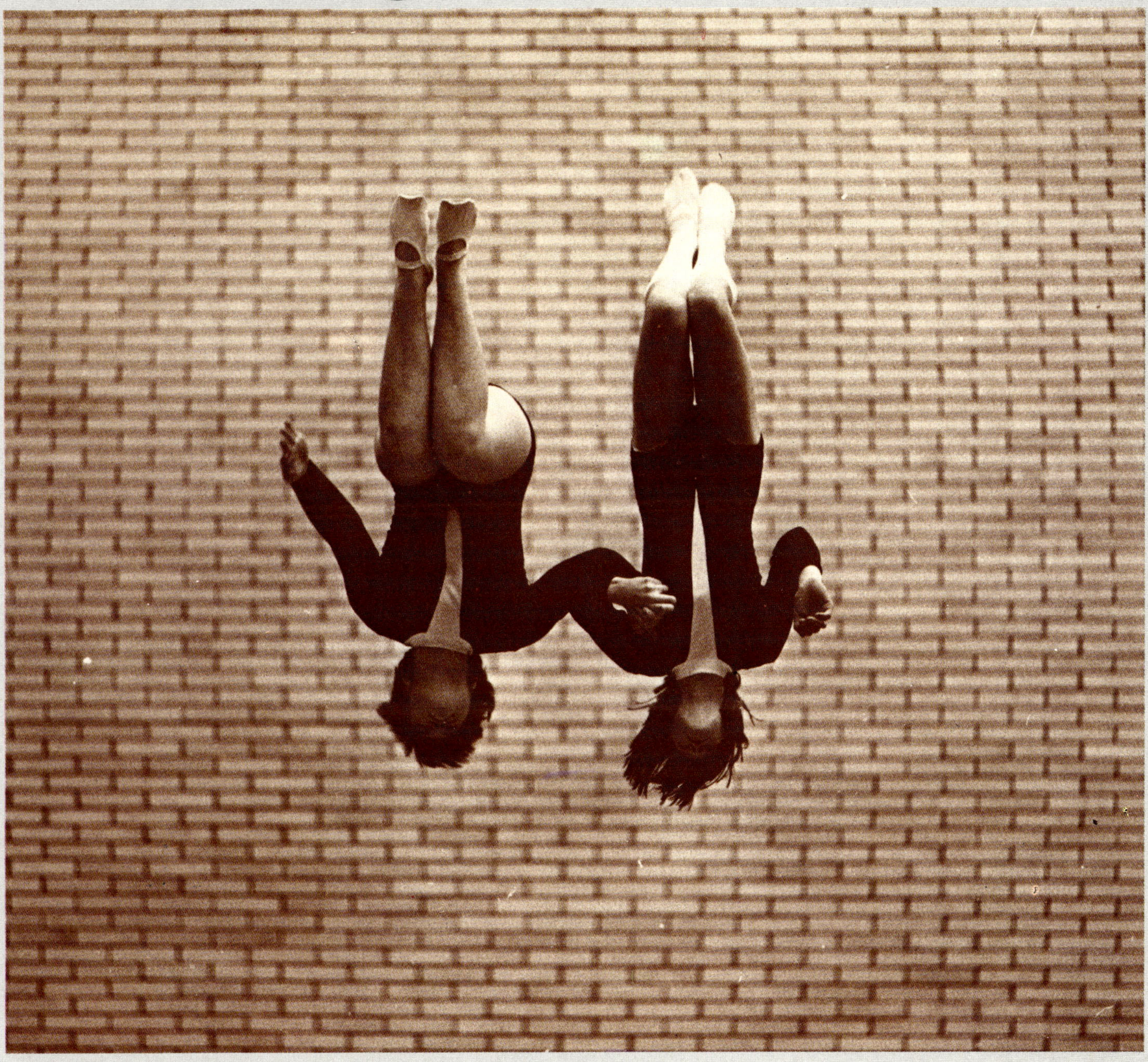

As a sporting and leisure activity, trampolining is a thrilling test of mobility, skill and agility, as well as an excellent training for other sports such as diving and gymnastics. The trampoline, a sprung nylon webbed bed, can project competitors up to 6m (20ft) in the air and enables them to go through routines consisting of somersaults and twists. It is very much an individual sport. The competitor has to put together combinations of moves and in training practises perfecting them. There is also synchronised trampolining. Here two trampolines are used side by side and two performers from the same team carry out exactly the same manoeuvres, keeping time with each other as much as possible.

Trampolining is common in Western Europe and the USA, and can be enjoyably practised by all age-groups and both sexes, who compete in their own divisions. It can take place outdoors, but serious events are staged inside since high winds and the sun could cause difficult and sometimes dangerous, conditions. The only equipment needed is the trampoline itself, which most large gymnasiums possess. Ordinary clothes for gymnastics are customarily worn. Some holiday resorts do have 'pit' trampolines set into the ground so that the top of the frame is level with the ground. Great agility is needed for trampolining and therefore is recommended for children. However its value to the heart and lungs is limited (as is gymnastics) and therefore aerobic work should be added to your work programme. Trampolining is often a pleasant and rewarding way to spend some minutes before and after an intensive session at another sport.

Thrills and spills on a trampoline are good practise for balance and mobility.

Coupled with an aerobic sport, it is good exercise

Volleyball

Most sports begin as a recreation and then graduate to competition level. Only later do they become recognized as a convenient way of keeping healthy. The curiosity of volleyball is that it was originated as a method of keeping businessmen fit. Only subsequently has it become an international sport with 50 million adherents in over 100 countries, and finally part of the Olympic programme. It was invented in Massachusetts in 1895 by W.G. Morgan, because the middle-aged men at Holyoke Y.M.C.A. found basketball too rigorous. Morgan wrote later: 'There was a need for a game which all age-groups could play, and above all, I felt that this game should be enjoyable. To begin with we use a basketball and batted it up with the hands; then we placed a net between the teams'. From this strange birth volleyball has grown into a vigorous team game for men and women, customarily with two teams of six players. It can be played indoors or out but usually important competitions are staged inside on smooth surfaces. Most large gymnasiums have the 18m (17yd) and 9m (8yd) wide courts marked out on their floors. Mini-Volley is a smaller version of the game played by junior teams of only three players.

Volleyball demands tremendous team-work to benefit from the three touches that each side can have before hitting the ball over the net. Considerable agility is needed both to leap high enough so that the final hit can be smashed downwards with maximum penetration and to prevent the ball from hitting the ground, when a point would have to be conceded. However, volleyball has little strenuous effect on the heart and lungs unless it is continued for very long spells. It should be regarded as recreation.

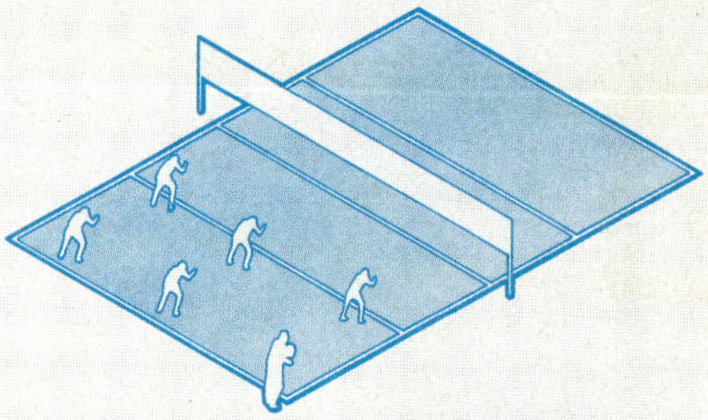

Moderate fitness can be obtained from the leaping and hitting in volleyball. A very enjoyable team game

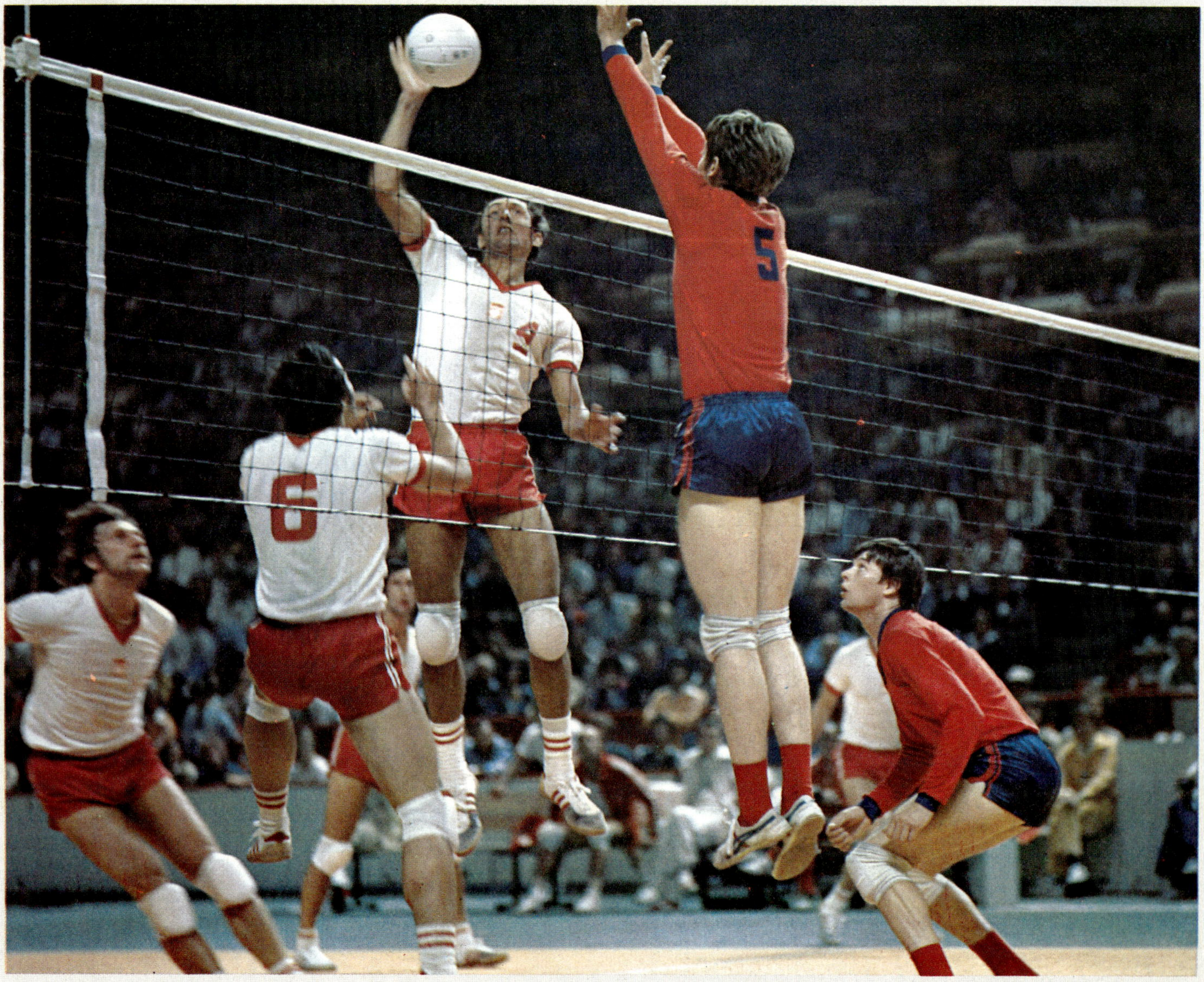

Water Skiing

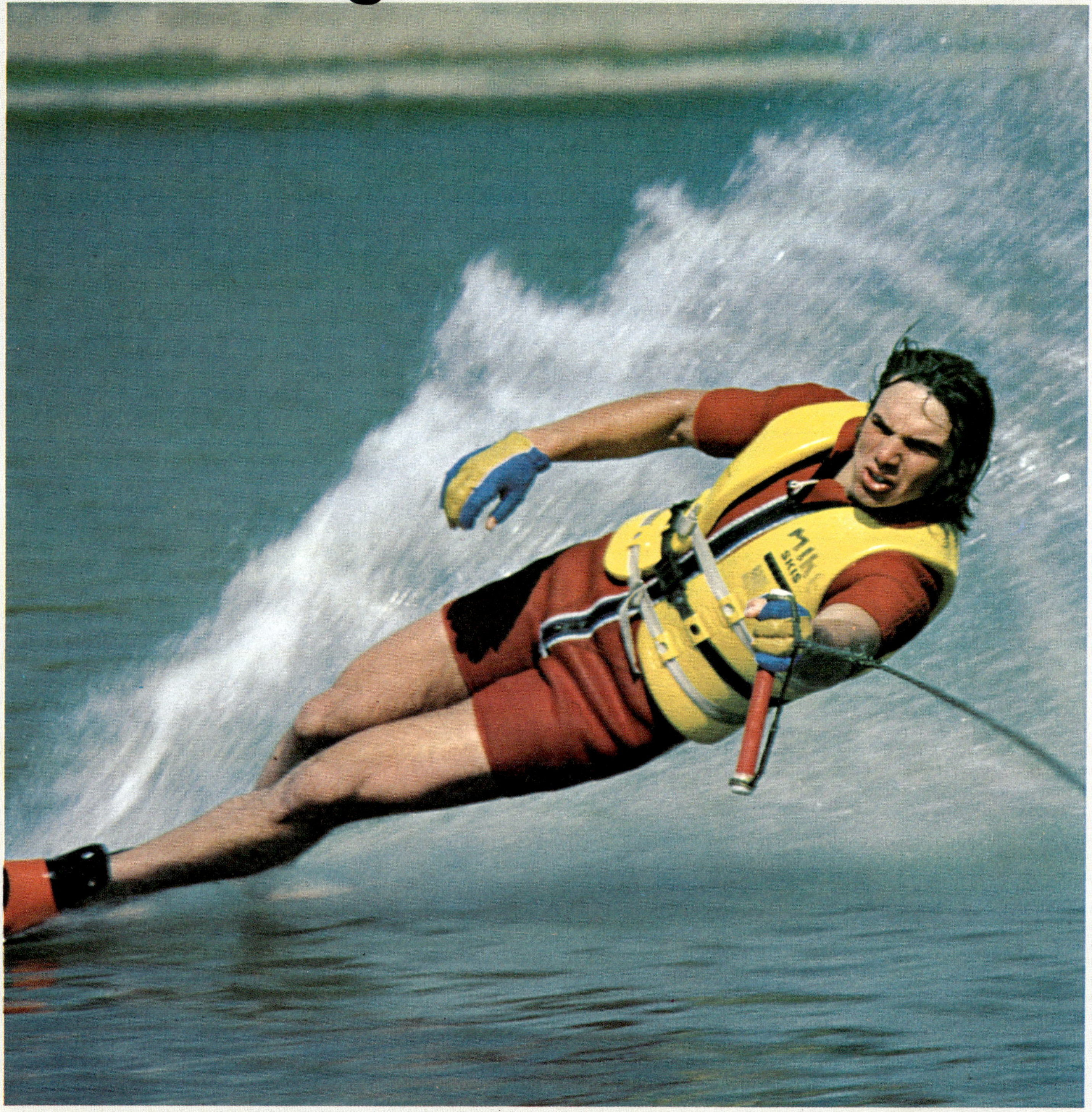

If you can swim, what better way to combine water and thrilling speed than water-skiing. Strong arm and leg muscles are developed and good balance is essential

Waterskiing is either a professional or leisure sport practiced throughout the world wherever a suitable stretch of calm water is available and the climate hospitable. Since its inception in France in the 1920s the water skiing fraternity has continued to grow at an ever increasing rate. It is a sport for the individual, group or the family – a great attraction. It calls for poise and balance and combined strength in the arms and legs. For most it is a recreation activity and not one in which a good degree of fitness can be gained.

The basic equipment is simple although at first may appear expensive. However, by joining a club or by pooling your resources the cost can be kept to a minimum. General purpose skis can be shared but regular performers tend to have their own. The powerboat could be very costly but here the advantage of joining a club is selfevident. Hardened skiers and the professionals competing in slalom events usually prefer to use the single ski which is tapered towards the end with both feet placed one behind the other in special rubber shoes which in the event of a fall allow the feet to come clear, thus preventing injury.

Wrestling

Amateur wrestling, which is an Olympic sport, should not be confused with professional wrestling, which is entertainment. The appeal of amateur wrestling is diversified because many countries have their own styles. These styles have local interest in their own right. Among the chief variants are: Cumberland and Westmorland, Devon and Cornwall in Britain; *schwingen* in Switzerland; *sumo* in Japan; *sambo* in Russia and *yagli* in Turkey. However, two styles – freestyle and Greco-Roman – are practised all over the world and are the only ones included in the Olympics. The main difference between them is that in Greco-Roman the use of the legs is not permitted for attack or defence.

Both demand a very high standard of strength, stamina and skill. It is a pity that such a basic sport is not used more as a training activity as well as for its own value. In particular, wrestling is a valuable means of developing the often neglected muscles of the neck which play such an important part in all body contact sports like soccer, rugby, American Football and boxing. Although women don't compete, boys can gain as much benefit as men from regular training sessions. Ideally a rubber mat between six and eight metres (19ft and 26ft) should be used, with leotards as costumes and light boots on the feet. However, provided the surface is reasonably soft and free from hazardous objects, any area will suffice and bathing costumes and bare feet are often used in training. Many gymnasiums, especially in America, have wrestling sections, but keen competitors can set up their own mat in their gardens. The only requirement is that there should be a number of wrestlers because people only develop their own styles if they can practise with a variety of opponents. For all-round physical development and fitness wrestling is ideal.

Demanding great physical exertion, body contact abounds in this exacting all-round exercise

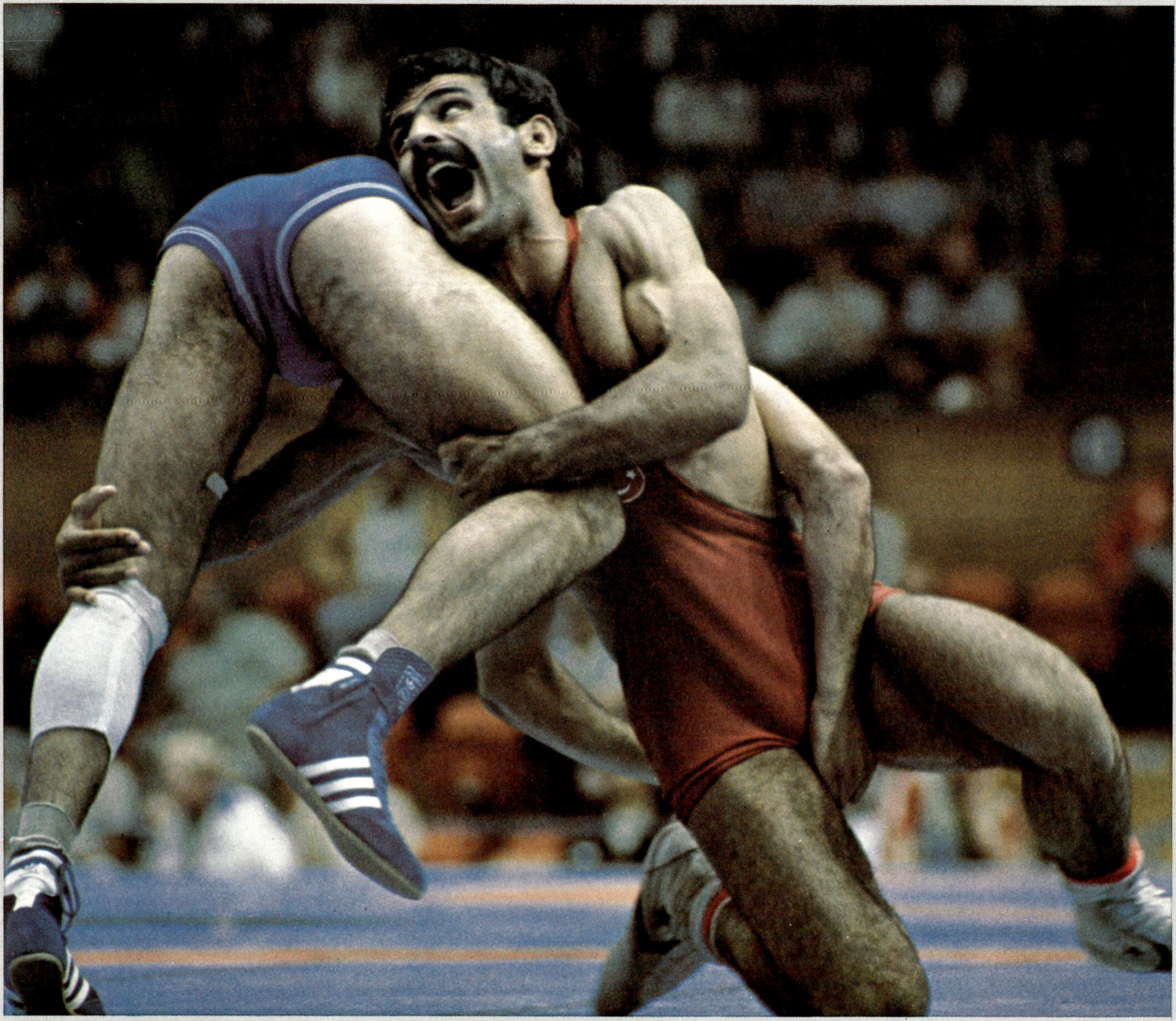

Yachting

Yachting has never completely cast off its reputation of being a sport either of the leisured rich or of those living close enough to the water to make it worthwhile to learning. This is a pity because yachting encourages a love of the water and basic nautical matters. In spite of all the sailing exploits of men like King Constantine of Greece, a gold medallist at the Tokyo Olympics, and Norway's King Olaf and Crown Prince Harald, yachting can cater for the less wealthy through the medium, for instance, of 4m (14ft) long racing dinghies.

Yachting is essentially a participation sport. An owner may enter a race simply by being a member of the club organizing it, or by belonging to a sailing club affiliated to the national racing organisation of his country, and by having a yacht eligible by size or type for the particular race. Anyone with enough sailing experience to make himself a useful member may be invited to join the crew of a yacht by her owner so that the amateur spirit is strongly maintained.

There is no need for the sport to be competitive; it can be active recreation. Sailing is, indeed, an ideal family activity because children can be instructed while assisting in the actual sailing. In this way, they acquire experience while hopefully enjoying themselves amongst the people they know best. Its main disadvantage is that there is usually only time to pursue it at week-ends unless you live near a large stretch of water.

Clearly the handling of the boat puts a premium on skill but some members of the serious crews taking part in international racing need a considerable amount of strength and stamina. Despite its manifold advantages otherwise, yachting for the week-end enthusiast should be regarded as a relaxation rather than as a strenuous and demanding exercise.

Nautical skills, fresh air and relaxation give yachting a particular attraction. It does not though, provide overall exercise for the body

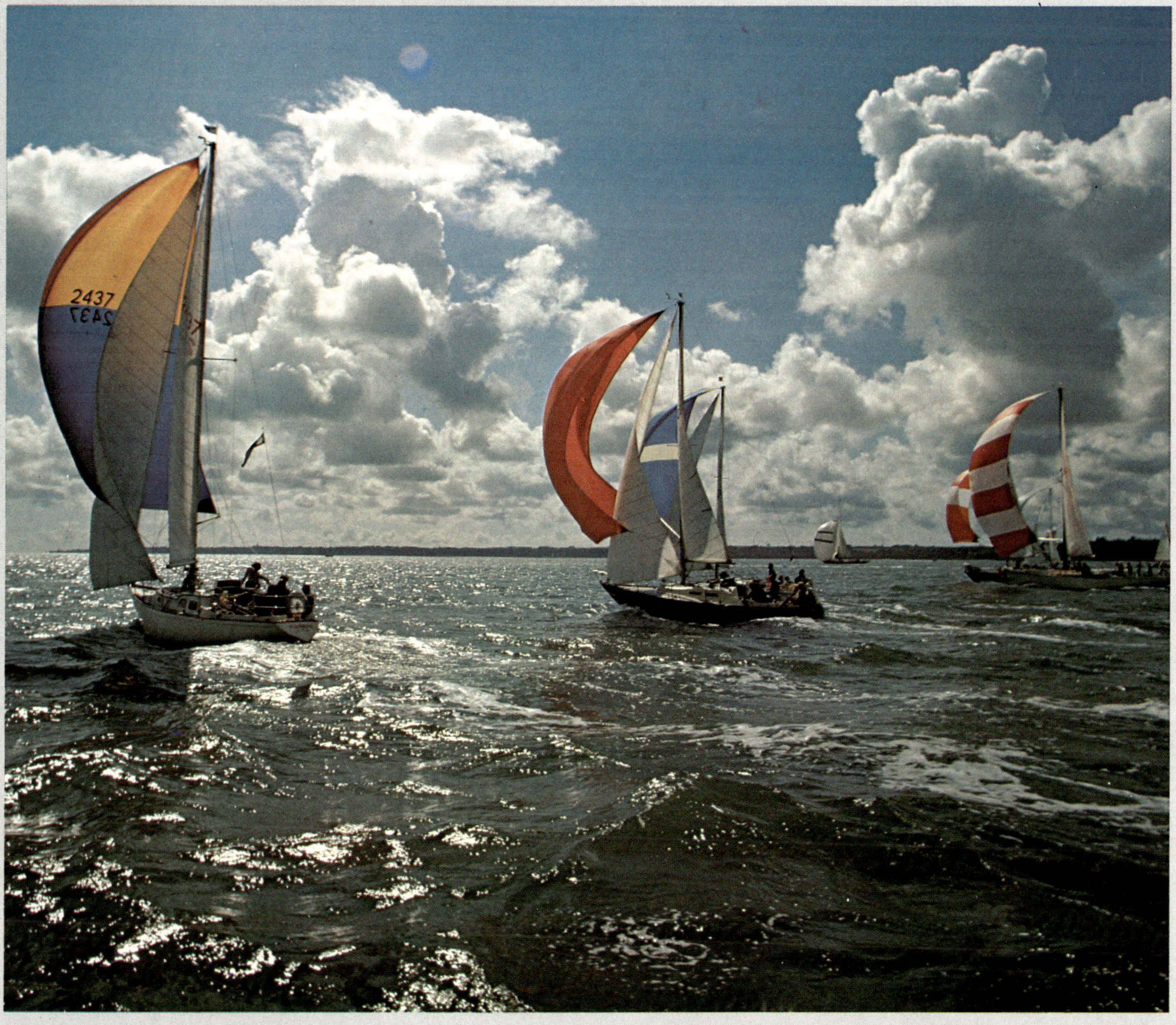

Preparing for Exercise

We are rapidly approaching a new era in medicine partly as a result of the fact that during the next few decades, one of the major problems facing mankind will be the employment of leisure. Increasing mechanization and industrial efficiency must ultimately leave everyone with time on their hands. Already more and more people are playing sport and the risk of physical injury associated with all sorts of recreations new demands attention.

Just as certain trades and occupations are subject to particular injuries and diseases, sports pose special medical problems. These may be general, like designing an optimum schedule of exercise or diet and avoiding overtraining, or specific, like injuries on the field.

Exercise schedules are designed to bring body and mind into optimum efficiency. This is achieved by the sportsman's gradual adaptation to a particular exercise, or set of exercises by means of a regular, systematic and increasingly demanding programme. General training is simply a toning-up of the mind and the body to improve condition and coordination of the various organs and systems. Specific training tones and improves the working of muscle groups involved in a particular sport.

The ideal state has these three distinct components: general fitness, specific fitness for the chosen sport and a high morale and confidence. The degree of training which can be described as the efficiency of the body as a machine, can be measured by functional and laboratory tests mainly involving the heart, circulation and respiration. The progress of training can be judged by such tests.

Excessive Exercise

One of the major problems of intensive training is the risk of producing a quite sudden loss of physical and psychological form. The symptoms are complex and progressive, and include loss of appetite, dyspepsia and loss of weight. Also, the increase in heart rate and blood pressure which follows exertion is excessive and takes longer than usual to return to normal. Respiration is also affected; breathlessness is more marked and takes longer to subside. These physical reactions to excessive exercise produce a tendency to psychic exhaustion; anxiety, depression, loss of concentration and will-power.

Laboratory tests show that excessive exercise results in actual physical changes, particularly in the body's absorption and use of oxygen and in the composition of body fluids. The muscles also become more susceptible to fatigue and strain.

Fatigue

The feeling of fatigue is a useful signal of the need to rest and rebuild strength. At the lower end of the scale there is simple tiredness which passes quickly and without trouble. If demands are greater, the fatigue experienced may include feelings of exhaustion and a loss of coordination. A really all-out effort can produce full-scale exhaustion and the risk of permanent injury. Fatigue does not only affect the muscles; it also makes demands on some of the internal organs, particularly the liver, and can disturb the nervous system, the endocrine glands and, of course, mental outlook.

Diet

The calorific value of your diet should meet your energy expenditure, but avoid excesses which can be a hindrance. As energy consumption varies, both with the size of the body and the individual metabolism, and since your diet must provide for activities outside of sport, it is seldom possible to calculate precisely how much food an individual needs. As a general guide, the energy consumption per day in athletics is not particularly high and calls for a diet of approximately 3000–5000 calories. For mountaineers and skiers, however, higher levels are needed amounting to something over 6000 calories a day for a man of average size and build.

Carbohydrates (sugar, bread and so on) should provide about 60–70 per cent of the calories required. This allows for the best replenishment of reserve energy, in the form of glycogen deposits in the liver and the muscles; up to 15 per cent of the total calories should be in the form of proteins.

The remainder of the calories should be provided by fats which can comprise up to 20–25 per cent of the total. The target in feeding sportsmen is easier to define than to meet; it is to supply their quite considerable energy requirements, without allowing a surplus which could spoil their condition.

Eating Before a Game

Probably one of the most overrated aspects of nutrition for athletic performance is the necessity to eat before a game. It is a well-known fact that the intake of food is not followed by an increase in physical efficiency and yet certain people have said that the special meals they have used throughout the years benefit their physical performance. Many coaches and trainers have ideas about eating before a game which are not in accordance with scientific information and although the choice of a particular meal is not likely to influence performance, there are certain principles to keep in mind when taking a meal prior to any sporting event. Two major points are timing and size. Long periods between meals may give rise to hunger which is often associated with feelings of nervousness and weakness. On the other hand, pre-game emotional tension or anxiety may contribute to possible indigestion and a feeling of nausea and may be very uncomfortable if the meal is too close to the time of the event.

A number of different foods which have been eaten before games have been criticized over the years. There are many diverse individual preferences and most of the scientific work done in this field in athletics, apart from the work done on long-distance endurance events, has been inconclusive.

It is wise to avoid liquids or foods which give rise to gaseous distention of the stomach such as pork, gravy, pickles, mustard, chips, chilli, cola or lemonade. Recent work has shown that heavy meals even up to five hours before a game, were still undergoing digestion in the bowel at game time. Some 20–25 per cent of the food was still in the stomach three hours after eating. You should really avoid a large meal, eating only a small, easily digested meal 3–4 hours prior to any event.

Fat and protein intake should be restricted, but carbohydrate content should be stressed. For instance, a simple carbohydrate meal with up to 1000 calories and a small amount of protein is to be recommended. This could consist of a toasted sandwich, honey and a banana; a number of carbohydrate substitutes could be made. The fat content should be restricted due to its slowing effect upon stomach-emptying time and slow absorption. As far as is known, except in long-distance endurance events such as marathon running, the ingestion of liquid glucose drinks during the event has no real benefit.

Prior to an important race, long-distance athletes store up glucose in their body muscles in the form of glycogen. They achieve this by eating no carbohydrates up to 24 hours before an event thus completely using up their reserve glycogen in their muscles. Having done this, they take in large quantities of carbohydrates on the day before an event, thus replenishing the glycogen storage in the muscle tissue. A light meal is then taken a few hours before the athletic activity.

Prevention and After-Care of Injury

There are many facts that one should consider regarding personal hygiene, fitness and protection. In this era of preventive medicine, it is imperative that all sportsmen, especially those involved in physical contact sport, should be immunized against tetanus. As regards personal hygiene, one of the most annoying problems which occurs is athlete's foot or groin. This is a highly infectious fungus-type disease which is spread through shower floors, swimming pools, bath mats and other moist surfaces. Much could be done to prevent it spreading by the proper cleaning and disinfecting of shower rooms. The treatment consists of washing the feet and changing socks and underpants daily, as well as the application of anti-fungal powders and ointment.

When it comes to personal protection, it is important that all clothing should be of a good fit. All rings should be removed before playing physical contact sport. Shoes or boots should be of a good fit and well padded.

In recent years, some near fatal injuries have occurred in physical contact sports due to the chewing of gum, because the gum obstructed the air passage. This is, therefore, to be avoided. Also, in some sports such as boxing and rugby, more players have taken to wearing a mouth guard in recent years. These reduce concussion, dental and facial injuries.

Soft-tissue injuries are the most common form of disability encountered in sports medicine and include damage to skin, muscles, ligaments and tendons. Prevention of 'pul-

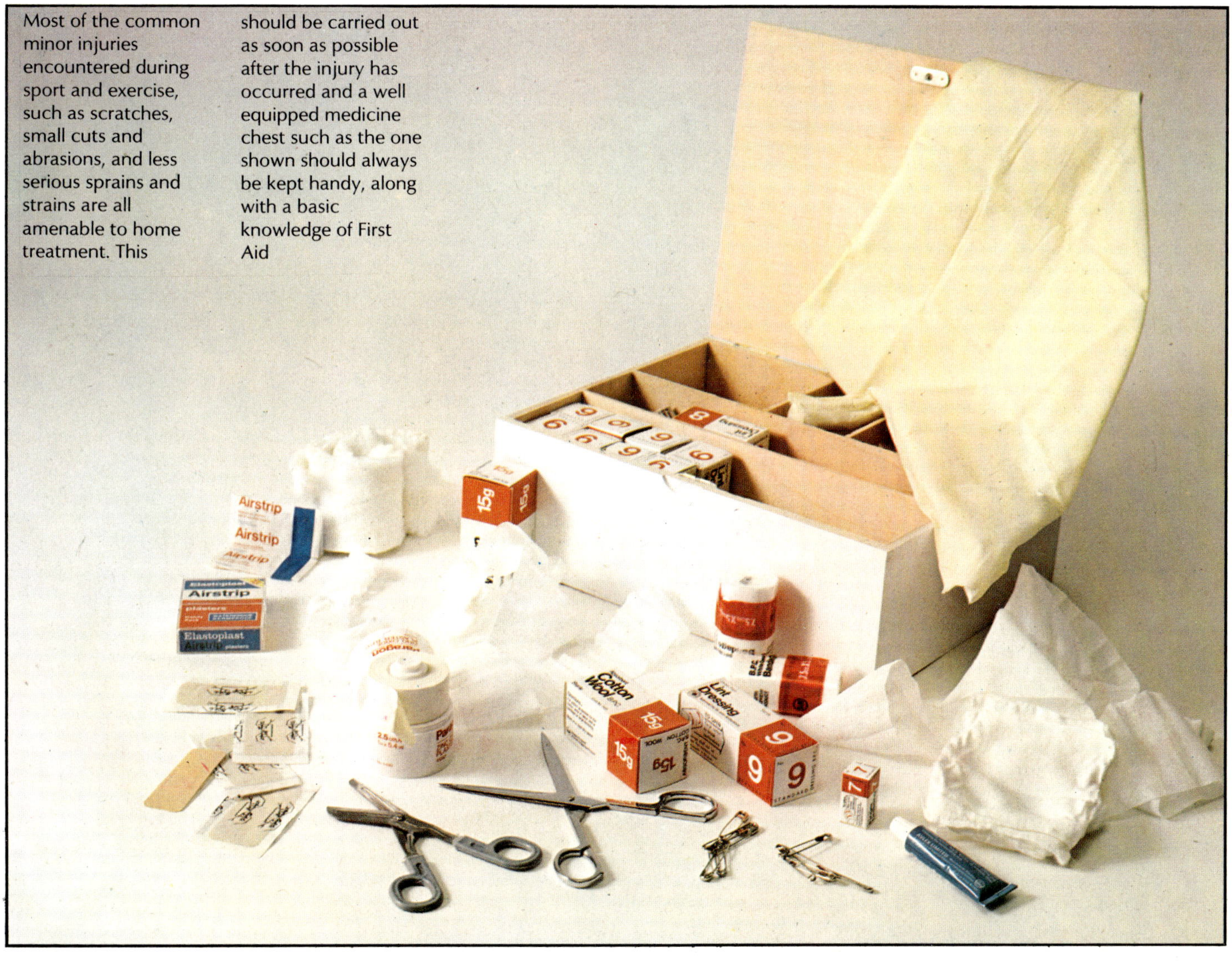

Most of the common minor injuries encountered during sport and exercise, such as scratches, small cuts and abrasions, and less serious sprains and strains are all amenable to home treatment. This should be carried out as soon as possible after the injury has occurred and a well equipped medicine chest such as the one shown should always be kept handy, along with a basic knowledge of First Aid

TREATMENT OF INJURIES			
Type of injury	**Immediate treatment**	**Next day**	**Towards fitness again**
Pulled muscles Leg (eg Hamstring)	Application of ice, elevation of leg	Gentle isometrics and stretching eg touching toes for a hamstring	Continue the isometrics and begin isotonics (weights). Begin a graduated running programme with jogging. After several days sprinting should be accomplished, and some weight lifting begun for full recovery. Remember always to warm-up well
Sprains Ankle	Cryotherapy i.e. application of ice for as long as possible over 24 hours. Strap with bandages and keep elevated as much as possible	Begin to move the foot, rotating and pushing against a wall. Pain permitting a long walk is a good idea, keeping the ankle strapped	Gentle jogging leading to running again after a few days, when running in a figure of 8 is particularly useful. Wobble-board exercise with the ankle unstrapped helps to strengthen the muscle and bring back neuromuscular coordination

led' muscles in any sport can usually be assured by adequate warming up prior to any programme of exercise.

Muscle injuries can result in either pulled or torn muscle. A common example of pulled muscle is the hamstring group of muscles at the back of the thigh. This happens when the player has not adequately warmed up and usually occurs at the musculo-tendinous junctions in the lower and upper part of the back of the thigh. Most affected are soccer players, joggers and sprinters. If it is not a severe muscle pull and all the player complains of is a niggle in the thigh, then gradual passive stretching of the muscle will aid recovery in 1–3 weeks. A severe pull may result in full activity being out for six weeks.

A torn muscle is when a muscle is damaged by a direct blow. It bleeds with a resulting *haematoma* formation, i.e. clotting. The commonest torn muscle is on the front of the thigh and is called the quadriceps muscle. If there is pain and swelling, then ice should be applied immediately, the limb should be rested in a firm bandage and elevated. (I – Ice C – Compression E – Elevation). The limb should be rested for 24 hours, then passive exercises started, but stopped if they produce pain. After the first 24 hours a graduated programme of exercises should be undertaken together with some form of heat. After seven days, weights should be introduced until the muscle bulk returns to normal and a full range of movement and power has been obtained.

Inflammation of a tendon is known as tendinitis. Examples occur in the Achilles tendon of the heel and the very common tennis elbow. It usually occurs as a result of what is known as an over-use injury.

With an Achilles tendinitis, a heel pad worn in the shoe and boot will often take the loading strain off the tendon and together with a form of physiotherapy known as ultrasonic therapy, will speed up the healing process.

Partial and complete tears of tendons require surgery and immobilization in plaster for up to six weeks.

Ligaments are found on either side of joints and are partly concerned with the stability of joints, e.g. as in the knee and ankle. These can be sprained, which is easily diagnosed by tenderness over a ligament with some slight swelling and loss of full movement in the joint. One of the commonest injuries in footballers and athletes is to the lateral outer ligament on the outside of the ankle joint. It is treated initially with rest, ice and strapping until the swelling subsides and the pain disappears when mobilizing exercises can then begin. Repeated contrast bathing in hot and cold water will also help to speed up the swelling loss in the affected joint.

When the signs are a bit more severe indicating a partial tear and the ligament allows increased movement of the joint, the treatment is rest in plaster for three weeks followed by intensive exercises to the affected limb. A complete tear requires surgical repair.

Over-Use Injuries

Many of the injuries affecting sportsmen come into this category. Repeated trauma such as continued running on hard surfaces or repetitious movements using one part of the anatomy, can lead to an over-use injury.

In the former, one can have stress fractures occurring in the small bones of the feet and in the tibia or fibula in the front of the lower leg, which may go undiagnosed for many weeks before an X-ray confirms the suspected diagnosis. With the repeated movements in rowing, an oarsman may develop an inflammation in the tendon sheaths of his forearms. Many athletes suffer from shin splints. This makes itself felt as pain in the front part of the lower leg as a result of inflammation at the musculo-tendinous junction.

There are, of course, many other injuries peculiar to sport, but what is terribly important to the individual sportsman, is the ability to get back to his sport as soon as possible, before he loses the fitness that he has worked so hard to obtain.

As previously stated, in soft-tissue injuries, i.e. the sprains and strains, the advent of cryotherapy (ice therapy) in the last few years, together with specialist use of hydrocortisone injections, has resulted in vast improvements in management. Along with the education of the sportsman regarding his diet, training methods and personal hygiene, it is an important adjunct towards ensuring that he remains completely fit.

Index

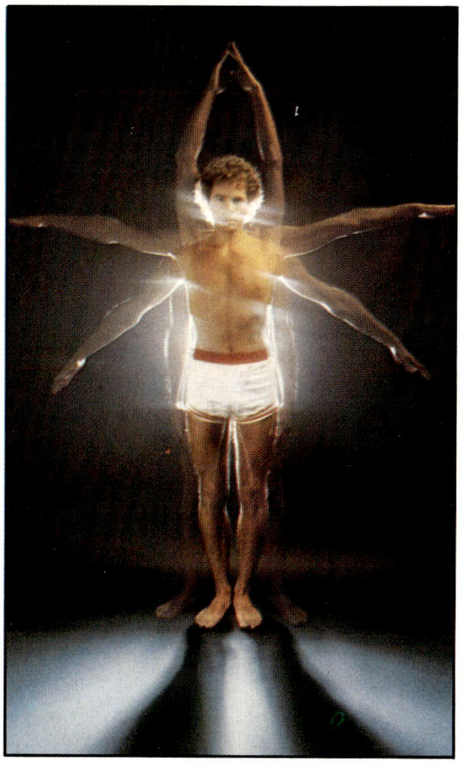

Page numbers in italics refer to illustration captions

Acknowledgements

The publishers would like to thank all of the organizations and individuals who generously gave advice and materials during the preparation of this book, especially Coppermine Ltd; Debenham's Ltd; Gus Arcon at Gym and Tonic, Midas (Shoes); and The Order of St John.

Photography by Michael Busselle

Additional photographs by kind permission of:
All-Sport (Tony Duffy) 8, 185 above, 188 below, 195 inset, 200, 203 below, 205 inset, 213, (John Starr) 176-177, 184, 193 above; Associated Press Ltd, 139 below; Theo Bergstrom 16; Rodney Bond 185 centre, 190; Camera Press Ltd 211, (Jon Blau) 146, (J. Bruell) 203 above, (K. Lambert) 210, (Leo Mason) 209, (Orion Press) 141 below inset; Colorsport 186 left and right, 187, 193 inset, 197, 202 inset, 207; Simon de Courcy-Wheeler 12-13, 15 below, 20 below, 62, 90-91 above and below right, 125 below, 181; Craftsmen Potters Association 127 above; Gerry Cranham 190 inset, 192, 196 inset, 199, 214, 215; Tony Duffy 201 inset, 202; Robert Estall 206 above and below; Melvin Grey 19, 114-115, 118-119, 122, 123 above, 131, 134-135, 135 above and below; Paul Kemp 114 left; John Lee 115 right, 123 below; Leo Mason 180, 189 inset, 191, 194, 196 below right, 204, 212; Ken Moreman 52 below left and right, 75 above and below; Norman Nicholls 133 inset; Roger Phillips 126-127, 130-131; Popperfoto 139 above right; Rex Features 90-91 below left, (Fotos International) 141 above inset, (J. Beas Gamma) 153, (Sipa Press) 139 above left, 143 above; Spectrum Colour Library 105 above and below, 143 below, 147 above; Sporting Pictures 185 below, 195 above, 208 left; R. Vente 205; Andrew Wagg 162, 208 inset; ZEFA (B. Benjamin) 140-141, (E. M. Bordis) 198 above, (W. L. Hamilton) 189, (A. Hubrich) 198, (M. Thornig) 201.

The following artists supplied illustrations:
John Carrod 88, 92, 96, 100, 101; Barry Glynn 83; Barry Jackson 26, 44, 45, 77; Tom Stimpson 27, 28-29, 30, 31, 32, 33, 34-35, 38, 50, 86, 98, 102, 144-145, 188, 190, 197, 200, 208, 209, 212.

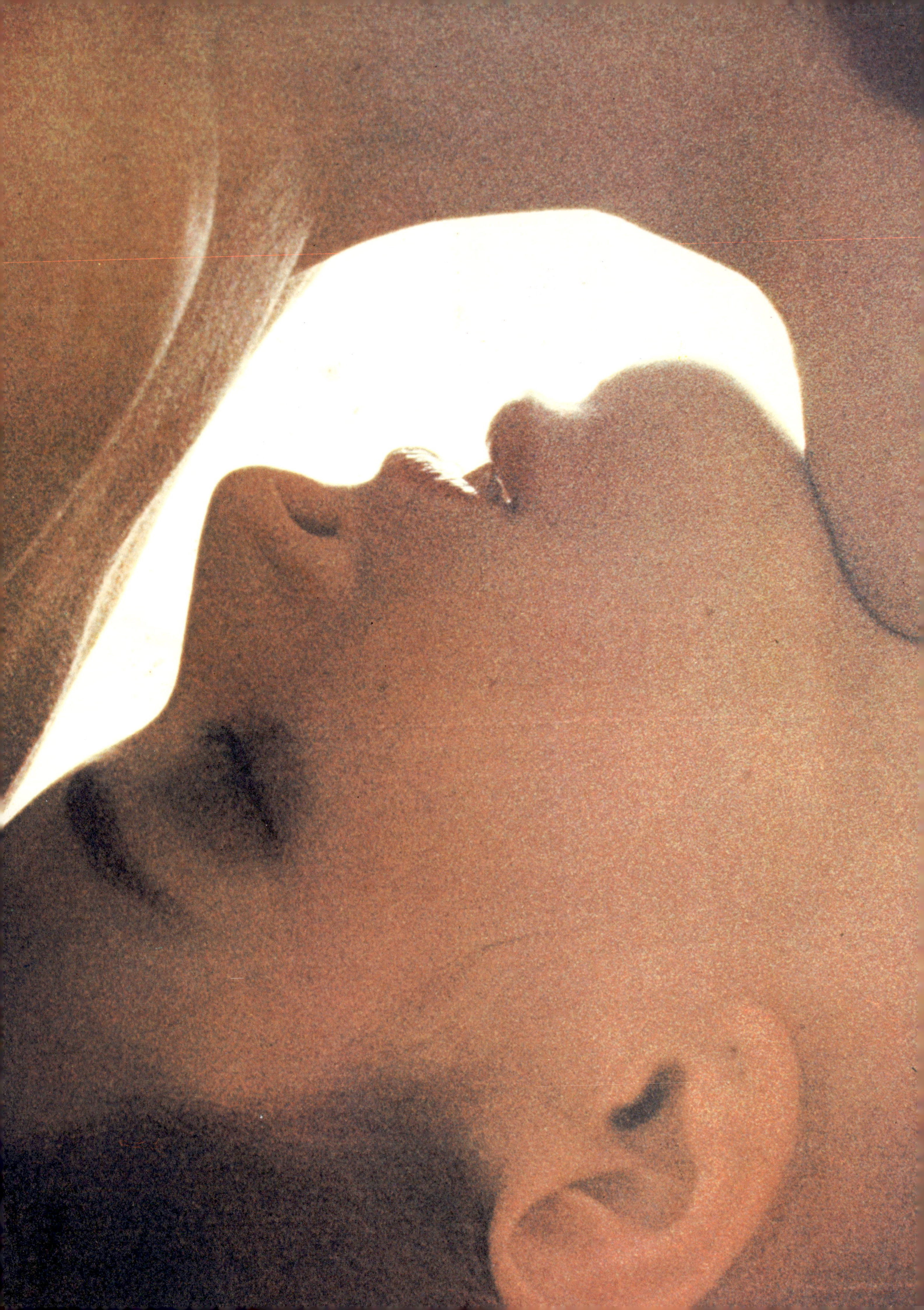